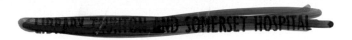

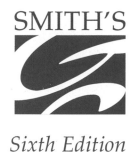

SMITH'S

Sixth Edition

Recognizable Patterns of Human Malformation

Kenneth Lyons Jones, MD

Professor of Pediatrics
Chief, Division of Dysmorphology and Teratology
University of California, San Diego
School of Medicine
La Jolla, California

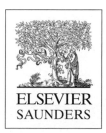

ELSEVIER
SAUNDERS

ELSEVIER
SAUNDERS

1600 John F. Kennedy Blvd.
Ste. 1800
Philadelphia, Pennsylvania 19103-2899

SMITH'S RECOGNIZABLE PATTERNS OF HUMAN MALFORMATION

NOTICE

Knowledge and best practice in this field are constantly changing. As new research and experience broaden
our knowledge, changes in practice, treatment, and drug therapy may become necessary or appropriate.
Readers are advised to check the most current information provided (i) on procedures featured or (ii) by the
manufacturer of each product to be administered, to verify the recommended dose or formula, the method
and duration of administration, and contraindications. It is the responsibility of the practitioners, relying on
their own experience and knowledge of the patient, to make diagnoses, to determine dosages and the best
treatment for each individual patient, and to take all appropriate safety precautions. To the fullest extent of
the law, neither the Publisher nor the Author assumes any liability for any injury and/or damage to persons
or property arising out of or related to any use of the material contained in this book.

Previous editions copyrighted 1997, 1988, 1982, 1976, 1970

Library of Congress Cataloging-in-Publication Data
Jones, Kenneth Lyons.
    Smith's recognizable patterns of human malformation/Kenneth Lyons Jones.—6th ed.
      p. ; cm.
    Includes bibliographical references and index.
  ISBN-13: 978-0-7216-0615-6   ISBN-10: 0-7216-0615-6
     1. Abnormalities, Human. I. Title: Recognizable patterns of human malformation. II.
Smith, David W., 1926–1981. III. Title.
    [DNLM: 1. Abnormalities. QS 675 J77s 2006]
  RG627.5.S58 2006
  616′.043—dc22

  ISBN-13: 978-0-7216-0615-6   2005049968
  ISBN-10: 0-7216-0615-6

Acquisitions Editor: *Todd Hummel*
Developmental Editor: *Kim J. Davis*
Publishing Services Manager: *Joan Sinclair*
Project Manager: *Joan Sinclair*
Design Direction: *Karen O'Keefe Owens*

Printed in the United States of America

Last digit is the print number: 9 8 7 6 5 4 3 2

Dedication of the First Edition

To my wife, Ann, beloved inspirational companion

To my father, William H. Smith, accomplished engineer and would-be physician

To my teachers Dr. Lawson Wilkins, molder of clinicians and humanist, and Professor Dr. Gian Töndury, complete anatomist, who brings embryology into living perspective

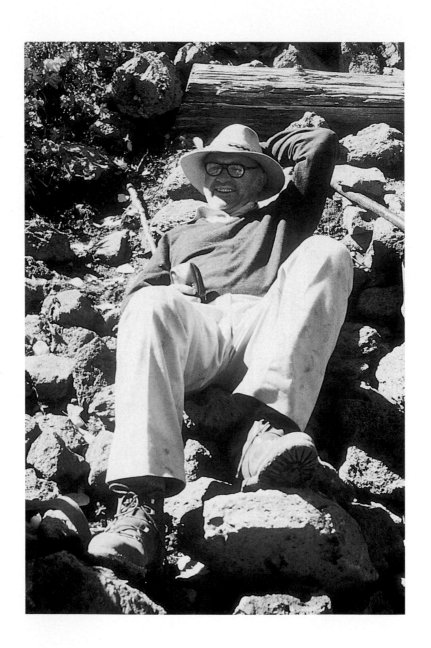

Dedicated to the Memory of

David W. Smith, MD

1926–1981

"Far better it is to dare mighty things, to win glorious triumphs, even though checkered by failure, than to take rank with those poor spirits who neither enjoy much nor suffer much, because they live in the great twilight that knows neither victory nor defeat."

Theodore Roosevelt, in a speech before the Hamilton Club, Chicago, April 10, 1899

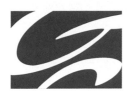 # Acknowledgments

The information set forth in this book represents an amalgamation of the knowledge, commitment, and hard work of many individuals. I would like to acknowledge a number of those who have made significant contributions to the development of the sixth edition:

Dr. Kurt Benirschke's breadth of knowledge, intellectual curiosity, creativity, and enthusiasm have acted as a continuing stimulus for me.

Dr. Marilyn C. Jones has tirelessly contributed her knowledge, advice, patience, writing skills, and love. She has made it possible for life to go on during the preparation of this edition.

Dr. Christina D. Chambers's wisdom, creativity, and understanding of epidemiology have made me aware of a totally new approach to understanding the causes of birth defects.

I am grateful to the following fellows in dysmorphology at the University of California, San Diego: Dr. Marilyn C. Jones, University of California, San Diego; Dr. H. Eugene Hoyme, Stanford University, Palo Alto; Dr. Luther K. Robinson, State University of New York, Buffalo; Dr. Ronald Lacro, Children's Hospital of Boston; Dr. Christopher Cuniff, University of Arizona, Tucson; Dr. Rick Martin, Washington University, St. Louis; Dr. Leah W. Burke, University of Vermont, Burlington; Dr. Stephen R. Braddock, University of Missouri, Columbia; Dr. Lynne M. Bird, University of California, San Diego; Dr. Kenjiro Kosaki, Keio University, Tokyo; Dr. Miguel del Campo, Universitat Pompeu Fabra, Barcelona; and Dr. Keith Vaux, University of California, San Diego. Each has made his or her own significant contribution to the development of this edition, and each has been a great inspiration to me.

Many colleagues have contributed photos, information, and expertise. Especially helpful have been Dr. John Carey, University of Utah School of Medicine, Salt Lake City; Dr. John Opitz, University of Utah School of Medicine, Salt Lake City; Dr. Robert Gorlin, University of Minnesota Medical and Dental School, Minneapolis; Dr. Michael Cohen, Jr., Dalhousie University, Halifax, Nova Scotia; Dr. Judith Hall, University of British Columbia, Vancouver; Dr. David Rimoin, Cedars-Sinai Medical Center, Los Angeles; Dr. Jaime Frias, Centers for Disease Control and Prevention, Atlanta; Dr. Jon Aase, University of New Mexico, Albuquerque; Dr. Bryan Hall, University of Kentucky, Lexington; Dr. James Hanson, National Institute of Child Health and Human Development, Rockville, Maryland; Dr. Sterling Clarren, University of Washington School of Medicine, Seattle; Dr. John Graham, Cedars-Sinai Medical Center, Los Angeles; Dr. Margot Van Allen, University of British Columbia, Vancouver; Dr. Cynthia Curry, University of California, San Francisco; Dr. Roger Stevenson, Greenwood Genetic Center, Greenwood, South Carolina; Dr. Buzz Chernoff, Sacramento; Dr. Jeffrey Golden, The Children's Hospital of Philadelphia; Dr. Mike Bamshad, University of Utah School of Medicine, Salt Lake City; Dr. David Weaver, Indiana University School of Medicine, Indianapolis; Dr. Jules Leroy, Gent University Hospital, Gent, Belgium; and Dr. Mark Stephan, University of Washington School of Medicine, Seattle.

Brian Chen has worked tirelessly to prepare most of the color photographs that appear in this edition. His considerable skill, patience, and good humor are immeasurable.

I am particularly grateful to Kathleen A. Johnson, my administrative assistant at the University of California, San Diego, for the past 25 years; Kim Davis, developmental editor at Elsevier; and Joan Vidal, production editor, each of whom has had a significant impact on the successful completion of this edition.

The invaluable assistance of Robert Felix, Kelly Kao, Lyn Dick, Sonya Alvardo, Carmen Chavez, Diana Johnson, and Lela Prewitt is also greatly appreciated.

Contents

Introduction

Dysmorphology Approach and Classification

We ought not to set them aside with idle thoughts or idle words about "curiosities" or "chances." Not one of them is without meaning; not one that might not become the beginning of excellent knowledge, if only we could answer the question—why is it rare? or being rare, why did it in this instance happen?

JAMES PAGET, *Lancet* 2:1017, 1882

The questions set forth by Paget are still applicable today. Every structural defect represents an inborn error in morphogenesis. Just as the study of inborn metabolic errors has extended our understanding of normal biochemistry, so the accumulation of knowledge concerning defects in morphogenesis may assist us in further unraveling the story of structural development. The major portion of this text is devoted to patterns of malformation, as contrasted with patterns of deformation due to mechanical factors, which is the subject of a separate text, *Smith's Recognizable Patterns of Human Deformation*. You will also find relevant chapters on normal and abnormal morphogenesis, genetics and genetic counseling, minor anomalies and their relevance, a clinical approach toward a specific diagnosis for certain categorical problems, and normal standards of measurement for a variety of features. It is hoped that the design of the book will lend itself to practical clinical application, as well as provide a basic text for the education of those interested in a better understanding of alterations in morphogenesis. Furthermore, many of the charts have been developed for direct use in the counseling of patients and parents.

Accurate diagnosis of a specific syndrome among the 0.7% of babies born with multiple malformations is a necessary prerequisite of providing a prognosis and plan of management for the affected infant, as well as genetic counseling for the parents.

DYSMORPHOLOGY APPROACH

The following is the author's approach toward the evaluation of an individual with multiple defects:

I. Gather information. The family history is an essential aspect of such an evaluation. A question such as "Are there any individuals in the family with a similar type of problem?" may be helpful. The early history should usually include information about the onset and vigor of fetal activity, gestational timing, indications of uterine constraint, mode of delivery, size at birth, neonatal adaptation, and problems in postnatal growth and development. The physical examination should be complete, with the physician searching for minor as well as major anomalies. When possible, measurements should be taken to determine whether a given feature, such as apparent ocular hypertelorism or a small-appearing ear, is truly abnormal. The charts of normal measurements in Chapter 6 are provided for this purpose. An unusual feature ideally should be interpreted in relation to the findings in other family members before its relevance is determined.

II. Interpret the patient's anomalies from the viewpoint of developmental anatomy and strive to answer the following questions:

A. Which anomaly in the individual represents the earliest defect in morphogenesis? A table for this purpose is found in Chapter 3 (see Table 3-1). From such information one can determine that the problem in development must have existed *before* a particular

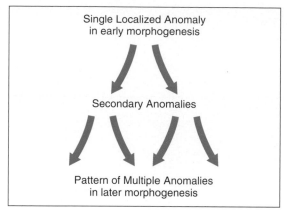

FIGURE 1. Sequence designates a single localized anomaly plus its subsequently derived structural consequences.

prenatal age and any factor *after* that time could not be the cause of that structural defect.

B. Can all the anomalies in the patient be explained on the basis of a single problem in morphogenesis that leads to a cascade of subsequent defects, as shown in Figure 1? These types of patterns of structural defects, referred to as *sequences*, may be divided into four categories from the developmental pathology viewpoint, as summarized in Figure 2. The first category is the *malformation sequence*, in which there has been a single localized poor formation of tissue that initiates a chain of subsequent defects. Malformation sequences occur in all gradation, the manifestations ranging from nearly normal to more severe, and have a recurrence risk that is most commonly in the 1% to 5% range.

The second category is the *deformation sequence,* in which there is no problem in the embryo or fetus (collectively referred to as fetus in this text), but mechanical forces such as uterine constraint result in altered morphogenesis, usually of the molding type. One example is the oligohydramnios deformation sequence, due to chronic leakage of amniotic fluid; another is the breech deformation sequence, the manifold effects of prolonged breech position late in fetal life. The deformations and deformation sequences are the subject of a separate text entitled *Smith's Recognizable Patterns of Human Deformation*. Most deformations have a very good to excellent prognosis in contrast with many malformations. The recurrence risk for deformation is usually of very low magnitude, unless the cause of the deformation problem is a persisting one, such as a bicornuate uterus.

The third category is the *disruption sequence*, in which the normal fetus is subjected to a destructive problem and its consequences. Such disruptions may be of vascular, infectious, or even mechanical origin. One example of this is disruption of normally developing tissues by amniotic bands. The spectra of consequences are set forth under *Amnion Rupture Sequence* in Chapter 1. In the final category, the *dysplasia sequence*, the primary defect is a lack of normal organization of cells into tissues. One example is the lack of migration of melanoblastic precursors from the neural crest. The spectra of consequences is referred to as the *neurocutaneous melanosis sequence* (see Chapter 1), in which melanocytic hamartomas of the skin occur in conjunction with similar changes in the pia and arachnoid.

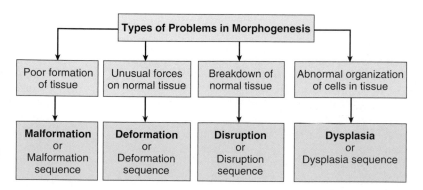

FIGURE 2. Four types of structural defects that can result in a chain of defects (sequence) by the time of birth.

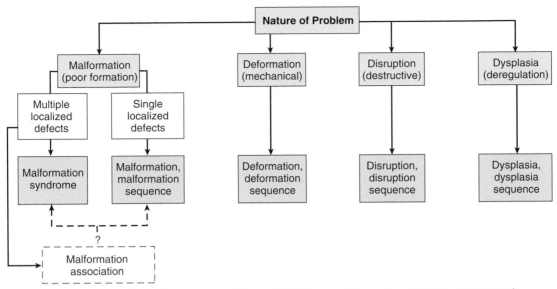

FIGURE 3. Most patients with multiple structural defects will fall into one of these six categories. The prognosis, management, and recurrence risk counseling may vary considerably among these categories.

C. Does the patient have multiple structural defects that cannot be explained on the basis of a single initiating defect and its consequences but rather appear to be the consequence of multiple defects in one or more tissues? These are referred to as *malformation syndromes* and are most commonly thought to be due to a single cause. The known modes of etiology for malformation syndromes include chromosomal abnormalities, mutant gene disorders, and environmental teratogens. However, there are still many for which the mode of etiology has not been resolved.

III. Attempt to arrive at a specific overall diagnosis within the six categories shown in Figure 3, confirm when possible, and counsel accordingly. When possible, counseling should include the following: an understanding of how the altered structures came to be as they are, the natural history of the condition and what measures can be used to assist the child, and the mode of etiology and genetic counseling (recurrence risk).

IMPORTANT GENERAL PRINCIPLES

The following are some of the important principles and information that should be appreciated in the evaluation of a patient with multiple defects.

Nonspecificity of Individual Defects

With rare exceptions, a clinical diagnosis of a pattern of malformation cannot be made on the basis of a single defect, as is evident in the differential diagnosis in the appendix. Even a rare defect may be a feature in several syndromes of variant etiology. A specific diagnosis usually depends on recognition of the overall *pattern of anomalies*, and the detection of minor defects may be as helpful as the detection of major anomalies in this regard.

Variance in Expression

Variance in extent of abnormality (expression) among individuals with the same etiologic syndrome is a usual phenomenon. Except for such nonspecific general features as mental deficiency and small stature, it is unusual to find a given anomaly in 100% of patients with the same etiologic syndrome. For example, in full 21 trisomy Down syndrome, only mental deficiency is ubiquitous; hypotonia is a frequent feature, but most of the other individual clinical features are found in less than 80% of such patients. However, a specific diagnosis of Down syndrome can generally be rendered, based on the *total pattern of anomalies*. It is especially important to appreciate that the environmentally determined disorders occur in all gradations of severity. Thus, as one example, prenatal exposure to alcohol leads to a spectrum of defects including spontaneous abortion, the pattern of structural defects referred to as the fetal alcohol syndrome, growth deficiency, and mental retardation.

Intraindividual variability in expression is also frequent, with variance in the degree of abnormality on the left versus the right side of the individual.

Heterogeneity

Similar phenotypes (overall physical similarity) may result from different etiologies. Only by finer discrimination of the phenotype or mode of etiology can such similar entities be distinguished. For example, the Marfan syndrome and homocystinuria were initially discriminated on the basis of homocystinuria, next by a difference in mode of etiology (autosomal dominant for the Marfan syndrome and autosomal recessive in homocystinuria), and finally by closer scrutiny of the phenotype. As another example, achondroplasia is frequently misdiagnosed among individuals who have chondrodystrophies that only superficially resemble true achondroplasia. A diagnosis should be rendered only when there is close resemblance in the overall pattern of malformation between the patient and the disorder under consideration.

Etiology

Most of the disorders herein set forth have a genetic basis. Chapter 4 provides the background information relative to genetic counseling for these conditions.

Beyond the following established disorders, roughly one half of the individuals with multiple defects have conditions that have not yet been recognized as specific disorders. A small percentage of such patients have a structural chromosomal abnormality. In such cases, genetic counseling should be withheld until it has been determined whether either parent is a balanced translocation carrier of the chromosomal abnormality. In the absence of an evident chromosomal abnormality or familial data suggesting a particular mode of etiology, it is generally impossible to state any accurate risk of recurrence for unknown patterns of multiple malformation. It is presumptuous to inform the parents that "this is a rare condition and therefore unlikely to recur in your future children." Under these circumstances, the author's present approach is to inform the parents that the lowest

recurrence risk is zero and the highest risk with each pregnancy would be 25%. This figure is predicated on the possibility of recessive inheritance or a nondetectable chromosomal abnormality from a patient who carries a balanced translocation.

Nomenclature

Some of the recommendations of an international committee on "Classification and Nomenclature of Morphologic Defects," published in *Lancet* 1:513, 1975, are used in this text. The recommendations of a more recent international group, which met in Mainz, Germany, under the direction of Professor Jurgen Spranger in November 1979 and again in Seattle in February 1980, have also been used.

Most of the nomenclature has already been alluded to; the following recommendations pertain to the naming of single defects and patterns of malformation.

Naming of Single Malformations

An adjective or descriptive term should be used with the name of the structure or the classic equivalent in common use (e.g., small mandible or micrognathia).

Naming of Patterns of Malformations

1. When the etiology is known and easily remembered, the appropriate term should be used to designate the disorder.
2. Time-honored designations should be continued unless there is good reason for change.
3. In the absence of a reasonably descriptive designation, eponyms, some of them multiple, may be used until the basic defect for the disorder is recognized. However, use of an eponym should thereafter be limited to one proper name.
4. The use of the possessive form of an eponym should be discontinued, because the author neither had nor owned the disorder.
5. Designation of a disorder by one or more of its manifestations does not necessarily imply that they are either specific or consistent components of that disorder.
6. Names that may have an unpleasant connotation for the family or affected individual should be avoided.

7. The syndrome should not be designated by the initials of the originally described patients.
8. Names that are too general for a specific syndrome should be avoided.
9. Unless acronyms are extremely pertinent or appropriate, they should be avoided.

Nomenclature Used to Describe Chromosomal Syndromes

Many of the disorders set forth in this book are the result of chromosomal abnormalities. This section is intended to familiarize readers who are not versed in cytogenetics with some of the basic nomenclature used in describing chromosomal syndromes. Several shorthand systems have been devised. The examples shown use the "short system," which is the one most commonly used in the recent literature. By comparing the karyotype examples with those in the text, the reader can decipher the cytogenetic shorthand. No attempt has been made to include every possible abnormality. For a comprehensive discussion of nomenclature, the reader is referred to the following source: Mitelman M (ed): *ISCN (1995): An International System for Human Cytogenetic Nomenclature.* Basel: S Karger, 1995.

METHOD AND UTILITY OF PRESENTATION OF PATTERNS OF MALFORMATION

The arrangement of the disorders in this book is predominantly based on the similarity in overall features or in one major feature among the patterns of malformation, as set forth in the table of contents. Thus, the order of presentation is designed to be of assistance in the diagnosis of the patient for whom a firm diagnosis has not been established. With the exception of the chromosomal abnormality syndromes, which share many features, and the disorders determined by an environmental agent, the conditions are not arranged in accordance with the mode of etiology. Each disorder has a listing of anomalies. The features that together tend to distinguish the syndrome from other known disorders are set forth in italic print. The main list consists of defects that occur in at least 25% and usually more than 50% of patients. Sometimes the actual percentage or number is stated for each anomaly. Below these are listed the occasional defects that occur with a frequency of 1% to 25%,

most commonly 5% to 10%. The occurrence of these "occasional abnormalities" is of interest and has been loosely ascribed to "developmental noise." In other words, an adverse influence that usually causes a particular pattern of malformation may occasionally cause other anomalies as well. Possibly it is differences of genetic background, environment, or both that allow some individuals to express these "occasional" anomalies. The important feature is that they are not random for a particular syndrome. For example, clinicians who have seen a large number of children with the Down syndrome are not surprised to see "another" Down syndrome baby with duodenal atresia, webbed neck, or tetralogy of Fallot.

The references listed for each disorder have been selected as those that give the best account of that disorder, provide recent additional knowledge, or represent the initial description. They are arranged in chronological order.

A word of caution is indicated. This book does not contain a number of very rare syndromes. Furthermore, information that appeared after June 2004, regarding the identification of specific genes responsible for disorders set forth in this book, is not always included.

OTHER SOURCES OF INFORMATION

Information about parent support groups for specific disorders as well as other general information that could be helpful to families is available on the following website: http://www.alliance.org.

Information on genetic testing and its use in diagnosis, management, and genetic counseling is available at http://genetests.org, and McKusick's Mendelian Inheritance in Man is available online at http://www.ncbi.nlm.nih.gov/entrez/query.fcgi?db =OMIM.

In addition to this text, many of the texts listed in the References may be of value in the recognition, management, and counseling of particular problems and patterns of malformation.

References
General
Benirschke K, Kaufmann P: Pathology of the Human Placenta, 4th ed. New York: Springer-Verlag, 2000.
Cassidy SB, Allison JE: Management of Genetic Conditions, 2nd ed. New York: Wiley-Liss, 2004.
Epstein CJ, Erickson RP, Wynshaw-Boris A: Inborn Errors of Development: The Molecular Basis of Clinical Disorders of Morphogenesis. New York: Oxford University Press, 2004.

Gorlin RJ, Cohen MM Jr, Hennekam RCM: Syndromes of the Head and Neck, 4th ed. New York: Oxford University Press, 2001.

Graham JM: Smith's Recognizable Patterns of Human Deformation, 2nd ed. Philadelphia: WB Saunders, 1988.

Rimoin DL, Connor JM, Pyeritz RE, Korf BR: Emery and Rimoin's Principles and Practice of Medical Genetics, 4th ed. New York: Churchill Livingstone, 2002.

Stevenson RE, Hall JG, Goodman RM: Human Malformations and Related Anomalies. New York: Oxford University Press, 1993.

Stevenson RE, Schwartz CE, Schroer RJ: X-Linked Mental Retardation. New York: Oxford University Press, 2000.

Warkany J: Congenital Malformations. Chicago: Year Book Medical Publishers, 1971.

Chromosomal Abnormalities

Borgaonkar DS: Chromosomal Variations in Man: A Catalog of Chromosomal Variants and Anomalies. New York: Wiley-Liss, 1997. Available at: http://www.wiley.com/legacy/products/subject/life/borgaonkar/.

de Grouchy J, Turleau C: Clinical Atlas of Human Chromosomes. New York: John Wiley & Sons, 1984.

Schinzel A: Catalogue of Unbalanced Chromosome Aberrations in Man. New York: Walter de Gruyter, 2001.

Connective Tissue, and Skeletal Dysplasias

Beighton P: McKusick's Heritable Disorders of Connective Tissue, 5th ed. St. Louis: Mosby, 1993.

Ornoy A, Borochowitz A, Lachman R et al: Atlas of Fetal Skeletal Radiology. Chicago: Year Book, 1988.

Spranger JW, Brill PW, Poznanski AK: Bone Dysplasias: An Atlas of Genetic Disorders of Skeletal Development, 2nd ed. New York: Oxford University Press, 2002.

Staheli LT, Hall JG, Jaffe KM et al: Arthrogryposis: A text atlas. New York: Cambridge University Press, 1998.

Wynne-Davies R, Hall CM, Apley AG: Atlas of Skeletal Dysplasias. New York: Churchill Livingstone, 1985.

Hereditary Deafness with Associated Anomalies

Toriello HV, Reardon W, Gorlin RJ: Hereditary Hearing Loss and Its Syndromes, 2nd ed. New York: Oxford University Press, 2004.

Overgrowth

Cohen MM, Neri G, Weksberg R: Overgrowth Syndromes. New York: Oxford University Press, 2002.

Craniosynostosis

Cohen MM, MacLean RE: Craniosynostosis: Diagnosis, Evaluation, and Management, 2nd ed. New York: Oxford University Press, 2000.

Teratology

Briggs GG, Freeman RK, Yaffe SJ: Drugs in Pregnancy and Lactation, 6th ed. Baltimore: Lippincott, Williams & Wilkins, 2002.

Shepard TH: Catalog of Teratogenic Agents, 9th ed. Baltimore: Johns Hopkins University Press, 1998.

1 Recognizable Patterns of Malformation

A Chromosomal Abnormality Syndromes

DOWN SYNDROME
(TRISOMY 21 SYNDROME)

Hypotonia, Flat Facies, Slanted Palpebral Fissures, Small Ears

Down's report of 1866 on the ethnic classification of idiots stated that a "large number of congenital idiots are typical Mongols," and he set forth the clinical description of the Down syndrome. The textbook by Penrose and Smith provides an overall appraisal of this disorder that has an incidence of 1 in 660 newborns, making it the most common pattern of malformation in man.

ABNORMALITIES

General. Hypotonia with tendency to keep mouth open and protrude the tongue, diastasis recti, hyperflexibility of joints, relatively small stature with awkward gait, increased weight in adolescence.

Central Nervous System. Mental deficiency.

Craniofacial. Brachycephaly with relatively flat occiput and tendency toward midline parietal hair whorl; mild microcephaly with up-slanting palpebral fissures; thin cranium with late closure of fontanels; hypoplasia to aplasia of frontal sinuses, short hard palate; small nose with low nasal bridge and tendency to have inner epicanthal folds.

Eyes. Speckling of iris (Brushfield spots) with peripheral hypoplasia of iris; fine lens opacities by slit lamp examination (59%); refractive error, mostly myopia (70%); nystagmus (35%); strabismus (45%); blocked tear duct (20%); acquired cataracts in adults (30% to 60%).

Ears. Small; overfolding of angulated upper helix; sometimes prominent; small or absent earlobes; hearing loss (66%) of conductive, mixed, or sensorineural type; fluid accumulation in middle ear (60% to 80%).

Dentition. Hypoplasia, irregular placement, fewer caries than usual. Periodontal disease.

Neck. Appears short.

Hands. Relatively short metacarpals and phalanges; fifth finger: hypoplasia of midphalanx of fifth finger (60%) with clinodactyly (50%), a single crease (40%), or both; simian crease (45%); distal position of palmar axial triradius (84%); ulnar loop dermal ridge pattern on all digits (35%).

Feet. Wide gap between first and second toes, plantar crease between first and second toes, open field dermal ridge patterning in hallucal area of sole (50%).

Pelvis. Hypoplasia with outward lateral flare of iliac wings and shallow acetabular angle.

Cardiac. Anomaly in approximately 40%; endocardial cushion defect, ventricular septal defect, patent ductus arteriosus, auricular septal defect, and aberrant subclavian artery, in decreasing order of frequency; mitral valve prolapse with or without tricuspid valve prolapse and aortic regurgitation by 20 years of age; risk for regurgitation occurs after 18 years of age.

Skin. Loose folds in posterior neck (infancy); cutis marmorata, especially in extremities (43%); dry, hyperkeratotic skin with time (75%);

infections in the perigenital area, buttocks, and thighs that begin as follicular pustules in 50% to 60% of adolescents.

Hair. Fine, soft, and often sparse; straight pubic hair at adolescence.

Genitalia. Relatively small penis and decreased testicular volume; primary gonadal deficiency is common, is progressive from birth to adolescence, and is definitely present in adults; although fertility has rarely been reported in females, no male has reproduced.

OCCASIONAL ABNORMALITIES.

Seizures (less than 9%); keratoconus (6%); congenital cataract (3%); low placement of ears; webbed neck; two ossification centers in manubrium sterni; funnel or pigeon breast; tracheal stenosis with hourglass trachea and midtracheal absence of tracheal pars membranacea; gastrointestinal tract anomalies (12%) including tracheoesophageal fistula; duodenal atresia; omphalocele, pyloric stenosis, annular pancreas, Hirschsprung disease, and imperforate anus. Incomplete fusion of vertebral arches of lower spine (37%); only 11 ribs; atlantoaxial instability (12%); posterior occipitoatlantal hypermobility (8.5%); abnormal odontoid process (6%); hypoplastic posterior arch C1 (26%). Hip abnormality (8%) including dysplasia, dislocation, avascular necrosis, or slipped capital femoral epiphyses; syndactyly of second and third toes; prune belly anomaly. The incidence of leukemia is approximately 1 in 95, or close to 1%. Thyroid disorders are more common, including athyreosis, simple goiter, and hyperthyroidism. Fatal perinatal liver disease has been reported.

PRINCIPAL FEATURES IN THE NEONATE.

The diagnosis can generally be made shortly after birth, and therefore, the following ten features of Down syndrome in the neonate are presented as set forth by Hall, who found at least four of these abnormalities in all of 48 neonates with Down syndrome and six or more in 89% of them.

Hypotonia	80%
Poor Moro reflex	85%
Hyperflexibility of joints	80%
Excess skin on back of neck	80%
Flat facial profile	90%
Slanted palpebral fissures	80%
Anomalous auricles	60%
Dysplasia of pelvis	70%
Dysplasia of midphalanx of fifth finger	60%
Simian crease	45%

NATURAL HISTORY.

Muscle tone tends to improve with age, whereas the rate of developmental progress slows with age. For example, 23% of a group of Down syndrome children under 3 years had a developmental quotient above 50, whereas none of those in the 3- to 9-year group had intelligence quotients above 50. Though the IQ range is generally said to be 25 to 50 with an occasional individual above 50, the mean IQ for older patients is 24. Fortunately, social performance is usually beyond that expected for mental age, averaging $3\frac{1}{3}$ years above mental age for the older individuals. Generally "good babies" and happy children, individuals with Down syndrome tend toward mimicry, are friendly, have a good sense of rhythm, and enjoy music. Mischievousness and obstinacy may also be characteristics, and 13% have serious emotional problems. Coordination is often poor, and the voice tends to be harsh. Early developmental enrichment programs for Down syndrome children have resulted in improved rate of progress during the first 4 to 5 years of life. Whether such training programs will appreciably alter the ultimate level of performance remains to be determined.

Sleep-related upper airway obstruction occurs in approximately one third of cases.

Growth is relatively slow, and during the first 8 years, secondary centers of ossification are often late in development. However, during later childhood, the osseous maturation is more "normal," and final height is usually attained around 15 years of age. Adolescent sexual development is usually somewhat less complete than normal. Because thyroid dysfunction is common and can be easily missed, periodic thyroid function studies should be performed.

The median age at death increased from 25 years in 1983 to 49 years in 1997. The major cause for early mortality is congenital heart defects. Mortality from respiratory disease, mainly pneumonia, as well as other infectious diseases is much higher than in the general population. Although leukemia has frequently appeared on death certificates of affected individuals, other neoplasms were listed less than one-tenth as often as expected. Low-grade problems that occur frequently are chronic rhinitis, conjunctivitis, and periodontal disease, none of which are easy to "cure." Immunologic dysfunction including both T-cell and B-cell derangement, has been demonstrated, as has the frequent occurrence of hepatitis B surface antigen carrier state. Therefore, HBV vaccination is advised.

Although asymptomatic atlantoaxial dislocation occurs in 12% to 20% of individuals with Down syndrome, symptoms referable to compression of the spinal cord are rare. Unfortunately, the literature regarding radiographic screening for this finding is controversial. No study to date has documented that radiographic findings can predict which children will develop neurologic problems. Any child with Down syndrome who develops changes in bowel or bladder function, neck posturing, or loss of ambulatory skills should be evaluated carefully with plain roentgenograms of the cervical spine. The majority of patients develop symptoms before 10 years of age, when the ligamentous laxity is most severe. The Committee on Genetics of the American Academy of Pediatrics has published health supervision guidelines for children with Down syndrome that offer recommendations for follow-up of affected children.

ETIOLOGY.

The etiology of Down syndrome is trisomy for all or a large part of chromosome 21. The combined results of 11 unselected surveys totaling 784 cases showed the following relative frequencies of particular types of chromosomal alteration for Down syndrome:

Full 21 trisomy	94%
21 Trisomy/normal mosaicism	2.4%
Translocation cases (with about equal occurrence of D/G and G/G translocations)	3.3%

Faulty chromosome distribution leading to Down syndrome is more likely to occur at older maternal age, as shown in the following figures of incidence for Down syndrome at term delivery for particular maternal ages: 15 to 29 years, 1 in 1500; 30 to 34 years, 1 in 800; 35 to 39 years, 1 in 270; 40 to 44 years, 1 in 100; and over 45 years, 1 in 50.

Though the general likelihood for recurrence of Down syndrome is 1%, the principal task in giving recurrence risk figures to parents is to determine whether the Down syndrome child is a translocation case with a parent who is a translocation carrier and thereby has a relatively high risk for recurrence. The likelihood of finding a translocation in the Down syndrome child of a mother under 30 years of age is 6%, and of such cases only one out of three will be found to have a translocation carrier parent. Therefore, the estimated probability that either parent of a Down syndrome patient born of a mother under 30 years is a G/D or G/G translocation carrier is 2% versus 0.3% when the Down syndrome patient is born of a mother over 30 years of age. Having excluded a translocation carrier parent, the risk for recurrence may be stated as about 1%. Although a low figure, it is enough to justify prenatal diagnosis for any future pregnancy. The recurrence risk for the rare translocation carrier parent will depend on the type of translocation and the sex of the parent. Mosaicism usually leads to a less severe phenotype. Any degree of intellectual ability from normal or nearly normal to severe retardation is found, and this does not always correlate with the clinical phenotype. Patients with the features of Down syndrome and relatively good performance are likely to have mosaicism (which is not always easy to demonstrate).

References

Down JLH: Observations on an ethnic classification of idiots. Clinical Lecture Reports, London Hospital 3:259, 1866.

Richards BW et al: Cytogenetic survey of 225 patients diagnosed clinically as mongols. J Ment Defic Res 9:245, 1965.

Hall B: Mongolism in newborn infants. Clin Pediatr 5:4, 1966.

Penrose LS, Smith GF: Down's Anomaly. Boston: Little, Brown, 1966.

Smith DW, Wilson AC: The Child with Down's Syndrome. Philadelphia: WB Saunders, 1973.

Baird PA, Sadovnick AD: Life expectancy in Down syndrome. J Pediatr 110:849, 1987.

Davidson RG: Atlantoaxial instability in individuals with Down syndrome: A fresh look at the evidence. Pediatrics 81:857, 1988.

Pueschel SM: Atlantoaxial instability and Down syndrome. Pediatrics 81:879, 1988.

Pueschel SM: Clinical aspects of Down syndrome from infancy to adulthood. Am J Med Genet Suppl 7:52, 1990.

Ugazio AG et al: Immunology of Down syndrome: A review. Am J Med Genet Suppl 7:204, 1990.

Pueschel SM et al: A longitudinal study of atlantodens relationships in asymptomatic individuals with Down syndrome. Pediatrics 89:1194, 1992.

Cremers MJG et al: Risks of sports activities in children with Down's syndrome and atlantoaxial instability. Lancet 342:511, 1993.

American Academy of Pediatrics. Health supervision for children with Down syndrome. Pediatrics 107:442, 2001.

Yang et al: Mortality associated with Down's syndrome in the USA from 1983 to 1997: a population-based study. Lancet 359:1019, 2002.

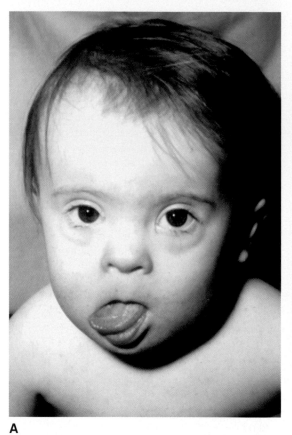

A

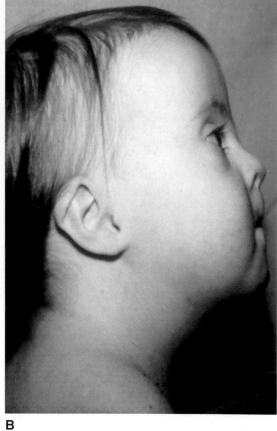

B

C

FIGURE 1. Down syndrome. **A–C,** Young infant. Flat facies, straight hair, protrusion of tongue, single crease on inturned fifth finger.

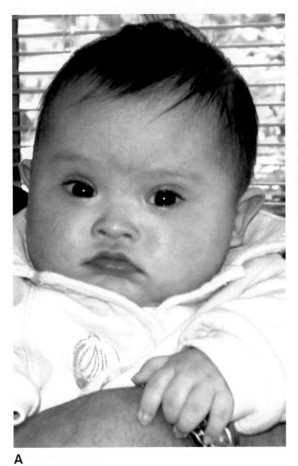

A

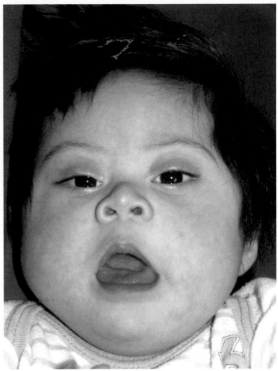

B

FIGURE 2. **A** and **B,** Upslanting palpebral fissures. Low nasal bridge with upturned nares. (Courtesy of Dr. Lynne M. Bird, Children's Hospital, San Diego.)

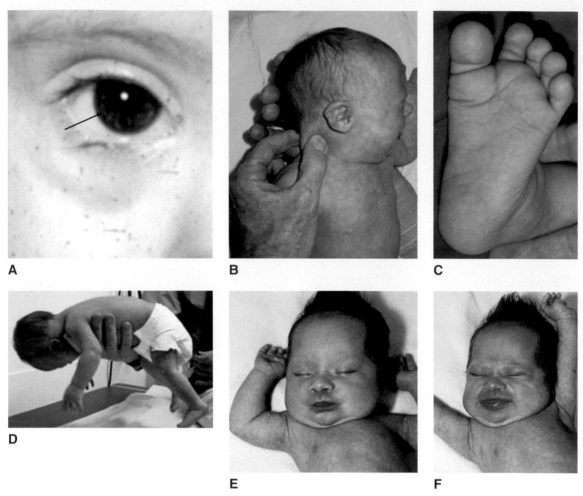

FIGURE 3. **A,** Brushfield spots. **B,** Loose nuchal skin. **C,** Wide space between toes 1 and 2. **D,** Poor tone. **E** and **F,** Accentuation of typical face when crying. (**E** and **F,** Courtesy of Dr. Marilyn C. Jones, Children's Hospital, San Diego.)

TRISOMY 18 SYNDROME

Clenched Hand, Short Sternum, Low Arch Dermal Ridge Patterning on Fingertips

This condition was first recognized as a specific entity in 1960 by discovery of the extra 18 chromosome in babies with a particular pattern of malformation (Edwards et al., Patau et al., and Smith et al.). It is the second most common multiple malformation syndrome, with an incidence of approximately 0.3 per 100 newborn babies. There has been a 3:1 preponderance of females to males. Several good reviews set forth a full appraisal of this syndrome. More than 130 different abnormalities have been noted in the literature on patients with the 18 trisomy syndrome, and therefore the listing of abnormalities has been divided into those that occur in 50% or more of patients, in 10% to 50% of patients, and in less than 10% of patients.

ABNORMALITIES FOUND IN 50% OR MORE OF PATIENTS

General. Feeble fetal activity, weak cry, altered gestational timing; one third premature, one third postmature; polyhydramnios, small placenta, single umbilical artery, growth deficiency; mean birth weight, 2340 g; hypoplasia of skeletal muscle, subcutaneous and adipose tissue; mental deficiency, hypertonicity (after neonatal period); diminished response to sound.

Craniofacial. Prominent occiput, narrow bifrontal diameter; low-set, malformed auricles; short palpebral fissures; small oral opening, narrow palatal arch; micrognathia.

Hands and Feet. Clenched hand, tendency for overlapping of index finger over third, fifth finger over fourth; absence of distal crease on fifth finger with or without distal creases on third and fourth fingers; low arch dermal ridge pattern on six or more fingertips; hypoplasia of nails, especially on fifth finger and toes; short hallux, frequently dorsiflexed.

Thorax. Short sternum, with reduced number of ossification centers; small nipples.

Abdominal Wall. Inguinal or umbilical hernia and/or diastasis recti.

Pelvis and Hips. Small pelvis, limited hip abduction.

Genitalia. Male: cryptorchidism.

Skin. Redundancy, mild hirsutism of forehead and back, prominent cutis marmorata.

Cardiac. Ventricular septal defect, auricular septal defect, patent ductus arteriosus.

ABNORMALITIES FOUND IN 10% TO 50% OF CASES

Craniofacial. Wide fontanels, microcephaly, hypoplasia of orbital ridges; inner epicanthal folds, ptosis of eyelid, corneal opacity; cleft lip, cleft palate, or both.

Hands and Feet. Ulnar or radial deviation of hand, hypoplastic to absent thumb, simian crease; equinovarus, rocker-bottom feet, syndactyly of second and third toes.

Thorax. Relatively broad, with or without widely spaced nipples.

Genitalia. Female: hypoplasia of labia majora with prominent clitoris.

Anus. Malposed or funnel-shaped anus.

Cardiac. Bicuspid aortic and/or pulmonic valves, nodularity of valve leaflets, pulmonic stenosis, coarctation of aorta.

Lung. Malsegmentation to absence of right lung.

Diaphragm. Muscle hypoplasia with or without eventration.

Abdomen. Meckels diverticulum, heterotopic pancreatic and/or splenic tissue, omphalocele. Incomplete rotation of colon.

Renal. Horseshoe defect, ectopic kidney, double ureter, hydronephrosis, polycystic kidney.

ABNORMALITIES FOUND IN LESS THAN 10% OF CASES

Central Nervous System. Facial palsy, paucity of myelination, microgyria, cerebellar hypoplasia, defect of corpus callosum, hydrocephalus, meningomyelocele.

Craniofacial. Wormian cranial bones, shallow elongated sella turcica; slanted palpebral fissures, hypertelorism, colobomata of iris, cataract, microphthalmos; choanal atresia.

Hands. Syndactyly of third and fourth fingers, polydactyly, short fifth metacarpals, ectrodactyly.

Other Skeletal. Radial aplasia, incomplete ossification of clavicle, hemivertebrae, fused vertebrae, short neck, scoliosis, rib anomaly, pectus excavatum, dislocated hip.

Genitalia. Male: hypospadias, bifid scrotum; female: bifid uterus, ovarian hypoplasia.

Cardiovascular. Anomalous coronary artery, transposition, tetralogy of Fallot, coarctation of aorta, dextrocardia, aberrant subclavian artery, intimal proliferation in arteries with arteriosclerotic change and medial calcification.

Abdominal. Pyloric stenosis, extrahepatic biliary atresia, hypoplastic gallbladder, gallstones, imperforate anus.

Renal. Hydronephrosis, polycystic kidney (small cysts), Wilms tumor.

Endocrine. Thyroid or adrenal hypoplasia.

Other. Hemangiomata, thymic hypoplasia, tracheoesophageal fistula, thrombocytopenia.

NATURAL HISTORY.
Babies with the trisomy 18 syndrome are usually feeble and have a limited capacity for survival. Resuscitation is often performed at birth, and they may have apneic episodes in the neonatal period. Poor sucking capability may necessitate nasogastric tube feeding, but even with optimal management, they fail to thrive. Fifty percent die within the first week and many of the remaining die in the next 12 months. Median survival time is 14.5 days. Only 5% to 10% survive the first year as severely mentally defective individuals. Although most children who survive the first year are unable to walk in an unsupported fashion and verbal communication is usually limited to a few single words, it is important to realize that some older children with trisomy 18 smile, laugh, and interact with and relate to their families. All achieve some psychomotor maturation and continue to learn. There are at least ten reports of affected children older than 10 years of age. Once the diagnosis has been established, limitation of extraordinary medical means for prolongation of life should be seriously considered. However, the personal feelings of the parents and the individual circumstances of each infant must be taken into consideration. Baty and colleagues documented the natural history of this disorder. For children who survive, the average number of days in the neonatal intensive care unit was 16.3, the average number of days on a ventilator was 10.1, and 13% had surgery in the neonatal period. There was no evidence for an increase in adverse reactions to immunizations. Growth curves for length, weight, and head circumference are provided in that study.

ETIOLOGY.
The etiology of this disorder is trisomy for all or a large part of the number 18 chromosome. The great majority of cases have full 18 trisomy, the result of faulty chromosomal distribution, which is most likely to occur at older maternal age; the mean maternal age at birth of babies with this syndrome is 32 years. Translocation cases, the result of chromosomal breakage, can be excluded only by chromosomal studies. When such a case is found, the parents should also have chromosomal studies to determine whether one of them is a balanced translocation carrier with high risk for recurrence in future offspring. No recurrence occurred in 170 women with a full 18 trisomy offspring who underwent amniocentesis. It seems safe with a full 18 trisomy to presume that the recurrence risk would be even lower than the 1% for full 21 trisomy syndrome cases. This statement is predicated on the indication that most 18 trisomic individuals die in embryonic or fetal life, as suggested by the chromosomal findings in spontaneous abortuses.

Mosaicism for an additional chromosome 18 leads to a partial clinical expression of the pattern of trisomy 18, with longer survival and any degree of variation between nearly normal and the full pattern.

Partial trisomy 18: Trisomy of the short arm causes a very nonspecific clinical picture and mild or no mental deficiency. Cases with familial trisomy of the short arm, centromere, and proximal one third of the long arm show features of trisomy 18, although not the full pattern. Trisomy for the entire long arm is clinically indistinguishable from full trisomy 18. Trisomy for the distal one third to one half of the long arm leads to a partial picture of trisomy 18 with longer survival and less profound mental deficiency. In early childhood, the patients resemble trisomy 18 cases, whereas adolescents and adults display a more nonspecific pattern of malformation, including prominent orbital ridges, broad and prominent nasal bridge, everted upper lip, receding mandible, poorly modeled ears, short neck, and long, hyperextendible fingers. Muscular tone tends to be decreased, mental deficiency is severe, and about one third of the patients suffer from seizures.

References
Edwards JH et al: A new trisomic syndrome. Lancet 1:787, 1960.

Patau K et al: Multiple congenital anomaly caused by an extra autosome. Lancet 1:790, 1960.

Smith DW et al: A new autosomal trisomy syndrome. J Pediatr 57:338, 1960.

Smith DW.: Autosomal abnormalities. Am J Obstet Gynecol 90:1055, 1964.

Taylor A, Polani PE: Autosomal trisomy syndromes, excluding Down's. Guys Hosp Rep 13:231, 1964.

Warkany J, Passarge E, Smith LB: Congenital malformations in autosomal trisomy syndromes. Am J Dis Child 112:502, 1966.

Weber WW: Survival and the sex ratio in trisomy 17–18. Am J Hum Genet 19:369, 1967.

Rasmussen S, Wong LY, Yang Q, et al: Population-based analysis of mortality in trisomy13 and trisomy 18. Pediatrics 111:777, 2003.

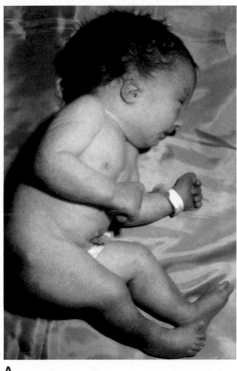

A

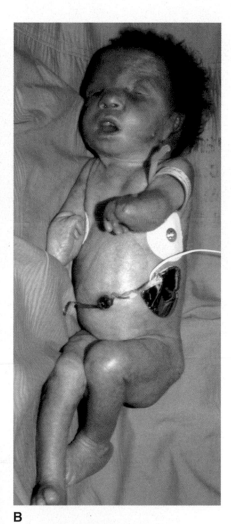

B

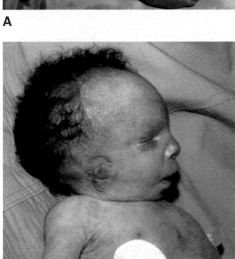

C

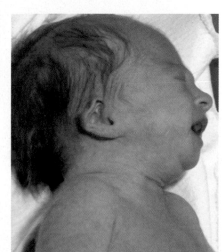

D

FIGURE 1. Trisomy 18 syndrome. **A** and **B,** Note hypertonicity evident in the clenched hands and crossed legs; note the narrow pelvis. **C** and **D,** Hypoplastic supraorbital ridges; prominent occiput; low-set, slanted, malformed auricle.

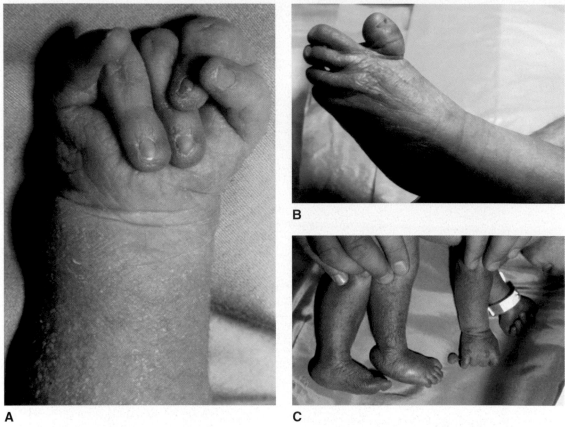

A

C

FIGURE 2. **A,** Clenched hand with index finger overlying third; hypoplasia of fingernails. **B,** Dorsiflexed short hallux. **C,** Prominent calcaneous and postaxial polydactyly.

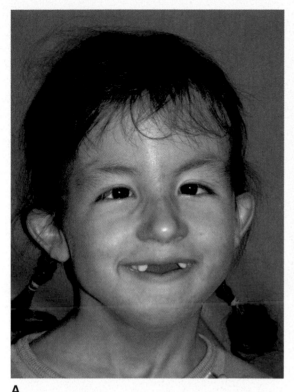

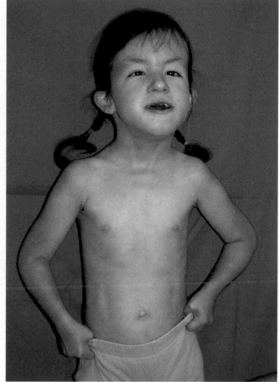

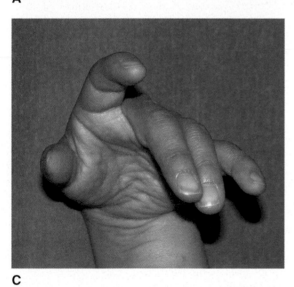

FIGURE 3. **A–C,** Older child with Trisomy 18 syndrome. (Courtesy of Dr. Lynne M. Bird, Children's Hospital, San Diego.)

TRISOMY 13 SYNDROME
(D₁ Trisomy Syndrome)

Defects of Eye, Nose, Lip, and Forebrain of Holoprosencephaly Type; Polydactyly; Narrow Hyperconvex Fingernails; Skin Defects of Posterior Scalp

Apparently described by Bartholin in 1657, this syndrome was not generally recognized until its trisomic etiology was discovered by Patau and colleagues in 1960. The incidence is approximately 1 in 5000 births.

ABNORMALITIES FOUND IN 50% OR MORE OF PATIENTS

Central Nervous System. Holoprosencephaly type defect with varying degrees of incomplete development of forebrain and olfactory and optic nerves; minor motor seizures, often with hypsarrhythmic electroencephalography (EEG) pattern; apneic spells in early infancy; severe mental retardation.

Hearing. Apparent deafness (defects of organ of Corti in the two cases studied).

Cranium. Moderate microcephaly with sloping forehead, wide sagittal suture and fontanels.

Eyes. Microphthalmia, colobomata of iris, or both; retinal dysplasia, often including islands of cartilage.

Mouth. Cleft lip (60% to 80%), cleft palate, or both.

Auricles. Abnormal helices with or without low-set ears.

Skin. Capillary hemangiomata, especially forehead; localized scalp defects in parieto-occipital area; loose skin, posterior neck.

Hands and Feet. Distal palmar axial triradii, simian crease, hyperconvex narrow fingernails, flexion of fingers with or without overlapping and camptodactyly, polydactyly of hands and sometimes feet, posterior prominence of heel.

Other Skeletal. Thin posterior ribs with or without missing rib, hypoplasia of pelvis with shallow acetabular angle.

Cardiac. Abnormality in 80% with ventricular septal defect, patent ductus arteriosus, auricular septal defect, and dextroposition, in decreasing order of frequency.

Genitalia. Male: cryptorchidism, abnormal scrotum; female: bicornuate uterus.

Hematologic. Increased frequency of nuclear projections in neutrophils, unusual persistence of embryonic and/or fetal type hemoglobin.

Other. Single umbilical artery, inguinal or umbilical hernia.

ABNORMALITIES FOUND IN LESS THAN 50% OF PATIENTS

Growth. Prenatal onset of growth deficiency; mean birth weight, 2480 g.

Central Nervous System. Hypertonia, hypotonia, agenesis of corpus callosum, hydrocephalus, fusion of basal ganglia, cerebellar hypoplasia, meningomyelocele.

Eyes. Shallow supraorbital ridges, upslanting palpebral fissures, absent eyebrows, hypotelorism, hypertelorism, anophthalmos, cyclopia.

Nose, Mouth, and Mandible. Absent philtrum, narrow palate, cleft tongue, micrognathia.

Hands and Feet. Retroflexible thumb, ulnar deviation at wrist, low arch digital dermal ridge pattern, fibular S-shaped hallucal dermal ridge pattern, syndactyly, cleft between first and second toes, hypoplastic toenails, equinovarus, radial aplasia.

Cardiac. Anomalous pulmonary venous return, overriding aorta, pulmonary stenosis, hypoplastic aorta, atretic mitral and/or aortic valves, bicuspid aortic valve.

Abdominal. Omphalocele, heterotopic pancreatic or splenic tissue, incomplete rotation of colon, Meckel's diverticulum.

Renal. Polycystic kidney (31%), hydronephrosis, horseshoe kidney, duplicated ureters.

Genitalia. Male: hypospadias; female: duplication and/or anomalous insertion of fallopian tubes, uterine cysts, hypoplastic ovaries.

Other. Thrombocytopenia, situs inversus of lungs, cysts of thymus, calcified pulmonary arterioles, large gallbladder, radial aplasia, flexion deformity of large joints, diaphragmatic defect.

NATURAL HISTORY.
The median survival for children with this disorder is 7 days. Ninety-one percent died within the first year. Survivors have severe mental retardation, often seizures, and fail to thrive. Only one adult, 33 years of age, has been reported. Because of the high infant mortality, surgical or orthopedic corrective procedures should be withheld in early infancy to await the outcome of the first few months. Furthermore, because of the severe brain defect, limitation of extraordinary medical means to prolong the life of individuals with this syndrome should be seriously considered. However, it is important to emphasize that each case must be taken on an individual basis. The individual circumstances of each child as well as the personal feelings of the parents must be acknowledged. Baty and colleagues documented the natural history of this disorder. For children who survived in their study, the average number of days in the neonatal intensive care unit was 10.8, average days on a ventilator was 13.3, and 23% had surgery in the neonatal period. There was no evidence for an increase in adverse reactions to immunizations. Growth curves are provided in that study.

ETIOLOGY.
The etiology for this disorder is trisomy for all or a large part of chromosome 13. Older maternal age has been a factor in the occurrence of this aneuploidy syndrome. Although no accurate empiric recurrence risk data are presently available, it is presumed that the likelihood for recurrence is of very low magnitude for the full 13 trisomy cases. As with Down syndrome, chromosomal studies are indicated on 13 trisomy syndrome babies in order to detect the rare translocation patient having a balanced translocation parent for whom the risk of recurrence would be of major concern.

Cases with *trisomy 13 mosaicism* most often show a less severe clinical phenotype with every degree of variation, from the full pattern of malformation seen in trisomy 13 to a near-normal phenotype. Survival is usually longer. The degree of mental deficiency is variable.

Partial trisomy for the proximal segment (13pter→q14) is characterized by a nonspecific pattern, including a large nose, short upper lip, receding mandible, fifth finger clinodactyly, and usually severe mental deficiency. The overall picture shows little similarity to that of full trisomy 13, and survival is not significantly reduced.

Partial trisomy for the distal segment (13q14→ qter) has a characteristic phenotype associated with severe mental deficiency. The facies is marked by frontal capillary hemangiomata, a short nose with upturned tip, and elongated philtrum, synophrys, bushy eyebrows and long, incurved lashes, and a prominent antihelix. Trigonocephaly and arrhinencephaly have occasionally been seen. Approximately one fourth of the patients die during early postnatal life.

COMMENT.
The defects of midface, eye, and forebrain, which occur in variable degree as a feature of this syndrome, appear to be the consequence of a single defect in the early (3 weeks) development of the prechordal mesoderm, which is not only necessary for morphogenesis of the midface but also exerts an inductive role on the subsequent development of the prosencephalon, the forepart of the brain. This type of defect has been referred to as holoprosencephaly or arrhinencephaly and varies in severity from cyclopia to cebocephaly to less severe forms.

References
Patau K et al: Multiple congenital anomaly caused by an extra chromosome. Lancet 1:790, 1960.
Warburg M, Mikkelsen M: A case of 13–15 trisomy or Bartholin-Patau's syndrome. Acta Ophthalmol 41:321, 1963.
Smith DW: Autosomal abnormalities. Am J Obstet Gynecol 90:1055, 1964.
Warkany J, Passarge E, Smith LB: Congenital malformations in autosomal trisomy syndromes. Am J Dis Child 112:502, 1966.
Schinzel A: Autosomale Chromosomenaberationen. Arch Genet 52:1, 1979.
Goldstein H, Nielsen KG: Rates and survival of individuals with trisomy 13 and 18: Data from a 10-year period in Denmark. Clin Genet 34:366, 1988.
Baty BJ et al: Natural history of trisomy 18 and trisomy 13: I. Growth, physical assessment, medical histories, survival and recurrence risk. Am J Med Genet 49:175, 1994.
Baty BJ et al: Natural history of trisomy 18 and trisomy 13: II. Psychomotor development. Am J Med Genet 49:189, 1994.
Rasmussen SA et al: Population-based analysis of mortality in trisomy 13 and trisomy 18. Pediatrics 111:777, 2003.

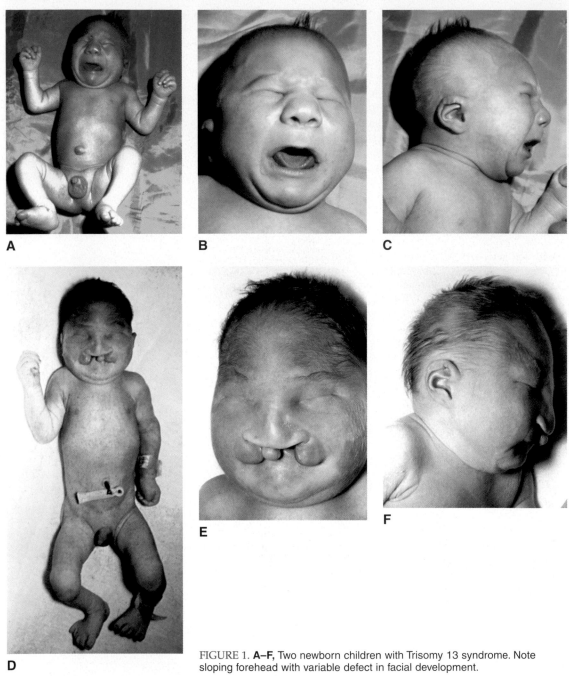

FIGURE 1. **A–F,** Two newborn children with Trisomy 13 syndrome. Note sloping forehead with variable defect in facial development.

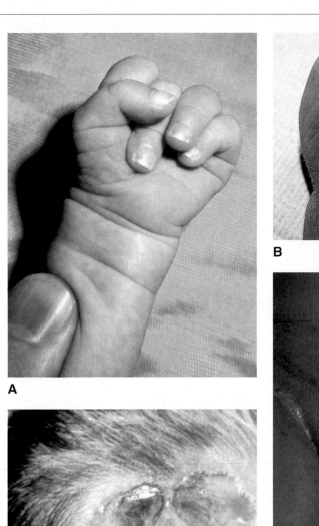

A

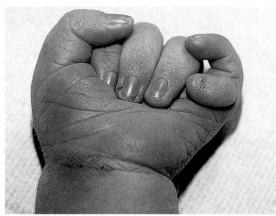

B

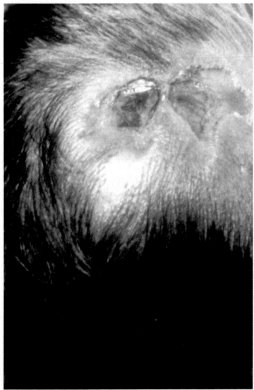

C

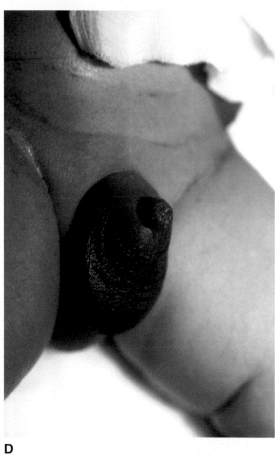

D

FIGURE 2. **A** and **B,** Note hyperconvex nails and postaxial polydactyly. **C,** Aplasia cutis congenita over posterior occiput. **D,** Scrotalization of the phallus.

TRISOMY 8 SYNDROME
(Usually Trisomy 8/Normal Mosaicism)

Thick Lips, Deep-Set Eyes, Prominent Ears, Camptodactyly

Patients with trisomy for a C-group autosome have been recognized since 1963. Most of them have been mosaics of trisomy C/normal. The phenotype tends to be similar, and, more recently, chromosomal banding techniques have identified the extra chromosome as number 8. More than 100 cases have been reported.

ABNORMALITIES

Growth. Variable, from small to tall.

Performance. Mild to severe mental deficiency with tendency to poor coordination.

Craniofacial. Tendency toward prominent forehead, deep-set eyes, strabismus, hypertelorism with broad nasal root and prominent nares, full lips, everted lower lip, micrognathia, high-arched palate, cleft palate, and prominent cupped ears with thick helices.

Limbs. Camptodactyly of second through fifth fingers and toes; limited elbow supination; deep creases, palms and soles; single transverse palmar crease; major joint contracture; abnormal nails.

Other. Long, slender trunk; abnormal scapula, abnormal sternum, short or webbed neck; narrow pelvis; hip dysplasia; widely spaced nipples; ureteral-renal anomalies; cardiac defects.

OCCASIONAL ABNORMALITIES. Absent patellae, pili bifurcati, conductive deafness, seizures, vertebral anomaly (bifid vertebrae, extra lumbar vertebra, spina bifida occulta), scoliosis, cryptorchidism, jejunal duplication, agenesis of corpus callosum, hypoplastic anemia, leukopenia, coagulation factor VII deficiency, mediastinal germ cell tumor, gastric leiomyosarcoma.

NATURAL HISTORY. The natural history is largely dependent on the severity of mental deficiency. There appears to be a lack of correlation between the phenotype and the percentage of trisomic cells.

ETIOLOGY. The etiology for this disorder is trisomy 8, the majority of patients being mosaics. Apparently, full trisomy 8 is usually an early lethal disorder.

References

Stalder GR, Buhler EM, Weber JR: Possible trisomy in chromosome group 6–12. Lancet 1:1379, 1963.

Schinzel A et al: Trisomy 8 mosaicism syndrome. Helv Pediatr Acta 29:531, 1974.

Riccardi VM: Trisomy 8: An international study of 70 patients. Birth Defects XIII(3C):171, 1977.

Kurtyka ZE et al: Trisomy 8 mosaicism syndrome. Clin Pediatr 27:557, 1988.

Breslau-Siderius LJ et al: Pili bifurcati occurring in association with the mosaic trisomy 8 syndrome. Clin Dysmorph 5:275, 1996.

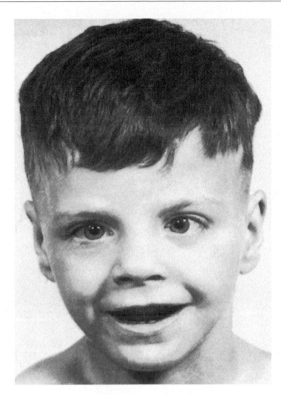

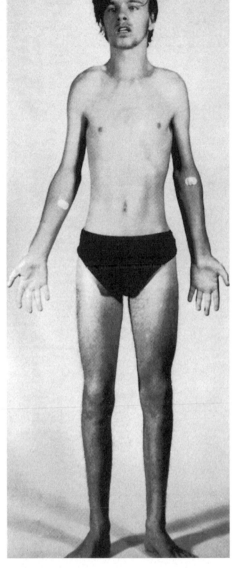

FIGURE 1. Amiable, tall individual at 4 years and at 16 years who has trisomy 8/normal mosaicism, with a normal karyotype from cultured leukocytes but trisomy 8 in skin fibroblast cells. He has a moderate hearing deficit and an IQ estimated in the 70s. He is quite active and skates, swims, and bowls. Note the facies, the small, widely spaced nipples, and the general body stance. There is some limitation of full extension of the fingers, which are partially webbed, and limited extension of the right elbow. There is hypoplasia of the supraspinatus, trapezius, and upper pectoral musculature. (Courtesy of Dr. G. Howard Valentine, War Memorial Children's Hospital, London, Ontario.)

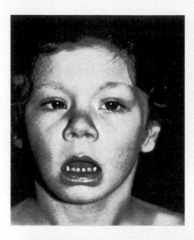
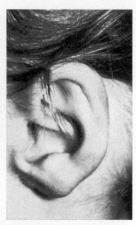
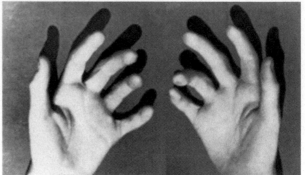

FIGURE 2. Boy with trisomy 8/normal mosaicism. (From Riccardi, VM et al: J Pediatr 77:664, 1970, with permission.)

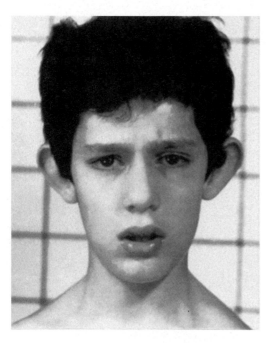

FIGURE 3. Mentally deficient 10-year-old boy with trisomy 8/normal mosaicism. Note the prominent ears. (From De Grouchy J et al: Ann Genet 14:69, 1971, with permission.)

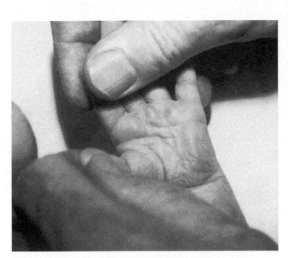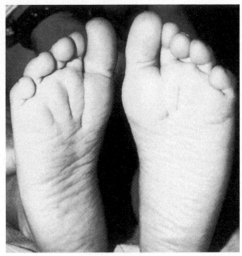

FIGURE 4. Note deep creases on palms and soles.

TRISOMY 9 MOSAIC SYNDROME

Joint Contractures, Congenital Heart Defects, Low-Set Malformed Ears

In 1973, Haslam and colleagues reported the first case of trisomy 9 mosaicism. In the same year, Feingold and colleagues reported the first example of a child with full trisomy 9 using blood lymphocytes.

ABNORMALITIES

Growth. Prenatal onset of growth deficiency.
Performance. Severe mental retardation.
Craniofacial. Sloping forehead with narrow bifrontal diameter; upslanting, short palpebral fissures, deeply set eyes; prominent nasal bridge with short root, small fleshy tip, and slit-like nostrils; prominent lip covering receding lower lip; micrognathia, low-set, posteriorly rotated, and misshapen ears.
Skeletal. Joint anomalies including abnormal position and/or function of hips, knees, feet, elbows, and digits; kyphoscoliosis; narrow chest; hypoplasia of sacrum, iliac wings, and pubic arch; hypoplastic phalanges of toes.
Other. Congenital heart defects in approximately two thirds of cases.

OCCASIONAL ABNORMALITIES.

Subarachnoid cyst, choroid plexus cyst, cystic dilatation of fourth ventricle with lack of midline fusion of cerebellum, hydrocephalus, lack of gyration of cerebral hemispheres, meningocele, microphthalmia, corneal opacities, Peters anomaly, absence of optic tracts, preauricular tags, short neck, cleft lip and/or palate, velopharyngeal insufficiency, bile duct proliferation in absence of a demonstrable stenosis or atresia, gastroesophageal reflux, punctate mineralization in developing cartilage, 13 ribs and 13 thoracic vertebrae. Diaphragmatic hernia. Nonpitting edema of legs, simian crease, nail hypoplasia, genitourinary anomalies including hypoplastic external genitalia, cryptorchidism, cystic dilatation of renal tubules, diverticulae of bladder, hydronephrosis, and hydroureter.

NATURAL HISTORY. The majority of patients die during the early postnatal period. In those that survive, failure to thrive and severe motor and mental retardation are the rule. Some patients remain bedridden throughout their lives, whereas others achieve the ability to walk and develop minimal speech.

ETIOLOGY. The etiology of this disorder is trisomy for chromosome 9. The incidence and severity of malformations and mental deficiency correlate with the percentage of trisomic cells in the different tissues.

References

Feingold M et al: A case of trisomy 9. J Med Genet 10:184, 1973.
Haslam RHA et al: Trisomy 9 mosaicism with multiple congenital anomalies. J Med Genet 10:180, 1973.
Bowen P et al: Trisomy 9 mosaicism in a newborn infant with multiple malformations. J Pediatr 85:95, 1974.
Akatsuka A et al: Trisomy 9 mosaicism with punctate mineralization in developing cartilages. Eur J Pediatr 131:271, 1979.
Frohlich GS: Delineation of trisomy 9. J Med Genet 19:316, 1982.
Kamiker CP et al: Mosaic trisomy 9 syndrome with unusual phenotype. Am J Med Genet 22:237, 1985.
Levy I et al: Gastrointestinal abnormalities in the syndrome of mosaic trisomy 9. J Med Genet 26:280, 1989.

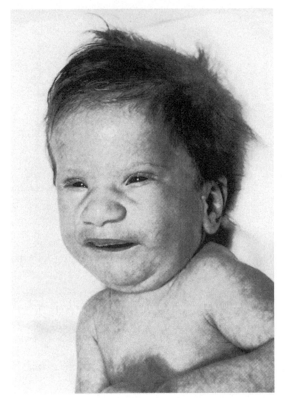
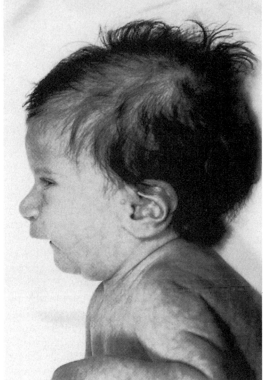
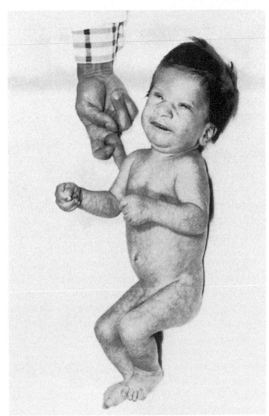

FIGURE 1. Trisomy 9 mosaic syndrome in a 2-month-old boy. Long and narrow face with narrow eyelids in mongoloid position, broad and bulbous nose with a broad and prominent bridge, short upper lip covering the receding lower lip, small mandible, left preauricular pit, cutis marmorata, inability to lie on the back because of congenital thoracic kyphosis, and flexion position of hands and fingers. (From Schinzel A et al: Humangenetik 25:171, 1974, with permission.)

TRIPLOIDY SYNDROME AND DIPLOID/TRIPLOID MIXOPLOIDY SYNDROME

Large Placenta with Hydatidiform Changes, Growth Deficiency, Syndactyly of Third and Fourth Fingers

Triploidy, a complete extra set of chromosomes, is estimated to occur in approximately 2% of conceptuses. Most are lost as miscarriages, accounting for approximately 20% of all chromosomally abnormal spontaneous abortuses. Triploid pregnancies may be accompanied by varying degrees of toxemia. Fetal wastage may be due to hydatidiform placental changes or to specific cytogenetic characteristics, with only 3% of 69XYY conceptuses surviving to be recognized. Partial hydatidiform moles are usually associated with a triploid fetus and very rarely undergo malignant changes. Classic moles show more pronounced trophoblastic hyperplasia in the absence of a fetus. These moles show a diploid karyotype and are totally androgenic in origin.

Infrequently, triploid infants survive to be born after 28 weeks' gestation with severe intrauterine growth retardation. Instances of diploid/triploid mixoploidy are less frequent. Asymmetric growth deficiency with mild syndactyly and occasional genital ambiguity in 46XX/69XXY individuals are the important diagnostic features in mixoploid individuals.

ABNORMALITIES FOUND IN 50% OR MORE OF CASES

Placenta. Large, with tendency toward hydatidiform changes.

Growth. Disproportionate prenatal growth deficiency that affects the skeleton more than the cephalic region; in mixoploid individuals, skeletal growth may be asymmetric.

Craniofacial. Dysplastic calvaria with large posterior fontanel, ocular hypertelorism with eye defects ranging from colobomata to microphthalmia, low nasal bridge, low-set, malformed ears, micrognathia.

Limbs. Syndactyly of third and fourth fingers, simian crease, talipes equinovarus.

Cardiac. Congenital heart defect (atrial and ventricular septal defects).

Genitalia. Male: hypospadias, micropenis, cryptorchidism, Leydig cell hyperplasia.

Other. Brain anomalies, including hydrocephalus and holoprosencephaly; adrenal hypoplasia; and renal anomalies, including cystic dysplasia and hydronephrosis.

ABNORMALITIES FOUND IN LESS THAN 50% OF CASES.

Aberrant skull shape; choanal atresia; cleft lip and/or palate; iris heterochromia; patchy cutaneous hyperpigmentation, hypopigmentation or a mixture of both referred to as pigmentary dysplasia; meningomyelocele; macroglossia; omphalocele or umbilical hernia; biliary tract anomalies, including aplasia of the gallbladder; incomplete rotation of colon; proximally placed thumb; clinodactyly of fifth finger; splayed toes.

NATURAL HISTORY.

Partial hydatidiform molar pregnancies associated with a triploid fetus should not raise concern regarding the development of choriocarcinoma. All cases of full triploidy either have been stillborn or have died in the early neonatal period, with 5 months being the longest recorded survival. Individuals with diploid/triploid mixoploidy usually survive and manifest some degree of psychomotor retardation. Because of body asymmetry, patients with mixoploidy may require a heel lift for the shorter leg to prevent compensatory scoliosis, and some of these people may resemble those having Russell-Silver syndrome. Diagnosis of mixoploidy usually requires skin fibroblast cultures, since the triploid cell line may have disappeared from among peripheral blood leukocytes. The degree of skeletal asymmetry does not appear to correspond to the proportions of triploid cells present, and triploid cells in culture grow with the same variability as diploid cells, except for those with the XYY complement, which grow much more slowly.

ETIOLOGY.

In 69% of cases, the extra set of chromosomes is paternally derived. However, the two most common mechanisms of origin are attributable to maternal factors: first, dispermy or double fertilization due to failure of the zone reaction, which normally prevents polyspermy, and second, a failure of meiosis II leading to a diploid egg. Approximately 60% of the cases have been XXY, with most of the remainder being XXX. It is not unusual for more than one X chromosome to remain active in triploidy. Older maternal age has not been a factor, and there are no data to indicate an increased recurrence risk, such as that seen for chromosomal disorders due to nondisjunction. In several instances, a triploid pregnancy has been followed or preceded by a molar pregnancy.

References

Book JA, Santesson B: Malformation syndrome in man associated with triploidy (69 chromosomes). Lancet 1:858, 1960.

Ferrier P et al: Congenital asymmetry associated with diploid-triploid mosaicism and large satellites. Lancet 1:80, 1964.

Niebular E: Triploidy in man: Cytogenetical and clinical aspects. Humangenetik 21:103, 1974.

Wertelecki W, Graham JM, Sergovich FR: The clinical syndrome of triploidy. Obstet Gynecol 47:69, 1976.

Jacobs PA et al: The origin of human triploids. Ann Hum Genet 42:49, 1978.

Poland BJ, Bailie DL: Cell ploidy in molar placental disease. Teratology 18:353, 1978.

Jacobs PA et al: Late replicating X chromosomes in human triploidy. Am J Hum Genet 31:446, 1979.

Graham JM et al: Diploid-triploid mixoploidy: Clinical and cytogenetic aspects. Pediatrics 68:23, 1981.

Wulfsberg EA et al: Monozygotic twin girls with diploid/triploid chromosome mosaicism and cutaneous pigmentary dysplasia. Clin Genet 39:370, 1991.

Zaragoza MV et al: Parental origin and phenotype of triploidy in spontaneous abortions: Predominance of diandry and association with the partial hydatidiform mole. Am J Hum Genet 66:1807, 2000.

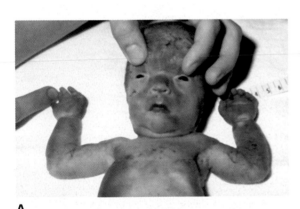
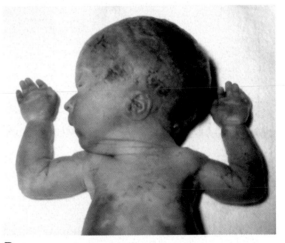

A   **B**

FIGURE 1. **A** and **B,** Stillborn infant with triploidy showing relatively large-appearing upper head in relation to very small face and 3-4 syndactyly of the fingers.

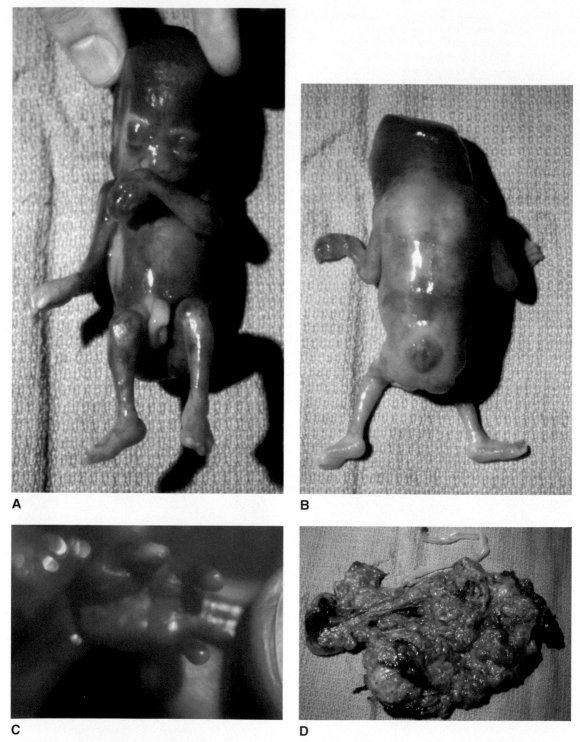

A

B

C

D

FIGURE 2. **A–D,** Severely growth-retarded 20-week fetus with 69XXY karyotype. Note the meningomyelocele and 3-4 syndactyly. This phenotype is consistent with two paternal and one maternal chromosomal copies. It is the most common form of triploidy and typically results in a growth-retarded fetus with a large hydatidiform placenta.

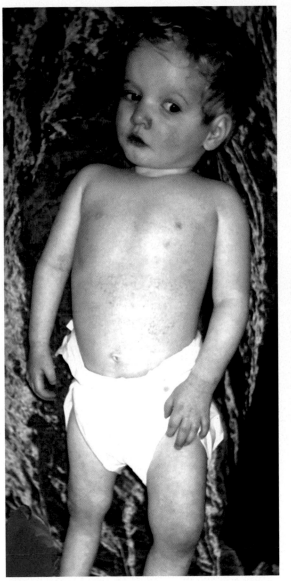

A

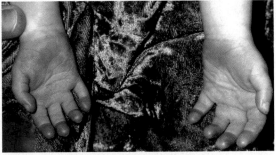

B

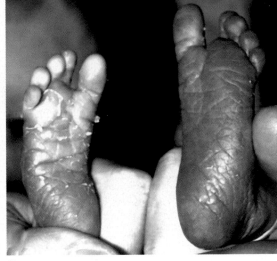

C

FIGURE 3. **A–C,** Infant with asymmetric growth deficiency (*right side smaller*), syndactyly of third and fourth fingers, and mild developmental delay who has triploid/diploid mixoploidy syndrome that is evident only in cultured fibroblasts. (Courtesy of Dr. John M. Graham, Cedars-Sinai Medical Center, Los Angeles.)

DELETION 3p SYNDROME

Mental and Growth Deficiency, Ptosis, Postaxial Polydactyly

Partial deletion of the distal part of the short arm of chromosome 3 was first reported by Verjaal and De Nef in 1978. Subsequently, 15 patients were reported. In all cases, the deleted segment has been 3p25→pter.

ABNORMALITIES

Growth. Prenatal onset of growth deficiency, most striking postnatally.

Performance. Severe to profound mental retardation, hypotonia.

Craniofacial. Microcephaly with flat occiput, synophrys, epicanthal folds, ptosis, short palpebral fissures, prominent nasal bridge, small nose with anteverted nares, long philtrum, malformed ears, micrognathia, downturned corners of mouth.

Other. Postaxial polydactyly of hands and less frequently the feet.

OCCASIONAL ABNORMALITIES.

Trigonocephaly with prominent metopic sutures, agenesis of corpus callosum, upslanting palpebral fissures, ocular hypertelorism, preauricular pits or fistula, cleft palate, cardiac defects including ventricular septal defect (two patients) and one patient with double mitral valve, atrioventricular canal and tricuspid atresia; inguinal and/or umbilical hernia, hiatal hernia, common mesentery, anteriorly placed anus, renal anomalies including pelvic and cystic kidney, cryptorchidism, scoliosis.

NATURAL HISTORY. Nasogastric tube feeding because of poor suck is often required. Persistent central and obstructive apnea is common with frequent pneumonia. Gastroesophageal reflux and profound failure to thrive often occur. Two children died, one at 3 days of age with a complex cardiac defect and the other at 3 months of age of aspiration pneumonia. The survivors, the oldest of which is 24 years old, all have severe mental retardation. Many are blind and deaf and interact only minimally with their environment.

ETIOLOGY. The cause of this disorder is partial deletion of the short arm of chromosome 3, del(3p25→pter). In all but one case the deletion has occurred de novo.

References

Verjaal M, De Nef J: A patient with a partial deletion of the short arm of chromosome 3. Am J Dis Child 132:43, 1978.

Higginbottom MC et al: A second patient with partial deletion of the short arm of chromosome 3: Karyotype 46XY, del(3) (p25). J Med Genet 19:71, 1982.

Tolmie JL et al: Partial deletion of the short arm of chromosome 3. Clin Genet 29:538, 1986.

Schwyzer U et al: Terminal deletion of the short arm of chromosome 3, del(3pter-p25): A recognizable syndrome. Helv Paediatr Acta 42:309, 1987.

Nienhaus H et al: Infant with del(3)(p25-pter): Karyotype-phenotype correlation and review of previously reported cases. Am J Med Genet 44:573, 1992.

Mowrey PN et al: Clinical and molecular analysis of deletion 3p25-pter syndrome. Am J Med Genet 46:623, 1993.

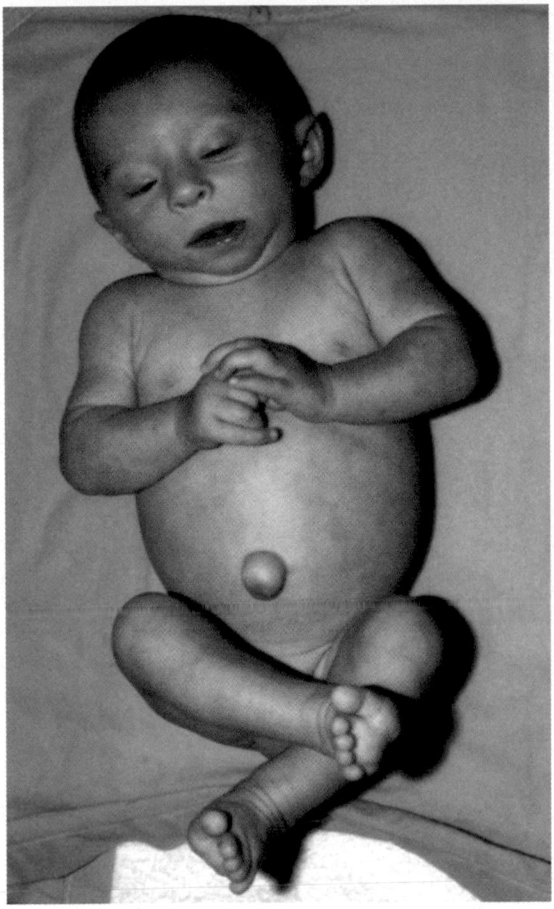

FIGURE 1. Deletion 3p syndrome. **A–C,** Photograph of affected 5-month-old boy. Note the bilateral ptosis, long philtrum, micrognathia, and umbilical hernia. (From Higginbottom MC et al: J Med Genet 19:71, 1982, with permission.)

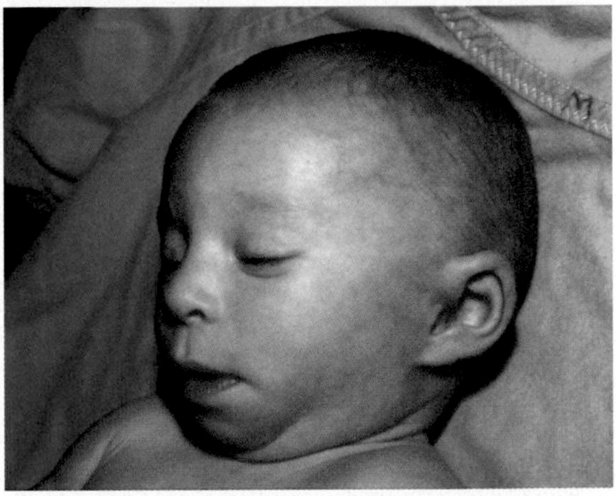

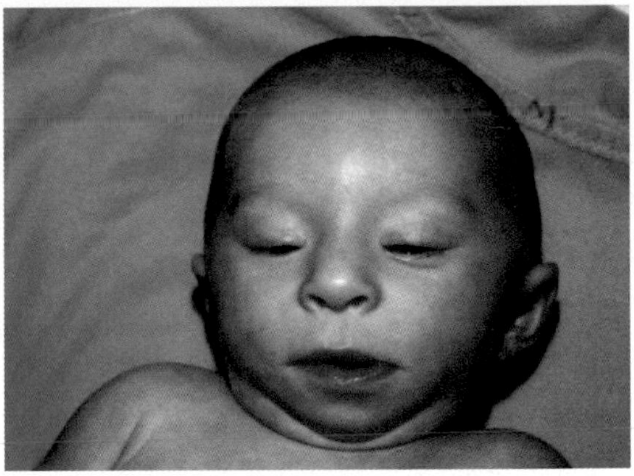

DUPLICATION 3Q SYNDROME

Mental and Growth Deficiency, Broad Nasal Root, Hypertrichosis

First described by Falek and colleagues in 1966, this disorder initially was confused with the Brachmann–de Lange syndrome. Hirschhorn and colleagues performed chromosome banding studies in 1973 that associated duplication of the 3q21→qter region with a distinct phenotype that Francke and Opitz subsequently emphasized can be clinically distinguished from Brachmann–de Lange. More than 40 cases of the duplication 3q syndrome now have been reported.

ABNORMALITIES

Growth. Severe postnatal growth deficiency (100%).

Performance. Severe mental deficiency (100%) with brain anomalies/seizures (83%).

Craniofacial. Abnormal head shape frequently due to craniosynostosis (92%); hypertrichosis and synophrys (86%); upslanting palpebral fissures (56%); broad nasal root (100%); anteverted nares (91%); prominent maxilla (86%); long philtrum (85%); downturned corners of mouth (82%); high-arched palate (100%); cleft palate (79%); micrognathia (100%); malformed ears (79%); short webbed neck (93%).

Limbs. Fifth finger clinodactyly (90%); hypoplastic nails (64%); simian crease (74%); talipes equinovarus (64%); arch dermal ridge pattern or digital pattern with low ridge counts (86%).

Other. Cardiac defects (75%); chest deformities (89%); renal or urinary tract anomalies (48%); genital anomalies in 61% (primarily cryptorchidism); umbilical hernia (50%).

OCCASIONAL ABNORMALITIES.

Microphthalmia, glaucoma, cataract, coloboma, strabismus, syndactyly, polydactyly, camptodactyly, short limbs, cubitus valgus, dislocated radial head, ulnar or fibular deviation of hands or feet, omphalocele, hemivertebrae.

NATURAL HISTORY. Death before 12 months has occurred in 36% of cases. For survivors, prognosis is grim with severe mental deficiency, growth retardation, and pulmonary infections the rule.

ETIOLOGY. The etiology of this disorder is duplication for 3q21→qter. In the majority of cases, duplication of 3q occurs concurrently with monosomy of another chromosomal region, frequently 3p. However, the clinical phenotype of duplication 3q is the same irrespective of the accompanying monosomy. Seventy-five percent of cases have arisen from segregation of parental rearrangements. A gene or genes at 3q26.31-q27.3 are most likely essential for the characteristic phenotype.

COMMENT. Although superficial resemblance exists between the duplication 3q syndrome and the Brachmann–de Lange syndrome, they are clearly distinct disorders that can be differentiated clinically.

References
Falek A et al: Familial de Lange syndrome with chromosome abnormalities. Pediatrics 37:92, 1966.

Hirschhorn K et al: Precise identification of various chromosomal abnormalities. Ann Hum Genet 36:3875, 1973.

Francke U, Opitz J: Chromosome 3q duplication and the Brachmann–de Lange syndrome (BDLS). J Pediatr 95:161, 1979.

Steinbach P et al: The dup (3q) syndrome: Report of eight cases and review of the literature. Am J Med Genet 10:159, 1981.

Wilson GN et al: Further delineation of the dup (3q) syndrome. Am J Med Genet 22:117, 1985.

Van Essen AJ et al: Partial 3q duplication syndrome and assignment of D3S5 to 3q25→3q28. Hum Genet 87:151, 1991.

Aqua M et al: Duplication 3q syndrome: Molecular delineation of the critical region. Am J Med Genet 55:33, 1995.

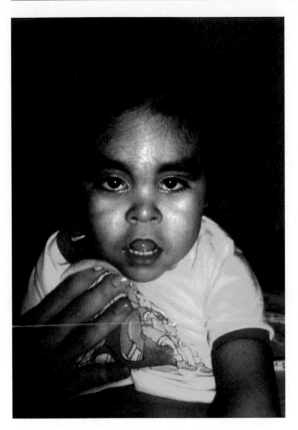

FIGURE 1. Duplication 3q syndrome. An affected 3-month-old boy. Note the hypertrichosis, long philtrum, and downturned corners of the mouth.

DELETION 4p SYNDROME
(CHROMOSOME NUMBER 4 SHORT-ARM
DELETION SYNDROME, 4p– SYNDROME)

Ocular Hypertelorism with Broad or Beaked Nose; Microcephaly and/or Cranial Asymmetry; and Low-Set, Simple Ear with Preauricular Dimple

After delineation of the cri du chat syndrome, occasional patients with deletions of the short arm of a B-group chromosome were found who lacked the typical cry and some other features of that condition. Autoradiographic labeling studies revealed that the deficit chromosome was a number 4 rather than a number 5. More than 100 cases have been published.

ABNORMALITIES

Growth. Marked growth deficiency, of prenatal onset, microcephaly.
Performance. Feeble fetal activity, hypotonia, severe mental deficiency, seizures.
Craniofacial. Strabismus, iris deformity, ocular hypertelorism, highly arched eyebrows, epicanthal folds, prominent glabella, cleft lip and/or palate, downturned "fishlike" mouth, short upper lip and philtrum, micrognathia, posterior midline scalp defects, cranial asymmetry, preauricular tag or pit.
Extremities. Hypoplastic dermal ridges, low dermal ridge count, simian creases, talipes equinovarus, hyperconvex fingernails.
Other. Hypospadias, cryptorchidism, sacral dimple or sinus, cardiac anomaly, primarily atrial septal defect, scoliosis.

OCCASIONAL ABNORMALITIES.
Exophthalmos, ptosis, Rieger anomaly, nystagmus, glaucoma, fused teeth, taurodontism, defect of the medial half of the eyebrows, hearing loss, hypodontia of permanent teeth, low hairline with webbed neck, metatarsus adductus, polydactyly, ectrodactyly, clinodactyly, hip dislocation, accessory ossification centers in proximal metacarpals, absence of pubic rami, bladder exstrophy, delayed bone age, abnormalities in sternal ossification centers, "bottle opener" deformity of clavicles, precocious puberty, renal anomaly, malrotation of small bowel, cavum septum pellucidum, absent septum pellucidum, interventricular cysts, myelodysplastic syndrome.

NATURAL HISTORY. Although profound mental retardation is the rule, 40% of patients in one study became ambulatory, 20% were able to perform simple household tasks, and 10% became toilet trained. Seizures, initially difficult to control, tend to disappear with age. Major feeding difficulties often requiring gastrostomy, are a major problem in infancy. Routine care in infancy should include cardiac, ophthalmologic, and audiologic evaluations, renal ultrasound, EEG, swallowing studies, and developmental testing. In childhood, continued developmental testing, appropriate school placement and follow-up EEG are indicated.

ETIOLOGY. The cause of this disorder is partial deletion of the short arm of chromosome 4. Approximately 87% of cases represent de novo deletions, while in 13% of cases, one of the parents is a balanced translocation carrier. In the cases in which there is a familial translocation, there is a two to one excess of maternally derived 4p deletions, while in the de novo deletions, the origin of the deleted chromosome is paternal in approximately 80% of cases. The phenotype does not differ based on the size of the deletion, which can vary from almost one half of the short arm to so small as to be cytogenetically undetectable. In those cases in which the disorder is suspected clinically but standard chromosome studies are normal, a molecular deletion on the short arm of chromosome 4 at 4p16.3, the critical region for determination of the phenotype, often can be detected using fluorescent in situ hybridization (FISH) analysis.

References
Leao JC et al: New syndrome associated with partial deletion of short arms of chromosome no. 4. JAMA 202:434, 1967.

Wolf U, Reinwein H: Klinische und cytogenetische Differentialdiagnose der Defizienzen an den kurzen Armen der B-Chromosomen. Z Kinderheilkd 98:235, 1967.

Guthrie RD et al: The 4p– syndrome. Am J Dis Child 122:421, 1971.

Lurie IW et al: The Wolf-Hirschhorn syndrome. Clin Genet 17:375, 1980.

Katz DS, Smith TH: Wolf syndrome. Pediatr Radiol 21:369, 1991.

Quarrell OWJ et al: Paternal origin of the chromosomal deletion resulting in Wolf-Hirschhorn syndrome. J Med Genet 28:256, 1991.

Estabrooks LL et al: Molecular characterisation of chromosome 4p deletions resulting in Wolf-Hirschhorn syndrome. J Med Genet 31:103, 1994.

Fagan-Bagric K et al: A practical application of fluorescent in situ hybridization to the Wolf-Hirschhorn syndrome. Pediatrics 93:826, 1994.

Battaglia A, Carey JC: Health supervision and anticipatory guidance of individuals with Wolf-Hirshhorn syndrome. Am J Med Genet 89:111,1999.

Battaglia A et al: Natural history of Wolf-Hirschhorn syndrome: Experience with 15 cases. Pediatrics 103:830, 1999.

Sharathkumar et al: Malignant hematological disorders in children with Wolf-Hirschhorn syndrome. Am J Med Genet 119:164, 2003.

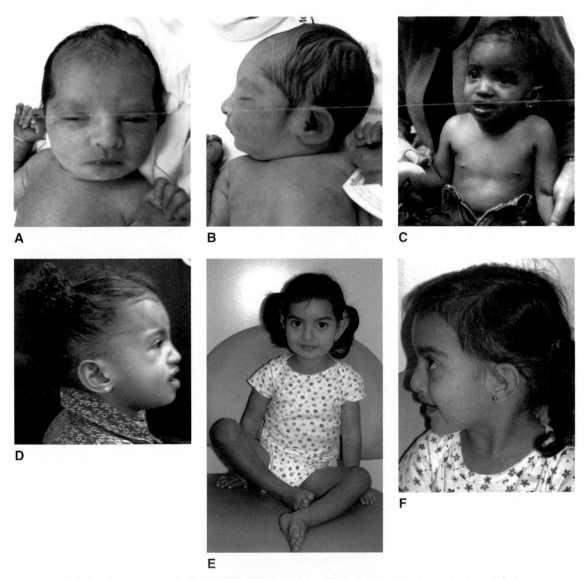

FIGURE 1. Deletion 4p syndrome. **A–F,** Affected children at three different ages. Note the ocular hypertelorism, prominent glabella, supraorbital ridge continuous with the nasal bridge, short philtrum, micrognathia, and simple ears. (**E** and **F,** Courtesy of Dr. Lynne M. Bird, Children's Hospital, San Diego.)

DELETION 4Q SYNDROME

Mental and Growth Deficiency, Cleft Palate, Limb Anomalies

Partial deletion of the long arm of chromosome 4 was initially reported by Ockey and colleagues in 1967. Townes and colleagues proposed the existence of a 4q– syndrome in 1981. The phenotype was further delineated by Mitchell and colleagues in 1981 and by Lin and colleagues in 1988.

ABNORMALITIES

Growth. Postnatal onset of growth deficiency (83%).
Performance. Moderate to severe mental deficiency (92%), hypotonia (28%), seizures (17%).
Craniofacial. Ocular hypertelorism (56%); short nose (67%); broad nasal bridge (94%); cleft palate (94%); micrognathia (94%); low-set, posteriorly rotated ears (56%); abnormal pinnae (67%).
Limbs. Fifth finger clinodactyly (44%), tapering fifth finger (50%), pointed/duplicated fifth fingernail (33%), absent to hypoplastic flexion creases on fifth fingers (56%), abnormal thumb/hallux implantation (44%), simian crease (61%), overlapping toes (22%).
Other. Cardiac defects (61%) including ventricular septal defect, patent ductus arteriosus, peripheral pulmonic stenosis, aortic stenosis, tricuspid atresia, atrial septal defect, aortic coarctation, tetralogy of Fallot; genitourinary defects (50%); gastrointestinal defects (22%).

OCCASIONAL ABNORMALITIES.

Asymmetric face (17%), small, upslanting palpebral fissures (22%), epicanthal folds (39%), anteverted nares (33%), cleft lip (39%), Robin sequence (28%), camptodactyly (17%), missing digits (11%).

NATURAL HISTORY. Fifty percent of patients with a terminal deletion (q31→qter) died before 15 months of age of cardiopulmonary difficulties including asphyxia, apnea, and congestive heart failure. Of those who survived, moderate to severe mental retardation occurred in the vast majority. One child who is at least 15 years old has profound mental deficiency, behavioral disorder, and seizures.

ETIOLOGY. The cause of this disorder is deletion of 4q31→qter. Virtually all cases represent de novo defects.

COMMENT. Deletions of 4q32 seem to be similar to 4q31. More distal deletions at 4q33 and 4q34 are associated with a less severe clinical phenotype. Patients with interstitial deletion of 4q differ completely from those with terminal deletions.

References
Ockey CH et al: A large deletion of the long arm of chromosome no. 4 in a child with limb abnormalities. Arch Dis Child 42:428, 1967.
Townes PL et al: 4q– syndrome. Am J Dis Child 133:383, 1979.
Davis JM et al: Brief clinical report: The del (4) (q31) syndrome—a recognizable disorder with atypical Robin malformation sequence. Am J Med Genet 9:113, 1981.
Mitchell JA et al: Deletions of different segments of the long arm of chromosome 4. Am J Med Genet 8:73, 1981.
Lin AE et al: Interstitial and terminal deletions of the long arm of chromosome 4: Further delineation of phenotypes. Am J Med Genet 31:533, 1988.

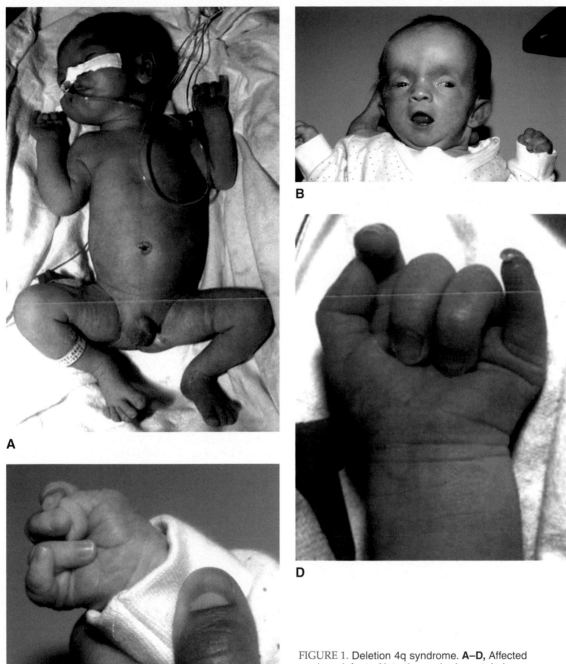

FIGURE 1. Deletion 4q syndrome. **A–D,** Affected newborn infants. Note the ocular hypertelorism, abnormal pinnae, and pointed fifth fingernail. (Courtesy of Dr. Marilyn C. Jones, Children's Hospital, San Diego.)

DELETION 5p SYNDROME
(CRI DU CHAT SYNDROME, PARTIAL DELETION
OF THE SHORT ARM OF CHROMOSOME
NUMBER 5 SYNDROME, 5p– SYNDROME)

Cat-Like Cry in Infancy, Microcephaly, Downward Slant of the Palpebral Fissures

Lejeune and colleagues first described this condition in 1963. Further reports have raised to over 100 the number of cases described.

ABNORMALITIES

General
Low birth weight (less than 2.5 kg)	72%
Slow growth	100%
Cat-like cry	100%

Performance
Mental deficiency	100%
Hypotonia	78%

Craniofacial
Microcephaly	100%
Round face	68%
Hypertelorism	94%
Epicanthal folds	85%
Downward slanting of the palpebral fissures	81%
Strabismus, often divergent	61%
Low-set and/or poorly formed ears	58%
Facial asymmetry	—

Cardiac
Congenital heart disease (variable in type)	30%

Hands
Simian crease	81%
Distal axial triradius	40%
Slightly short metacarpals	—

OCCASIONAL ABNORMALITIES.
Cleft lip and cleft palate, myopia, optic atrophy, preauricular skin tag, bifid uvula, dental malocclusion, short neck, clinodactyly, inguinal hernia, cryptorchidism, absent kidney and spleen, hemivertebra, scoliosis, flat feet, premature graying of hair.

NATURAL HISTORY. As babies, the patients tend to be unusually squirmy in their activity. The mewing cry, ascribed to abnormal laryngeal development, becomes less pronounced with the increasing age of the patient, thus making the diagnosis more difficult in older patients. A study by Wilkins and colleagues of 65 children with cri du chat syndrome reared in the home suggests that a much higher level of intellectual performance can be achieved than was previously suggested from studies performed on institutionalized patients. With early special schooling and a supportive home environment, some affected children attained the social and psychomotor level of a normal 5- to 6-year-old child. One half of the children older than 10 years had a vocabulary and sentence structure adequate for communication. Scoliosis is a frequent occurrence.

ETIOLOGY. The underlying chromosomal aberration is partial deletion of the short arm of chromosome number 5. Approximately 85% of cases result from sporadic de novo deletions, while 15% arise secondary to unequal segregation of a parental translocation. Although the size of the deletion is variable, a critical region for the high-pitched cry maps to 5p15.3, while the chromosomal region involved in the remaining features maps to 5p15.2. Thus individuals with deletion involving just 5p15.3 have the cat-like cry, but the facial features and degree of developmental delay are much less severe. The deleted chromosome is of paternal origin in 80% of cases in which the syndrome is the result of a de novo deletion.

References
Lejeune J et al: Trois cas de deletion partielle du bras court du chromosome 5. C R Acad Sci [D] (Paris) 257:3098, 1963.
Berg JM et al: Partial deletion of short arm of a chromosome of the 4 and 5 group (Denver) in an adult male. J Ment Defic Res 9:219, 1965.
Breg WR et al: The cri-du-chat syndrome in adolescents and adults. J Pediatr 77:782, 1970.
Wilkins LE, Brown JA, Wolf B: Psychomotor development in 65 home-reared children with cri-du-chat syndrome. J Pediatr 97:401, 1980.

Overhauser J et al: Parental origin of chromosome 5 deletions in the cri-du-chat syndrome. Am J Med Genet 37:83, 1990.

Overhauser J et al: Molecular and phenotypic mapping of the short arm of chromosome 5: Sublocalization of the critical region of the cri-du-chat syndrome. Hum Mol Genet 3:247, 1994.

Gersh M et al: Evidence for a distinct region causing a cat-like cry in patients with 5p deletions. Am J Med Genet 56:1404, 1995.

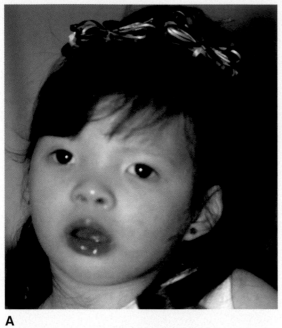

A

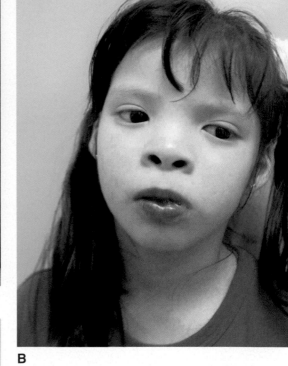

B

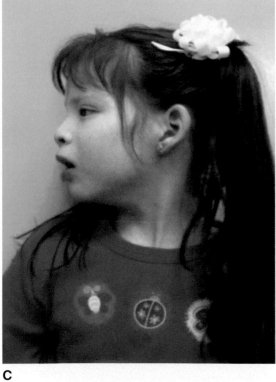

C

FIGURE 1. Deletion 5p syndrome. **A–C,** Affected child at 3 and 5 years of age. Note the round face, ocular hypertelorism, and epicanthal folds. (Courtesy of Dr. Lynne M. Bird, Children's Hospital, San Diego.)

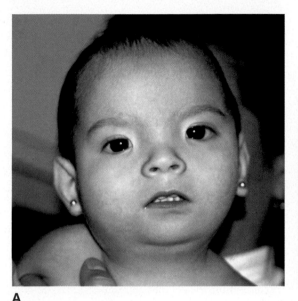
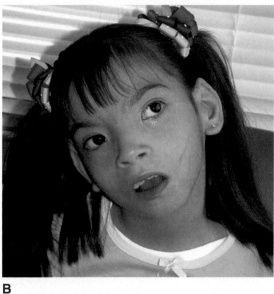

A

B

FIGURE 2. **A** and **B,** Affected child at 13 months and 8 years of age. Note the round face, ocular hypertelorism, and epicanthal folds. (Courtesy of Dr. Lynne M. Bird, Children's Hospital, San Diego.)

DELETION 9p SYNDROME
(9p MONOSOMY, 9p– SYNDROME)

Craniostenosis with Trigonocephaly, Upslanting Palpebral Fissures, Hypoplastic Supraorbital Ridges

Since the initial delineation of this disorder in 1973 by Alfi and colleagues, approximately 100 similarly affected patients with 9p– as the sole chromosomal anomaly have been reported.

ABNORMALITIES

Growth. Usually normal.

Performance. Mean intelligence quotient (IQ) is 49 with a range from 33 to 73; social adaptation is often good.

Craniofacial. Craniostenosis involving the metopic suture leading to trigonocephaly; flat occiput; upslanting palpebral fissures; epicanthal folds, prominent eyes secondary to hypoplastic supraorbital ridges; highly arched eyebrows; midfacial hypoplasia with a short nose, depressed nasal bridge, anteverted nares, and long philtrum; small mouth, micrognathia; posteriorly rotated, poorly formed ears with hypoplastic, adherent ear lobes; short broad neck with low hairline.

Limbs. Long middle phalanges of the fingers with extra flexion creases; short distal phalanges with short nails; excess in whorl patterns on fingertips; foot positioning defects; simian crease.

Cardiovascular. Ventricular septal defects, patent ductus arteriosus, and/or pulmonic stenosis in one third to one half of patients.

Other. Scoliosis, widely spaced nipples, diastasis recti, inguinal and/or umbilical hernia, micropenis and/or cryptorchidism in males; hypoplastic labia majora in females.

OCCASIONAL ABNORMALITIES. Ptosis; cleft palate; choanal atresia; postaxial polydactyly; diaphragmatic hernia; hydronephrosis; radiographic anomalies of ribs, clavicles, and vertebrae.

ETIOLOGY. Deletion of the distal portion of the short arm of chromosome 9. In most cases, the breakpoint is located at band 9p22 and the deletion is de novo.

COMMENT. In cases in which the 9p deletion is associated with another unbalanced chromosome segment, the breakpoint usually occurs at 9p24. Most of them are inherited from a balanced translocation carrier parent. Mean IQ in those cases is 46 with a range from 33 to 57. Trigonocephaly, long philtrum, digital anomalies, and hernias are all usually present despite the variability of the associated unbalanced chromosome segment.

References
Alfi OS et al: Deletion of the short arm of chromosome 9(46,9p–): A new deletion syndrome. Ann Genet 16:17, 1973.
Alfi OS et al: The 9p– syndrome. Ann Genet 19:11, 1976.
Mattei JF et al: Pericentric inversion, inv(9)(p22q32), in the father of a child with a duplication-deletion of chromosome 9 and gene dosage effect for adenylate kinase-I. Clin Genet 17:129, 1980.
Huret JL et al: Eleven new cases of del (9p) and features from 80 cases. J Med Genet 25:741, 1988.
Shashi V et al: Choanal atresia in a patient with the deletion (9p) syndrome. Am J Med Genet 49:88, 1994.

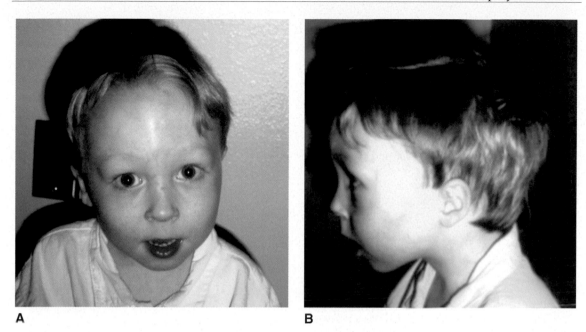

A **B**

FIGURE 1. Deletion 9p syndrome. **A** and **B,** Note the prominent forehead with metopic ridge, trigonocephaly, frontal hair upsweep, short nose with anteverted nares, and low-set ears.

DUPLICATION 9p SYNDROME
(TRISOMY 9p SYNDROME)

Distal Phalangeal Hypoplasia, Delayed Closure of Anterior Fontanel, Ocular Hypertelorism

First reported in 1970 by Rethoré and colleagues, the pattern of malformation was set forth by Centerwall and Beatty-DeSana in 1975. Over 130 individuals with complete or partial dup9p have been reported.

ABNORMALITIES

Growth. Growth deficiency, primarily of postnatal onset; delayed puberty such that some patients continue to grow up to the middle of their third decade.

Performance. Severe mental deficiency; language tends to be most significantly delayed.

Craniofacial. Microcephaly, hypertelorism, downslanting palpebral fissures, deep-set eyes, prominent nose, downturned corners of the mouth, cup-shaped ears.

Limbs. Short fingers and toes with small nails and short terminal phalanges; fifth finger clinodactyly with single flexion crease; single palmar crease.

Other Skeletal. Kyphoscoliosis, usually developing during the second decade; hypoplasia of periscapular muscles with deep acromial dimples; defective ossification of the pubic bone, broad ischial tuberosity; pseudoepiphysis of metacarpals, metatarsals, and middle phalanges of fifth fingers; delayed closure of cranial sutures and fontanels.

OCCASIONAL ABNORMALITIES.

Micrognathia; epicanthal folds, short or webbed neck; partial 2-3 syndactyly of toes and 3-4 syndactyly of fingers, congenital heart defects in 5% to 10% of cases and cleft lip and/or palate in 5%; hydrocephalus, agenesis of corpus callosum, renal malformations, micropenis, cryptorchidism, hypospadias, talipes equinovarus, and congenital hip dislocation.

NATURAL HISTORY. Approximately 5% to 10% of reported patients have died in early childhood.

ETIOLOGY. The degree of clinical severity correlates with the extent of triplicated material. However, mental retardation occurs in virtually all patients. Partial trisomy 9pter→p21 is associated with mild craniofacial features and rare skeletal or visceral defects. Partial trisomy 9pter→p11 is associated with the typical craniofacial features, while partial trisomy 9pter→q11-13 is associated not only with the typical craniofacial features but also skeletal and cardiac defects. Partial trisomy 9pter→q22-32 is associated with the typical craniofacial features, intrauterine growth deficiency, cleft lip/palate, micrognathia, cardiac anomalies, and congenital hip dislocation. If the trisomic segment is larger than that (9pter→9q31 or 32), the clinical findings no longer fit into the trisomy 9p syndrome but rather resemble trisomy 9 mosaic syndrome.

References

Rethoré MO et al: Sur quatre cas de trisomie pour le bras court du chromosome 9. Individualisation d'une nouvelle entité morbide. Ann Genet 13:217, 1970.

Centerwall WR, Beatty-Desana JW: The trisomy 9p syndrome. Pediatrics 56:748, 1975.

Centerwall WR et al: Familial "partial 9p" trisomy: Six cases and four carriers in three generations. J Med Genet 13:57, 1976.

Schinzel A: Trisomy 9p, a chromosome aberration with distinct radiologic findings. Radiology 130:125, 1979.

Wilson GN et al: The phenotypic and cytogenetic spectrum of partial trisomy 9. Am J Med Genet 20:277, 1985.

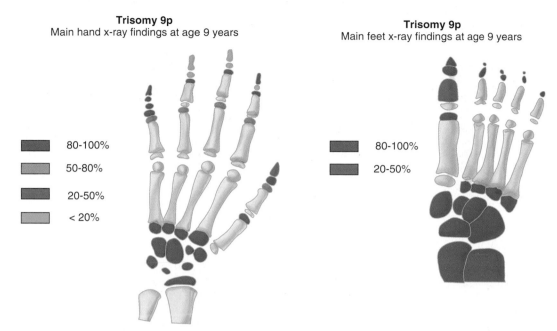

Trisomy 9p
Main hand x-ray findings at age 9 years

80-100%
50-80%
20-50%
< 20%

Trisomy 9p
Main feet x-ray findings at age 9 years

80-100%
20-50%

FIGURE 1. Duplication 9p syndrome. Diagram of major radiologic findings in hand and foot of a 9-year-old patient. Pseudoepiphyses on metacarpals and metatarsals 2 to 5; notches on metacarpal 1, metatarsal 1, and proximal and middle phalanges of fingers; hypoplasia of the middle phalanx of fifth finger, terminal phalanges of fingers, and middle and terminal phalanges of toes; thick epiphyses, especially of terminal phalanges of big toe, thumb, and little finger; and clinodactyly of fifth finger. (From Schinzel A: Radiology 130:125, 1979, with permission.)

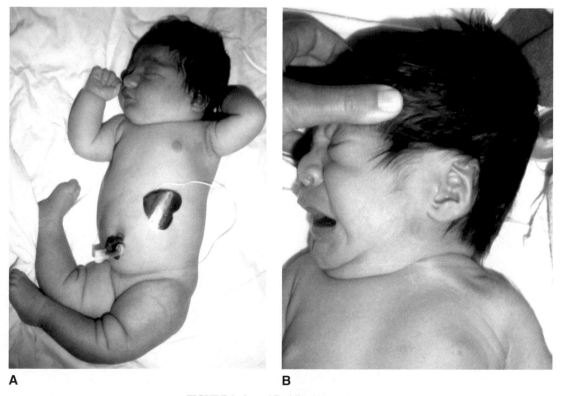

A **B**

FIGURE 2. **A** and **B**, Affected newborn.

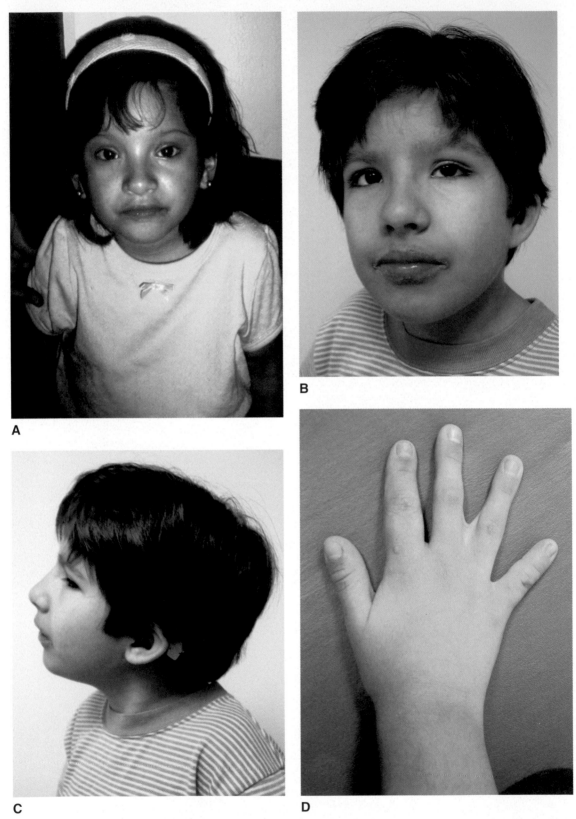

FIGURE 3. **A–D,** Note the ocular hypertelorism, prominent nose, downturned corners of mouth, cup-shaped ear, short fingers, and 3-4 syndactyly.

DUPLICATION 10Q SYNDROME

Ptosis, Short Palpebral Fissures, Camptodactyly

First set forth as a specific phenotype by Yunis and Sanchez in 1974, this disorder was further delineated by Klep-de Pater and colleagues in 1979.

ABNORMALITIES

Growth. Prenatal onset of growth deficiency; mean birth weight of 2.7 kg.

Performance. Severe to moderate mental retardation, hypotonia.

Craniofacial. Microcephaly; flat face with high forehead and high, arched eyebrows; ptosis; short downslanting palpebral fissures; microphthalmia; broad and depressed nasal bridge, anteverted nares, bow-shaped mouth with prominent upper lip; cleft palate; malformed posteriorly rotated ears.

Limbs. Camptodactyly, proximally placed thumbs, syndactyly between second and third toes, foot position anomalies, hypoplastic dermal ridge patterns.

Other. Heart and renal malformations—each occurs in approximately one half of affected patients; kyphoscoliosis; pectus excavatum; 11 pairs of ribs; congenital hip dislocation; cryptorchidism.

OCCASIONAL ABNORMALITIES.

Brain malformations, ocular anomalies, malrotation of the gut, hypospadias, vertebral malformations, postaxial polydactyly of hands, streak gonads.

NATURAL HISTORY. Approximately one half of reported patients died within the first year of life, usually from congenital heart defects and other malformations. Surviving children showed marked mental deficiency and usually are bedridden without the ability to communicate.

ETIOLOGY. This disorder is caused by duplication 10q24→qter; the distal segment of the long arm of chromosome 10. Individuals with dup10q25-qter lack major malformations and the prognosis is more favorable.

References

Yunis JJ et al: A new syndrome resulting from partial trisomy for the distal third of the long arm of chromosome 10. J Pediatr 84:567, 1974.

Klep-de Pater JM et al: Partial trisomy 10q. A recognizable syndrome. Hum Genet 46:29, 1979.

Briscioli V et al: Trisomy 10qter confirmed by in situ hybridization. J Med Genet 30:601, 1993.

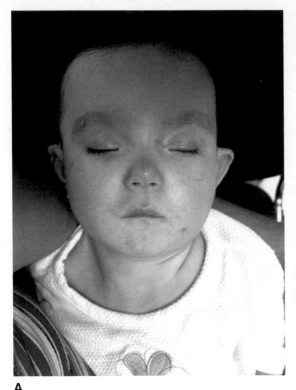

A

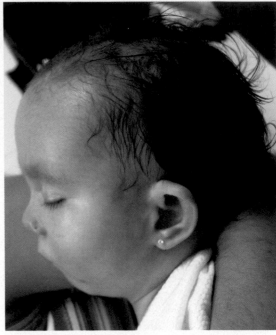

B

FIGURE 1. Duplication 10q syndrome. **A–C,** Photograph of 6-month-old infant. Note the flat face with high forehead; broad nasal bridge; anteverted nares; malformed, posteriorly rotated ears; camptodactyly; and proximally placed thumbs.

C

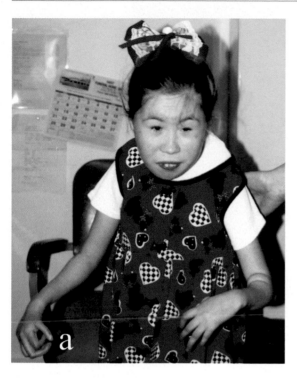

FIGURE 2. Note the ptosis, high-arched eyebrows, and proximally placed thumbs. (Courtesy of Dr. Bryan D. Hall, University of Kentucky, Lexington.)

ANIRIDIA–WILMS TUMOR ASSOCIATION
(WAGR Syndrome)

Numerous cases of the association of Wilms tumor and aniridia have been reported, and it is estimated that 1 in 70 patients with aniridia also has Wilms tumor. In 1978, Riccardi and colleagues identified an interstitial deletion of 11p in a group of patients with aniridia and Wilms tumor, who also had genitourinary anomalies and mental retardation, a pattern of malformation referred to as WAGR syndrome. The features of that disorder are set forth below.

ABNORMALITIES

Performance. Moderate to severe mental deficiency in most patients.
Growth. Growth deficiency and microcephaly in at least one half of the patients.
Craniofacial. Prominent lips, micrognathia, poorly formed ears.
Eyes. Aniridia in most patients; congenital cataracts, nystagmus, ptosis, blindness.
Genitalia. Cryptorchidism, hypospadias.
Other. Wilms tumor in one half of the patients.

OCCASIONAL ABNORMALITIES.
Glaucoma, anterior segment anomaly, microphthalmia, kyphoscoliosis, inguinal hernias, obesity, ambiguous external genitalia, cystic lesions of the kidney, streak gonads, gonadoblastoma, fifth finger clinodactyly, ventricular septal defects.

ETIOLOGY.
Most cases represent a de novo deletion of 11p13 that encompasses, among a number of contiguous genes, the aniridia gene, PAX6, and the Wilms tumor suppressor gene, WT1. Differences in the size of the deleted segment (especially distal to 11p13) in individual cases may account for the observed variability in concomitant features and in the degree of growth and mental deficiency. Deletions of segments in 11p, not including 11p13, do not cause the aniridia–Wilms tumor association. Familial occurrence resulting from unbalanced transmission of a balanced insertional translocation has been recorded. An interstitial deletion in 11p should be particularly sought in the cytogenetic investigation of mentally retarded patients with Wilms tumor and/or aniridia.

COMMENT.
It has been estimated that Wilms tumor develops in one third of patients with sporadic aniridia and in 50% of patients with aniridia, genitourinary anomalies, and mental retardation. The risk of Wilms tumor in patients with aniridia who have a cytogenetically detectable deletion of 11p13 increases to 60%. FISH using a probe spanning PAX6 and WT1 is available to determine if a risk for Wilms tumor exists for patients with sporadic aniridia for whom there are normal chromosomes and an otherwise normal phenotype. Although the risk for renal failure is less than 1% in patients with isolated unilateral Wilms tumor, at least 20% of patients with WAGR syndrome develop renal failure and thus should be followed throughout life.

References

Anderson SR et al: Aniridia, cataract and gonadoblastoma in a mentally retarded girl with deletion of chromosome 11. Ophthalmologica 176:171, 1978.

Riccardi VM et al: Chromosomal imbalance in the aniridia–Wilms' tumor association: 11p interstitial deletion. Pediatrics 61:604, 1978.

Francke U et al: Aniridia–Wilms' tumor association: Evidence for specific deletion of 11p13. Cytogenet Cell Genet 24:185, 1979.

Hittner HM, Riccardi VM, Francke U: Aniridia caused by a heritable chromosome 11 deletion. Ophthalmology 86:1173, 1979.

Yunis JJ, Ramsay NKC: Familial occurrence of the aniridia–Wilms tumor syndrome with deletion 11p13-14.1. J Pediatr 96:1027, 1980.

Clericuzio CL: Clinical phenotypes and Wilms' tumor. Med Pediatr Oncol 21:182, 1993.

Pavilack MA, Walton DS: Genetics of aniridia: The aniridia–Wilms' tumor association. Int Ophthalmol Clin 33:77, 1993.

Breslow NE et al: Renal failure in the Denys-Drash and Wilms tumor-anirida syndromes. Cancer Res 60:4030, 2000.

Gul D et al: Third case of WAGR syndrome with severe obesity and constitutional deletion of chromosome (11)(p12p14). Am J Med Genet 107:70, 2002.

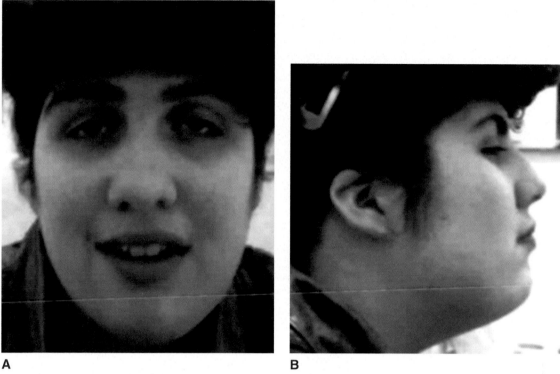

A

B

FIGURE 1. **A** and **B**, Prominent lips and poorly formed ears in a female with aniridia-Wilms tumor association. (Courtesy of Dr. Carol Clericuzio, University of New Mexico, Albuquerque.)

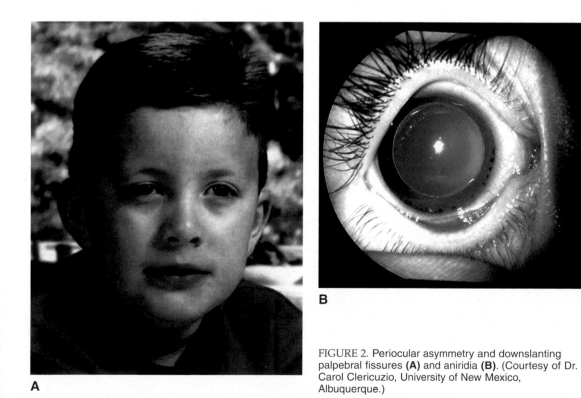

B

A

FIGURE 2. Periocular asymmetry and downslanting palpebral fissures **(A)** and aniridia **(B)**. (Courtesy of Dr. Carol Clericuzio, University of New Mexico, Albuquerque.)

DELETION 11Q SYNDROME

Ocular Hypertelorism; Large, Carp-Shaped Mouth; Cardiac Defects

Described initially by Jacobsen and colleagues in 1973, approximately 90 cases of this disorder have now been reported. In the majority of cases, the deletion involves band 11q23→qter. However, it appears that the clinical phenotype is due to deletion of sub-band 11q24.1.

ABNORMALITIES

Growth. Prenatal onset of growth deficiency (76%).

Performance. Mental retardation (96%). Although all degrees have been reported, approximately one half have been in the moderate range, and most of the remainder are more severely affected. A small percentage of children are in the normal range. Hypotonia in infancy, frequently progressing toward spasticity, hearing loss, speech impairment.

Craniofacial. Prominent forehead (62%), microcephaly (40%), epicanthal folds (60%), ocular hypertelorism (70%), ptosis (67%), strabismus (75%), depressed nasal bridge (93%), short nose with upturned nasal tip (91%) and long philtrum, large, carp-shaped mouth (78%) with thin upper lip, micrognathia (77.7%), low-set and/or malformed ears (85%).

Other. Joint contractures (65%); cardiac defect (60%), primarily ventricular septal defect and left-sided obstructive defect; hypospadias and/or cryptorchidism (50%); Paris-Trousseau syndrome (defect in platelet development characterized by neonatal thrombocytopenia and persistent platelet dysfunction).

OCCASIONAL ABNORMALITIES.

Trigonocephaly, macrocephaly, hydrocephalus, holoprosencephaly, seizures, cataract, ocular coloboma, optic atrophy, retinal reduplication, retinal dysplasia, cerebral atrophy, agenesis of corpus callosum, cerebellar hypoplasia, short neck, dental anomalies, digital anomalies including hammer position of great toes, 2-3 syndactyly of toes, fifth finger clinodactyly, brachydactyly, pyloric stenosis, imperforate anus, inguinal hernia, renal malformations, vesico-vaginal fistula, hypoplasia of labia and clitoris, eczema, hypoplastic left heart, IGF-1 deficiency.

NATURAL HISTORY. Life expectancy is unknown. Cardiac defects and bleeding are the major causes of morbidity and mortality. Feeding difficulties are common and chronic constipation occurs in almost one half. Recurrent episodes of otitis media and/or sinusitis are frequent, although no evidence of immunodeficiency has been demonstrated.

ETIOLOGY. Partial deletion of the long arm of chromosome 11 involving 11q23→qter; most commonly a simple deletion and occasionally as part of a ring-11 chromosome. Larger deletions extending into 11q23 or q24.1 are associated with moderate degrees of mental retardation and significant speech impairment while those with small terminal deletions are more mildly affected with some having normal intelligence.

References

Jacobsen PH et al: An (11;21) translocation in four generations with chromosome 11 abnormalities in the offspring. Hum Hered 23:568, 1973.

Schinzel A et al: Partial deletion of long arm of chromosome 11[del(11)(q23)]: Jacobsen syndrome. J Med Genet 14:438, 1977.

O'Hare AE et al: Deletion of the long arm of chromosome 11 [46,XX,del(11)(q24.1→qter)]. Clin Genet 25:373, 1984.

Fryns JP et al: Distal 11q monosomy. The typical 11q monosomy syndrome is due to deletion of subband 11q24.1. Clin Genet 30:255, 1986.

Wardinsky TD et al: Partial deletion of the long arm of chromosome 11[del(11)(q23.3→qter)] with abnormal white matter. Am J Med Genet 35:60, 1990.

Penny LA et al: Clinical and molecular characterization of patients with distal 11q deletions. Am J Med Genet 56:676, 1995.

Grossfeld PD et al: The 11q terminal deletion disorder: A prospective study of 110 cases. Am J Med Genet 129:51, 2004.

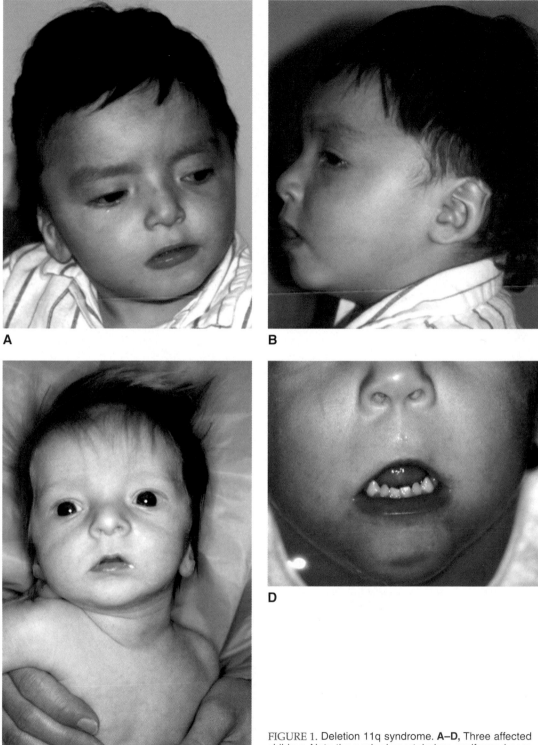

FIGURE 1. Deletion 11q syndrome. **A–D,** Three affected children. Note the ocular hypertelorism, malformed ears, and carp-shaped mouth.

DELETION 13Q SYNDROME
(13Q– SYNDROME)

Microcephaly with High Nasal Bridge, Eye Defect, Thumb Hypoplasia

Partial deletion of the long arm of one of the D-group chromosomes was initially reported in 1963 by Lele and colleagues in a mentally retarded and growth-deficient patient with retinoblastoma. Subsequently, well over 100 cases have been recorded, and the deleted chromosome has been considered number 13. The phenotype has been variable, but a pattern of malformation is emerging that should allow for suspicion of this disorder. A similar phenotype has been noted in 13 ring chromosome patients who are missing part of the short arm as well as part of the long arm of chromosome 13. The features listed below are those found in del(13q) patients.

ABNORMALITIES

Growth. Growth deficiency, usually of prenatal onset.
Central Nervous System. Mental deficiency, microcephaly with tendency toward trigonocephaly and holoprosencephaly-type of brain defects.
Facial. Prominent nasal bridge, hypertelorism, ptosis, epicanthal folds, microphthalmia, colobomata, retinoblastoma, usually bilateral; prominent maxilla, micrognathia, prominent ears, slanting, low placement.
Neck. Short, webbing.
Limbs. Small to absent thumbs, clinodactyly of fifth finger, fused metacarpal bones 4 and 5, talipes equinovarus, short big toe.
Cardiac. Cardiac defect.
Genitalia. Hypospadias, cryptorchidism.
Other. Focal lumbar agenesis.

OCCASIONAL ABNORMALITIES.
Optic nerve and retinal dysplasia, facial asymmetry, posterior auricular pits, narrow palate, imperforate anus, Hirschsprung disease, celiac disease, bifid scrotum, pelvic anomaly, renal anomaly.

ETIOLOGY. This disorder is caused by deletion of part of the long arm of a 13 chromosome.

Ring 13 chromosome individuals may have a similar pattern of malformation.

COMMENT. The natural history is dependent on the deleted segment. Patients with proximal deletions not extending into q32 have mild to moderate mental retardation, variable minor anomalies, and growth retardation. If the q14 region is involved, a significant risk exists for retinoblastoma. Patients with more distal deletions including at least part of q32 usually have severe mental retardation; growth deficiency; and major malformations including microcephaly and CNS defects, distal limb anomalies, eye defects, and gastrointestinal malformations. Patients with the most distal deletions, involving q33-q34, have severe mental retardation but usually lack growth deficiency or gross structural malformations.

Although the majority of patients with deletions of chromosome 13 involving the q14 region develop retinoblastoma, it is estimated that 13% to 20% remain unaffected. Chromosome studies would seem merited in all patients with retinoblastoma.

References
Lele KP, Penrose LS, Stallarf HB: Chromosome deletion in a case of retinoblastoma. Ann Hum Genet 27:171, 1963.
Allerdice PW et al: The 13q-deletion syndrome. Am J Hum Genet 21:499, 1969.
Taylor AI: Dq–, Dr and retinoblastoma. Humangenetik 10:209, 1970.
Yunis JJ, Ramsay N: Retinoblastoma and subband deletion of chromosome 13. Am J Dis Child 132:161, 1978.
Riccardi VM et al: Partial triplication and deletion of 13q: Study of a family presenting with bilateral retinoblastoma. Clin Genet 18:332, 1979.
Wilson WG et al: Deletion (13) (q14.1q14.3) in two generations: Variability of ocular manifestations and definition of the phenotype. Am J Med Genet 28:675, 1987.
Tranebjaerg L et al: Interstitial deletion 13q: Further delineation of the syndrome by clinical and high-resolution chromosome analysis of five patients. Am J Med Genet 29:739, 1988.
Brown S et al: Preliminary definition of a "critical region" of chromosome 13 in q32: Report of 14 cases with 13q deletions and review of the literature. Am J Med Genet 45:52, 1993.
Talvik I et al: Boy with celiac disease, malformations, and ring chromosome 13 with deletion 13q32-qter. Am J Med Genet 93:399, 2000.

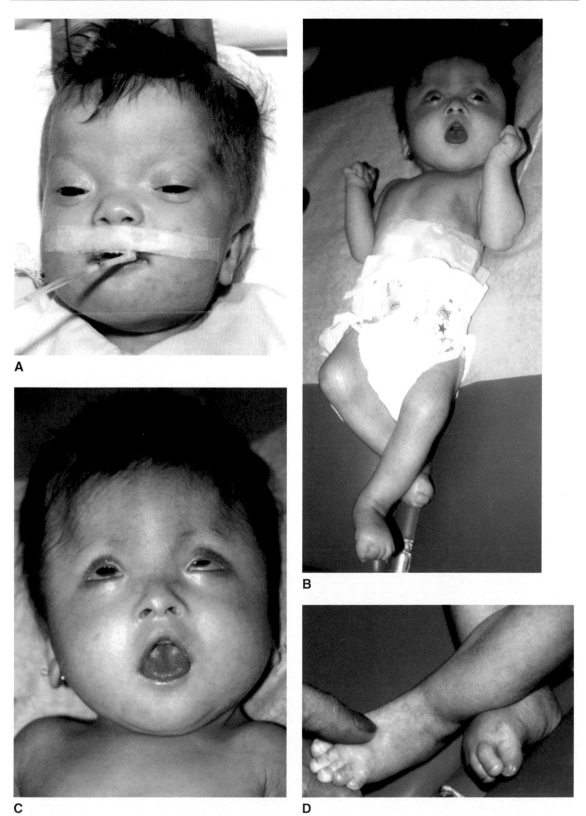

FIGURE 1. Deletion 13q syndrome. **A–D,** Two affected newborns. Note the ptosis, trigonocephaly, metopic ridge, and short big toe. (**A,** Courtesy of Dr. Bryan D. Hall, University of Kentucky, Lexington.)

DUPLICATION 15Q SYNDROME

Prominent Nose with Broad Nasal Bridge, Camptodactyly, Cardiac Defects

Initially described by Fujimoto and colleagues, duplication of distal 15q has been described now in at least 28 additional cases. The breakpoints have all been between bands 15q21 and 15q23 except for two families with breakpoints at 15q25 and two families with breakpoints at 15q15. The clinical phenotype is consistent and recognizable.

ABNORMALITIES

Growth. Prenatal growth deficiency (15%), post-natal growth deficiency (60%), tall stature (11%).

Performance. Severe to profound mental retardation (92%), two patients with duplication of 15q25→qter were only mildly retarded.

Craniofacial. Microcephaly (37%), sloping forehead (71%), short palpebral fissures (78%), downslanting palpebral fissures (71%), ptosis (56%), prominent nose with broad nasal bridge (96%), long, well-defined philtrum (77%); midline crease in lower lip (86%); micrognathia (88%); puffy cheeks (70%).

Skeletal. Pectus excavatum (46%); scoliosis (60%); short neck with or without vertebral anomalies (68%).

Hands. Arachnodactyly (75%); camptodactyly (100%).

Other. Cardiac defects (69%).

OCCASIONAL ABNORMALITIES.

Genital abnormalities including cryptorchidism and hypoplastic labia majora, preauricular pit.

NATURAL HISTORY.

Death primarily related to congenital heart defects, recurrent respiratory infections, and aspiration pneumonia has occurred in one third of patients. A 27-year-old mentally retarded male is the oldest known survivor.

ETIOLOGY.

The cause of this disorder is duplication of distal 15q. The majority of cases have resulted from unbalanced translocations, all but one of which were the offspring of a balanced carrier parent. Despite the fact that the second chromosome involved in the reciprocal translocation has varied, the clinical phenotype is consistent.

References

Fujimoto A, et al: Inherited partial duplication of chromosome no. 15. J Med Genet 11:287, 1974.

Lacro RV et al: Duplication of distal 15q: Report of five new cases from two different translocation kindreds. Am J Med Genet 26:19, 1987.

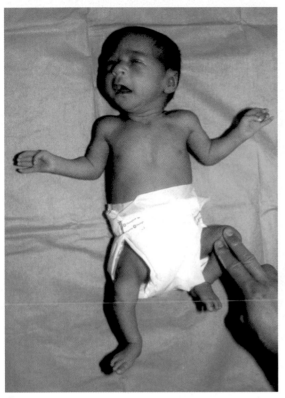

A

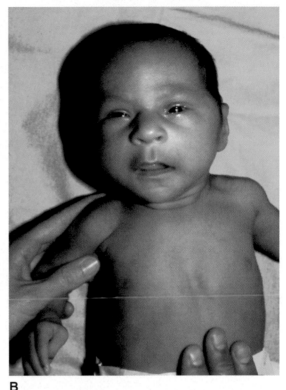

B

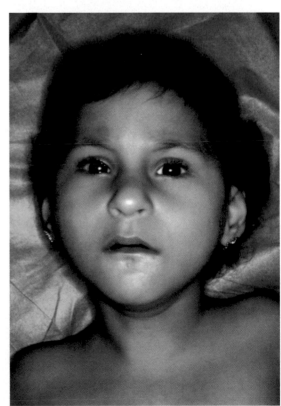

C

FIGURE 1. Duplication 15q syndrome. **A,** Affected newborn female infant. Note the sloping forehead, downslanting palpebral fissures, and prominent nose with broad nasal bridge. Affected girl at birth **(B)** and 41 months **(C)**. (**A–C,** From Lacro RV et al: Am J Med Genet 26:719, 1987. Reprinted with permission of Wiley-Liss, Inc., a subsidiary of John Wiley & Sons, Inc.)

DELETION 18p SYNDROME
(18p– SYNDROME)

Mental and Growth Deficiencies, Ptosis or Epicanthal Folds, Prominent Auricles

Deletion of the short arm of chromosome 18 was first noted by de Grouchy and colleagues in 1963. Subsequently, more than 100 cases have been reported. There is rather broad variability in the phenotype.

ABNORMALITIES. The most consistent features are listed below.

Growth. Mild to moderate growth deficiency.

Central Nervous System. Mental deficiency, tendency toward hypotonia, microcephaly (mild) (29%).

Facial. Ptosis (38%), epicanthal folds (40%), low nasal bridge, hypertelorism (41%), rounded facies, micrognathia (25%), wide mouth, downturning corners of mouth, large protruding ears.

Dental. High frequency of caries (29%).

Limbs. Relatively small hands and feet.

Other. Pectus excavatum.

OCCASIONAL ABNORMALITIES

Immunologic. IgA absence or deficiency, usually asymptomatic.

Central Nervous System and Facial. Holoprosencephaly arrhinencephaly-type defect (12%).

Skin and Hair. Alopecia (three cases), hypopigmentation.

Other. Cataract, strabismus (15%), webbed neck, broad chest, cleft palate, kyphoscoliosis, clinodactyly of fifth fingers (21%), syndactyly (11%), simian crease, cubitus valgus, pectus excavatum (17%), inguinal hernia, dislocation of hip (9%), talipes equinovarus (13%), genital anomalies (18%), development of rheumatoid arthritis–like signs and symptoms, polymyositis, cardiac defects (10%), ulerythema ophryogenes (i.e., reticular erythema, small horny papules, atrophy, and permanent loss of hairs in outer halves of eyebrows sometimes extending to adjacent skin, scalp, and cheeks), growth hormone deficiency.

NATURAL HISTORY. There is a mild to severe mental deficiency. IQs range from 25 to 75, with an average of approximately 45 to 50. There is a dissociation between language ability and practical performance; many do not speak even simple sentences before 7 to 9 years of age. Restlessness, emotional lability, fear of strangers, and lack of ability to concentrate are features of this disorder. These patients can best be helped in small groups intended especially for the mentally deficient. The prognosis is poor for those patients with holoprosencephaly-type defect. Otherwise, life expectancy does not seem to be impaired. Alopecia, when a problem, develops during infancy. Adequate adaptation has occurred in some patients, and they are capable of reproduction.

ETIOLOGY. The cause of this disorder is short arm 18 deletion, sometimes as part of the deficiency in a ring 18 chromosome. Parents should undergo chromosome analysis to determine whether either is a balanced translocation carrier or has the unbalanced 18p– deletion.

Sex ratio (female:male) is 3:2. The mean parental ages of 32 years for the mothers and 38 for the fathers are older than average.

References

de Grouchy J et al: Dysmorphie complexe avec oligophrénie: Délétion des bras courts d'un chromosome 17–18. D R Acad Sci 256:1028, 1963.

Uchida IA et al: Familial short arm deficiency of chromosome 18 concomitant with arhinencephaly and alopecia congenita. Am J Hum Genet 17:410, 1965.

Reinwein H et al: Defizienz am kurzen Arm eines Chromosoms Nr. 18 (46,XX,18p–): Ein einheitliches Missbildungs syndrom. Monatsschr Kinderheilkd 116:511, 1968.

Schinzel A et al: The 18p– syndrome. Arch Genetik 47:1, 1974.

Movahhedian HR et al: Heart disease associated with deletion of the short arm of chromosome 18. Del Med J 63:285, 1991.

Tsukahara M et al: Familial del(18p) syndrome. Am J Med Genet 99:67, 2001.

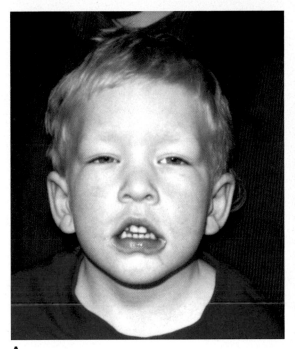
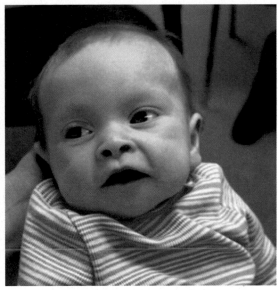

A   **B**

FIGURE 1. Deletion 18p syndrome. **A** and **B,** Two affected children. Note the ptosis, hypertelorism, round facies, and wide mouth with downturning corners. (**A,** Courtesy of Dr. Bryan D. Hall, University of Kentucky, Lexington; **B,** courtesy of Dr. Cynthia Curry, University of California, San Francisco.)

DELETION 18Q SYNDROME
(LONG ARM 18 DELETION SYNDROME, 18Q– SYNDROME)

Midfacial Hypoplasia, Prominent Antihelix, Whorl Digital Pattern

Initially described by de Grouchy and colleagues in 1964, this disorder has been documented in more than 100 cases and occurs in approximately 1 of 40,000 live births.

ABNORMALITIES. The most consistent features are listed subsequently.

Growth. Postnatal onset of growth deficiency with disproportionate short stature secondary to decreased lower segment.

Performance. Mental retardation with hypotonia, poor coordination, nystagmus, conductive deafness, seizures.

Craniofacial. Microcephaly, midfacial hypoplasia with deep-set eyes, short palpebral fissures, carp-shaped mouth, narrow palate.

Ears. Prominent antihelix, antitragus, or both; narrow or atretic external canal.

Limbs. Long hands, tapering fingers, short first metacarpal with proximal thumb, high-frequency whorl digital pattern, distal axial triradius, simian crease, fifth finger clinodactyly, abnormal toe placement, vertical talus with or without talipes equinovarus, short feet.

Genitalia. Female: hypoplastic labia minora; male: cryptorchidism with or without small scrotum and penis, hypospadias.

Other. Skin dimples over acromion and knuckles, cardiac defect.

OCCASIONAL ABNORMALITIES

Eyes. Inner epicanthal folds, slanted palpebral fissures, ocular hypertelorism, microphthalmia, corneal abnormality, iris hypoplasia, coloboma, cataract, retinal defect, abnormal optic disk, myopia, optic atrophy.

Ears. Atretic middle ear, low-set ears, microtia.

Other. Cleft palate (30%), cleft lip, short frenulum, widely spaced nipples, prominent venous pattern on the abdomen, extra rib, horseshoe kidney, celiac disease, lipomata at lateral border of feet, hemihypertrophy, scoliosis, vertebral anomalies, femoral head abnormalities, choreoathetotic movements, eczema, decreased to absent IgA, growth hormone deficiency, atrophy of olfactory and optic nerves, poor myelination of central white matter tracts with relatively normal myelination of corpus callosum, hydrocephalus, porencephaly, cerebellar hypoplasia.

NATURAL HISTORY. Ureteral reflux and urinary tract infection can be a significant problem. Mental deficiency, with IQs from 40 to 85, and growth deficiency, coupled with various visual and hearing problems, may leave these individuals seriously handicapped. Behavioral problems, including obnoxious or autistic behavior, may be features. However, some patients with this deletion have not been severely affected. For example, a 10-year-old child studied by Wertelecki and Gerald was not obviously debilitated.

ETIOLOGY. Variable deletions of part of the long arm of chromosome 18 from 18q21.3 or 18q22.2 to qter. In general, the size of the deletion correlates with the severity of the phenotype.

References

de Grouchy J et al: Délétion partielle du bras long du chromosome 18. Pathol Biol (Paris) 12:579, 1964.

Wertelecki W, Gerald PS: Clinical and chromosomal studies of the 18q– syndrome. J Pediatr 78:44, 1971.

Miller G et al: Neurologic manifestations in 18q– syndrome. Am J Med Genet 37:128, 1990.

Kline AD et al: Molecular analysis of the 18q– syndrome and correlation with phenotype. Am J Hum Genet 52:895, 1993.

Cody JD et al: Congenital anomalies and anthrometry of 42 individuals with deletion of chromosome 18q. Am J Med Genet 85:455, 1999.

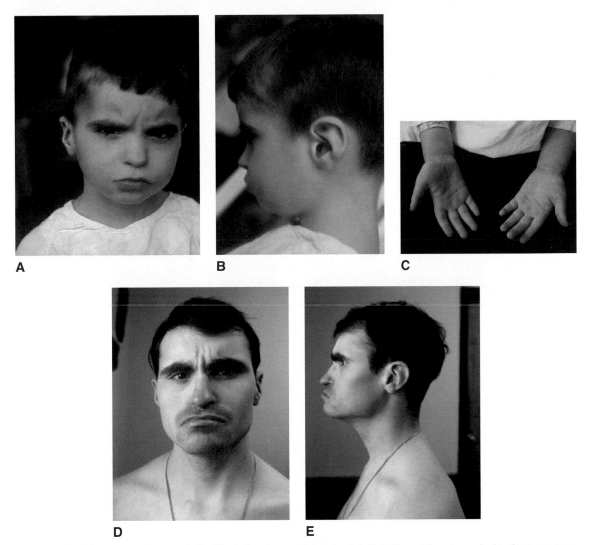

FIGURE 1. Deletion 18q syndrome. **A–E,** Affected male as child and adult. Note the midface hypoplasia, deep-set eyes, carp-shaped mouth, and prominent antihelix. (Courtesy of Dr. Wladimir Wertelecki, University of South Alabama, Birmingham.)

CAT-EYE SYNDROME
(COLOBOMA OF IRIS–ANAL ATRESIA SYNDROME)

Coloboma of Iris, Downslanting Palpebral Fissures, Anal Atresia

Anal atresia and colobomata of the iris, initially considered the hallmarks of this disorder, are present in combination in only a minority of affected patients. Greater than 100 cases have been reported, only 9% of which showed all the major clinical features.

ABNORMALITIES

Performance. Usually mild mental retardation, some patients have been of normal intelligence but emotionally retarded.

Growth. Normal in the majority of cases.

Craniofacial. Mild hypertelorism; downslanting palpebral fissures; inferior coloboma of iris, choroid, and/or retina; micrognathia, preauricular pits, and/or tags.

Cardiac. Cardiac defects in more than one third of cases, including total anomalous pulmonary venous return, persistence of the left superior vena cava, VSD, and ASD.

Anus. Anal atresia with rectovestibular fistula.

Urogenital. Hypospadias, renal agenesis, hydronephrosis, vesicoureteral reflux.

OCCASIONAL ABNORMALITIES.

Severe mental retardation (7%); microcephaly; microphthalmos; ocular motility problems; hearing loss; ventricular dilatation; abnormal EEG; seizures; spasticity; cerebral or cerebellar atrophy; ataxia; facial nerve palsy; low-set, malformed ears with stenotic external canals; biliary atresia; dislocation of hip; radial aplasia; scoliosis; vertebral defects; rib or sternal anomaly; cleft palate; malrotation of gut; agenesis of uterus and fallopian tubes; dysplastic or polycystic kidney; bladder defects; aganglionosis of small and large intestine; ectopic anus; volvulus; Meckel diverticulum.

ETIOLOGY. Usually the result of an extra chromosome derived from two identical segments of chromosome 22, consisting of the satellites, the entire short arm, the centromere, and a tiny piece of the long arm (22pter→q11). That segment is thus present in quadruplicate.

The phenotype can also result from an interstitial duplication of the 22q11 region. In this situation, the segment is present in triplicate, which may explain the few reported cases of cat-eye syndrome in which an extra chromosome is not present. Fluorescent in situ hybridization studies have been used successfully to document typical as well as atypical cases in which only a few of the features are present.

References

Schachenmann G et al: Chromosomes in coloboma and anal atresia. Lancet 2:290, 1965.

Darby CW, Hughes DT: Dermatoglyphics and chromosomes in cat-eye syndrome. BMJ 3:47, 1971.

Balci S et al: The cat-eye syndrome with unusual skeletal malformations. Acta Paediatr Scand 63:623, 1974.

Schinzel A et al: The "cat eye syndrome": Dicentric small marker chromosome probably derived from a No. 22 (tetrasomy 22pter q11) associated with a characteristic phenotype. Report of 11 patients and delineation of the clinical picture. Hum Genet 57:148, 1981.

McDermid HE et al: Characterization of the supernumerary chromosome in cat eye syndrome. Science 232:646, 1986.

Liehr T et al: Typical and partial cat eye syndrome: Identification of the marker chromosome by FISH. Clin Genet 42:91, 1992.

Rosias PPR et al: Phenotypic variability of the cat-eye syndrome, case report and review of the literature. Genet Counsel 12:273, 2001.

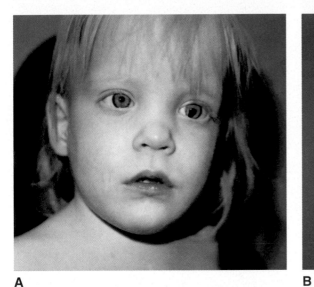 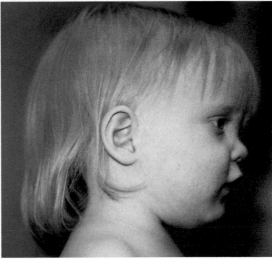

A   B

FIGURE 1. Cat-eye syndrome. **A** and **B,** Infant showing coloboma of iris and ocular hypertelorism. (Courtesy of Dr. Bryan D. Hall, University of Kentucky, Lexington.)

XYY SYNDROME
Tall Stature, Aberrant Behavior

Despite an incidence of 1 in 840 newborn males, the XYY individual is seldom detected during childhood or even in the adult. Based on studies of unselected newborns with sex chromosome anomalies who have been followed longitudinally, it is now recognized that the majority of XYY males are phenotypically normal. However, a pattern of variable abnormalities has come to be appreciated, which may allow for clinical suspicion of the XYY syndrome in childhood.

ABNORMALITIES. Variable features from among the following:

Growth. Acceleration in midchildhood.

Performance. Dull mentality; full-scale IQ is within normal limits although usually lower than siblings (range, 80 to 140); relative weakness, with poor fine motor coordination and sometimes a fine intentional tremor; speech delay common; learning disabilities (50%).

Dentition. Large teeth.

Facies. Prominent glabella, asymmetry, long ears.

Skeletal. Increased length versus breadth; evident in cranial vault, hands, and feet; mild pectus excavatum.

Skin. Severe nodulocystic acne at adolescence.

OCCASIONAL ABNORMALITIES

Skeletal. Radioulnar synostosis.

Genital. Cryptorchidism, small penis, hypospadias.

Other. EEG abnormality, electrocardiogram showing prolonged PR interval, Dandy-Walker malformation, agenesis of corpus callosum, enlarged lateral ventricles.

NATURAL HISTORY. Although affected patients are occasionally long at birth, the tendency toward tall stature is usually not evident until they reach 5 to 6 years of age. Despite the large size, these boys are usually not strong or well coordinated and tend to have poor development of the pectoral and shoulder girdle musculature. Behavioral problems, especially distractibility, hyperactivity, and temper tantrums are present in childhood and early adolescence. Aggressive behavior is not usually a problem and they learn to control anger as they get older. Onset of puberty is approximately 6 months delayed. Heterosexual activity is normal. The majority of 47XYY males are fertile and have chromosomally normal offspring. However, an increased risk for offspring with chromosomal abnormalities as well as miscarriage and perinatal death has been suggested.

Although early reports suggested that there existed an overrepresentation of 47XYY individuals among institutionalized male juvenile delinquents, prospective longitudinal studies of unselected 47XYY males suggest that behavior disorders are not a significant problem for these individuals in childhood and adolescence.

COMMENT. Based on normal testicular biopsies on seven men with 47XYY to look for carcinoma in situ, it is concluded that men with a 47XYY karyotype are not at increased risk of developing gonadal tumors.

ETIOLOGY. The diagnosis is confirmed by chromosomal analysis revealing a 47XYY karyotype.

References

Sandberg AA et al: XYY human male. Lancet 2:488, 1961.

Daly RF: Neurological abnormalities in XYY males. Nature 221:472, 1969.

Sundequist U, Hellstrome E: Transmission of 47,XYY karyotype. Lancet 2:1367, 1969.

Nielsen J, Friedrich U, Zeuthen E: Stature and weight in boys with the XYY syndrome. Humangenetik 14:66, 1971.

Voorhees JJ et al: Nodulocystic acne as a phenotypic feature of the XYY genotype. Report of five cases, review of all known XYY subjects with severe acne, and discussion of XYY cytodiagnosis. Arch Dermatol 105:913, 1972.

Grass F et al: Reproduction in XYY males: Two new cases and implications for genetic counseling. Am J Med Genet 19:533, 1984.

Muller J, Skakkeback ND: Gonadal malignancy in individuals with sex chromosome anomalies. Birth Defects 26(4):247, 1991.

Robinson A et al: Sex chromosome aneuploids: The Denver prospective study. Birth Defects 26(4):59, 1991.

Robinson A ct al: Summary of clinical findings in children and young adults with sex chromosome anomalies. Birth Defects 26(4):225, 1991.

Maymon R et al: Brain anomalies associated with 47XYY karyotype detected on a prenatal scan. Prenat Diagn 22:487, 2002.

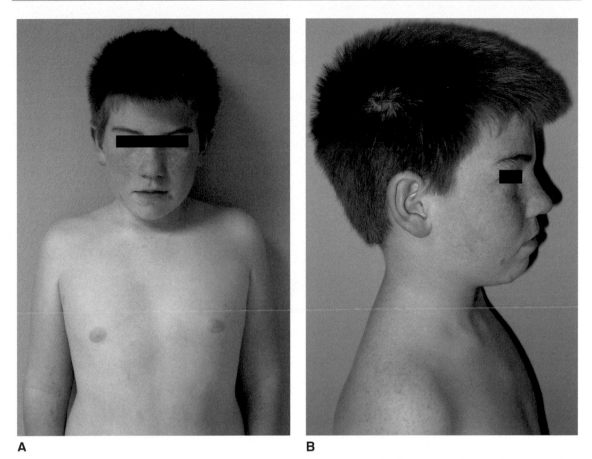

A   B

FIGURE 1. XYY syndrome. **A** and **B,** An 8-year-old boy, evaluated because of behavioral problems and poor school performance. Note the relatively long face and large ears.

XXY SYNDROME, KLINEFELTER SYNDROME

Hypogenitalism and Hypogonadism, with or without Long Legs, Dull Mentality, and/or Behavioral Problems

This disorder, initially described by Klinefelter and colleagues in 1942, is now appreciated as being the most common single cause of hypogonadism and infertility, affecting approximately 1 in 500 males.

ABNORMALITIES. Variable features relating to timing and amount of androgen deficiency.

Performance. Although a wide range of IQs has been noted from well below to well above average, mean full-scale IQ is between 85 and 90. Verbal IQ is usually higher than performance, with significant problems in expressive language, auditory processing abilities, and auditory memory, leading to decreased ability to read and spell. Between 20% and 50% have a fine to moderate intention tremor. Tendency toward behavior problems, especially immaturity, insecurity, shyness, poor judgment, and unrealistic boastful and assertive activity; formation of peer relationships is difficult. Problems with psychosocial adjustment are increased, although significant psychiatric difficulties are not often encountered.

Growth. Tendency from childhood toward long limbs, with low upper to lower segment ratio and relatively tall and slim stature; height ranges from the 25th to 99th percentile with a mean at the 75th percentile; weight and head circumference at the 50th percentile.

Hypogonadism with Hypogenitalism. Childhood: Relatively small penis and testes. Adolescence and adulthood: Testes remain small, usually less than 2.5 cm in length. With rare exception, testosterone production is inadequate, with the average serum testosterone values in the adult being less than one half the normal value. Infertility is the rule, with hyalinization and fibrosis of the seminiferous tubules because of excess gonadotropin leading to firm testes. Virilization is partial and inadequate, with gynecomastia occurring in one third of adolescents.

Other. Mild elbow dysplasia, fifth finger clinodactyly, taurodontism (enlargement of pulp with thinning of tooth surface).

OCCASIONAL ABNORMALITIES. Severe acne; genital: cryptorchidism, hypospadias; central precocious puberty; scoliosis during adolescent years; as adults, diabetes mellitus (8%) and chronic bronchitis are more common; mild to moderate ataxia occasionally occurs, and ulcerative breakdown of the skin over the anterior lower legs may develop; varicose veins; deep vein thrombosis; extragonadal germ cell tumors; breast cancer; lung cancer; osteoporosis; autoimmune disease.

NATURAL HISTORY. Most 47XXY boys enter puberty normally. Testosterone levels decrease in late adolescence and early adulthood. The majority of affected individuals require some help in school, particularly in reading and spelling. Some have been placed in full-time special education programs. A significant number of affected individuals can be expected to complete a college degree. Although the incidence of breast cancer is 20 times more common in Klinefelter syndrome than in the normal male population, it occurs in only 1 case in 5000 affected men providing no rationale for screening mammography. The average age of presentation for extragonadal germ cell tumors ranges from 15 to 30 years.

ETIOLOGY AND DIAGNOSIS. The diagnosis is confirmed by chromosomal analysis revealing a 47XXY karyotype. Paternal meiosis I errors account for about one half of 47XXY males while the remainder are due to maternal meiosis I errors, maternal meiosis II errors, and in a very small number of cases to a postzygotic mitotic error. Initial studies documented no increase in paternal age associated with paternally derived 47XXY karyotypes, but a marked increase in maternal age associated with maternally derived 47XXY males, the increase associated with maternal meiosis I but not meiosis II errors. However, more recent evidence suggests that older fathers produce a higher frequency of XY sperm, placing them at higher risk of fathering boys with Klinefelter syndrome. Individuals with XXY/XY mosaicism have a better potential prognosis for testicular function, while those with XXYY are more likely to be mentally retarded and have behavioral problems.

MANAGEMENT. Diagnosis during childhood of XXY (or XXYY or XXXY) syndrome is helpful in allowing for prospective testosterone replacement therapy beginning at the age of 11 to 12 years, if and when studies show deficient testosterone and elevated gonadotropin values for maturational age. This will bring about a more masculine physique, increase in facial and pubic hair, more goal-directed thinking, improved self-esteem, less fatigue and irritability, and increased libido, strength, and bone mineral density.

References

Klinefelter HF Jr, Reifenstein EC Jr, Albright F: Syndrome characterized by gynecomastia, aspermatogenesis without aleydigism and increased secretion of follicle-stimulating hormone (gynecomastia). J Clin Endocrinol Metab 2:615, 1942.

Caldwell PD, Smith DW: The XXY syndrome in childhood: Detection and treatment. J Pediatr 80:250, 1972.

Baughman FH, Higgin JV, Mann J: Sex chromosome anomalies and essential tremor. Neurology 23:623, 1973.

Graham JM et al: Oral and written language abilities of XXY boys: Implications for anticipatory guidance. Pediatrics 81:795, 1988.

Jacobs PA et al: Klinefelter's syndrome: An analysis of the origin of the additional sex chromosome using molecular probes. Ann Hum Genet 52:93, 1988.

Mandocki MW, Summer GS: Klinefelter syndrome: The need for early identification and treatment. Clin Pediatr 30:161, 1991.

Muller J, Skakkeback NE: Gonadal malignancy in individuals with sex chromosome anomalies. Birth Defects 26(4):247, 1991.

Robinson A et al: Summary of clinical findings in children and young adults with sex chromosome anomalies. Birth Defects 26(4):225, 1991.

Smyth CM, Bremner WJ: Klinefelter syndrome. Arch Intern Med 158:1309, 1998.

Lowe X et al: Frequency of XY sperm increases with age in fathers of boys with Klinefelter syndrome. Am J Hum Genet 69:1046, 2001.

Swerdlow AJ et al: Mortality and cancer incidence in persons with chromosome abnormalities: A cohort study. Ann Hum Genet 65:177, 2001.

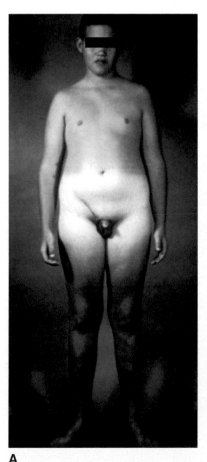
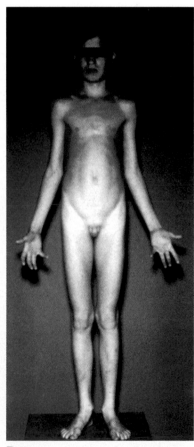

A   **B**

FIGURE 1. XXY syndrome. **A,** A 16-year-old untreated XXY adolescent; note the gynecomastia. **B,** A 9-year-old child; note the small penis, long arms and legs. (**A** and **B,** Courtesy of Dr. Mark Stephan, Madigan General Hospital, Tacoma, Washington.)

XXXY AND XXXXY SYNDROMES

Hypogenitalism, Limited Elbow Pronation,
Low Dermal Ridge Count on Fingertips

The greater the aneuploidy, from XXY to XXXXY, the more severe the growth deficiency, mental retardation, hypogenitalism, and other features. The abnormalities listed subsequently are for XXXXY syndrome, and the findings for XXXY syndrome extend from the milder XXY features toward this more severe end of the spectrum.

ABNORMALITIES

Performance. Mental deficiency; IQ 20 to 78, mean IQ 35; speech impairment; hypotonia, joint laxity, or both, in about one third.

Growth
Tendency to low birth weight, shortness of stature, retarded osseous maturation	53%

Craniofacial
Sclerotic cranial sutures	57%
Wide-set eyes	80%
Upward slant to palpebral fissures	79%
Inner epicanthal folds	82%
Strabismus	59%
Low nasal bridge; wide, upturned nasal tip	95%
Mandibular prognathism	50%
Auricular anomaly (large, low-set, malformed)	70%

Neck
Short	72%

Limbs
Limited pronation at elbow	95%
Radioulnar synostosis	42%
Clinodactyly of fifth finger	90%
Coxa valga	25%
Genu valgum	50%
Pes planus	73%
Epiphyseal dysplasia, usually mild	—

Other Skeletal
Thick, undersegmented sternum	75%
Congenital hip dislocation	—
Early degeneration of articular cartilage	—

Genitalia
Small penis	80%
Small testes, hypoplastic tubules, diminished Leydig cells	94%
Cryptorchidism	28%
Hypoplastic scrotum	80%

OCCASIONAL ABNORMALITIES. Obesity, flat occiput, microcephaly, arrhinencephaly, hypoplasia of corpus callosum, seizures, antimongoloid slant to palpebral fissures, Brushfield speckled iris, myopia, cleft palate, cleft lip, small peg-shaped teeth, delayed eruption of teeth, taurodontism and enamel defects leading to premature loss of deciduous anterior teeth, webbed neck (12%), preauricular pit, pectus excavatum, cervical rib, gynecomastia, congenital heart defect (14%) most commonly patent ductus arteriosus, umbilical and/or inguinal hernia, scoliosis, simian creases, talipes, abnormal toes, wide gap between first and second toes, intravesical ureterocele, hypospadias, bifid scrotum, growth hormone deficiency.

NATURAL HISTORY. Perinatal problems in adaptation have been frequent; linear growth is generally slow, with moderately short final height attainment. Infertility and inadequate virilization may be anticipated. Depending on the overall life situation, testosterone replacement therapy should be considered at 11 to 12 years of age. A decline in intellectual performance occurs with advancing age. Behavioral problems including irritability and agitation, hyperactivity, and noncompliance, and inappropriate speech occur. Poor language development has been documented with a significant discrepancy between expressive ability and comprehension.

ETIOLOGY. The diagnosis is confirmed by chromosomal analysis revealing an XXXY or XXXXY karyotype. Molecular methods have indicated that the X chromosomes are maternally derived. There is no association with older maternal age.

COMMENT. The mean IQ of 35 may be inappropriately low. Several patients with IQs in the borderline to low normal range recently have been reported.

References

Fraccaro M, Kaijser K, Lindsten J: A child with 49 chromosomes. Lancet 2:899, 1960.

Zaleski WA et al: The XXXXY chromosome anomaly: Report of three new cases and review of 30 cases from the literature. Can Med Assoc J 94:1143, 1966.

Schmid R, Pajewski M, Rosenblatt M: Epiphyseal dysplasia: A constant finding in XXXXY syndrome. J Med Genet 15:282, 1978.

Borghgraef M et al: The 49 XXXXY syndrome: Clinical and psychological follow-up data. Clin Genet 33:429, 1988.

Plaha DS et al: Origin of the X chromosomes in a patient with the 49 XXXXY syndrome. J Med Genet 27:203, 1990.

Lomelino CA, Reiss AL: 49 XXXXY syndrome: Behavioral and developmental profiles. J Med Genet 28:609, 1991.

Peet J et al: 49XXXXY: A distinct phenotype: Three new cases and review. J Med Genet 35:420, 1998.

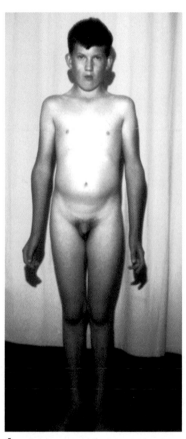

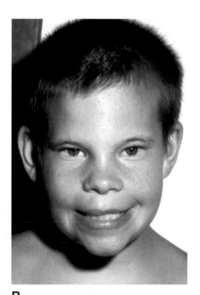

A   **B**

FIGURE 1. **A** and **B,** Adolescent and preadolescent boys with XXXY syndrome; both are short and of dull mentality. Note the facial dysmorphia, elbow aberrations, and hypogonadism.

XXX AND XXXX SYNDROMES

Initially described by Jacobs and colleagues in 1959 in a woman of normal intelligence who had secondary amenorrhea, the XXX syndrome is recognized to occur in 1 in 1000 newborn females. There is no pattern of malformation associated with this karyotype. Based on studies of unselected newborns with sex chromosome anomalies who have been followed longitudinally, the following can be stated relative to females with a 47XXX karyotype: Affected individuals are usually tall with average height of 172 cm. Mean occipitofrontal circumference is approximately the 20th percentile. Pubertal development is normal with an average age of menarche of 12 (range, 8 to 12) years. Fertility is probably normal. Delay in achievement of motor milestones, poor coordination, and awkwardness are common. IQ scores cluster in the 85 to 90 range (generally lower than that in their siblings). Problems with verbal learning and expressive language are frequent. Special education classes in high school are required in 60%. Behavior problems, including mild depression, conduct disorder, or being undersocialized, occur in 30%. However, most cope well and adapt as young adults without major problems.

This is in contrast to the XXXX syndrome, initially described by Carr and colleagues in 1961, in which only 40 cases have been reported. Individuals with the XXXX syndrome have a variable phenotype with the facies suggestive of the Down syndrome in several cases.

ABNORMALITIES IN THE XXXX SYNDROME. For other than mental retardation, all of the other features are variable. The patients are usually of normal to tall stature.

Performance. IQ of 30 to 80, average of 55; speech development is most prominently affected.

Facies. Midfacial hypoplasia, upward slanting palpebral fissures, mild hypertelorism, epicanthal folds, mild micrognathia.

Limbs. Occasional fifth finger clinodactyly, radioulnar synostosis, reduced total finger ridge count.

Other. Tall stature, narrow shoulder girdle, taurodontism, variable amenorrhea, irregular menses.

OCCASIONAL ABNORMALITIES. Seizures, variable EEG abnormalities, mild ventricular enlargement on CT scan, webbed neck.

NATURAL HISTORY. Besides mental retardation, speech and behavioral problems are frequent in the XXXX syndrome. The patient initially reported by Carr and colleagues, now 56 years old, is in good physical health with no evidence of intellectual deterioration. Her full-scale IQ is 56. Although menstrual disorders are common and fertility is reduced, offspring of these individuals tend to be normal.

ETIOLOGY. The diagnosis is confirmed by chromosomal analysis revealing a XXX or XXXX karyotype. Nondisjunction at maternal meiosis I is the most common cause of 47XXX. Although not as striking an effect as is seen with trisomy 21, an increased maternal age effect has been seen for 47XXX females.

References

Jacobs PA et al: Evidence for the existence of the human "super female." Lancet 2:423, 1959.

Carr DH, Barr ML, Plunkett ER: An XXXX sex chromosome complex in two mentally defective females. Can Med Assoc J 84:131, 1961.

Telfer MA et al: Divergent phenotypes among 48,XXXX and 47,XXXX females. Am J Hum Genet 22:326, 1970.

Gardner RJM, Veale AMO, Sands VE: XXXX syndrome: Case report, and a note on genetic counselling and fertility. Humangenetik 17:323, 1973.

Berg JM et al: Twenty-six years later: A woman with tetra-X chromosomes. J Mental Defic Res 32:67, 1988.

Robinson A et al: Sex chromosome aneuploidy: The Denver prospective study. Birth Defects 26(4):59, 1991.

Robinson A et al: Summary of clinical findings in children and young adults with sex chromosome anomalies. Birth Defects 26(4):225, 1991.

Liebezeit BU et al: Tall stature as presenting symptom in a girl with triple X syndrome. J Pediatr Endocrinol Metab 16:233, 2003.

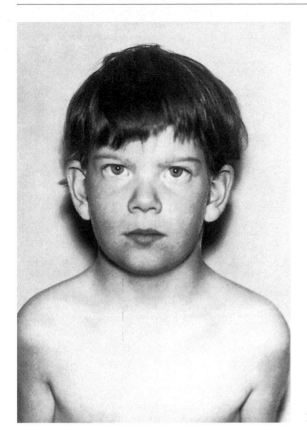

FIGURE 1. A 6½-year-old girl with XXXX syndrome.

XXXXX SYNDROME
(PENTA X SYNDROME)

Upward Slant to Palpebral Fissures, Patent Ductus Arteriosus, Small Hands with Clinodactyly of Fifth Fingers

The first description of an individual with XXXXX was by Kesaree and Wooley in 1963.

ABNORMALITIES. Mental retardation, moderate to severe; prenatal onset of growth deficiency, failure to thrive, short stature; microcephaly; mild upward slant (mongoloid) to palpebral fissures; low nasal bridge, short neck; hypertelorism; epicanthal folds; low hairline; dental malocclusion; taurodontism and enamel defects leading to premature loss of deciduous anterior teeth; small hands with mild clinodactyly of fifth fingers; congenital heart defect (patent ductus arteriosus or ventricular septal defect).

OCCASIONAL ABNORMALITIES. Dandy-Walker malformation; colobomata of iris; low-set ears; preauricular tags; macroglossia; cleft palate; micrognathia; high-frequency, low-arch dermal ridge patterns; simian creases; equinovarus; overlapping toes; multiple joint dislocations including shoulder, elbow, hips, wrists, and fingers; renal dysplasia; horseshoe kidney; ovarian agenesis.

NATURAL HISTORY. IQ varies from 20 to 75. The oldest known affected individual, a 16-year-old girl, had small nipples, prepubertal external genitalia, and an atrophic vaginal smear. Information on fertility is lacking.

COMMENT AND ETIOLOGY. Of interest is the occurrence in these XXXXX individuals of many of the nonspecific anomalies found in Down syndrome, a diagnosis that was initially considered in some of the patients. The diagnosis is confirmed by chromosomal analysis revealing an XXXXX karyotype. Molecular methods have indicated that the X chromosomes are maternally derived.

References

Kesaree N, Wooley PV: A phenotypic female with 49 chromosomes, presumably XXXXX: A case report. J Pediatr 63:1099, 1963.

Sergovich F, Uilenberg C, Pozsonyi J: The 49,XXXXX condition. J Pediatr 78:285, 1971.

Dryer FR et al: Pentasomy X with multiple dislocations. Am J Med Genet 4:313, 1979.

Funderburk SJ et al: Pentasomy X: Report of a patient and studies of X-inactivation. Am J Med Genet 8:27, 1981

Deng HX et al: Parental origin and mechanism of formation of polysomy X: An XXXXX case and four XXXXY cases determined with RFLPs. Hum Genet 86:541, 1991.

Myles TD et al: Dandy-Walker malformation in a fetus with pentasomy X (49XXXXX) prenatally diagnosed by fluorescent in situ hybridization technique. Fetal Diag Ther 10:333, 1995.

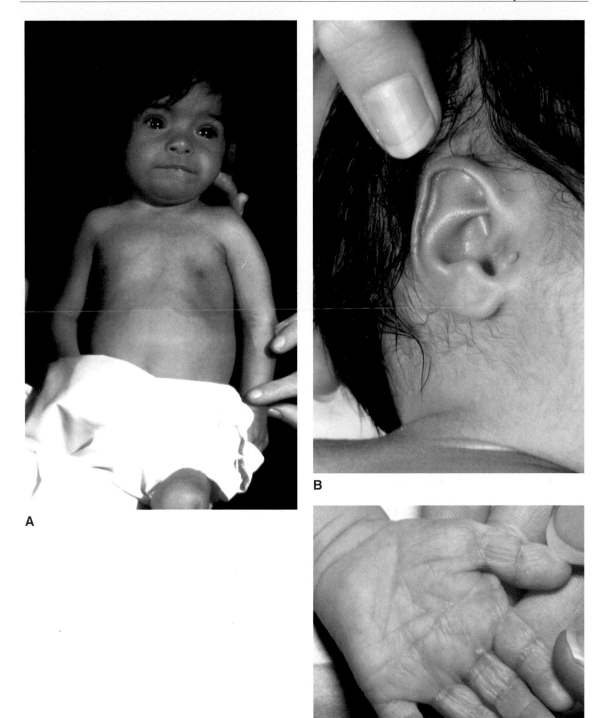

FIGURE 1. XXXXX syndrome. **A–C,** Note the ocular hypertelorism, preauricular tags, simian crease, and fifth finger clinodactyly.

45X SYNDROME
(XO Syndrome, Turner Syndrome)

Short Female, Broad Chest with Wide Spacing of Nipples, Congenital Lymphedema or Its Residua

An association between small stature and defective ovarian development had been noted as early as 1922 by Rossle, who classified the disorder under "sexagen dwarfism." A more expanded syndrome of small stature, sexual infantilism, webbed neck, and cubitus valgus in seven females was described by Turner in 1938. Most 45X conceptuses die early. It is estimated that approximately 1 in 2500 live-born phenotypic females are affected. Recommendations for diagnosis, treatment, and management of affected individuals have been established and published by Rosenfeld and colleagues.

ABNORMALITIES. The following list of abnormalities, with the approximate percentage for each anomaly, includes those of the full monosomic X syndrome. Patients with mosaicism (XX/X mosaics, XY/X mosaics with varying degrees of male-type genitalia) or in whom only a part of one X is missing (X-isochromosome X or X-deleted X) generally have a lesser degree of malformation. The most consistent features for the entire group are small stature and gonadal dysgenesis. Because the latter feature is not evident during childhood, a chromosomal study is indicated in any girl with short stature of unknown cause whose clinical phenotype is not incompatible with the 45X syndrome. In addition, any adolescent with absent breast development by 13 years of age, pubertal arrest, or primary or secondary amenorrhea with elevated follicle-stimulating hormone should undergo karyotype analysis.

Growth. Small stature, often evident by birth; tendency to become obese.

Performance. Mean IQ approximately 90 with performance usually below verbal scores. Although early development is usually normal, delays in motor skills are common, as is poor coordination. Specific neuropsychological deficits are as follows: Visual-spatial organization deficits such as difficulty driving; deficits in social cognition such as failure to appreciate subtle social cues; problems with nonverbal problem solving such as math; psychomotor deficits, such as clumsiness; a tendency for low self-esteem and depression in teenagers and young adults.

Gonads. Ovarian dysgenesis with hypoplasia to absence of germinal elements (90+%).

Lymph Vessels. Congenital lymphedema with residual puffiness over the dorsum of the fingers and toes (80+%). Can be seen at any age; often associated with initiation of growth hormone and/or estrogen therapy.

Thorax. Broad chest with widely spaced nipples that may be hypoplastic, inverted, or both (80+%); often mild pectus excavatum.

Auricles. Anomalous auricles, most commonly prominent (80+%).

Facies. Narrow maxilla (palate) (80+%), relatively small mandible (70+%), inner canthal folds (40+%).

Neck. Low posterior hairline, appearance of short neck (80+%), webbed posterior neck (50%).

Extremities. Cubitus valgus or other anomaly of elbow (70+%); knee anomalies, such as medial tibial exostosis (60+%); short fourth metacarpal, metatarsal, or both (50+%).

Other Skeletal. Bone dysplasia with coarse trabecular pattern, most evident at metaphyseal ends of long bones (50+%); dislocation of hip.

Nails. Narrow, hyperconvex, and/or deep-set nails (70+%).

Skin. Excessive pigmented nevi (50+%); distal palmar axial triradii (40+%); loose skin, especially around the neck in infancy; tendency toward keloid formation.

Renal. Most commonly horseshoe kidney, double or cleft renal pelvis, and minor alterations (60+%).

Cardiac. Cardiac defects, the majority of which are bicuspid aortic valve (30%), coarctation of aorta (10%), valvular aortic stenosis, mitral valve prolapse, and aortic dissection later in life.

Central Nervous System. Perceptive hearing impairment (50+%).

OCCASIONAL ABNORMALITIES

Skeletal. Abnormal angulation of radius to carpal bones, Madelung deformity, short midphalanx of fifth finger, short third to fifth metacarpals and/or metatarsals, scoliosis, kyphosis, spina bifida, vertebral fusion, cervical rib, abnormal sella turcica.

Eyes. Ptosis (16%), strabismus, amblyopia, blue sclerae, cataract.

Central Nervous System. Mental retardation. Agenesis or reduced areas of the genu of the corpus callosum, pons, and lobules VI and VII of the cerebellar vermis and increased area of the fourth ventricle.

Other. Hemangiomata, rarely of the intestine; long hair on arms; idiopathic hypertension; diabetes mellitus; ulcerative colitis; celiac disease; Crohn disease; primary hypothyroidism (10% to 30%); agenesis of corpus callosum (two cases); partial anomalous pulmonary venous return; hypoplastic left heart; persistent left superior vena cava.

NATURAL HISTORY.

The congenital lymphedema usually recedes in early infancy, leaving only puffiness of the dorsum of the fingers and toes, although there may be recrudescence of the lymphedema with growth hormone or estrogen replacement therapy. At birth, the skin tends to be loose, especially in the posterior neck where excess skin may persist as the pterygium colli. Small size is often evident at birth, the mean birth weight being 2900 g. From birth up to 3 years of age the growth rate is normal, although there is a delay in bone maturation. Between 3 and 12 years, bone age progression is normal, but height velocity decreases. After 12 years of age, there is a decreased growth rate, deceleration of bone age progression, and relative increase in weight. Mean final height of untreated women with Turner syndrome is 143 cm (4 feet, 8 inches), 20 cm (8 inches) less than the general female population. Regarding treatment for short stature, 99 females with Turner syndrome were enrolled in a U.S. Multicenter Trial of growth hormone and low dose estrogen. Significant growth hormone–induced improvement in height was demonstrated (individuals who received 0.36 mgm/kg per week with or without estrogen achieved near-final heights of 149.9 ± 6.0 cm and 150 ± 6.0 cm, respectively). Factors that influenced the response to therapy included younger age, lower bone age to chronologic age ratio, lower baseline weight, and greater baseline height at initiation of therapy. Even at low doses, estrogen therapy did not affect near final height.

Studies of XO abortuses have disclosed near-normal development of the ovaries in early fetal life. Apparently, they usually do not make primary follicles, and the ovary degenerates rather rapidly. In the majority of affected individuals, by adolescence there is seldom any functional ovarian tissue remaining. However, it is important to recognize that 10% to 20% will have spontaneous pubertal development and 2% to 5% will have spontaneous menses, although this is generally transient; at least several 45X individuals have been fertile. Estrogen replacement therapy is indicated, beginning between 13 and 14 years in hypogonadotropic girls. Treatment before 12 years of age may compromise final adult height. At some time between 8 years and adolescence, these patients should be told that their ovaries are probably incompletely developed and that they should plan on adopting children and taking "the same kind of medicine the ovary makes" at adolescence.

The actual incidence of early mortality due to congenital heart defects is unknown. An increased risk for dissection of the aorta has been documented in adults. Aortic root dilatation occurs with a prevalence estimated to be between 8% and 42%. Therefore, affected females with normal echocardiograms should be imaged every 5 years and those with abnormal echocardiograms should be followed yearly. In addition, increased morbidity secondary to diabetes mellitus, hypertension, ischemic heart disease, and stroke has been documented. The types of renal anomalies that occur generally pose no problem to health. However, an increased risk of osteoporosis, autoimmune thyroid disease, and chronic liver disease has been reported with increasing age. Enhancement of physical appearance by plastic surgery for prominent inner canthal folds, protruding auricles, and especially for webbed neck should be given serious consideration before school age. However, there is a markedly increased incidence of keloid formation that must be taken into account.

Approximately 6% of females with Turner syndrome have 45X/46XY mosaicism. In those cases, an exploratory laparotomy in childhood seems indicated to remove any gonadoblastoma, which such patients have an increased risk of developing.

If the child is mentally retarded, a careful search should be made for a chromosome abnormality in addition to that of the sex chromosome. For example, patients with X-autosome translocation are more likely to be mentally deficient. Mental retardation has also been seen more frequently in individuals with a small ring X chromosome.

ETIOLOGY.

Faulty chromosomal distribution leading to 45X individual. The paternal X chromosome is the one more likely to be missing. There has been no significant older maternal age factor for this aneuploidy syndrome. It is generally a sporadic event in a family, although there are as yet no adequate data on risk for recurrence.

Mosaicism does not ensure survival to term. However, the incidence of sex chromosome mosaicism is higher in live born than in aborted 45X fetuses.

References

Rossle RI: Wachstum und Altern. München, 1922.

Turner HH: A syndrome of infantilism, congenital webbed neck, and cubitus valgus. Endocrinology 23:566, 1938.

Weiss L: Additional evidence of gradual loss of germ cells in the pathogenesis of streak ovaries in Turner's syndrome. J Med Genet 8:540, 1971.

Kastrup KW: Oestrogen therapy in Turner's syndrome. Acta Paediatr Scand Suppl 343:43, 1988.

Rosenfeld RG: Update on growth hormone therapy for Turner's syndrome. Acta Paediatr Scand Suppl 356:103, 1989.

Chang HJ et al: The phenotype of 45X/46XY mosaicism: An analysis of 92 prenatally diagnosed cases. Am J Hum Genet 46:156, 1990.

Robinson A et al: Sex chromosome aneuploidy: The Denver prospective study. Birth Defects 26(4):59, 1991.

Hassold T et al: Molecular studies of parental origin and mosaicism in 45X conceptuses. Hum Genet 89:647, 1992.

Rosenfeld RG et al: Recommendations for diagnosis, treatment and management of individuals with Turner syndrome. Endocrinologist 4:351, 1994.

Gravholt CH et al: Morbidity in Turner syndrome. J Clin Epidemiol 51:147, 1998.

Guarneri MP et al: Turner's syndrome. J Pediatr Endocrinol Metab 14(Suppl 2):959, 2001.

Elsheikh M et al: Turner's syndrome in adulthood. Endocr Rev 23:120, 2002.

Quigley CA et al: Growth hormone and low dose estrogen in Turner syndrome: Results of a United States multicenter trial to near-final height. J Clin Endocrinol Metab 87:2033, 2002.

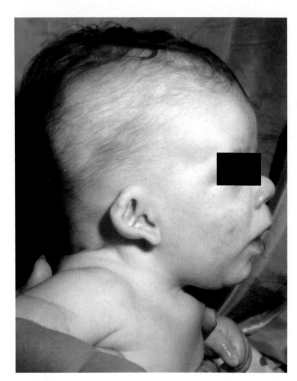

FIGURE 1. Baby with 45X syndrome. Note the protuberant ears and loose nuchal skin.

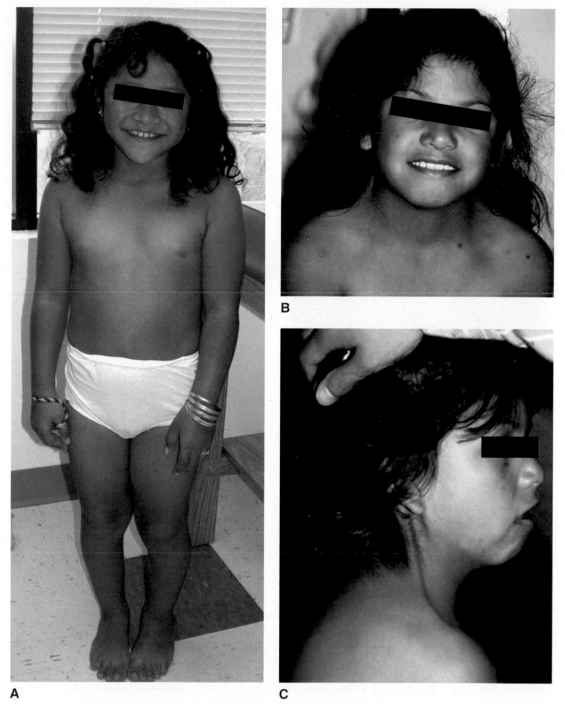

FIGURE 2. Turner syndrome. **A–C,** Note prominent ears, loose folds of skin in posterior neck with low hairline, broad chest with widely spaced nipples. (Courtesy of Dr. Lynne M. Bird, Children's Hospital, San Diego.)

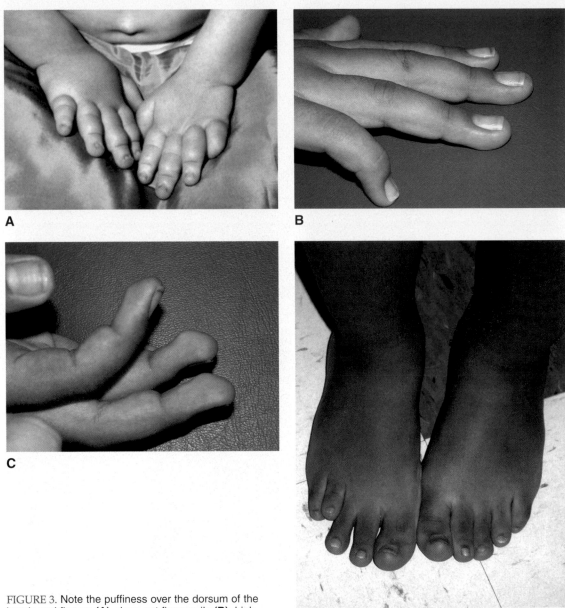

FIGURE 3. Note the puffiness over the dorsum of the hands and fingers **(A)**, deep-set fingernails **(B)**, high fingertip pads **(C)**, and short fourth metatarsals **(D)**.

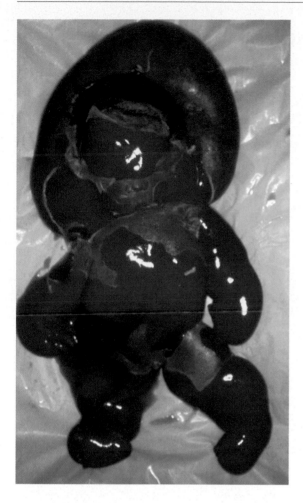

FIGURE 4. Twenty-week fetus with 45X Turner syndrome. Note the massive edema.

Very Small Stature,
Not Skeletal Dysplasia

BRACHMANN–DE LANGE SYNDROME
(CORNELIA DE LANGE SYNDROME, DE LANGE SYNDROME)

Synophrys, Thin Downturning Upper Lip, Micromelia

The syndrome was originally reported in 1933 by Cornelia de Lange. Brachmann described a child with similar features at autopsy in 1916.

ABNORMALITIES

Growth. Prenatal onset growth deficiency with respect to length and weight.

Retarded osseous maturation	100%
Low-pitched, weak, growling cry in infancy	74%

Performance. Mental retardation and sluggish physical activity. Average intelligence quotient (IQ) ranges from below 30 to 86 with an average of 53. Those with higher IQs tend to have a higher birth weight and head circumference.

Initial hypertonicity	100%
Low-pitched, weak, growling cry in infancy	74%

Cranium

Microbrachycephaly	93%

Eyes

Bushy eyebrows and synophrys	98%
Long, curly eyelashes	99%

Nose

Depressed nasal bridge	83%
Anteverted nares	85%

Mouth

Long philtrum, thin upper lip, and downturned angles of mouth	94%
High-arched palate	86%
Late eruption of widely spaced teeth	86%

Mandible

Micrognathia	84%
Spurs in the anterior angle of the mandible, prominent symphysis	66%

Skin

Hirsutism	78%

Cutis marmorata and perioral pale "cyanosis"	56%
Hypoplastic nipples and umbilicus	50%

Hands and Arms

Micromelia	93%
Phocomelia and oligodactyly	27%
Clinodactyly of fifth fingers	74%
Simian crease	51%
Proximal implantation of thumbs	72%
Flexion contracture of elbows	64%

Feet

Micromelia	93%
Syndactyly of second and third toes	86%

Male Genitalia

Hypoplasia	57%
Undescended testes	73%
Hypospadias	33%

Radiographic. Mandibular spur present up to 3 months of age, dislocated/hypoplastic radial head, hypoplastic first metacarpal and fifth middle phalanx, short sternum with precocious fusion and 13 ribs.

Other. Ocular abnormalities including myopia, ptosis, and nystagmus in 57%; low posterior hairline (92%); short neck (66%); gastrointestinal problems including gastroesophageal reflux (30%) and various forms of obstruction including duplication of gut, malrotation of colon with volvulus, and pyloric stenosis; hearing loss (60%).

OCCASIONAL ABNORMALITIES.
Seizures (23%), microcornea, astigmatism, optic atrophy, coloboma of the optic nerve, strabismus, proptosis, choanal atresia, low-set ears, cleft palate, congenital heart defect most commonly ventricular septal defect, hiatus hernia, diaphragmatic hernia, brachyesophagus, inguinal hernia, small labia majora, radial hypoplasia, absent second to third interdigital triradius, thrombocytopenia.

NATURAL HISTORY AND MANAGEMENT.

These patients show a marked retardation of growth, evident by the time of birth, and as a rule, they fail to thrive. Feeding difficulties, including regurgitation, projectile vomiting, chewing, and swallowing difficulties, often continue beyond 6 months. Although a high percentage of affected children have severe mental retardation, a significant number have a much higher potential relative to performance than earlier studies have suggested. Hearing loss associated with speech delay occurs frequently. Their gait tends to be broad-based. They sometimes show autistic behavior, including self-destructive tendencies. The patients may avoid and reject social interactions and physical contact. Although rapid movement may be pleasurable, they show infrequent facial emotion and tend to have stereotypic behavior. The majority of patients followed beyond 13 years had onset of puberty, with normal menses documented in several women. Episodes of aspiration in infancy, apnea, complications related to bowel obstruction, and cardiac defects appear to constitute the major hazards for survival in these patients.

ETIOLOGY.

This disorder has an autosomal dominant inheritance; mutations in *Nipped-B homolog (Drosophila)* (NIPBL), which is located at 5p13, are responsible. The *Drosophila Nipped-B* gene is a facilitator of enhancer-promoter communication that plays a role in Notch signaling and other developmental pathways in *Drosophila*. Most cases are sporadic. The observed low recurrence risk most likely represents the inability of more severely affected individuals to reproduce. As with other autosomal dominant disorders, marked variability of expression has been observed.

References

Brachmann W: Ein Fall von symmetrischer Monodaktylie durch ulnadefekt mit symmetrischer Flughautbildung in den Ellenbeugen, sowie anderen Abnormitaten (Zwerghaftigheit, Halsrippen, Behaarung). Jahrb Kinderkeilk 84:224, 1916.

de Lange C: Sur un type nouveau de génération (typus Amstelodamensis). Arch Med Engant 36:713, 1933.

Ptacek LJ et al: The Cornelia de Lange syndrome. J Pediatr 63:1000, 1963.

Vischer D: Typus degenerativus Amstelodamensis (Cornelia de Lange syndrome). Helv Paediatr Acta 20:415, 1965.

Johnson HG et al: A behavioral phenotype in the de Lange syndrome. Pediatr Res 10:843, 1976.

Robinson LK, Wolfsberg E, Jones KL: Brachmann–de Lange syndrome: Evidence for autosomal dominant inheritance. Am J Med Genet 22:109, 1985.

Jackson L et al: de Lange syndrome: A clinical review of 310 individuals. Am J Med Genet 47:940, 1993.

Braddock SR et al: Radiological features in Brachmann–de Lange syndrome. Am J Med Genet 47:1006, 1993.

Berney TP et al: Behavioral phenotype of Cornelia de Lange syndrome. Arch Dis Child 81:333, 1999.

Krantz ID et al: Cornelia de Lange syndrome is caused by mutations in NIPBL, the human homolog of the Drosophila *Nipped-B* gene. Nat Genet 36:631, 2004.

Gillis LA et al: NIPBL mutational analysis in 120 individuals with Cornelia de Lange syndrome and evaluation of genotype-phenotype correlations. Am J Hum Genet 75:610, 2004.

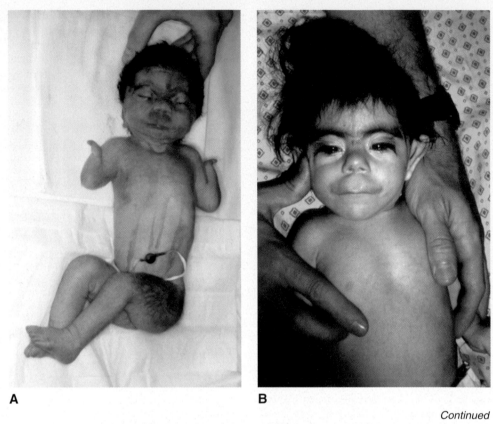

A   B

Continued

FIGURE 1. De Lange syndrome. **A–D,** Four different affected individuals. Note the synophrys, thin downturned upper lip, long philtrum, hirsutism, small hands and feet, and severe limb defects.

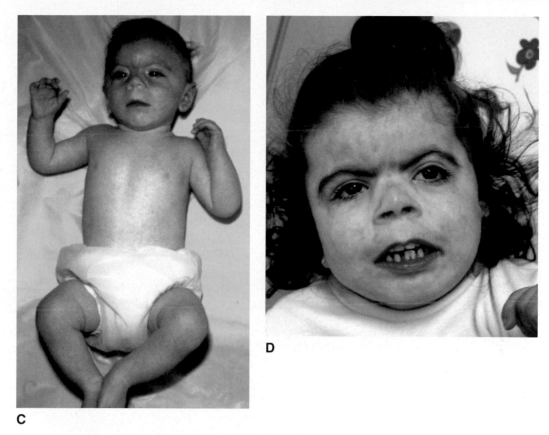

C

D

Fig. 1, cont'd.

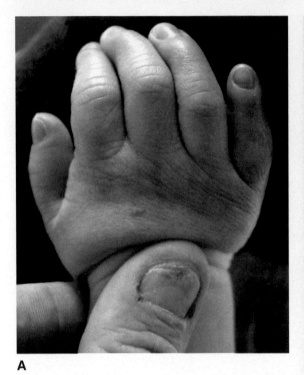

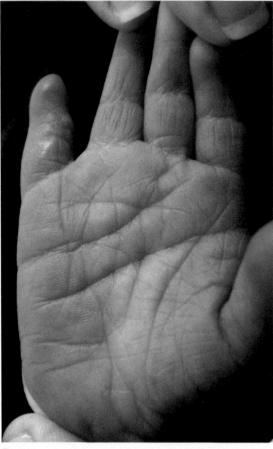

FIGURE 2. **A** and **B,** Note the fifth finger clinodactyly and proximal implantation of the thumb.

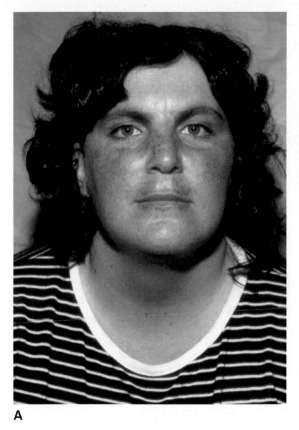

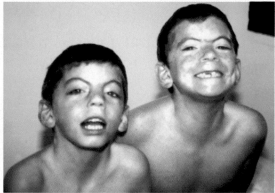

FIGURE 3. **A** and **B,** Mildly affected mother and her severely affected sons.

A

RUBINSTEIN-TAYBI SYNDROME

*Broad Thumbs and Toes, Slanted Palpebral
Fissures, Hypoplastic Maxilla*

Rubinstein and Taybi set forth this clinical entity in
1963. More than 550 cases have been reported.

ABNORMALITIES

Growth. Postnatal onset of growth deficiency; in
adults, average height of 153 cm in males
and 147 cm in females; average weight of 48
kg in males and 55 kg in females.

Retarded osseous maturation	74%

Performance. IQ 30 to 79 with an average of 51;
52% have an IQ less than 50.

Speech difficulties	90%
EEG abnormality	57%
Seizures	23%
Stiff, unsteady gait	85%
Hypotonia	67%
Hyperreflexia	40%

Cranium

Microcephaly	35%
Large anterior fontanel	41%
Delayed closure of fontanel	24%
Frontal bossing	33%

Facies

Palpebral fissures slant downward (50% below age 5 years)	88%
Hypoplastic maxilla with narrow palate	100%
Small opening of mouth	56%
Prominent or beaked nose with or without nasal septum extending below alae nasi and short columella	90%
Deviated nasal septum	71%
Frontal hair up-sweep	20%
Auricles low-set, malformed, or both	84%
Low anterior hairline	24%
Low posterior hairline	42%
Micrognathia	49%

Ocular

Heavy eyebrows	76%
Highly arched eyebrows	73%
Long eyelashes	87%
Stenosis nasolacrimal duct	43%
Ptosis	36%
Epicanthal folds	55%
Strabismus	69%
Enophthalmos	22%

Hands and Feet

Broad thumbs with radial angulation	87%
Broad great toes	100%
Other fingers broad	87%
Fifth finger clinodactyly	62%
Persistent fetal fingertip pads	31%
Deep plantar crease between first and second toes	33%
Flat feet	72%

Other Skeletal

Scoliosis	42%
Spina bifida occulta	47%
Cervical hyperkyphosis	37%
Small, flared iliac wings	26%

Genitourinary

Cryptorchidism	78% of males
Renal anomalies	52%

Skin

Hirsutism	75%
Capillary hemangioma	25%
Keloid formation	22%

Cardiac. Defects, most frequent of which are
patent ductus arteriosus, ventricular septal
defect, and atrial septal defect, occur in
approximately one third of cases.

OCCASIONAL ABNORMALITIES

Skeletal. Large foramen magnum, parietal foramina, micrognathia, sternal anomalies, syndactyly, polydactyly.

Other. Cataract, glaucoma, ocular coloboma, ptosis
of eyelid, nystagmus, myopia, Duane retraction syndrome, exophthalmia, cardiac conduction defects, camptodactyly, polydactyly,
simian crease, distal axial triradius, duplicated
halluces, patellar dislocation, dislocation of
radial head, Perthes disease, bifid uterus,
paratubal cystadenoma, pectus excavatum,
angulated penis, hypospadias, shawl scrotum,
Hirschsprung disease, absence of corpus
callosum, café au lait spots, stereotypic
movements, mirror movements, tethered cord,
mediastinal vascular ring, premature thelarche.

NATURAL HISTORY.

Respiratory infections, obstipation, and feeding difficulties are frequent problems in infancy. Aggressive assessment and treatment of gastroesophageal reflux is warranted. Constipation occurs in 40% to 74%. Average ages for childhood milestones are as follows: crawl, 15 months; sit up, 11 months; walk, 30 months; say first word, 25 months; and toilet trained, 62 months. In addition to speech therapy, the majority of affected children require physical therapy; 67% of patients 6 years of age or older can read, although for the majority it does not progress beyond the first-grade level. Recurrent ear infections with mild hearing loss and dental problems primarily associated with overcrowding of the teeth occur frequently. Hand and/or foot surgery frequently improves grasp, oppositional function, and comfort. Unusual reactions to anesthesia (respiratory distress and cardiac arrhythmias) have been reported. In addition, airway anomalies, skeletal anomalies, and increased risk of aspiration occur. Obstructive sleep apnea may contribute to hypertension. Management of ingrown toenails and early treatment of paronychia are warranted.

ETIOLOGY.

The majority of cases are sporadic. The locus for this disorder is at 16p13.3, a region that contains the gene for the human CREB binding protein (CBP), a nuclear protein participating as a co-activator in cyclic-AMP-regulated gene expression. Four percent to 25% of cases are due to submicroscopic deletions detectable by fluorescent in situ hybridization. Point mutations in the CBP gene, a transcriptional co-activator that mediates cyclic adenosine monophosphate–regulated gene expression have been demonstrated.

References

Rubinstein JH, Taybi H: Broad thumbs and toes and facial abnormalities: A possible mental retardation syndrome. Am J Dis Child 105:588, 1963.

Rubinstein JH: The broad thumbs syndrome—progress report 1968. Birth Defects 5:25, 1969.

Simpson NE, Brissenden JE: The Rubinstein-Taybi syndrome: Familial and dermatoglyphic data. Am J Hum Genet 25:225, 1973.

Hannekam RCM et al: Rubinstein-Taybi syndrome in the Netherlands. Am J Med Genet Suppl 6:17, 1990.

Stevens CA et al: Growth in Rubinstein-Taybi syndrome. Am J Med Genet Suppl 6:51, 1990.

Stevens CA et al: Rubinstein-Taybi syndrome: A natural history study. Am J Med Genet Suppl 6:30, 1990.

Breuning MJ et al: Rubinstein-Taybi syndrome caused by submicroscopic deletions within 16p13.3 Am J Med Genet 52:249, 1993.

Petrij F et al: Rubinstein-Taybi syndrome caused by mutations in the transcriptional co-activator CBP. Nature 346:348, 1995.

Allanson JE, Hennekam RCM: Rubinstein-Taybi syndrome: Objective evaluation of craniofacial structure. Am J Med Genet 71:414, 1997.

Wiley S et al: Rubinstein-Taybi syndrome medical guidelines. Am J Med Genet 119:101, 2003.

RUSSELL-SILVER SYNDROME
(SILVER SYNDROME)

Short Stature of Prenatal Onset, Skeletal Asymmetry, Small Incurved Fifth Finger

This pattern of malformation was independently described by Silver and colleagues and by Russell in 1953 and 1954. Silver emphasized the skeletal asymmetry as a feature of the disorder. This was a variable finding in the patients described by Russell. Diagnostic criteria for this disorder are inconsistent, most likely reflecting etiologic heterogeneity.

ABNORMALITIES

Growth and Skeletal. Small stature, of prenatal onset; immature osseous development in infancy and early childhood, with late closure of anterior fontanel; asymmetry, most commonly of limbs; short or incurved fifth finger.

Facies. Small, triangular facies with frontal prominence and a normal head circumference (relative macrocephaly); downturned corners of mouth; the sclerae may be bluish in early infancy; micrognathia.

Skin. Café au lait spots.

Other. Tendency toward excess sweating, especially on the head and upper trunk, during infancy; liability to fasting hypoglycemia from about 10 months until 2 to 3 years of age.

OCCASIONAL ABNORMALITIES.
Developmental delay; syndactyly of second to third toes; camptodactyly; Sprengel deformity; renal anomaly; posterior urethral valves; hypospadias; inguinal hernia; cardiac defects; malignancy including craniopharyngioma, testicular seminoma, hepatocellular carcinoma, and Wilms tumor; gastrointestinal abnormalities including gastroesophageal reflux, esophagitis, and food aversion; growth hormone deficiency.

NATURAL HISTORY.
The patients are usually slim and underweight for length during early childhood. There tends to be a gradual improvement in growth in weight and appearance during childhood and especially during adolescence. As a result, the adult usually appears more normal than the infant with this disorder. Final height attainment can be up to 5 feet. During infancy, patients tend to be weak, have feeding difficulties, and may be slow in major motor progress. Approximately one third have learning disabilities. Because of the small facies, the upper head may *appear* large, although head circumference is well within the normal range. This appearance, plus the relatively large fontanels in early infancy, may give rise to a false impression of hydrocephalus—which they do not have. Somewhat frequent feedings and adequate glucose intake during illnesses should be ensured from 6 months of age until 3 years, the period of enhanced liability to fasting hypoglycemia. Growth hormone deficiency should be considered if the linear growth rate reaches a plateau.

ETIOLOGY.
The etiology of this disorder is unknown. The majority of cases are sporadic. A study by Saal and colleagues indicates the marked heterogeneity of this disorder. Maternal uniparental disomy (UPD)7 has been documented with a frequency of approximately 10%. In addition, abnormalities of chromosome 8, 15, 17, and 18 may initially resemble Russell-Silver syndrome.

COMMENT.
Children with Russell-Silver syndrome with matUPD(7) comprise a mild phenotype distinct from nonmatUPD(7) cases. Characteristic are pre- and postnatal growth deficiency; absence of (or mild) craniofacial features consisting of slight or absent facial triangularity, micrognathia, and downturned corners of mouth; speech delay; poor feeding; excessive sweating without episodes of hypoglycemia; and increased paternal age.

References

Silver HK et al: Syndrome of congenital hemihypertrophy, shortness of stature and elevated urinary gonadotrophins. Pediatrics 12:368, 1953.

Russell A: A syndrome of "intra-uterine" dwarfism recognizable at birth with craniofacial dysostosis, disproportionately short arms and other anomalies. Proc R Soc Med 47:1040, 1954.

Silver HK: Asymmetry, short stature, and variations in sexual development: A syndrome of congenital malformations. Am J Dis Child 107:495, 1964.

Garesis FJ, Smith DW, Summitt RL: The Russell-Silver syndrome without asymmetry. J Pediatr 79:775, 1971.

Haslam RHA, Berman W, Heller RM: Renal abnormalities in the Russell-Silver syndrome. Pediatrics 51:216, 1973.

Nishi Y et al: Silver-Russell syndrome and growth hormone deficiency. Acta Paediatr Scand 71:1035, 1982.

Saal HM, Pagon RA, Pepin MG: Reevaluation of Russell-Silver syndrome. J Pediatr 107:733, 1985.

Price SM et al: The spectrum of Silver-Russell syndrome: A clinical and molecular genetic study and new diagnostic criteria. J Med Genet 36:837, 1999.

Hannula K et al: Do patients with maternal uniparental disomy for chromosome 7 have a distinct mild Silver-Russell phenotype? J Med Genet 38:273, 2001.

Anderson J et al: Gastrointestinal complications of Russell-Silver syndrome: A pilot study. Am J Med Genet 113:15, 2002.

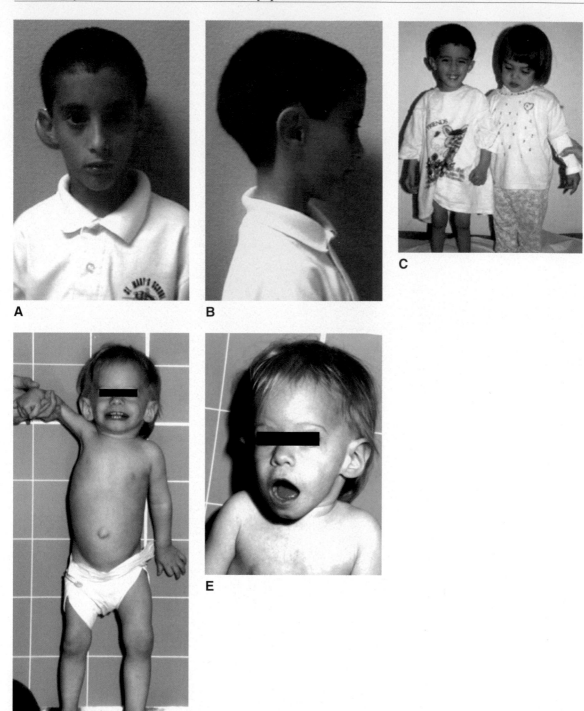

FIGURE 1. Russell-Silver syndrome. **A** and **B,** Note the small triangular face with frontal prominence. **C,** A 3½-year-old boy with his 2-year-old unaffected sister. (**C,** Courtesy of Dr. Lynne M. Bird, Children's Hospital, San Diego.) **D** and **E,** A 2-year-old boy. Note the small facies, slimness, and "loose" posture.

SHORT SYNDROME

First reported in 1975 by Gorlin and colleagues and by Sensenbrenner and colleagues, the acronym SHORT refers to the principle features, which include *S*hort stature, *H*yperextensibility of joints or *H*ernia (inguinal) or both, *O*cular depression, *R*ieger anomaly, and *T*eething delay. Approximately 15 cases have been reported.

ABNORMALITIES

Growth. Mild intrauterine growth retardation, postnatal growth deficiency, delayed bone age.
Performance. Delay in speech development with normal mental and motor development.
Craniofacies. "Triangular-shaped" face, prominent ears, broad nasal bridge, telecanthus (lateral displacement of medial canthi), deeply set eyes, hypoplastic ala nasi, micrognathia.
Skeletal. Hyperextensible joints; fifth finger clinodactyly; radiologic findings including large epiphyses, gracile diaphyses, and cone-shaped epiphyses.
Other. Delayed dental eruption, Rieger anomaly, inguinal hernia.

OCCASIONAL ABNORMALITIES.

Sensorineural hearing loss, congenital glaucoma, chin dimple, microcephaly.

NATURAL HISTORY. Although IUGR occurs in the majority of affected children, the growth retardation, involving both height and weight, is most severe postnatally. Illnesses including chronic vomiting, diarrhea, and feeding problems are frequent throughout the first 2 years of life, and hospitalization for failure to thrive is common in infancy. Decreased subcutaneous fat in the face has been noted as early as 3 months. Onset of speech has been delayed to 36 months. Diabetes mellitus secondary to insulin resistance has occurred in two patients, at 16 and 13 years of age, respectively, the latter while receiving growth hormone therapy.

ETIOLOGY. Although autosomal dominant inheritance is most likely, affected siblings born to normal parents have been described.

References
Gorlin et al: Rieger anomaly and growth retardation (The SHORT syndrome). Birth Defects Orig Artic Ser 11(2):464, 1975.
Sensenbrenner et al: CC—A low birthweight syndrome, Rieger syndrome. Birth Defects Orig Artic Ser 11(2): 423, 1975.
Toriello HV et al: Report of a case and further delineation of the SHORT syndrome. Am J Med Genet 22:311, 1985.
Lipson et al: The SHORT syndrome: further delineation and natural history. J Med Genet 26:473, 1989.
Schwingshandl et al: SHORT syndrome and insulin resistance. Am J Med Genet 407:907, 1993.

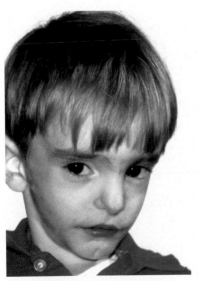
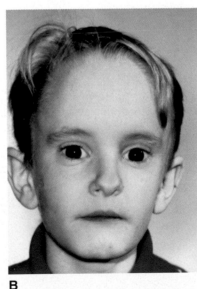

A **B**

FIGURE 1. SHORT syndrome. **A** and **B,** Brothers with "triangular-shaped" face, deeply set eyes, hypoplastic ala nasi, and micrognathia. (From Gorlin RJ et al: Birth Defects 11:46, 1975.)

3-M SYNDROME

Prenatal and Postnatal Growth Deficiency, Short Neck, Slender Long Bones

Initially described by Fuhrmann and colleagues in 1972, this disorder was designated the 3-M syndrome after the initials of the first three authors by Miller and colleagues in 1975. Over 30 cases have been reported.

ABNORMALITIES

Growth. Prenatal growth deficiency with mean birth length of 40.5 cm and mean birth weight of 2120 g at full-term; severe post-natal linear growth deficiency with weight below the third percentile for chronological age, but increased for height; slightly increased upper/lower segment ratio; delayed bone age.

Craniofacial. Dolichocephaly; frontal bossing; triangular-shaped face; malar hypoplasia; full, pointed chin; fleshy nasal tip; short nose with anteverted nares; long philtrum; full lips.

Skeletal. Short neck with prominent trapezius muscles and horizontal clavicles giving appearance of square shoulders, short thorax with pectus (carinatum or excavatum), hyperextensible joints, lumbar hyperlordosis, short fifth fingers.

Radiographic. Slender shafts of long bones and ribs, tall vertebral bodies with reduced anterior-posterior diameter particularly in lumbar region, small pelvis, small iliac wings, short femoral necks.

OCCASIONAL ABNORMALITIES.

Mild mental deficiency; full eyebrows; prominent, dysplastic ears; V-shaped dental arch with anterior crowding and malocclusion; dental caries; prominent scapulae; diastasis recti; joint dislocation; decreased elbow extension; congenital hip dislocation; frequent fractures; fifth finger clinodactyly; transverse grooves of anterior chest; pes planus; prominent heels; supernumerary nipple; hypospadias; intracerebral aneurysm.

NATURAL HISTORY. Feeding problems are common during the first year. Although female gonadal function is usually normal with menarche occurring at the usual time, males may have gonadal dysfunction and subfertility or infertility. Final adult height in six affected individuals averaged between 4 and 5 standard deviations below the mean.

ETIOLOGY. This disorder has an autosomal recessive inheritance pattern.

References

Fuhrmann W et al: Familiärer Minderwuchs mit unproo-portioniert hohen Wirbeln. Humangenetik 16:271–282, 1972.

Miller JD et al: The 3-M syndrome: A heritable low birth weight dwarfism. Birth Defects Orig Artic Ser 11(5):39–47, 1975.

Hennekam RCM et al: Further delineation of the 3-M syndrome with review of the literature. Am J Med Genet 28:195–209, 1987.

van der Wal G et al: 3-M syndrome: Description of six new patients with review of the literature. Clin Dysmorphology 10:241–252, 2001.

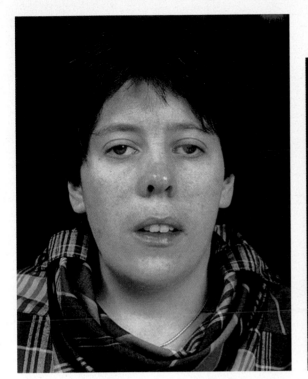
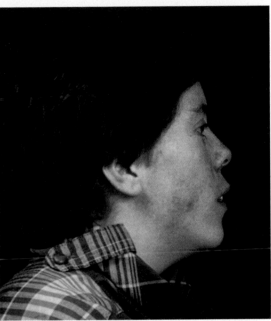

FIGURE 1. 3-M syndrome. Note the full eyebrows, flattened malar region, fleshy nasal tip, upturned nares, and long philtrum. (Courtesy of Dr. Raoul Hennekam, University of Amsterdam.)

MULIBREY NANISM SYNDROME
(PERHEENTUPA SYNDROME)

Small Stature, Pericardial Constriction, Yellow Dots in Fundus

Perheentupa and colleagues described this disorder in 1970, and more than 50 cases have been reported. The term "mulibrey" is an acronym used to denote the organs most frequently involved: *mu*scle, *li*ver, *br*ain, and *ey*es.

ABNORMALITIES

Growth. Prenatal onset of growth deficiency; mean birth weight and length at term are 2.4 kg and 45 cm, respectively; adult height ranges from 136 to 161 cm for males and from 126 to 151 cm for females; hands and feet appear relatively large in relation to body.

Craniofacial. Dolichocephaly with J-shaped sella turcica, triangular facies with frontal bossing, depressed nasal bridge, relatively small tongue, dental crowding, missing or small frontal and/or sphenoidal sinuses.

Eye. Decreased retinal pigmentation with dispersion and clusters of pigment and yellowish dots in the midperipheral region, choroidal hypoplasia.

Other. Development of thick adherent pericardium with hepatomegaly and prominent neck veins; variable fibrous dysplasia, especially in tibia; muscle hypotonia; high-pitched voice; hypodontia of second bicuspid; cutaneous nevi.

OCCASIONAL ABNORMALITIES.

Cortical thickening of long bones; strabismus; mild mental retardation; large cerebral ventricles; high-set hyoid bones; eosinophilia; edema of vocal cords; iris coloboma; dental enamel hypoplasia; hydrops fetalis; Wilms tumor; ovarian tumor; hypoglycemia; hyperammonemia; humoral immunodeficiency consisting of disturbed antibody response and impaired opsonization; delayed puberty; hypothyroidism; growth hormone deficiency; hypoadrenocorticism.

NATURAL HISTORY. Normal intelligence in majority of cases; onset of pericardial constrictive problems from infancy to late childhood; whether the hepatomegaly is secondary to pericardial constriction remains to be resolved; pulmonary infections and early heart failure occur, the latter secondary to pericardial constriction, subendocardial fibrosis, or myocardial infarction.

ETIOLOGY. This disorder has an autosomal recessive pattern. The gene, located at 17q22-q23, encodes a new member of the RING-B-box-Coiled-coil (RBCC) family of zinc-finger proteins whose members are involved in developmental patterning and oncogenesis.

References

Perheentupa J et al: Mulibrey-nanism: Dwarfism with muscle, liver, brain and eye involvement. Acta Paediatr Scand 50(Suppl. 206):74, 1970.

Voorhees ML, Husson GS, Blackman MS: Growth failure with pericardial constriction. Am J Dis Child 130:1146, 1976.

Tarkkanen A, Raitta C, Perheentupa J: Mulibrey nanism: An autosomal recessive syndrome with ocular involvement. Acta Ophthalmol 60:628, 1982.

Lapunzina P et al: Mulibrey nanism: Three additional patients and a review of 39 cases. Am J Med Genet 55:349, 1995.

Avela A et al: Gene encoding a new RING-B-box-coiled-coil protein is mutated in mulibrey nanism. Nat Genet 25:298, 2000.

Karlberb N et al: Mulibrey nanism: Clinical features and diagnostic criteria. J Med Genet 41:92, 2004.

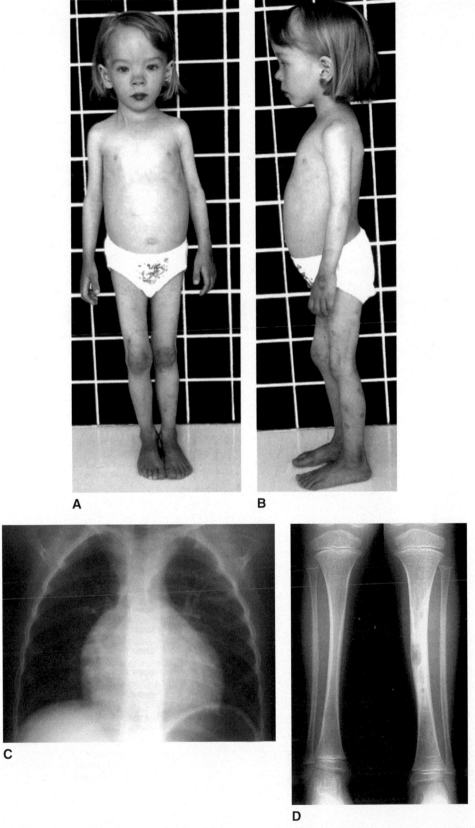

FIGURE 1. **A–D,** Girl with Mulibrey Nanism syndrome. Note the triangular face with frontal bossing, the aberrant cardiac silhouette and enlarged liver relating to constriction of the pericardium, and the fibrous dysplasia of the femur. (Courtesy of Dr. M. Lipsanen-Nyman, University of Helsinki.)

DUBOWITZ SYNDROME

*Peculiar Facies, Infantile Eczema,
Small Stature, Mild Microcephaly*

This disorder was initially reported by Dubowitz in 1965, and Wilroy and colleagues summarized 21 cases, eight of their own, in 1978. More than 140 cases have now been described.

ABNORMALITIES

Growth. Prenatal growth deficiency in the majority of cases, with average birth weight of 2.3 kg, birth length of 44 cm, and head circumference of 30.6 cm; retarded osseous maturation; postnatal growth deficiency (86%).

Performance. Mental retardation (72%) ranging from mild (51%) to moderate (14%) to severe (10%), hyperactivity (67%), short attention span, stubbornness, and shyness, high-pitched, hoarse cry, speech delay (67%), muscular hypotonia (40%).

Craniofacial. Microcephaly, sloping forehead, broad nasal bridge, small facies, shallow supraorbital ridge with nasal bridge at about same level as forehead, broad nasal tip, short palpebral fissures with telecanthus and appearance of hypertelorism, variable ptosis and blepharophimosis, epicanthal folds, prominent or mildly dysplastic ears, micrognathia.

Skin and Hair. Eczema-like skin disorder on face and flexural areas, sparseness of lateral eyebrows and scalp hair.

Dentition. Lag in eruption, caries, missing teeth.

Other. Brachyclinodactyly of fifth fingers; syndactyly of second and third toes; cryptorchidism; ocular abnormalities including strabismus, microphthalmia, hyperopia, megalocornea, hypoplasia of iris, and coloboma; abnormalities of the ocular fundus include abnormal veins, tapetoretinal degeneration, and ocular albinism.

OCCASIONAL ABNORMALITIES.

Normal intelligence; submucous cleft palate; large mouth; velopharyngeal insufficiency; pes planus; metatarsus adductus; hyperextensible joints; hypospadias; pilonidal dimple; delayed bone age; hypoparathyroidism; bone marrow hypoplasia; cryptorchism; hypospadias; inguinal hernia; vesicoureteral reflux; malignancies including lymphoma, neuroblastoma, and acute lymphatic leukemia; fatal aplastic anemia; cardiac defect; seizures; large anterior fontanel; broad thumbs; scoliosis.

NATURAL HISTORY. Eczema, noted in approximately one half of the patients, usually clears by 2 to 4 years. Approximately one third of the patients have poor feeding. Vomiting and chronic constipation occur. Respiratory and gastrointestinal infections occur frequently, raising the possibility of immunodeficiency. Teeth tend to become carious, and rhinorrhea and otitis media are frequent problems. Behavioral aberrations with lag in development of speech pose problems in function.

ETIOLOGY. The inheritance of this disorder is autosomal recessive, based on affected male and female siblings from unaffected parents.

COMMENT. The facies may appear similar to that of the fetal alcohol syndrome.

References

Dubowitz V: Familial low birth weight dwarfism with an unusual facies and a skin eruption. J Med Genet 2:12, 1965.

Opitz JM et al: The Dubowitz syndrome: Further observations. Z Kinderheilkd 116:1, 1973.

Kuster W, Majewski F: Dubowitz syndrome. Eur J Pediatr 144:574, 1986.

Winter RM: Dubowitz syndrome. J Med Genet 23:11, 1986.

Tsukahara M, Opitz JM: Dubowitz syndrome: Review of 141 cases including 36 previously unreported patients. Am J Med Genet 63:277, 1996.

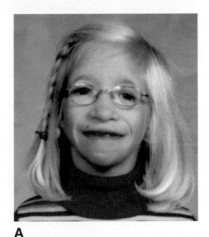

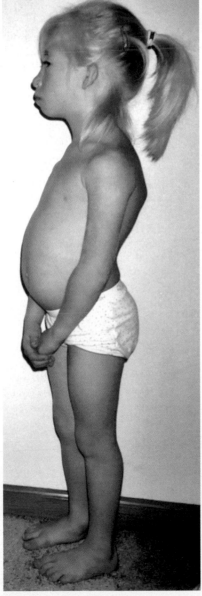

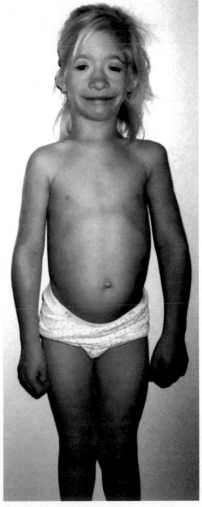

FIGURE 1. Dubowitz syndrome. **A–C,**
Note the short palpebral fissures,
asymmetric ptosis, shallow supraorbital
ridges, and mild micrognathia. (Courtesy
of Dr. John M. Opitz, University of Utah,
Salt Lake City.)

BLOOM SYNDROME

Short Stature, Malar Hypoplasia, Telangiectatic Erythema of the Face

Since Bloom's original description in 1954, more than 130 patients with this disorder have been reported.

ABNORMALITIES

Growth. Prenatal onset of growth deficiency; average adult male height, 151 cm, and adult female height, 144 cm.

Craniofacial. Mild microcephaly with dolichocephaly; malar hypoplasia, with or without small nose.

Skin. Facial telangiectatic erythema involves the butterfly midface region and is exacerbated by sunlight, usually develops during the first year; small and large areas of hyperpigmentation and hypopigmentation.

OCCASIONAL ABNORMALITIES.

Mild mental deficiency; short attention span during childhood and learning difficulties, including reading disabilities; telangiectatic erythema of the dorsa of the hands and forearms; high-pitched voice; colloid-body–like spots in Bruch membrane of the eye; absence of upper lateral incisors; prominent ears; ichthyotic skin, hypertrichosis, pilonidal cyst, sacral dimple; syndactyly, polydactyly, clinodactyly of fifth finger, short lower extremity, talipes; café au lait spots; immunoglobulin deficiency, with decreased serum levels of immunoglobulins and an impaired lymphocyte proliferation response to mitogens; propensity to develop malignancy; non–insulin-dependent diabetes mellitus.

NATURAL HISTORY.

These patients show a consistently slow pace of growth. Feeding problems are frequent during infancy. Susceptibility to infection decreases with age. However, chronic lung disease has been responsible for three deaths, at ages 18, 19, and 24 years. The facial erythema is very seldom present at birth, usually appearing during infancy following exposure to sunlight; it may excoriate, but improves after childhood. Non–insulin-dependent diabetes mellitus occurs in approximately 8% of patients in late adolescence or early adulthood. Although learning disabilities occur, the majority of patients are within the normal range for intelligence.

Malignancy has been the major known cause of death. Malignancy develops in approximately one in four patients. Although leukemia occurs frequently, solid tumors with a variety of histologic types and sites of origin are the most common type of neoplasia. Of those with malignancy, the mean age at diagnosis is 24.8 years, with a range from 4 to 44 years. Gastrointestinal malignancy is common after the age of 30. Infertility due to lack of spermatogenesis is the rule in males. Subfertility in females may be common.

An increased rate of chromosomal breakage and sister chromatid exchange is found in cultured leukocytes and fibroblasts from all patients studied, but not reliably so in the heterozygotes.

ETIOLOGY.

The inheritance of this disorder is autosomal recessive, with the majority of individuals being of Ashkenazic Jewish ancestry. The gene has been mapped to chromosome 15q26.1 and the gene product is homologous to RecQ helicases. The frequency of the gene carrier in the Ashkenazic Jewish population is estimated at a minimum of 1:100. The excess of affected males to females is probably more apparent because of underdiagnosis of the disorder in females, in whom the skin lesion tends to be milder.

COMMENT.

The relation of the in vitro chromosomal breakage and the development of malignancies is not well understood at present.

References

Bloom D: Congenital telangiectatic erythema resembling lupus erythematosus in dwarfs. Am J Dis Child 88:754, 1954.

Bloom D: The syndrome of congenital telangiectatic erythema and stunted growth. J Pediatr 68:103, 1966.

Sawitsky A, Bloom D, German J: Chromosomal breakage and acute leukemia in congenital telangiectatic erythema and stunted growth. Ann Intern Med 65:487, 1966.

German J, Bloom D, Passarge E: Bloom's syndrome VII: Progress report for 1978. Clin Genet 15:361, 1979.

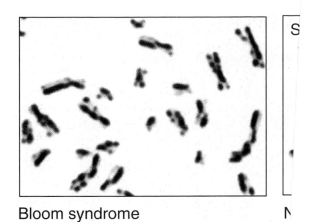

Bloom syndrome

FIGURE 2. Photograph of increased sister chromatin exchange in the control on the right. (From Passarge E: Color Atlas of Genetic 1995, p 338. Reprinted by permission.)

German J, Bloom D, Passarge E: Bloom's syndrome XI: Progress report for 1983. Clin Genet 25:166, 1984.

German J, Passage E: Bloom's syndrome XII: Report from the Registry for 1987. Clin Genet 35:57, 1989.

German J et al: Bloom syndrome: An analysis of con-sanguineous families assigns the locus mutated to chromosome band 15q26.1. Proc Natl Acad Sci USA 91:6669, 1994.

Ellis NA: The Bloom's syndrome gene product is homologous to RecQ Helicases. Cell 83:655, 1995.

FIGURE 1. Bloom syndrome. Note the facial telangiectatic erythema involving the butterfly midface region. (From Passarge E: Color Atlas of Genetics. New York: George Thieme Medical Publishers, 1995, p 338. Reprinted by permission.)

SECKEL SYNDROME

Severe Short Stature, Microcephaly, Prominent Nose

Reported by Mann and Russell in 1959, this condition was extensively studied by Seckel in 1960. More precise criteria for diagnosis have recently been set forth.

ABNORMALITIES

Growth. Prenatal onset of marked growth deficiency; average birth weight at term is 1543 g (1000 to 2005 g); mean postnatal growth deficiency is −7.1 SD ± 2.08, one adult was 104 cm; delayed bone age.

Central Nervous System. Mental retardation, nearly one half with IQ less than 50.

Craniofacial. Microcephaly with secondary premature synostosis; in one half of cases, head circumference is more retarded than height, while for the remainder it is consistent with height age; receding forehead; prominent nose; micrognathia; low-set, malformed ears with lack of lobule; relatively large eyes with downslanting palpebral fissures.

Upper Extremities. Clinodactyly of fifth finger, simian crease, absence of some phalangeal epiphyses, hypoplasia of proximal radius with dislocation of radial head.

Lower Extremities. Dislocation of hip, hypoplasia of proximal fibula, gap between first and second toes, inability to completely extend at knees.

Thorax. Only 11 pairs of ribs.

Genitalia. Male: cryptorchidism.

OCCASIONAL ABNORMALITIES.
Facial asymmetry, strabismus, cataract, seizures, agenesis of corpus callosum, dysgenetic cerebral cortex, dorsal cerebral cyst, pachygyria, partial anodontia, enamel hypoplasia, sparse hair, scoliosis, talipes, pes planus, hypoplastic external genitalia, hypoplastic anemia, chromosome breakage, cleft palate, delayed puberty, osteosarcoma, ventricular septal defect.

NATURAL HISTORY. Gestational timing may be prolonged. Although moderate to severe mental retardation occurs, early motor progress may be near normal. The cerebrum is small, with a simple primitive convolutional pattern resembling that of a chimpanzee. Though they tend to be friendly and pleasant, these patients are often hyperkinetic and easily distracted. Poor joint development and support may be evident by dislocations of the hip, elbow, or both, and by later development of scoliosis, kyphosis, or both. Survival to an age of 75 years has been recorded.

ETIOLOGY. This disorder has an autosomal recessive inheritance pattern. Two different disease loci, one at 3q22.1-q24 and the other at 18p11.31-q11.2, have been mapped indicating genetic heterogeneity for this disorder.

References

Mann TP, Russell A: Study of microcephalic midget of extreme type. Proc R Soc Med 52:1024, 1959.

Seckel HPG: Bird-Headed Dwarfs. Springfield, Ill: Charles C Thomas, 1960.

Harper RG, Orti E, Baker RK: Bird-headed dwarfs (Seckel's syndrome): A familial pattern of developmental, dental, skeletal, genital, and central nervous system anomalies. J Pediatr 70:799, 1967.

McKusick VA et al: Seckel's bird-headed dwarfism. N Engl J Med 277:279, 1967.

Majewski F, Goecke T: Studies of microcephalic primordial dwarfism I: Approach to a delineation of the Seckel syndrome. Am J Med Genet 12:7, 1982.

Shanske A et al: Central nervous system anomalies in Seckel syndrome: Report of a new family and review of the literature. Am J Med Genet 70:155, 1997.

Faivre L et al: Clinical and genetic heterogeneity of Seckel syndrome. Am J Med Genet 112:379, 2002.

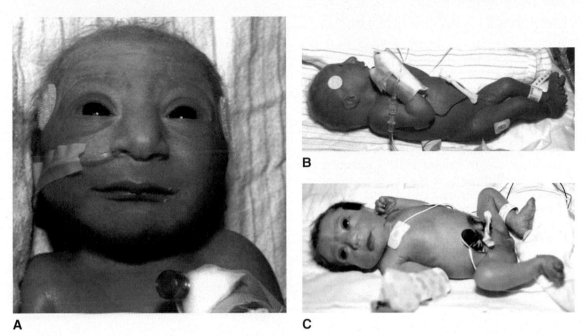

A

B

C

FIGURE 1. Seckel syndrome. **A** and **B,** Newborn at 38 weeks' gestation with birth weight of 1651 g, birth length of 41 cm, and OFC of 28 cm. **C,** Her sibling. Note the disproportion of nose size to the size of the face and mandible, whereas general body proportions and adiposity are near normal for age. (**A–C,** Courtesy of Dr. Marilyn C. Jones, Children's Hospital, San Diego.)

HALLERMANN-STREIFF SYNDROME
(OCULOMANDIBULODYSCEPHALY
WITH HYPOTRICHOSIS SYNDROME)

Microphthalmia, Small Pinched Nose, Hypotrichosis

The first report of this disorder was by Audry, who described an incomplete case in 1893. Hallermann, in 1948, and Streiff, in 1950, independently described three cases, recognizing this syndrome as a separate entity. In 1958, Francois collected all the previously published cases and emphasized the cardinal features of the condition. Approximately 150 cases have been reported in the literature.

ABNORMALITIES

Growth. Prematurity, low birth weight, or both in one third; proportionate small stature; postnatal growth deficiency in two thirds with mean final height of 152 cm in females and 155 to 157 cm in males.

Craniofacial. Brachycephaly with frontal and parietal bossing, thin calvarium, and delayed ossification of the sutures; malar hypoplasia; micrognathia, with hypoplasia of the rami and anterior displacement of the temporomandibular joint; nose is thin, small, and pointed, with hypoplasia of the cartilage, becoming parrot-like with age; narrow and high-arched palate; dentition: hypoplasia or malimplantation of the teeth, neonatal teeth, and partial anodontia; atrophy of the skin, most prominent over the nose and sutural areas of the scalp; thin and light hair with hypotrichosis, especially of the scalp, eyebrows, and eyelashes.

Ocular. Bilateral microphthalmia (80%); cataracts (94%), total or incomplete, which may resorb spontaneously; nystagmus; strabismus.

Radiologic. Large poorly ossified skull with decreased ossification in sutural areas; wormian bones; obtuse or straight gonial angle; thin, gracile long bones with widening at the metaphyseal ends; thin ribs; small vertebral bodies; decreased number of sternal ossification centers; thin, gracile metacarpals.

OCCASIONAL ABNORMALITIES.
Scaphocephaly, microcephaly, platybasia, shallow sella turcica, absence of the mandibular condyles, tracheomalacia, double cutaneous chin, microstomia, blue sclerae, downward slant to palpebral fissures, optic disk colobomata, glaucoma, persistence of pupillary membrane, various chorioretinal pigment alterations, ear anomalies, syndactyly, winging of the scapulae, lordosis, scoliosis, spina bifida, funnel chest, cardiac defects, mental retardation (15%), hyperactivity, choreoathetosis, generalized tonic-clonic seizures, hypogenitalism and cryptorchidism in the male, renal anomalies, hepatic defects, immunodeficiency, hematopoietic abnormalities.

NATURAL HISTORY. The patients' narrow upper airway associated with the craniofacial configuration can lead to serious complications including severe early pulmonary infection, respiratory embarrassment, obstructive sleep apnea, and anesthetic complications. During early infancy, patients with this disorder may have feeding and respiratory problems, even necessitating tracheostomy. Respiratory infections may contribute to the cause of death. Laryngoscopy and endotracheal intubation at the time of anesthesia may be difficult because of the upper airway obstruction. The major handicap is the ocular defect, which usually culminates in blindness despite surgery. Though the majority of the reported patients have been of normal intelligence, motor and mental deficits, even to severe degree, have been reported.

ETIOLOGY. All cases have been sporadic occurrences.

References

Audry C: Variété d'alopécia congénitale; alopécie suturale. Ann Dermatol Syph (Ser. 3), 4:899, 1893.

Hallermann W: Vogelgesicht und cataracta congenita. Klin Monatsbl Augenheilkd 113:315, 1948.

Streiff EB: Dysmorphie mandibulo-faciale (tête d'oiseau) et alterations oculaires. Ophthalmologica 120:79, 1950.

Francois J: A new syndrome: Dyscephalis with bird face and dental anomalies, nanism, hypotrichosis, cutaneous atrophy, microphthalmia and congenital cataract. Arch Ophthalmol 60:842, 1958.

Hoefnagel D, Bernirschke K: Dyscephalia mandibulo-oculofacialis (Hallermann-Streiff syndrome). Arch Dis Child 40:57, 1965.

Judge C, Chalcanovskis JF: The Hallermann-Streiff syndrome. J Ment Defic Res 15:115, 1971.

Golomb RS, Porter PS: A distinct hair shaft abnormality in the Hallermann-Streiff syndrome. Cutis 16:122, 1975.

Christian CL et al: Radiological findings in Hallermann-Streiff syndrome: Report of five cases and a review of the literature. Am J Med Genet 41:508, 1991.

Cohen MM: Hallermann-Streiff syndrome: A review. Am J Med Genet 41:488, 1991.

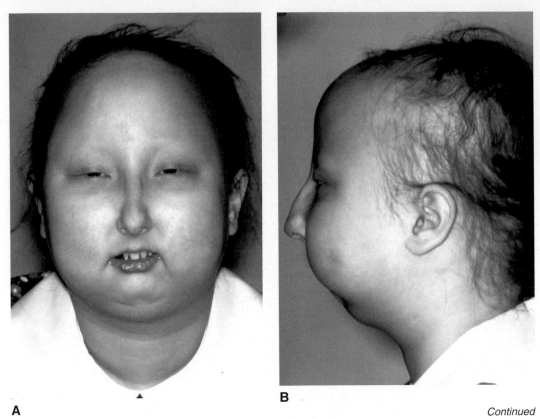

A

B

Continued

FIGURE 1. Hallermann-Streiff syndrome. **A–D,** Two affected children. Note the brachycephaly with frontal and parietal bossing, malar hypoplasia, micrognathia, thin nose, microphthalmia, and hypotrichosis. (**A** and **B,** From Cohen M: Am J Med Genet 41:488, 1991, with permission; **C** and **D,** courtesy of Dr. Michael Cohen, Dalhousie University, Halifax, Nova Scotia.)

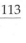

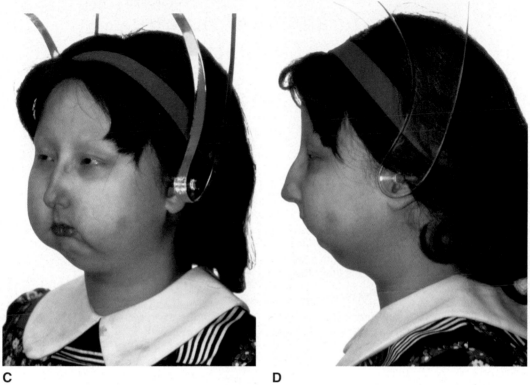

C   D

Fig. 1, cont'd.

C Moderate Short Stature, Facial, ± Genital

SMITH-LEMLI-OPITZ SYNDROME

Anteverted Nostrils, Ptosis of Eyelids, or Both; Syndactyly of Second and Third Toes; Hypospadias and Cryptorchidism in Male

Four patients with this disorder were described by Smith and colleagues in 1964. Its birth prevalence has been estimated by Opitz to be 1 in 20,000, placing it third behind cystic fibrosis and phenylketonuria among the North American white population. Tint and colleagues in 1993 identified an abnormality in cholesterol biosynthesis in patients with this disorder that appears to explain much of the clinical phenotype.

ABNORMALITIES

Growth. Moderately small at birth, with subsequent failure to thrive; final height between 143 and 170 cm.

Performance. Moderate to severe mental deficiency, with variable altered muscle tone; approximately 10% of biochemically diagnosed cases have intelligence quotients (IQs) between 50 and 70.

Craniofacial. Microcephaly with narrow frontal area, auricles slanted or low-set, ptosis of eyelids, inner epicanthal folds, strabismus, broad nasal tip with anteverted nostrils, broad maxillary secondary alveolar ridges, micrognathia.

Limb. Simian crease; high frequency of digital whorl dermal ridge patterning; "Y-shaped" syndactyly of second and third toes; short, proximally placed thumb; postaxial polydactyly of hand and less often feet.

Genitourinary. Genital abnormalities (70%) including hypospadias, cryptorchidism, micropenis, hypoplastic scrotum, bifid scrotum, and microurethra; upper tract anomalies (57%) including ureteropelvic junction obstruction, hydronephrosis, renal cystic dysplasia, renal duplication, renal agenesis, reflux.

Cardiac. Defect in 50% particularly endocardial cushion defect, hypoplastic left heart, atrial septal defect, patent ductus arteriosus, membranous ventricular septal defect.

OCCASIONAL ABNORMALITIES

Central and Peripheral Nervous Systems. Seizures; abnormal EEG; demyelination found in cerebral hemispheres, cranial nerves, and peripheral nerves; enlarged ventricles; agenesis of corpus callosum; cerebellar hypoplasia; holoprosencephaly (5%).

Optic. Cataract, sclerosis of lateral geniculate bodies, lack of visual following, opsoclonus, nystagmus, sclerocornea, iris coloboma, heterochromia iridis, posterior synechiae, glaucoma, optic atrophy, microphthalmia.

Limb. Flexed fingers, asymmetrically short finger(s), radial agenesis, clinodactyly, camptodactyly, ectrodactyly, short first toes, metatarsus adductus, vertical talus, dislocation of hip.

Other. Ocular hypertelorism, absent lacrimal puncta, cleft palate, macrostomia, microglossia, bifid tongue, small larynx and vocal cords, sensorineural hearing loss, abnormal pulmonary lobation, hypoplasia of thymus, adrenal enlargement, inguinal hernia, hepatic dysfunction, pancreatic islet cell hyperplasia, deep sacral dimple, rectal atresia, pyloric stenosis, gallbladder aplasia, cholestatic liver disease, intestinal malrotation, diaphragmatic hernia, anal stenosis, Hirschsprung disease, pit anterior to anus, unusually blond hair, short neck.

NATURAL HISTORY. Many of these babies are born in a breech presentation. Stillbirth and early neonatal death are not uncommon. Feeding difficulty and vomiting have been frequent problems in early infancy. Oral tactile defensive-

114

ness and failure to progress to textured food is common resulting in the need for nasogastric tube feeding in 50%. Gastroesophageal reflux is common because of small stomach, intestinal dysmotility, and milk or soy protein allergy. Of those who survive, 20% die during the first year. Death appeared to be related to pneumonia in most of them, one of whom had a hemorrhagic necrotizing pneumonia with varicella, suggesting an impaired immune response. Irritable behavior with shrill screaming may pose a problem during infancy. Muscle tone, which may be hypotonic in early infancy, tends to become hypertonic with time. Diminished amount of sleep is common in early infancy. The degree of mental deficiency is usually moderate to severe. However, affected children are sociable, have better receptive than expressive language, and may be mechanically adept. Behavioral characteristics of autism, self-injurious and aggressive behavior, and forceful backward arching are common.

ETIOLOGY. This disorder has an autosomal recessive inheritance pattern. A severe defect in cholesterol biosynthesis has been identified leading to abnormally low plasma cholesterol levels and elevated concentrations of the cholesterol precursor 7-dehydrocholesterol, the result of a deficiency of 7-dehydrocholesterol reductase (DHCR7). The DHCR7 gene is localized to chromosome 11q12-13. Cholesterol is vitally important in normal development through its contribution to the cell membrane and outer mitochondrial membrane as well as its role in steroid, bile acid, and vitamin D metabolism, and myelination of the nervous system. Its relative deficiency explains many of the variable features of this disorder. Furthermore, it provides the potential for treatment. Although efficacy has not yet been determined, dietary trials are currently under way. Conventional colorimetric techniques to measure cholesterol will not invariably detect the cholesterol abnormalities in this condition. At present, only a chromatographic assay is suitable for measuring 7-dehydrocholesterol.

Prenatal diagnosis has been successfully accomplished at 16 weeks' gestation on an affected fetus on the basis of reduced amniotic fluid cholesterol, elevated 7-dehydrocholesterol with undetectable amniotic fluid unconjugated estriol.

COMMENT. A number of infants with female external genitalia and a 46XY karyotype who have multiple structural anomalies, including postaxial polydactyly, cleft palate, small tongue, eye anomalies, and cardiac defects, have died in the neonatal period. It is now clear that the difference between this severe phenotype, referred to as Smith-Lemli-Opitz type II, and the more mild type I can be explained by the severity of the mutations responsible. Patients with type II disease are either homozygotes or compound heterozygotes for mutations with no or severely reduced DHCR7 activity, while patients with type I disease are compound heterozygotes for a severe truncating mutation and a second missense mutation associated with residual enzyme activity.

References

Smith DW, Lemli L, Opitz JM: A newly recognized syndrome of multiple congenital anomalies. J Pediatr 64:210, 1964.

Gibson R: A case of the Smith-Lemli-Opitz syndrome of multiple congenital anomalies in association with dysplasia epiphysealis punctata. Can Med Assoc J 92:574, 1965.

Dallaire L, Fraser FC: The syndrome of retardation with urogenital and skeletal anomalies in siblings. J Pediatr 69:459, 1966.

Fierro M: Smith-Lemli-Opitz syndrome: Neuropathological and ophthalmological observations. Dev Med Child Neurol 19:57, 1977.

Lowry RB: Editorial comment: Variability in the Smith-Lemli-Opitz syndrome: Overlap with the Meckel syndrome. Am J Med Genet 14:429, 1983.

Curry CJR et al: Smith-Lemli-Opitz syndrome. Type II: Multiple congenital anomalies with male pseudohermaphroditism and frequent early lethality. Am J Med Genet 26:45, 1987.

Joseph DB et al: Genitourinary abnormalities associated with the Smith-Lemli-Opitz syndrome. J Urol 137:179, 1987.

Irons M et al: Abnormal cholesterol metabolism in the Smith-Lemli-Opitz syndrome: Report of clinical and biochemical findings in four patients and treatment in one patient. Am J Med Genet 50:347, 1994.

Opitz JM: RSH/SLO ("Smith-Lemli-Opitz") syndrome: Historical, genetic and developmental considerations. Am J Med Genet 50:344, 1994.

Opitz JM, de La Cruz F: Cholesterol metabolism in the RSH/Smith-Lemli-Opitz syndrome: Summary of an NICHD Conference. Am J Med Genet 50:326, 1994.

Tint GS et al: Defective cholesterol biosynthesis associated with the Smith-Lemli-Opitz syndrome. N Engl J Med 330:107, 1994.

Kelley RI, Hennekam RCM: The Smith-Lemli-Opitz syndrome. J Med Genet 37:321, 2000.

Tierney E et al: Behavior phenotype in the RSH/Smith-Lemli-Opitz syndrome. Am J Med Genet 98:191, 2001.

KABUKI SYNDROME

Initially reported in 1981 by Niikawa and colleagues and by Kuroki and colleagues in ten unrelated Japanese children, this disorder has now been reported in over 300 patients, many of them non-Japanese. Because of the facial resemblance of affected individuals to the make-up of actors in Kabuki, the traditional Japanese theater, this disorder has been referred to as the Kabuki syndrome.

ABNORMALITIES

Growth. Postnatal growth deficiency, with onset usually occurring in the first year, becomes more marked with increasing age; mean height in children 12 months of age or over was −2.3 SD.

Performance. Mean developmental quotient in infants and children was 52, and in older patients, mean IQ was 62; severe mental retardation is uncommon; IQ equal to or greater than 80 in 12%; hypotonia.

Craniofacial. Long palpebral fissures with eversion of the lateral portion of the lower eyelid; ptosis; arching of eyebrows with sparse lateral third; blue sclera; strabismus; epicanthal folds; short nasal septum; large protuberant ears; preauricular pit; cleft palate; tooth abnormalities; open mouth with tented upper lip giving myopathic appearance.

Skeletal. Anomalies in 88% including short, incurved fifth finger secondary to short fourth and fifth metacarpals; short middle phalanges; brachydactyly; rib anomalies; vertebral anomaly; hip dislocation; scoliosis, kyphosis, or both.

Cardiac. Defects occur in approximately 50% of patients and include malformations associated with altered hemodynamics such as coarctation of the aorta, bicuspid aortic valve, mitral valve prolapse, membranous ventricular septal defect, pulmonary, aortic, and mitral valve stenosis as well as tetralogy of Fallot, single ventricle with common atrium, double outlet right ventricle, and transposition of great vessels.

Other. Joint hyperextensibility (74%); persistent fetal finger pad (96%); excess digital ulnar loops; renal anomalies, urinary tract anomalies, or both (28%); hearing loss (32%).

OCCASIONAL ABNORMALITIES.

Microcephaly; polymicrogyria; subarachnoid cyst; hydrocephalus secondary to aqueductal stenosis; premature graying of hair; vitiligo; cleft lip; lower lip pits; Mondini dysplasias and ossicular anomalies; microtia; short nasal septum; broad nasal root; long eyelashes; preauricular pit; cutaneous syndactyly; nail hypoplasia; cryptorchidism; micropenis; imperforate anus; umbilical and inguinal hernias; malrotation of colon; premature thelarche; precocious puberty; obesity; seizures; pectus excavatum; diaphragmatic hernia, eventration, or both; biliary atresia; stenosis of bronchial tree; growth hormone deficiency.

NATURAL HISTORY.
Although many are present in neonates, the characteristic facial features become more obvious with age. Susceptibility to infection, particularly otitis media, upper respiratory tract, and pneumonia are common. Obesity often occurs at adolescence. Delays in speech and language acquisition with articulation errors are common.

ETIOLOGY.
The etiology of this disorder is unknown. Most cases are sporadic. Autosomal dominant inheritance with marked variability of expression has been suggested based on a few instances of parent to child transmission. That this represents a microdeletion syndrome is an alternative hypothesis.

References

Kuroki Y et al: A new malformation syndrome of long palpebral fissures, large ears, depressed nasal tip, and skeletal anomalies associates with postnatal dwarfism and mental retardation. J Pediatr 99:570, 1981.

Niikawa N et al: Kabuki make-up syndrome: A syndrome of mental retardation, unusual facies, large and protruding ears, and postnatal growth deficiency. J Pediatr 99:565, 1981.

Niikawa N et al: Kabuki make-up (Niikawa-Kuroki) syndrome: A study of 62 patients. Am J Med Genet 31:565, 1988.

Philip N et al: Kabuki make-up (Niikawa-Kuroki) syndrome: A study of 16 non-Japanese cases. Clin Dysmorph 1:63, 1992.

Burke LW, Jones MC: Kabuki syndrome: Underdiagnosed recognizable pattern in cleft palate patients. Cleft Palate Craniofac J 32:77, 1995.

Wessels MJ et al: Kabuki syndrome: A review study of three hundred patients. Clin Dysmorph 11:95, 2002.

Matsumoto N, Niikawa N: Kabuki make-up syndrome: A review. Am J Med Genet 117C:57, 2003.

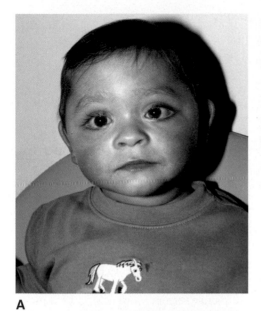

A

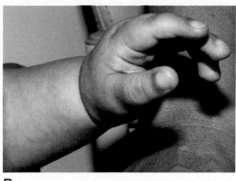

B

FIGURE 1. Kabuki syndrome. **A** and **B,** An 18-month-old boy. Note the long palpebral fissures, eversion of the lateral portion of the lower eyelid, and prominent fingertip pads. (Courtesy of Dr. Marilyn C. Jones, Children's Hospital, San Diego.)

A

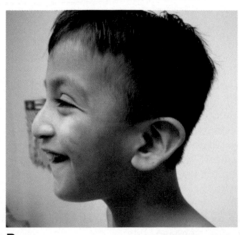

B

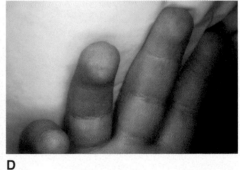

D

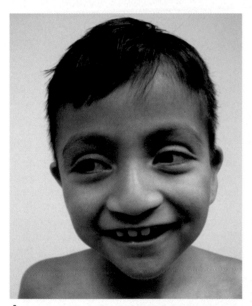

C

FIGURE 2. **A–D,** A 3-year-old boy and 4-year-old girl. Note the long palpebral fissures, large protruding ears, and prominent fingertip pads.

119

WILLIAMS SYNDROME

Prominent Lips, Hoarse Voice, Cardiovascular Anomaly

In 1961, Williams and colleagues described this disorder in four unrelated children with mental deficiency, an unusual facies, and supravalvular aortic stenosis. Subsequently, more than 100 cases have been described. Hypercalcemia has been an infrequent finding; cardiovascular anomalies, including supravalvular aortic stenosis, have been variable; and features such as aberrations of growth and performance and the unusual facies are more consistent relative to diagnosis.

ABNORMALITIES. Varying features from among the following:

Growth. Mild prenatal growth deficiency, postnatal growth rate approximately 75% of normal, mild microcephaly.

Performance. Average IQ of approximately 56, with a range from 41 to 80; friendly, loquacious personality; anxious; hoarse voice; hypersensitivity to sound; mild neurologic dysfunction; primarily mild spasticity manifest by tight heel cords and hyperactive deep tendon reflexes and poor coordination; hypotonia; perceptual and motor function more reduced (–3.0 to –3.9 SD) than verbal and memory performance (–2.0 SD); level of general language ability is much greater than general cognitive ability.

Facies. Medial eyebrow flare, short palpebral fissures; depressed nasal bridge; epicanthal folds; periorbital fullness of subcutaneous tissues; blue eyes; stellate pattern in the iris; anteverted nares; long philtrum; prominent lips with open mouth.

Limb. Hypoplastic nails, hallux valgus.

Cardiovascular. Supravalvular aortic stenosis, peripheral pulmonary artery stenosis, pulmonic valvular stenosis, ventricular and atrial septal defect, renal artery stenosis with hypertension, hypoplasia of the aorta, and other arterial anomalies.

Dentition. Partial anodontia, microdontia, enamel hypoplasia, malocclusion.

Musculoskeletal. Joint hypermobility, contractures, lordosis, scoliosis, kyphosis, extra sacral crease.

Urinary. Renal anomalies including nephrocalcinosis, asymmetry in kidney size, small solitary or pelvic kidney, bladder diverticula, urethral stenosis, vesicoureteral reflux.

Other. Soft lax skin, premature gray hair.

OCCASIONAL ABNORMALITIES. Ocular hypotelorism, amblyopia, strabismus, refractive errors, tortuousity of retinal vessels, high-frequency sensorineural hearing loss, vocal cord paralysis, malar hypoplasia, fifth finger clinodactyly, radioulnar synostosis, small penis, pectus excavatum, inguinal or umbilical hernia, colon diverticula, rectal prolapse, Chiari type I malformation, mucinous cystadenoma of ovary, portal hypertension, celiac disease, hypercalcemia, hypothyroidism, diabetes mellitus, obesity, early onset of puberty.

NATURAL HISTORY. In early infancy, these children tend to be fretful, have feeding problems, vomit frequently, are constipated, and are often colicky. During childhood, they tend to be outgoing and loquacious, easily approach strangers, and have a strong interest in others. However, almost two thirds of children older than 3 years of age display more difficult temperament characteristics than controls including higher activity, lower adaptability, greater intensity, more negative moods, less persistence, greater distractibility, and lower threshold arousal.

Progressive medical problems are the rule in adults. These include hypertension; progressive joint limitations; recurrent urinary tract infections; and gastrointestinal problems including obesity, chronic constipation, diverticulosis and cholelithiasis, and hypercalcemia. The vast majority live with their parents, in group homes, or in supervised apartments.

Sudden death has been documented in a number of children. Some deaths were associated with the administration of anesthesia. Health supervision guidelines have been established for children with Williams syndrome by the Committee on Genetics of the American Academy of Pediatrics.

ETIOLOGY. Although most individuals with this disorder represent sporadic cases within otherwise normal families, parent to child transmission has been documented. Studies using fluorescent in situ hybridization and quantitative Southern analysis indicate that both inherited and sporadic cases of Williams syndrome are caused by a deletion at 7q11.23, a region that includes approximately 17 genes. Hemizygosity for the elastin gene is responsible for supravalvular aortic stenosis as well as other vascular stenosis, and LIM-kinase 1 hemizygosity is a contributing factor to impaired visuospatial construction cognition in this disorder. Many of the other features must be the result of hemizygosity for other genes in the deleted region.

References

Joseph MC, Parrott D: Severe infantile hypercalcemia with special reference to the facies. Arch Dis Child 33:385, 1958.

Williams JCP, Barratt-Boyes BG, Lowe JB: Supravalvular aortic stenosis. Circulation 24:1311, 1961.

Jones KL, Smith DW: The Williams elfin facies syndrome: A new perspective. J Pediatr 86:718, 1975.

Jensen OA, Marborg M, Dupont A: Ocular pathology in the elfin face syndrome. Opthalmologica 172:434, 1976.

Bennett FC, LaVeck B, Sells CJ: The Williams elfin facies syndrome: The psychological profile as an aid in syndrome identification. Pediatrics 61:303, 1978.

Morris CA et al: The natural history of the Williams syndrome: Physical characteristics. J Pediatr 113:318, 1988.

Ewart AK et al: Hemizygosity at the elastin locus in a developmental disorder, Williams syndrome. Nat Genet 5:11, 1993.

Pober BR et al: Renal findings in 40 individuals with Williams syndrome. Am J Med Genet 46:271, 1993.

Bird LM et al: Sudden death in patients with supravalvular aortic stenosis and Williams syndrome. J Pediatr 129:926, 1996.

Frangiskakis JM et al: LIM-kinase 1 hemizygosity implicated in impaired visuospatial constructive cognition. Cell 86:59, 1996.

Donnai D, Karmiloff-Smith A: Williams syndrome: From genotype through to the cognitive phenotype. Am J Med Genet (Semin Med Genet) 97:164, 2000.

Committee on Genetics—American Academy of Pediatrics: Health care supervision for children with Williams syndrome. Pediatrics 107:1192, 2001.

Eronen M et al: Cardiovascular manifestations in 75 patients with Williams syndrome. J Med Genet 39:554, 2002.

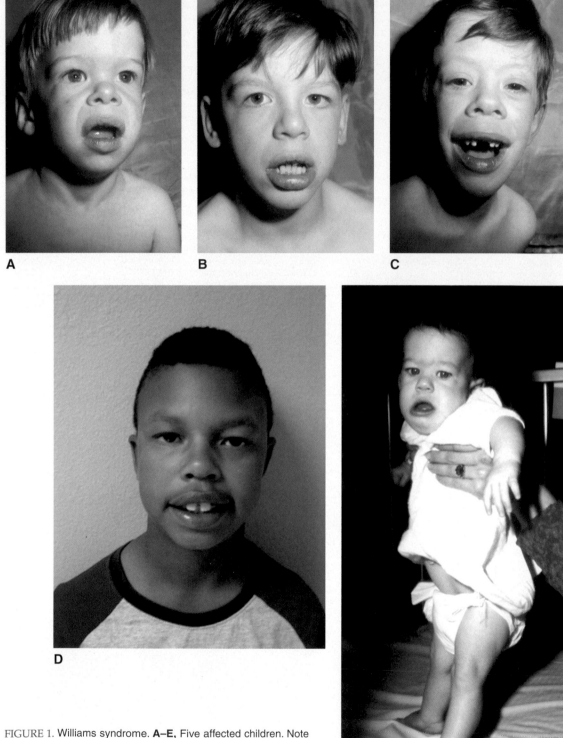

FIGURE 1. Williams syndrome. **A–E,** Five affected children. Note the depressed nasal bridge, epicanthal folds, periorbital fullness, anteverted nares, long philtrum, and prominent lips with large mouth. (**A–C,** From Jones KL, Smith DW: J Pediatr 86:718, 1975, with permission.)

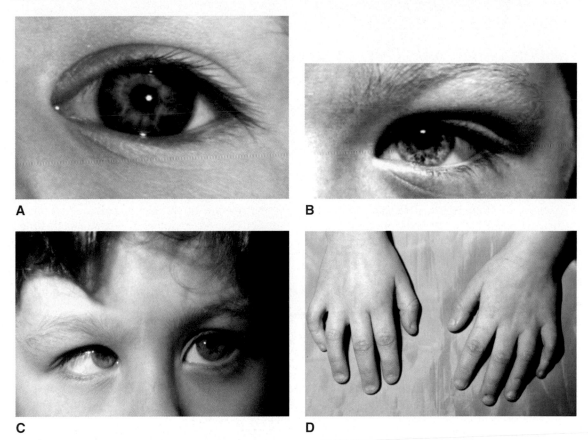

FIGURE 2. **A–D,** Note the typical stellate pattern of the iris in **A** and the less typical but also characteristic pattern in **B**; the medial eyebrow flare, short palpebral fissures, epicanthal folds, and strabismus in **C**; and the hypoplastic nails in **D**. (From Jones KL, Smith DW: J Pediatr 86:718, 1975, with permission.)

NOONAN SYNDROME

Webbing of the Neck, Pectus Excavatum, Cryptorchidism, Pulmonic Stenosis

Kobilinsky reported in 1883 a 20-year-old man with webbing of the neck, incomplete folding of the ears, and low posterior hairline, but no mention was made of other physical findings. The first complete description appears to be that of Weissenberg in 1928. In 1963, Noonan and Ehmke further delineated the clinical phenotype and documented its association with valvular pulmonic stenosis.

ABNORMALITIES

Growth. Short stature of postnatal onset in 50%.
Performance. Mean full-scale IQ ranges from 48 to 130 with a mean of 86, verbal IQ exceeding performance.
Facies. Epicanthal folds; ptosis of eyelids; hypertelorism; low nasal bridge; downslanting palpebral fissures; myopia; keratoconus; strabismus; nystagmus; low-set or abnormal auricles; anterior dental malocclusion; increased width of mouth; prominent, protruding upper lip; moderate retrognathia.
Neck. Low posterior hairline, short or webbed neck.
Thorax. Shield chest and pectus excavatum or pectus carinatum or both.
Other Skeletal. Cubitus valgus, scoliosis with thoracic lordosis, abnormalities of vertebral column.*
Heart. Pulmonary valve stenosis due to a dysplastic or thickened valve, hypertrophic cardiomyopathy, atrial septal defect, tetralogy of Fallot, aortic coarctation, mitral valve anomalies, atrioventricular canal.
Genitalia. Small penis, cryptorchidism.
Bleeding Diathesis. A variety of defects in the coagulation and platelet systems including abnormalities in the intrinsic pathway (partial factor XI:C, XII:C, and VIII:C deficiencies), von Willebrand disease, and thrombocytopenia in approximately one third of cases.

---

*Abnormal curvature of abnormal vertebrae (e.g., spina bifida occulta, hemivertebrae).

OCCASIONAL ABNORMALITIES. High-arched palate, large or asymmetric head, cerebral arteriovenous malformation, iridoretinal colobomas, nerve deafness, hypoplastic nipples, kyphosis, winging of scapula, cervical ribs, edema of the dorsum of the hands and feet, lymphatic vessel dysplasia, chylothorax, nonimmune hydrops, hepatosplenomegaly, simian creases, unusual wool-like consistency of the hair (curly), skin nevi, keloids, hyperelastic skin, hypogonadism, malignant hyperthermia, juvenile myelomonocytic leukemia.

NATURAL HISTORY. Poor feeding and symptoms of gastrointestinal dysfunction (vomiting, constipation, abdominal pain, and distention) often lead to failure to thrive and require nasogastric tube feeding. The degree of mental retardation is seldom severe. It has been suggested that those with more severe feeding problems in infancy, as well as those with a more severe phenotype, have more cognitive issues in childhood. Two thirds of those with pulmonic stenosis do not require surgery. Twenty percent with cardiomyopathy die in the first 2 years of life. Onset of the myelomonocytic leukemia has been in the first 2 months of life. Although impairment in fertility is present in some males, the major contributing factor is bilateral cryptorchidism. Fertility is normal in males with normally descended testes and in females.

Allanson and colleagues documented changes in the clinical phenotype from birth through adulthood. In teenagers and in young adults, the face becomes more triangular and facial features are sharper. There is a tendency toward normalization.

ETIOLOGY. This disorder usually occurs sporadically within families. Autosomal dominant inheritance has been documented. Mutations in PTPN11, a gene encoding the nonreceptor protein tyrosine phosphatase SHP-2, which maps to chromosome 12q24.1, is responsible for some cases of this disorder. However, nonlinkage has been documented, indicating genetic heterogeneity. Because of the variability in expression, careful evaluation of both parents must be undertaken before recurrence risk counseling.

COMMENT. The differential diagnosis for patients with the Noonan syndrome is extensive. In particular, Costello syndrome and cardio-facio-cutaneous syndrome, neither of which is associated with mutations of PTPN11, have similar phenotypes.

References

Kobilinsky O: Ueber eine flughautahnliche Ausbreitung am Halse. Arch Anthropol 14:343, 1883.

Weissenberg S: Eine eigentumliche Hautflatengildung am Halse. Anthropol Anz 5:141, 1928.

Noonan JA, Ehmke DA: Associated noncardiac malformations in children with congenital heart disease. J Pediatr 63:469, 1963.

Allanson JE et al: Noonan syndrome: The changing phenotype. Am J Med Genet 21:507, 1985.

Mendez HMM, Opitz JM: Noonan syndrome: A review. Am J Med Genet 21:493, 1985.

Witt DR et al: Bleeding diathesis in Noonan syndrome. A common association. Am J Med Genet 31:305, 1988.

Sharland M et al: Coagulation-factor deficiencies and abnormal bleeding in Noonan's syndrome. Lancet 339:19, 1992.

Lee C-K et al: Spinal deformities in Noonan syndrome. J Bone Joint Surg 83 A:1495, 2001.

Marino B et al: Congenital heart diseases in children with Noonan syndrome: An expanded cardiac spectrum with high prevalence of atrioventricular canal. J Pediatr 135:703, 1999.

Noonan JA: Noonan syndrome revisited. J Pediatr 135:667, 1999.

van der Burgt I et al: Patterns of cognitive functioning in school-aged children with Noonan syndrome associated with variability in phenotypic expression. J Pediatr 135:707, 1999.

Tartaglia M et al: PTPN11 mutations in Noonan syndrome: Molecular spectrum, genotype-phenotype correlation, and phenotypic heterogeneity. Am J Hum Genet 70:1555, 2002.

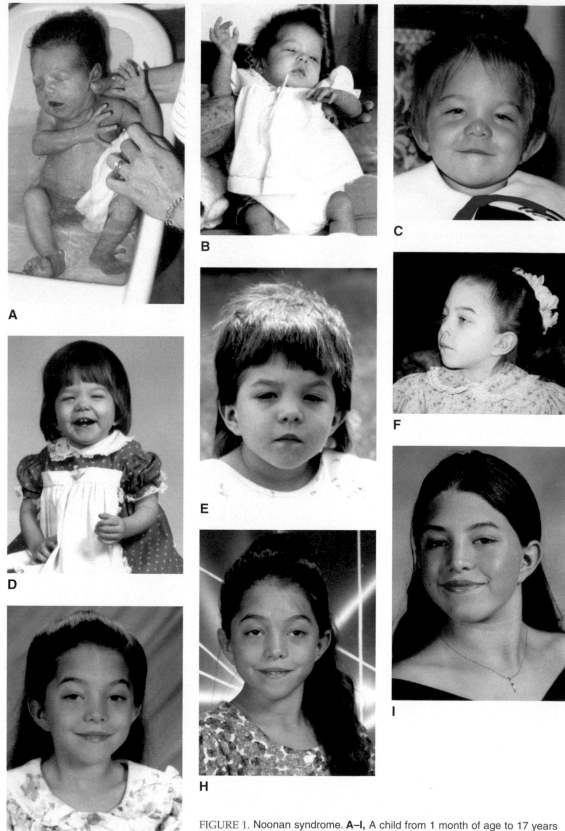

FIGURE 1. Noonan syndrome. **A–I,** A child from 1 month of age to 17 years of age shows the changing phenotype. (Courtesy of Dr. Jacqueline Noonan, University of Kentucky, Lexington.)

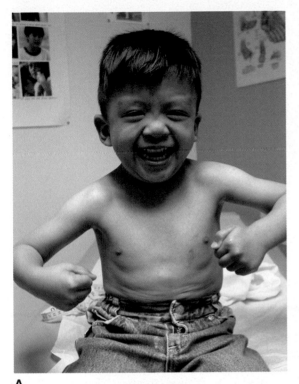

A

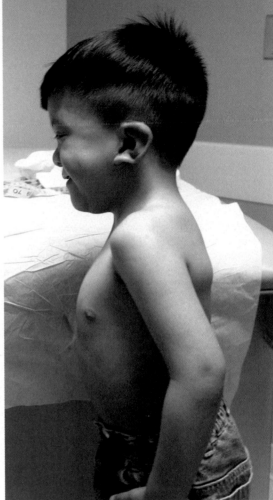

B

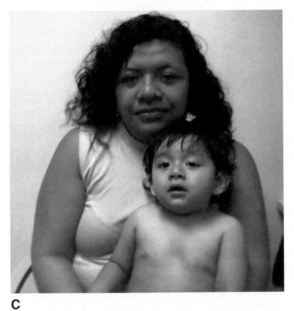

C

FIGURE 2. **A** and **B,** Affected male. Note the downslanting palpebral fissures, low-set ears, low posterior hairline, elevated left shoulder secondary to scoliosis, and wide-spaced nipples. **C,** Affected mother and daughter.

COSTELLO SYNDROME

This disorder initially was described by Costello in 1977. Subsequently, more than 100 cases have been reported.

ABNORMALITIES

Growth. Postnatal onset of growth deficiency, delayed bone age.

Performance. Mental deficiency with IQ ranging from 47 to 68; poor suck; hypotonia; seizures; sociable, warm personality.

Craniofacial. Macrocephaly; coarse face; low-set ears with thick lobes; epicanthal folds; downslanting palpebral fissures; strabismus; large mouth; thick lips; macroglossia; gingival hyperplasia; depressed nasal bridge; short bulbous nose; full cheeks.

Skin/Hair/Nails/Teeth. Thin, deep-set nails; cutis laxa (particularly hands and feet); dark skin pigmentation; thick eyebrows; curly, sparse hair; teeth abnormalities; deep plantar, palmar, creases; hyperkeratotic palms and soles.

Musculoskeletal. Short neck; tight Achilles tendon; hyperextensible fingers; foot positional defects; increased anteroposterior diameter of chest; defective range of elbow motion; broad distal phalanges.

Cardiac. Defects in 52% especially pulmonary valve stenosis, ventricular septal defect, atrial septal defect; thickening of the intraventricular septum and hypertrophic cardiomyopathy and dysrhythmia.

Other. Papillomas in the perioral, nasal, and anal regions, with variable age of onset ranging from 2 to 15 years; hoarse voice; hypertrophic cardiomyopathy; inguinal hernia; cerebral atrophy.

OCCASIONAL ABNORMALITIES.

Hypertrichosis, acanthosis nigricans, palmar nevi, hyperhidrosis, multiple hemangioma, hyperplastic nipples, supernumerary nipples, mammary fibroadenosis, epithelioma, ganglioneuroblastoma, bladder carcinoma, acoustic neuroma, neuroblastoma, embryonal rhabdomyosarcoma (abdomen, pelvis, or urogenital area occurring between 6 months and 6 years of age), cranial dermoid cyst.

NATURAL HISTORY. Polyhydramnios occurs and swallowing difficulties leading to failure to thrive frequently necessitate gavage feedings in the neonatal period. A disproportionate weight gain relative to linear growth has its onset in midchildhood when the facial changes become coarser. The cardiomyopathy can be associated with dysrhythmias and sudden death. The papillomas may undergo malignant change.

ETIOLOGY. This disorder has an autosomal dominant inheritance pattern. The fact that the majority of cases have occurred sporadically and that older mean paternal age has been documented suggests that a fresh gene mutation is the most likely cause of this disorder. The occurrence of the disorder in siblings in two families is most likely related to gonadal mosaicism.

References

Costello JM: A new syndrome: Mental subnormality and nasal papillomata. Aust Pediatr J 13:114, 1977.

Martin RA, Jones KL: Delineation of the Costello syndrome. Am J Med Genet 41:345, 1991.

Johnson JP et al: Costello syndrome: Phenotype, natural history, differential diagnosis, and possible cause. J Pediatr 133:441, 1998.

Lin AE et al: Further delineation of cardiac anomalies in Costello syndrome. Am J Med Genet 111:115, 2002.

Hennekam RCM et al: Costello syndrome: An overview. Am J Med Genet 117C:42, 2003.

Kawame H et al: Further delineation of the behavioral and neurological features in Costello syndrome. Am J Med Genet 118:8, 2003.

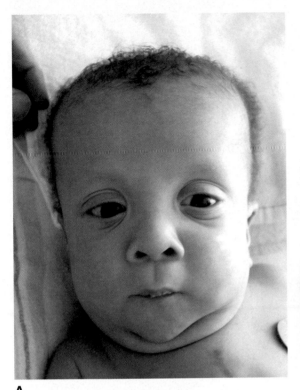

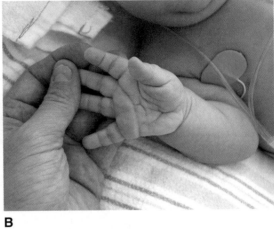

A

B

FIGURE 1. Costello syndrome. **A** and **B,** Newborn infant. Note the coarse face, epicanthal folds, depressed nasal bridge, and deep creases on the palm.

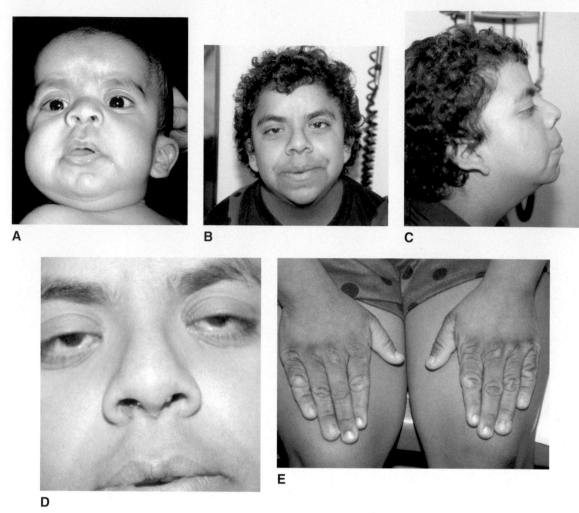

FIGURE 2. **A–E,** Note the coarse face; low-set ears with thick lobes; thick lips; nasal papillomas; and thin, deep-set nails with loose skin on the hands. (From Martin RA, Jones KL: Am J Med Genet 41:346, 1991, with permission. Reprinted with permission of Wiley-Liss, Inc., a subsidiary of John Wiley & Sons, Inc.)

CARDIO-FACIO-CUTANEOUS SYNDROME

Congenital Heart Defects, Ectodermal Anomalies, Frontal Bossing

Reynolds and colleagues reported eight patients with this disorder in 1986. More than 50 affected individuals have been reported.

ABNORMALITIES

Neurologic. Mild to severe mental retardation (80%); hypotonia; nystagmus; strabismus; brain anomalies on computed tomography, including mild hydrocephalus, cortical atrophy, hypoplasia of frontal lobes, and/or brainstem atrophy; abnormal electroencephalogram.

Growth. Postnatal growth deficiency (68%), delayed bone age.

Craniofacial. Relative macrocephaly (88%) with large prominent forehead (100%), bitemporal narrowing (100%), and shallow orbital ridges (100%); downslanting palpebral fissures (71%); epicanthal folds; hypertelorism (84%); ptosis (53%); exophthalmos (55%); short upturned nose (92%); prominent philtrum (82%); posteriorly rotated, low-set ears (95%); webbed neck.

Cardiac. Abnormalities in 77% of cases, atrial septal defects and pulmonic stenosis being most common.

Skin and Hair. Sparse, curly, or slow-growing hair (100%); lack of eyebrows and eyelashes; abnormalities of skin in 95% varying from severe atopic dermatitis to hyperkeratosis/ichthyosis-like lesions.

OCCASIONAL ABNORMALITIES.

Microcephaly, hydrocephalus, large ears, dental anomalies, seizures, hypertonia, hearing loss, optic nerve pallor, refractive errors, eyelid fluttering, cleft palate, photophobia, clinodactyly, joint hyperextensibility, pectus excavatum, hypertonia, hernia, cryptorchidism, splenomegaly, hepatomegaly, intestinal malrotation, cavernous hemangiomas, nail dysplasia, hyperelastic skin, eczema, seborrheic dermatitis, café au lait patches, cutis marmorata, polyhydramnios, chylothorax.

NATURAL HISTORY. Feeding difficulties with gastroesophageal reflux, vomiting, and oral aversion beginning in infancy are common, often requiring gastrostomy tube placement. Extensive neurologic problems often associated with defects of the cortex, brainstem, or ventricular system represent a major problem. Language dysfunction is common and has not been well characterized. Little information is available regarding long-term follow-up.

ETIOLOGY. The etiology of this disorder is unknown. All cases have been sporadic. An observed increase in paternal age has been noted, suggesting that all cases of this disorder have been due to an autosomal dominant mutation. However, no affected offspring of an affected parent has been documented.

References

Reynolds JF et al: New multiple congenital anomalies/mental retardation syndrome with cardio-facio-cutaneous involvement. The CFC syndrome. Am J Med Genet 25:413, 1986.

Bottani A et al: The cardio-facio-cutaneous syndrome: Report of a patient and review of the literature. Eur J Pediatr 150:486, 1991.

Borradori L et al: Skin manifestations of cardio-facio-cutaneous syndrome. J Am Acad Dermatol 28:815, 1993.

Sabatino G et al: The cardio-facio-cutaneous syndrome: A long term follow-up of two patients with special reference to the neurological features. Child Nerv Syst 13:238, 1997.

Grebe TA, Clericuzio C: Neurologic and gastrointestinal dysfunction in cardio-facio-cutaneous syndrome: Identification of a severe phenotype. Am J Med Genet 95:135, 2000.

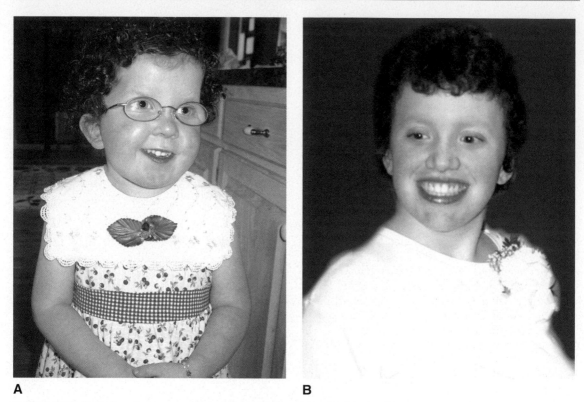

A   **B**

FIGURE 1. Cardio-facio-cutaneous syndrome. **A** and **B,** Prominent forehead, mild ocular hypertelorism, and curly hair in two affected individuals. (Courtesy of Dr. John M. Opitz, University of Utah, Salt Lake City.)

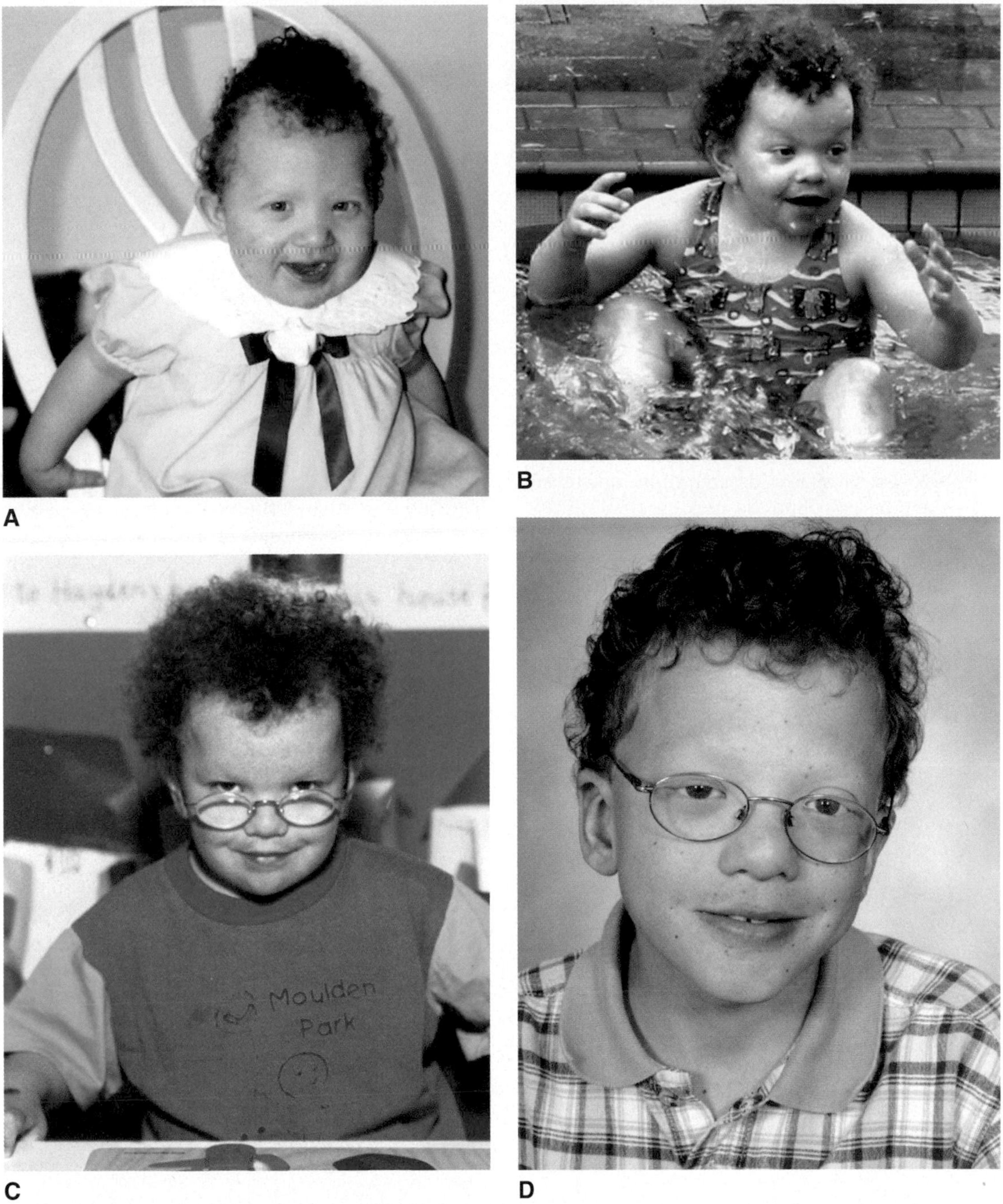

FIGURE 2. **A–D,** Note the somewhat sparse curly hair, relative macrocephaly with large prominent forehead, bitemporal narrowing, shallow orbits, and lack of eyebrows and eyelashes. The same girl is depicted in **B** and **C**. The boy in **D** is 11 years old. (Courtesy of Dr. John M. Opitz, University of Utah, Salt Lake City.)

AARSKOG SYNDROME

Hypertelorism, Brachydactyly, Shawl Scrotum

Set forth by Aarskog in 1970, there has been increasing recognition of this disorder. It can easily be misdiagnosed as the Noonan syndrome.

ABNORMALITIES

Growth. Slight to moderate short stature, final adult height between 160 and 170 cm, delayed bone age.

Facies. Rounded. Facial edema in children less than 4 years of age. Hypertelorism with variable ptosis of eyelids and slight downward slant to palpebral fissures; widow's peak; small nose with anteverted nares, broad philtrum, maxillary hypoplasia, slight crease below the lower lip; upper helices of ears incompletely outfolded; hypodontia, retarded dental eruption, broad central upper incisors (permanent dentition), orthodontic problems.

Limbs. Brachydactyly with clinodactyly of fifth fingers, unusual position of extended fingers, simian crease, mild interdigital webbing; broad thumbs and great toes.

Radiologic. Short long tubular bones with wide metaphysis; brachyphalangia; hypoplastic middle phalanges of fifth fingers; short, broad first metacarpals and metatarsals; pelvic hypoplasia.

Abdomen. Prominent umbilicus, inguinal hernias.

Genitalia. "Shawl" scrotum in 90%; cryptorchidism.

Other. Short neck with or without webbing; cervical vertebral anomalies, including hypoplasia and synostosis of one or more cervical vertebrae and spina bifida occulta; mild pectus excavatum; protruding umbilicus.

OCCASIONAL ABNORMALITIES

Ocular. Strabismus, amblyopia, hyperopia, astigmatism, latent nystagmus, inferior oblique overaction, blue sclerae, anisometropia, posterior embryotoxon, corneal enlargement.

Skeletal. Scoliosis, cubitus valgus, splayed toes with bulbous tips, metatarsus adductus.

Genitalia. Cleft scrotum, phimosis.

Other. Mild to moderate mental retardation, scalp defects, anomalous cerebral venous drainage, Hirschsprung disease, midgut malrotation, hypoplastic kidney, dental enamel hypoplasia, delayed eruption of teeth, cleft lip and/or cleft palate, cardiac defects.

NATURAL HISTORY. Growth deficiency may be of prenatal onset. Marked failure to thrive in the first year with feeding difficulties and recurrent respiratory infections in 35%. More commonly, mild growth deficiency is first evident at 1 to 3 years of age and may be associated with slow maturation and a late advent of adolescence. A positive effect of growth hormone treatment on growth and adult height has been suggested. Fertility is normal. Orthodontic correction is often necessary. IQ is normal in the majority of cases. However, hyperactivity and attention deficit disorders are common, particularly in those with mental retardation.

ETIOLOGY. The disorder has an X-linked recessive inheritance pattern, with carrier females often showing some minor manifestations of the disorder, especially in the facies and hands. The gene for this disorder, designated FGD1, has been mapped to Xp11.21.

References

Aarskog D: A familial syndrome of short stature associated with facial dysplasia and genital anomalies. J Pediatr 77:856, 1970.

Furukawa CT, Hall BD, Smith DW: The Aarskog syndrome. J Pediatr 81:1117, 1972.

Halse A, Bjorvatn K, Aarskog D: Dental findings in patients with the Aarskog syndrome. Scand J Dent Res 87:253, 1979.

Brodsky MC et al: Ocular and systemic findings in the Aarskog (facial-digital-genital) syndrome. Am J Ophthalmol 109:450, 1990.

Fryns JP: Aarskog syndrome: The changing phenotype with age. Am J Med Genet 43:420, 1992.

Teebi AS et al: Aarskog syndrome: Report of a family with review and discussion of nosology. Am J Med Genet 46:501, 1993.

Lizcano-Gil LA et al: The facio-digito-dental syndrome (Aarskog syndrome): A further delineation of the distinct radiological findings. Genet Counsel 5:387, 1994.

Pasteris NG et al: Isolation and characterization of the faciogenital dysplasia (Aarskog-Scott syndrome) gene: A putative Rho/Rac guanine nucleotide exchange factor. Cell 79:669, 1994.

Logie LG, Porteous MEM: Intelligence and development in Aarskog syndrome. Arch Dis Child 79:359, 1998.

Schwartz CE et al: Two novel mutations confirm FGD1 is responsible for the Aarskog syndrome. Eur J Hum Genet 8:869, 2000.

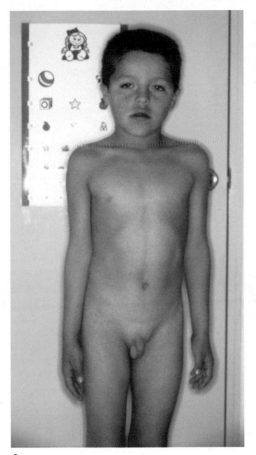

A

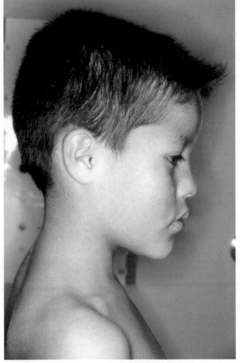

B

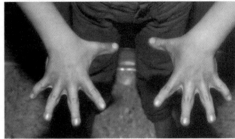

D

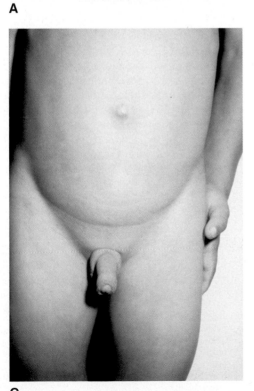

C

FIGURE 1. Aarskog syndrome. **A** and **B,** Photograph of a 7-year-old boy. Note the round face, hypertelorism, and downslanting palpebral fissures. **C,** "Pouting" umbilicus and "shawl" scrotum in an 8-year-old boy. **D,** Mild brachyclinodactyly with mild syndactyly.

ROBINOW SYNDROME
(FETAL FACE SYNDROME)

Flat Facial Profile, Short Forearms, Hypoplastic Genitalia

Initially reported by Robinow and colleagues in 1969, many additional cases of this disorder have been recognized.

ABNORMALITIES

Growth. Slight to moderate shortness of stature of postnatal onset (93%).

Craniofacial. Macrocephaly (44%); large anterior fontanel, frontal bossing (94%), hypertelorism (100%), prominent eyes (86%), downslanting palpebral fissures (80%), small upturned nose (100%), long philtrum (88%), triangular mouth with downturned angles (94%) and micrognathia (87%), hyperplastic alveolar ridges (66%), crowded teeth (96%), and posteriorly rotated ears (53%).

Limbs. Short forearms (100%), small hands with clinodactyly (88%), nail dysplasia (48%).

Other Skeletal. Hemivertebrae of thoracic vertebrae (70%); rib anomalies, primarily fusion of or absent ribs (40%); scoliosis (50%).

Genitalia. Small penis, clitoris, labia majora (94%); cryptorchidism (65%).

OCCASIONAL ABNORMALITIES

Oral-Facial. Nevus flammeus (23%), epicanthal folds, macroglossia, high-arched palate, absent or bifid uvula (18%), cleft lip and/or cleft palate (9%), short frenulum of tongue with cleft tongue tip, midline clefting of lower lip.

Limbs. Broad thumbs and toes, bifid terminal phalanges, clinodactyly of fifth finger, hyperextensible fingers, short metacarpals. Madelung-like anomaly of forearm, dislocation of hip, hypoplastic interphalangeal creases, single flexion creases on third and fourth fingers, hypoplastic middle and terminal phalanges of fingers and toes, transverse palmar crease, ectrodactyly.

Other. Seizures; developmental delay and mental retardation (18%); language deficiency; pectus excavatum (19%); superiorly positioned, broad, and poorly epithelialized umbilicus and inguinal hernia (20%); pilonidal dimple; renal anomalies (29%); vaginal atresia with hematocolpos; cardiac defects especially right ventricular outlet obstruction (13%).

NATURAL HISTORY. Early death secondary to pulmonary or cardiac complications occurs in 10% of patients. The penile hypoplasia may be sufficient to initially raise the question of sex of rearing. Although partial primary hypogonadism evidenced by elevated serum follicle-stimulating hormone levels was documented in four affected males, normal pubertal virilization occurred in all three patients older than 16 years. Two adult women are 4 feet 10 inches and 5 feet, respectively, and three adult men are 5 feet 3 inches, 5 feet 7 inches, and 5 feet 10 inches in height. The facial features become less pronounced with age owing to accelerated growth of the nose at adolescence. Performance has been normal in most individuals.

ETIOLOGY. Both an autosomal dominant and a more severe autosomal recessive type of this disorder have been described. The recessive type is distinguished by more severe mesomelic and acromelic dwarfism, multiple rib and vertebral anomalies, radioulnar dislocation, severe hypoplasia of the proximal radius and distal ulna, and a more triangular-shaped mouth. Mutations of ROR2, a gene located on chromosome 9q22, which encodes a receptor tyrosine kinase-like orphan receptor 2, are responsible for the recessive type.

References

Robinow M, Silverman FN, Smith HD: A newly recognized dwarfing syndrome. Am J Dis Child 117:645, 1969.

Wadlington WB, Tucker VL, Schimke RN: Mesomelic dwarfism with hemivertebrae and small genitalia (the Robinow syndrome). Am J Dis Child 126:202, 1973.

Bain MD, Winter RM, Burn J: Robinow syndrome without mesomelic brachymelia: A report of five cases. J Med Genet 23:350, 1986.

Butler MG, Wadlington WB: Robinow syndrome: Report of two patients and review of the literature. Clin Genet 31:77, 1987.

Afzal AR et al: Recessive Robinow syndrome, allelic to brachydactyly type B, is caused by mutations of ROR2. Nat Genet 25:419, 2000.

Patton MA, Afzal AR: Robinow syndrome. J Med Genet 39:305, 2002.

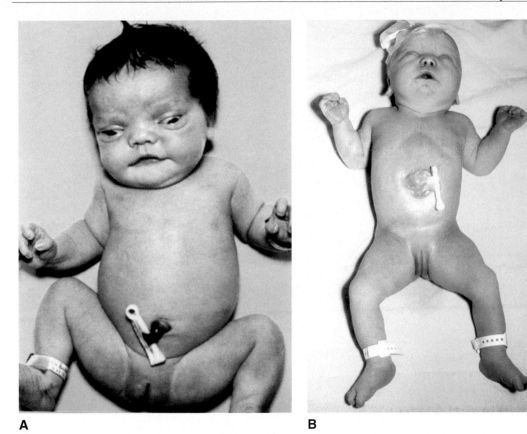

A   **B**

FIGURE 1. Robinow syndrome. **A,** A 2-day-old female with flat facies, hypertelorism, and minute clitoris. (From Robinow M et al: Am J Dis Child 117:645, 1969. Copyright 1969, American Medical Association.) **B,** Newborn female with small nose, hypertelorism, and omphalocele.

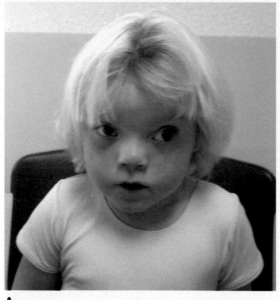

A

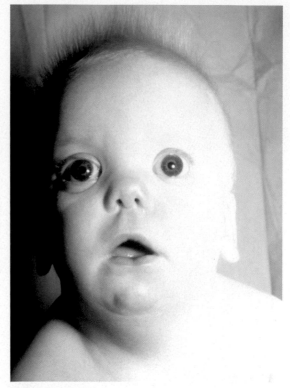

B

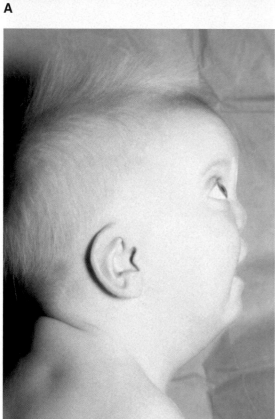

C

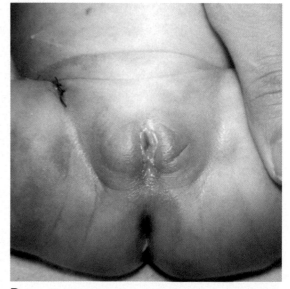

D

FIGURE 2. **A–D,** Note the relative macrocephaly; frontal bossing; hypertelorism; prominent eyes; small, upturned nose; long philtrum; triangular mouth with downturned angles; micrognathia; posteriorly rotated ears; and minute clitoris.

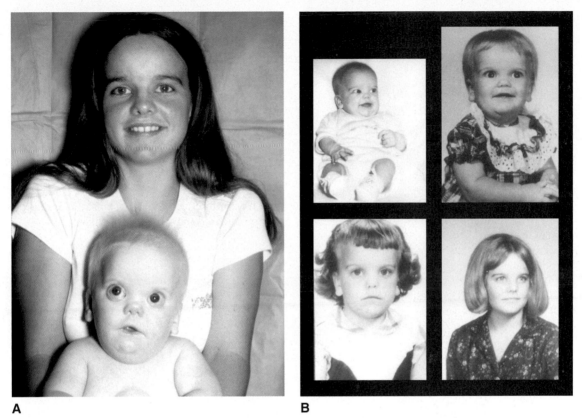

FIGURE 3. **A,** Affected mother and her daughter. **B,** Mother depicted in **A** from birth through 17 years of age shows progression of the phenotype in the autosomal dominant type.

OPITZ G/BBB SYNDROME
(Hypertelorism-Hypospadias Syndrome, Opitz-Frias Syndrome, Opitz Oculo-Genito-Laryngeal Syndrome)

Hypertelorism, Hypospadias, Swallowing Difficulties

In 1965 and again in 1969, Opitz, Smith, and Summitt reported this condition, previously referred to as the BBB syndrome, in three families in which affected males usually have apparent ocular hypertelorism and hypospadias and affected females have only hypertelorism. As the spectrum of defects in this disorder has evolved, it has become clear that the disorder described by Opitz and colleagues in 1969, previously referred to as the G syndrome or Opitz-Frias syndrome, is the same condition.

ABNORMALITIES

Performance. Mild to moderate mental deficiency in about two thirds of patients, hypotonia.

Facial. Prominent forehead, ocular hypertelorism, upward or downward slanting of palpebral fissures and epicanthal folds, broad flat nasal bridge with anteverted nostrils, cleft lip with or without cleft palate, short frenulum of tongue, posterior rotation of auricles, micrognathia.

Genital. In males, hypospadias, cryptorchidism, bifid scrotum; in females, splayed labia majora.

Laryngo-Tracheo-Esophageal. Laryngotracheal cleft, malformation of larynx, tracheoesophageal fistula, hypoplastic epiglottis, and high carina.

Other. Hernias.

OCCASIONAL ABNORMALITIES.
Cranial asymmetry, widow's peak, strabismus, grooving of nasal tip, flattened elongated philtrum, thin upper lip, bifid uvula, cleft tongue, dental anomalies; brain magnetic resonance imaging findings including agenesis or hypoplasia of corpus callosum, cerebellar vermal hypoplasia, cortical atrophy and ventriculomegaly, macro cisterna magna, pituitary macroadenoma, cranial osteoma, and wide cavum septum pellucidum; malformation of larynx, tracheoesophageal fistula, hypoplastic epiglottis, high carina, pulmonary hypoplasia; renal defect; cardiac defects, most commonly conotruncal lesions; agenesis of gallbladder; duodenal stricture; imperforate anus; hiatal hernia; diastasis recti; increased monozygotic twinning.

NATURAL HISTORY. Swallowing problems with recurrent aspiration, stridulous respirations, intermittent pulmonary difficulty, wheezing, and a weak, hoarse cry should raise concern about a potentially lethal laryngoesophageal defect. In those individuals, mortality is high unless vigorous efforts are made to repair the defect and protect the lungs with gastrostomy or jejunostomy. Although males tend to have more severe and more frequent laryngoesophageal defects, it is important to recognize that this disorder can express itself in both males and females with equal severity. Initial failure to thrive is followed by normal growth in survivors.

ETIOLOGY. Heterogeneity has been demonstrated with an autosomal dominant locus linked to 22q11.2 and an X-linked locus. The gene responsible for the X-linked form, MID1 maps to Xp22.3. MID1 encodes a protein which is highly expressed in tissues that are aberrant in this disorder. Although anteverted nares and posterior pharyngeal clefts have been seen only in the X-linked form, all other manifestations have been seen in both, making it difficult to distinguish between the two forms in an affected male who lacks a positive family history.

References
Opitz JM, Smith DW, Summitt RL: Hypertelorism and hypospadias (abst.) J Pediatr 67:968, 1965.

Opitz JM et al: The G syndrome of multiple congenital anomalies. Birth Defects 5:95, 1969.

Opitz JM, Summitt RL, Smith DW: The BBB syndrome: Familial telecanthus with associated anomalies. In Bergsma D (ed): First Conference on Clinical Delineation of Birth Defects, vol. 5. White Plains, NY: National Foundation, 1969, pp 86–94.

Gonzales CH, Hermann J, Opitz JM: The hypertelorism-hypospadias (BBB) syndrome. Eur J Pediatr 12:51, 1977.

Cordero JF, Holmes LB: Phenotypic overlap of the BBB and G syndromes. Am J Med Genet 2:145, 1978.

Brooks JK et al: Opitz (BBB/G) syndrome: Oral manifestations. Am J Med Genet 43:595, 1992.

MacDonald MR et al: Brain magnetic resonance imaging findings in the Opitz/G/BBB syndrome: Extension of the spectrum of midline brain anomalies. Am J Med Genet 46:706, 1993.

McDonald-McGinn DM: Autosomal dominant "Opitz" GBBB syndrome due to a 22q11.2 deletion. Am J Med Genet 59:103, 1995.

Robin NH et al: Opitz G/BBB syndrome: Clinical comparisons of families linked to Xp22 and 22q and a review of the literature. Am J Med Genet 62:305, 1996.

Quaderi NA et al: Opitz G/BBB syndrome, a defect of midline development, is due to mutations in a new RING finger gene mapped on Xp22. Nat Genet 17:285, 1997.

DeFalco F et al: X-linked Opitz syndrome: Novel mutations in the MID1 gene and redefinition of the clinical spectrum. Am J Med Genet 120:222, 2003.

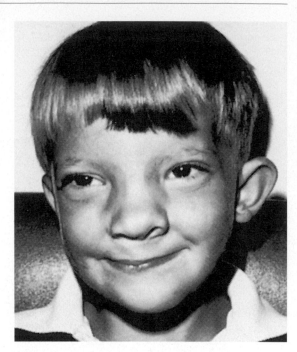

FIGURE 1. A 7-year-old boy with Opitz syndrome. Note hypertelorism, repaired cleft lips, and protruding auricle. Hypospadias was also present. (Courtesy of Dr. Robert Fineman.)

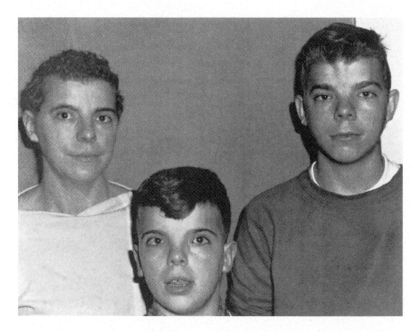

FIGURE 2. An affected mother (mild hypertelorism) and two of her affected boys who show hypertelorism and also have hypospadias. (From the B. O. family pedigree of Opitz JM et al: Birth Defects 5:86, 1969, with permission.)

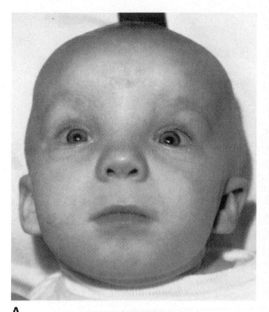

A

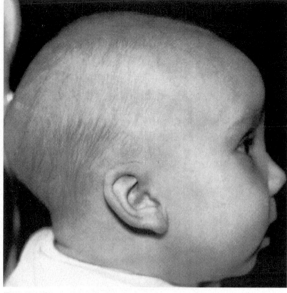

B

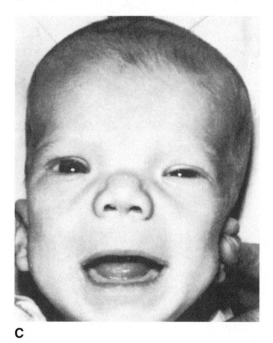

C

FIGURE 3. **A** and **B,** Photographs of a 1-month-old affected child. **C,** Photographs of a 7½-month-old affected child. (**A–C,** From Opitz JM et al: Birth Defects 5(2):95, 1969, with permission.)

FLOATING-HARBOR SYNDROME

*Postnatal Growth Deficiency, Bulbous Nose,
Speech Delay*

Pelletier and Feingold described the initial patient with this disorder in 1973. One year later, Leisti and colleagues reported a child with almost identical features and suggested the term "Floating-Harbor syndrome," an amalgam of the names of the hospitals where the initial two patients were evaluated (Boston Floating and Harbor General, Torrance, Calif.). Approximately 30 patients have been reported with this condition.

ABNORMALITIES

Growth. Birth weight and length at third percentile, striking postnatal growth deficiency, delayed bone age.

Performance. Significant speech delay, normal motor development, mild mental retardation (50%).

Craniofacial. Broad, bulbous nose with prominent nasal bridge and wide columella; short, smooth philtrum; wide mouth with thin lips; prominent eyes in infancy, which in older children give the appearance of being deep-set; posteriorly rotated ears.

Other. Low posterior hairline, short neck, fifth finger clinodactyly, brachydactyly, broad thumbs, joint laxity.

OCCASIONAL ABNORMALITIES.

Microcephaly, trigonocephaly due to metopic suture synostosis, abnormal electroencephalograph, pulmonary stenosis, tetralogy of Fallot with atrial septal defect, triangular face, rib anomalies, high-pitched voice, preauricular pit, delayed motor skills, accessory or hypoplastic thumb, subluxated hypoplastic radial head, cone-shaped epiphyses, Perthes disease, clavicular pseudoarthrosis, finger clubbing, celiac disease, abdominal distention, constipation, hirsutism, long eyelashes, growth hormone deficiency.

NATURAL HISTORY. The facial features are most recognizable in midchildhood. During childhood, height and weight tend to parallel the third percentile, but 4 to 6 SD below the mean. The speech problem is related to deficient expressive language skills.

ETIOLOGY. This disorder has a probable autosomal dominant inheritance pattern. The majority of cases occur sporadically and older mean paternal age has been reported. At least two cases of mother-to-daughter transmission have been reported.

References

Leisti J et al: Case report 12. Syndrome Identification 2:3, 1973.

Pelletier G, Feingold M: Case report 1. Syndrome Identification 1:8, 1973.

Robinson PL et al: A unique association of short stature, dysmorphic features and speech impairment (Floating-Harbor syndrome). J Pediatr 113:703, 1988.

Patton MR et al: Floating-Harbor syndrome. J Med Genet 28:201, 1991.

Houlston RS et al: Further observations on the Floating-Harbor syndrome. Clin Dysmorph 3:143, 1994.

Lacombe D et al: Floating-Harbor syndrome: Description of a further patient, review of the literature, and suggestion of autosomal dominant inheritance. Eur J Pediatr 154:658, 1995.

Hersh JH et al: Changing phenotype in Floating-Harbor syndrome. Am J Med Genet 76:58, 1998.

Rosen AC et al: A further report of Floating-Harbor syndrome in a mother and daughter. J Clin Exp Neuropsychol 20:483, 1998.

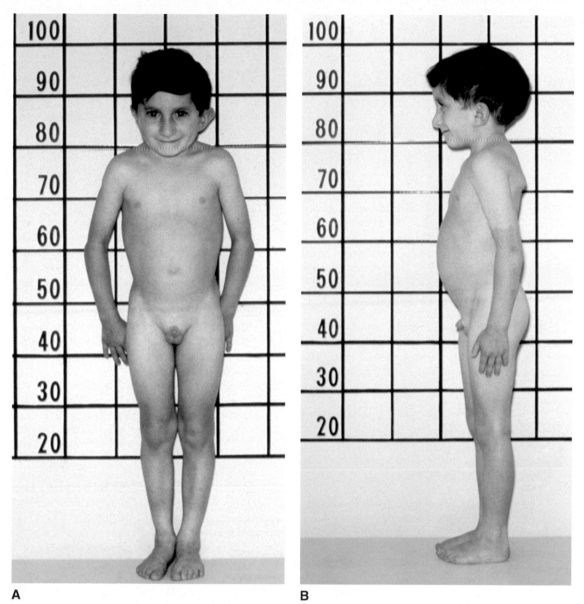

A **B**

FIGURE 1. Floating-Harbor syndrome. **A** and **B,** Affected male at 6½ years. Note the proportionate short stature, broad, bulbous nose, and short philtrum. (Courtesy of David L. Rimoin, Cedars-Sinai Medical Center, Los Angeles.)

D | Senile-Like Appearance

PROGERIA SYNDROME
(Hutchinson-Gilford Syndrome)

*Alopecia, Atrophy of Subcutaneous Fat,
Skeletal Hypoplasia and Dysplasia*

The following entry was recorded in the *St. James Gazette* in 1754: "March 19, 1754 died in Glamorganshire of mere old age and a gradual decay of nature at seventeen years and two months, Hopkins Hopkins, the little Welshman, lately shown in London. He never weighed more than 17 pounds but for three years past no more than twelve."

In 1886, Hutchinson described a similar patient. Later, Gilford studied this boy and another patient and termed the condition progeria, meaning premature aging. DeBusk summarized the findings in 60 cases.

ABNORMALITIES

Alopecia. Onset at birth to 18 months, with degeneration of hair follicles.

Skin. Thin with onset in early to midinfancy; prominent scalp veins; localized scleroderma-like areas over lower abdomen, upper legs, and buttocks appearing at birth or early infancy; irregular pigmentary changes over sun-exposed areas that become more prominent with age.

Nails. Hypoplastic with onset in infancy; nails may be brittle, curved, yellowish.

Subcutaneous Fat. Diminished with onset in infancy, last areas of adipose atrophy are cheeks and pubic areas.

Periarticular Fibrosis. Onset at 1 to 2 years; stiff or partially flexed prominent joints or both; leads to "horse-riding" stance.

Skeletal Hypoplasia, Dysplasia, and Degeneration. Deficient growth, which becomes evident between 6 and 18 months; subsequent growth rate one third to one half normal; facial hypoplasia and micrognathia; slim tubular bones and ribs with small thoracic cage; and thin calvarium with marked delay in ossification of fontanels; generalized osteoporosis; skeletal dysplasia evident in coxa valga; tendency toward ovoid vertebral bodies; in the long bones, sclerotic changes with thinned shafts, reduced corticomedullary ratio, and pathological fractures, particularly of the humerus; skeletal degeneration evident in loss of bone in clavicle and distal phalanges.

Dentition. Delayed eruption of deciduous and permanent dentition; crowding of teeth; anodontia and hypodontia, especially of permanent teeth; discoloration; high incidence of cavities.

Atherosclerosis. As early as 5 years, onset of generalized atherosclerosis, especially evident in coronary arteries, aorta, and mesenteric arteries; at later age, may have cardiac murmur, left ventricular hypertrophy.

OCCASIONAL ABNORMALITIES.
Perceptive hearing deficit, congenital or acquired cataract, microphthalmia, absent breast and nipple, upper radial metaphyseal changes consisting of a waist-like defect in the region of the proximal radial metaphysis, talus deformities of feet, dislocated hips, immunologic abnormalities, relatively large thymus, lymphoid and reticular hyperplasia.

NATURAL HISTORY.
Although the onset of disease manifestations is usually stated as 1 to 2 years, there may be subtle indicators of disease within the first year. The average birth weight for 17 patients was 2.7 kg. One patient whose scalp was shaved at 6 weeks had no regrowth of hair. The deficit of growth becomes severe after 1 year of age and there is absent sexual maturation. The tendency to fatigue easily is a factor that might limit full participation in childhood activities. The life span is shortened by the early advent of relentless arterial atheromatosis, and the usual cause of death is coronary occlusion. One instance of cerebral infarction has been reported. Renal

ischemia resulting in focal subcortical scars, diffuse glomerulosclerosis, tubular atrophy, and chronic interstitial nephritis occur in patients surviving into adolescence. In addition, an abnormal distribution of collagen in the mesangium with overexpression of collagen V and VI has been documented. The life expectancy for 13 patients was 7 to 27 years, with an average of 14.2 years. Because intelligence and brain development do not appear to be impaired, children with progeria should be allowed as normal a social life as possible.

At this time, there is no effective therapy. One affected child who suffered from severe angina pectoris underwent coronary angiography, saphenous and internal mammary artery–to–coronary artery bypass surgery, and percutaneous transluminal angioplasty at 14 years of age. At follow-up, 1 year after surgery, the child was having only infrequent episodes of chest pain. The use of a wig is recommended for cosmetic purposes.

ETIOLOGY. The etiology of this disorder is sporadic. All cases studied to date have been the result of a variety of different mutations in the paternal copy of the LMNA gene located on chromosome 1q. This results in a defective form of a protein called lamin A, which is a constituent of the membrane of the cell nucleus. Instances of affected siblings from normal parents are probably the result of gonadal mosaicism.

References

Hutchinson J: Congenital absence of hair and mammary glands with atrophic condition of the skin and its appendages in a boy whose mother had been almost wholly bald from alopecia areata from the age of six. Trans Med Chir Soc Edinb 69:473, 1886.

Gilford H: Progeria: A form of senilism. Practitioner 73:188, 1904.

DeBusk FL: The Hutchinson-Gilford progeria syndrome. J Pediatr 80:697, 1972.

Dyck JD et al: Management of coronary artery disease in Hutchinson-Gilford syndrome. J Pediatr 711:407, 1987.

Gillar PJ et al: Progressive early dermatologic changes in Hutchinson-Gilford progeria syndrome. Pediatr Dermatol 8:199, 1991.

Wagle WA et al: Cerebral infarction in progeria. Pediatr Neurol 8:476, 1992.

Delahunt B et al: Progeria kidney has abnormal mesangial collagen distribution. Pediatr Nephrol 15:279, 2000.

Eriksson M et al: Recurrent de novo point mutations in lamin A cause Hutchinson-Gilford syndrome. Nature 423:293, 2003.

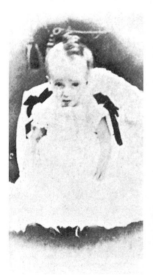 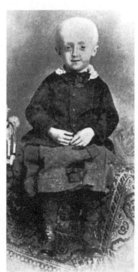 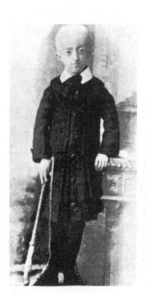 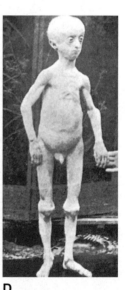

A   B   C   D

FIGURE 1. Progeria syndrome. **A–D**, Gilford's original patient. (From Gilford H: Practitioner, 73:188, 1904, with permission.)

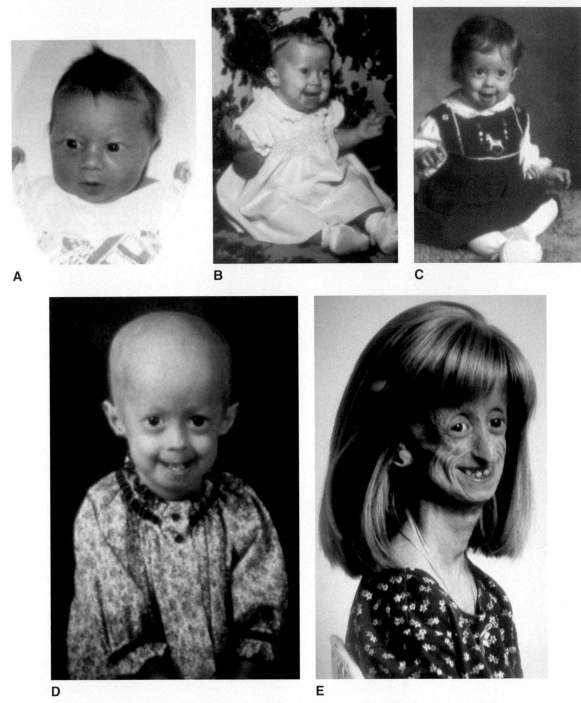

FIGURE 2. **A–E,** An affected child beginning in the neonatal period demonstrates the progression of the phenotype. (From Ackerman J, Gilbert E: Pediatr Pathol Molec Med 21:1, 2002, with permission.)

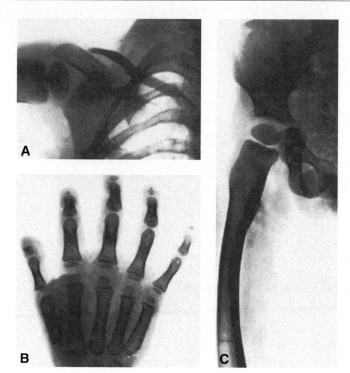

FIGURE 3. **A–C,** Radiographs of a 3-year-old child show loss of outer clavicle, distal phalanges, and straight femur. (From Macleod W: Br J Radiol 39:224, 1966, with permission.)

WIEDEMANN-RAUTENSTRAUCH SYNDROME

Decreased Subcutaneous Fat, Natal Teeth, Aged Face

ABNORMALITIES

General. Intrauterine growth retardation with respect to length and weight, postnatal growth deficiency.

Performance. Mental retardation ranging from severe (the majority of cases) to mild; three children are described as having normal development, one of whom was in regular school at 13 years of age.

Craniofacial. Frontal and parietal bossing with hypoplastic facial bones leading to a triangular-shaped face; aged face; large fontanels with wide sutures; sparse scalp hair, eyelashes, and eyebrows; prominent scalp veins; small, beak-shaped nose; upslanting palpebral fissures; lid entropion; natal teeth.

Skeletal. Apparently large hands and feet with long digits; large joint contractures; radiologic abnormalities, including partly ossified atlas, squared iliac bones, trident configuration of acetabula, and irregular end-plants of metaphyses.

OCCASIONAL ABNORMALITIES.

Congenital heart defects; laryngomalacia; low-set ears; neurosensory hearing loss; hypertonia; "sclerodermatous" skin; camptodactyly; large penis; hypoplastic prepuce; endocrine abnormalities, including hypothyroidism, hyperprolactinemia, and insulin resistance; disturbed lipid metabolism; central nervous system defects, including generalized demyelination of white matter, ventricular dilatation with cortical atrophy, and Dandy-Walker malformation.

NATURAL HISTORY. Although one severely mentally retarded patient is surviving at 16 years of age and a 13-year-old who attends regular school has been reported, the life expectancy of affected patients is approximately 7 months. Hypotonia, poor head control, intention tremors, and truncal ataxia are common. Feeding difficulties and respiratory infections occur frequently. The generalized decrease of subcutaneous fat is present in the newborn period in virtually all cases. During infancy, paradoxical fat accumulation occurs in approximately 50% of cases in the buttocks and lumbosacral region, and less frequently in the armpits, on the fingers, and in the suprapubic region. The radiologic abnormalities usually normalize by 1 year of age.

ETIOLOGY. This disorder has an autosomal recessive inheritance pattern.

References

Rautenstrauch T, Snigula F: Progeria: A cell culture study and clinical report of familial incidence. Eur J Pediatr 124:101–111, 1977.

Wiedemann H-R: An unidentified neonatal progeroid syndrome: Follow-up report. Eur J Pediatr 130:65–70, 1979.

Obregon MG et al: Radiographic findings in Wiedemann-Rautenstrauch syndrome. Pediatr Radiol 22:474–475, 2002.

Pivinick EK et al: Neonatal progeroid (Wiedemann-Rautenstrauch) syndrome: Report of five new cases and review. Am J Med Genet 90:131–140, 2000.

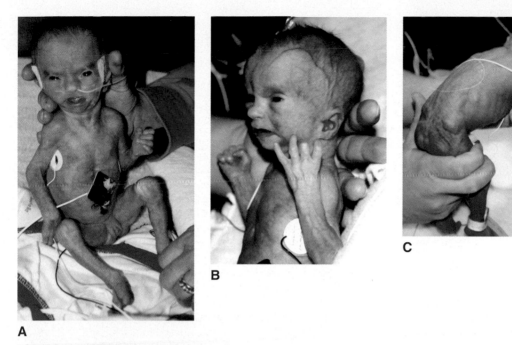

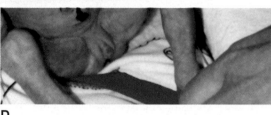

FIGURE 1. Wiedemann-Rautenstrauch syndrome. A–D, Note the generalized lipoatrophy, triangular face, relative macrocephaly, prominent scalp veins, high nasal bridge and full nasal tip, prominent chin, loculations of fat over buttocks, and enlarged buttocks due to fat deposition. (From Pivnick EK et al: Am J Med Genet 90:131, 2000, with permission.)

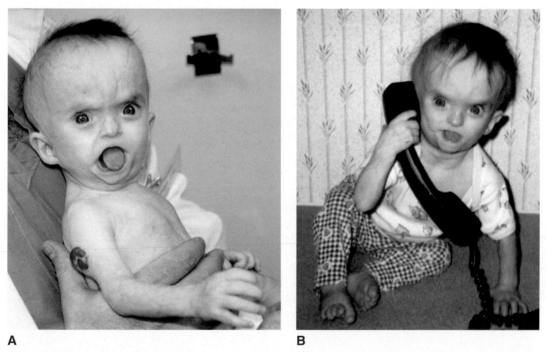

FIGURE 2. Same child as in Figure 1 at 7 months of age (A) and at 19 months of age (B). (From Pivnick EK et al: Am J Med Genet 90:131, 2000, with permission.)

WERNER SYNDROME

Early Adult—Cataract, Thin Skin with Thick Fibrous Subcutaneous Tissue, Gray Sparse Hair

The subject of Werner's doctoral thesis in 1904, this disease is usually not diagnosed until young adult life. More than 400 cases have been recorded.

ABNORMALITIES

Growth. Short stature; mean stature of affected males, 61 inches; females, 57.5 inches.

Deterioration. Loss of subcutaneous fat; slim, spindly extremities with small hands and feet; pinched facies with beak nose; irregular dental development; patches of stiffened skin, particularly on face and lower legs; skin ulcerations; atrophy of distal extremities; thick, fibrous subcutaneous tissue with thin dermis; osteoporosis, atherosclerosis with calcification; muscle hypoplasia with patchy areas of fibrosis; gray, sparse hair, premature balding; cataract, retinal degeneration; premature loss of teeth; hypogonadism, reduced fertility; high-pitched, hoarse voice secondary to vocal chord atrophy; liver atrophy; adult-type diabetes mellitus (44%); Mönckeberg sclerosis with organic brain syndrome; metastatic calcifications; excess urinary excretion of hyaluronic acid.

OCCASIONAL ABNORMALITIES.

Propensity toward malignancy (10%), especially sarcoma and meningioma; mild hyperthyroidism; adrenal atrophy; valvular sclerosis; hyperkeratosis of palms and soles.

NATURAL HISTORY.

Often noted to be slim with a slow rate of growth in later childhood, these individuals have no adolescent growth spurt and reach their final height at 10 to 18 years, usually at approximately 13 years. Gray hair develops at around 20 years. Thereafter follows skin changes, primarily atrophy involving the face and distal extremities, hair loss, development of a high-pitched or hoarse voice, visual symptoms, detection of cataracts, skin ulcers, and lastly, diabetes mellitus at an average age of 34 years. Old age appearance is evident by 30 to 40 years, with the mean age of survival being 47 years with a range of 31 to 63 years. Common causes of death are malignancy and myocardial infarction. A high representation of sarcomas of mesenchymal origin, occurring at unusual sites, has been documented. Atherosclerotic lesions are more extensive in arterioles than in major arteries. Calcification occurs not only in the atheromatous vessels but in the thick subcutaneous tissues as well. Hypertension occurs in approximately 50% of patients.

ETIOLOGY.

This disorder has an autosomal recessive inheritance pattern. The gene responsible for this disorder (WRN) has been mapped to 8p12. At least 35 different WRN mutations have been reported. Its product shows significant similarity to DNA helicases. As such, mutations of this gene could lead to abnormalities of DNA replication, recombination, chromosome segregation, DNA repair, transcription or other functions requiring DNA unwinding.

References

Werner O: Uber Katarakt in Verbindung mit Sklerodermie. (Doctoral dissertation, Kiel University.) Kiel, Schmidt and Klaunig, 1904.

Epstein CJ et al: Werner's syndrome. Medicine 45:177, 1966.

Fleischmajer R, Nedwich A: Werner's syndrome. Am J Med 54:111, 1973.

Murata K, Nakashima H: Werner's syndrome: 24 cases with a review of the Japanese literature. J Am Geriatr Soc 30:303, 1982.

Salk D: Werner's syndrome: A review of recent research with an analysis of connective tissue metabolism, growth control of cultured cells, and chromosome aberrations. Hum Genet 62:1, 1982.

Goto M et al: Genetic linkage of Werner's syndrome to five markers on chromosome 8. Nature 355:733, 1992.

Chang-En Y et al: Positional cloning of the Werner's syndrome gene. Science 272:258, 1996.

Chen L, Ochima J: Werner syndrome. J Biomed Biotechnol 2(2):46, 2002.

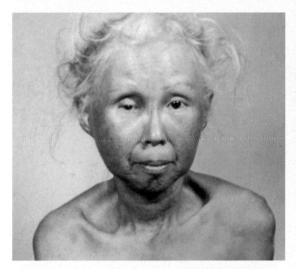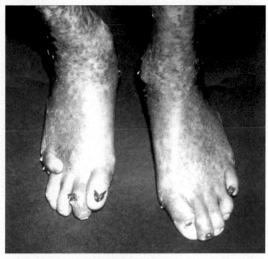

FIGURE 1. A 48-year-old woman with Werner syndrome. (From Epstein CJ et al: Medicine 45:177, 1966, with permission.)

COCKAYNE SYNDROME

Senile-Like Changes Beginning in Infancy, Retinal Degeneration and Impaired Hearing, Photosensitivity of Thin Skin

Cockayne reported this disorder in siblings in 1946. Subsequently, two forms of this condition have been described, the classic form described below (type I) and an early onset, more severe form (see comment).

ABNORMALITIES

Growth. Profound postnatal growth deficiency with loss of adipose tissue beginning in the first year of life; weight more affected than length; final height and weight are rarely greater than 115 cm and 20 kg, respectively.

Central and Peripheral Nervous Systems. Microcephaly by 2 years of age in almost 100%; mental deficiency (borderline in 14%; mild in 29%; moderate in 38%; severe in 19%); unsteady gait; ataxia, tremor, incoordination, dysarthric speech; weakness with peripheral neuropathy; sensorineural hearing loss (50%); seizures (5% to 10%); decreased lacrimation or sweating, miotic pupils; increased ventricular size, cerebral atrophy, or both; calcifications in basal ganglia; demyelination of subcortical white matter.

Ocular. Salt and pepper retinal pigmentation, optic atrophy, strabismus, hyperopia, corneal opacity, cataract, decreased lacrimation, nystagmus.

Facial. Relatively small cranium with radiographic evidence of a thickened calvarium; loss of facial adipose tissue with slender nose, moderately sunken eyes, and thin skin that is photosensitive; dental abnormalities including caries, delayed eruption of deciduous teeth, malocclusion, and absent/hypoplastic teeth.

Skin. Photosensitive dermatitis (75%); dry and sometimes scaly skin.

Extremities. Cool hands and feet, sometimes cyanotic; mild to moderate joint limitation.

Trunk. Relatively short, with biconvex flattening of vertebrae and tendency toward dorsal kyphosis.

Other. Hypertension; renal dysfunction (10%); cryptorchidism in one third of males; underdeveloped breasts and irregular menstrual cycles are frequent; thin, dry hair; sclerotic "ivory" epiphyses most obviously in the fingers; small, "squared off" pelvis with hypoplastic iliac wings.

OCCASIONAL ABNORMALITIES.

Intrauterine growth retardation, intracranial calcification, small sella turcica, micropenis, anhidrosis, cardiac arrhythmias, peripheral vascular disease, asymmetric fingers, short second toes, hepatomegaly, splenomegaly, osteoporosis.

NATURAL HISTORY.

Although prenatal growth deficiency occasionally has been documented, growth and development usually proceed at a normal rate in early infancy, and it is not until 2 to 4 years of age that the pattern of defect is clearly evident. Personality and behavior tend to correspond to the mental age, which is defective. No affected individual has fathered or given birth to a child. Photosensitivity of the skin may lead to problems with exposure to sunlight. The average age at death is $12\frac{1}{2}$ years; the major contributing factor being pneumonia.

ETIOLOGY.

This disorder has an autosomal recessive inheritance pattern. Type I is linked to mutations of the CSA gene located on chromosome 5p. A defect in DNA repair has been documented in fibroblasts. Following exposure to ultraviolet light, Cockayne syndrome cells show reduced survival, reduced recovery of DNA and RNA synthesis, hypermutability, and increased chromosome instability that are thought to be the consequence of a defect in transcription-coupled response. This process effects the rapid removal of damage from regions of DNA that are actively being transcribed into RNA.

COMMENT.

An early onset "severe form" of Cockayne syndrome, referred to as type II, has been reported in which death usually occurs by 6 or 7 years of age. Prenatal onset of growth deficiency, a lack of all neurologic development, early post-natal onset of congenital cataracts, and structural eye defects characterize this condition, which is linked to mutations of the CSB gene located on chromosome 10q11. In addition to this severe infantile variant of Cockayne syndrome, some cases of cerebro-oculo-facio-skeletal syndrome are due to mutations of the CSB gene. Finally, there exists a Xeroderma Pigmentosa–Cockayne syndrome (XP-CS) complex resulting from mutations in any one of three XP genes. Mutations in two result in a severe type II Cockayne syndrome phenotype and mutations in the third, in a mild type I phenotype.

References

Cockayne EA: Dwarfism with retinal atrophy and deafness. Arch Dis Child 21:52, 1946.

MacDonald WB, Fitch KD, Lewis IC: Cockayne's syndrome: An heredo-familial disorder of growth and development. Pediatrics 25:997, 1960.

Rainbow AJ, Howes M: A deficiency in the repair of UV and γ-ray damaged DNA in fibroblasts from Cockayne's syndrome. Mutat Res 93:235, 1982.

Patton MA et al: Early onset Cockayne's syndrome: Case reports with neuropathological and fibroblast studies. J Med Genet 26:154, 1989.

Nance MA, Berry SA: Cockayne syndrome: Review of 140 cases. Am J Med Genet 42:68, 1992.

Lehmann AR et al: Cockayne's syndrome: Correlation of clinical features with cellular sensitivity of RNA synthesis to UV irradiation. J Med Genet 30:679, 1993.

Stefanini M et al: Genetic analysis of 22 patients with Cockayne syndrome. Hum Genet 97:418, 1996.

Le Page F: Transcription-coupled repair of 8-oxoguanine: requirement for XPG, TFIIH, and CS and implications for Cockayne syndrome. Cell 101:159, 2000.

Rapin I: Cockayne syndrome and Xeroderma Pigmentosa: DNA repair disorders with overlaps and paradoxes. Neurology 55:1442, 2000.

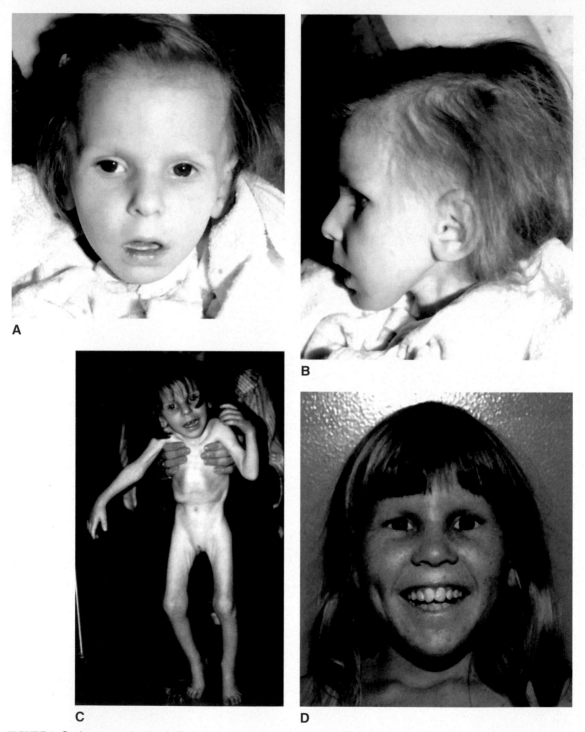

FIGURE 1. Cockayne syndrome. **A–C,** A 4-year-old girl. **D,** A 10-year-old girl. Note the loss of facial adipose tissue with slender nose; sunken eyes; thin, dry hair; and evidence of severe neurologic compromise. (**A–D,** Courtesy of Dr. Marilyn C. Jones, Children's Hospital, San Diego.)

ROTHMUND-THOMSON SYNDROME
(Poikiloderma Congenitale Syndrome)

Development of Poikiloderma, Cataract with or without Other Ectodermal Dysplasia

This condition was first described in 1868 by Rothmund, a Munich ophthalmologist who discovered multiple cases among an inbred group of people living in the nearby Alps. An excellent review of over 200 cases has been published by Vennos and colleagues.

ABNORMALITIES. Wide variance in expression, the most usual features being the following:

Growth. Small stature of prenatal onset in majority of cases.

Skin. Irregular erythema progressing to poikiloderma (i.e., telangiectasia, scarring, irregular pigmentation and depigmentation, atrophy); although most marked in sun-exposed areas, skin changes frequently occur on buttocks; hyperkeratotic lesions (33%) may be warty or verrucous; blister formation (20%) occurs before onset of poikiloderma; photosensitivity (35%).

Hair. Sparse, prematurely gray, and occasionally alopecia (80%); thinning of eyebrows and eyelashes occurs initially; scalp, facial, and pubic hair are often only thin.

Eyes. Juvenile zonular cataract (52%) in all cases bilateral; occasionally corneal dystrophy.

OCCASIONAL ABNORMALITIES

Skeletal. Small hands and feet (20%), hypoplastic to absent thumbs, syndactyly, forearm reduction defects, absence of patella, clubfeet, osteoporosis, areas of cystic or sclerotic change.

Facial. Frontal bossing, small saddle nose, prognathism.

Teeth. Microdontia and anodontia, ectopic eruption, dental caries (40%).

Nails. Small, dystrophic (32%).

Other Skin. Hyperkeratosis of palms and soles, nonmelanoma skin cancers.

Other. Mental deficiency (5% to 13%), microcephaly, hydrocephalus, craniosynostosis, cleft palate, hemihypertrophy, hypertension, hypercholesterolemia, hypothyroidism, scoliosis, osteogenic sarcoma (32%), hypogonadism or delayed sexual development (28%), cryptorchidism, irregular menses, anteriorly placed anus, annular pancreas, growth hormone deficiency, anhidrosis, neutropenia.

NATURAL HISTORY. Feeding or gastrointestinal problems often occur in infancy. Although skin changes have been present in six patients at birth, they usually occur between 3 months and 1 year of age. The progression toward irregular "marbled" hypoplasia, termed poikiloderma, is mainly noted in the first few years. Cataract most commonly becomes evident between 2 and 7 years of age. Alopecia progresses and may be complete by the second or third decade. Reduced fertility is frequent, although pregnancy has been reported on several occasions. Regarding management, avoidance of sun exposure and use of sunscreen are mandatory. Annual ophthalmologic exams to screen for cataracts is recommended and when initial diagnosis is made, parents should be counseled regarding signs of osteosarcoma, including bone pain, swelling, or an enlarging limb lesion. Radiographs should be performed by 5 years of age, and subsequent radiographs should be taken when merited by clinical signs.

ETIOLOGY. This disorder has an autosomal recessive inheritance pattern. Mutation in a RECQL4 helicase gene at 8q24.3 is responsible for some cases. Bloom syndrome and Werner syndrome, also due to RECQ helicase gene mutations, are characterized by growth deficiency, premature aging, and predisposition to site-specific malignancies.

References
Rothmund A: Ueber Cataracten in Verbindung miteiner eigenthümlichen Hautdegeneration. Arch Ophthalmol 14:159, 1868.

Rook A, Davis R, Stevanovic D: Poikiloderma congenitale: Rothmund-Thomson syndrome. Acta Derm Venereol (Stockh) 39:392, 1959.

Hall JG, Pagon RA, Wilson KM: Rothmund-Thomson syndrome with severe dwarfism. Am J Dis Child 134:165, 1980.

Starr DG, McClure JP, Connor JM: Non-dermatological complications and genetic aspects of the Rothmund-Thomson syndrome. Clin Genet 27:102, 1985.

Kaufman S et al: Growth hormone deficiency in the Rothmund-Thomson syndrome. Am J Med Genet 23:861, 1986.

Vennos EM et al: Rothmund-Thomson syndrome: Review of the world literature. J Am Acad Dermatol 27:750, 1992.

Kitao S: Mutations in RECQL4 cause a subset of cases of Rothmund-Thomson syndrome. Nat Genet 22:82, 1999.

Wang LL et al: Clinical manifestations in a cohort of 41 Rothmund-Thomson syndrome patients. Am J Med Genet 102:11, 2001.

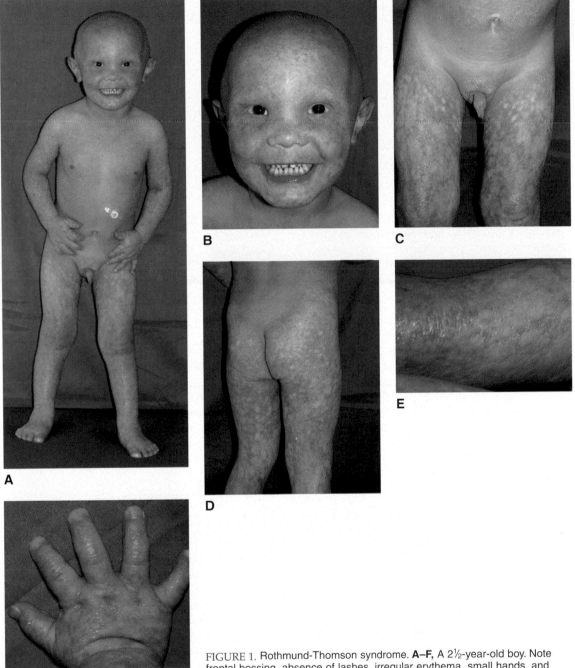

FIGURE 1. Rothmund-Thomson syndrome. **A–F,** A 2½-year-old boy. Note frontal bossing, absence of lashes, irregular erythema, small hands, and small nails. (Courtesy of Dr. Lynne M. Bird, Children's Hospital, San Diego.)

E Early Overgrowth with Associated Defects

FRAGILE X SYNDROME
(MARTIN-BELL SYNDROME, MARKER X SYNDROME)

Mental Deficiency, Mild Connective Tissue Dysplasia, Macro-Orchidism

This subgroup can now be differentiated from other types of X-linked mental retardation. In 1943, Martin and Bell published the first pedigree documenting a sex-linked form of mental retardation. Lubs in 1969 showed the presence of a fragile site on the long arm of the X chromosome in affected males and some carrier females in one family. Macro-orchidism without endocrinologic abnormalities was described by Turner and colleagues and Cantu and colleagues in the affected males of a number of families. However, it was not until Sutherland demonstrated that expression of the fragile site was dependent on the nature of the cell culture medium that the association between X-linked mental retardation, macro-orchidism, and the marker X chromosome was made.

The disorder appears to be common. Population-based studies suggest a prevalence of from 1 in 3717 to 1 in 8918 white males. Among populations of mentally handicapped individuals, fragile X–positive studies have been documented in up to 5.9% of males and up to 0.3% of females. The phenotype is most readily identified in the male.

ABNORMALITIES

Performance. Mild to profound mental retardation in males with intelligence quotients (IQs) of 30 to 55, but sometimes extending into the mildly retarded to borderline normal range. Hand flapping or biting (60%) and poor eye contact (90%). Cluttered speech in mildly retarded males, short bursts of repetitive speech in more severely retarded males, and complete lack of speech in severely and profoundly retarded males. Attention problems associated with hyperactivity are common. Sensitivity to stimuli leading to serious behavior problems in overstimulating situations. Autism (60%). IQ < 70 in approximately 30% to 50% of females with the full mutation and IQ < 85 in 50% to 70%.

Craniofacial. Macrocephaly in early childhood, prognathism usually not noted until after puberty, thickening of nasal bridge extending down to the nasal tip, large ears with soft cartilage, pale blue irides, epicanthal folds, dental crowding.

OCCASIONAL ABNORMALITIES.
Nystagmus, strabismus, epilepsy, myopia, hypotonia, hyperextensible fingers, mild cutis laxa, torticollis, pectus excavatum, kyphoscoliosis, flat feet, submucous cleft palate, mitral valve prolapse, aortic dilation. Early features may suggest cerebral gigantism.

NATURAL HISTORY.
Life span is normal. The patient's growth rate is slightly increased in the early years, with delayed motor milestones. Testicular size may be increased before puberty, but this increase becomes more obvious post-pubertally. A characteristic speech pattern, referred to as "cluttering," is observed in higher functioning individuals. Psychologic profile is characterized by hyperkinetic behavior, emotional instability, hand biting, and other autistic features. Higher levels of maternal psychological problems as well as less effective educational and therapeutic services are related to the extent of behavioral problems in boys but not girls.

ETIOLOGY.
X-linked inheritance. Expansions of a trinucleotide repeat (CGG) in the promoter region of the FMR1 gene located at Xq27.3 is responsible for the phenotype and is the basis for molecular diagnosis of this disorder. Normal individuals have from 6 to 54 repeats. Both male

and female premutation carriers have 54 to 200 repeats, while affected individuals have greater than 200. Female premutation carriers have a 20% risk for premature ovarian failure, mood and anxiety difficulties in a subset, and abnormalities on MRI. Male premutation carriers have evidence of anxiety, which increases with age, deficits in executive function, and cerebellar tremor in a sub-group of older males. Expansion of premutations to full mutations occurs only in female meiotic transmission and correlates with the size of the premutation. The risk that an individual will be affected clinically is dependent upon the position of that individual within the family. Thus the risk that the daughter of a phenotypically normal carrier male will be effected is zero. However, the risk that his daughter's son (his grandson) will be affected is 50%. Most likely based on the phenomenon of X-inactivation, the risk that the daughter of a pre-mutation carrier female will be clinically affected is smaller (approximately 15% to 30% depending on the number of CGG repeats, i.e., the size of the premutation allele). DNA-based molecular analysis allows for both identification of full mutations and permutation carriers.

References

Lubs HA: A marker X chromosome. Am J Hum Genet 21:231, 1969.

Turner G et al: X-linked mental retardation associated with macro-orchidism. J Med Genet 12:367, 1975.

Cantu JM et al: Inherited congenital normofunctional testicular hyperplasia and mental deficiency. Hum Genet 33:23, 1976.

Sutherland GR: Fragile sites on human chromosomes: Demonstration of their independence on the type of tissue culture medium. Science 197:265, 1977.

Turner G et al: Conference report: Second international workshop on the fragile X and on X-linked mental retardation. Am J Med Genet 23:11, 1986.

Chudley AE, Hagerman RJ: Fragile X syndrome. J Pediatr 10:821, 1987.

Fu Y et al: Variation of the CGG repeat at the fragile X site results in genetic instability: Resolution of the Sherman paradox. Cell 67:1047, 1991.

Verkerk AJMH et al: Identification of a gene (FMR-1) containing a CGG repeat coincident with a breakpoint cluster region exhibiting length variation in fragile X syndrome. Cell 67:905, 1991.

Crawford DC et al: FMR1 and the fragile X syndrome: Human genome epidemiology review. Genet Med 3:359, 2001.

Hagerman RJ, Hagerman PJ: Fragile X syndrome: A model of gene-brain-behavior relationships. Mol Genet Metab 74:89, 2001.

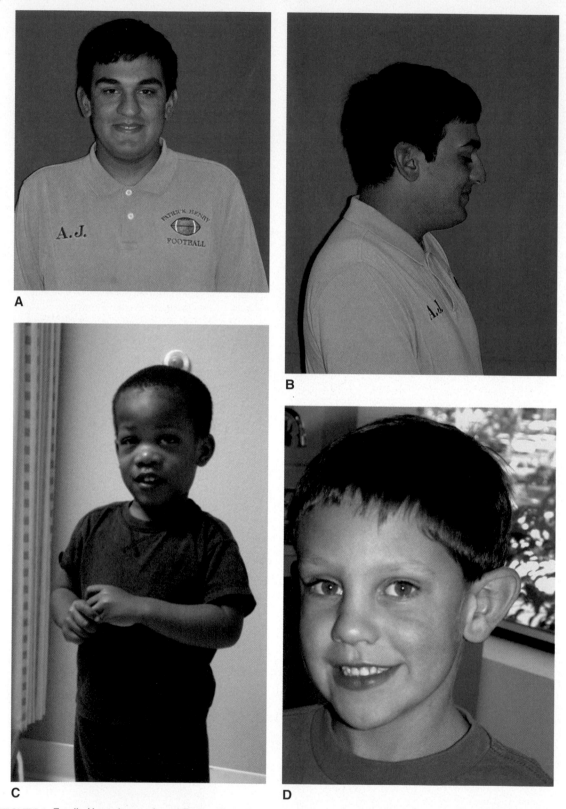

FIGURE 1. Fragile X syndrome. **A** and **B,** An affected 18-year-old male. **C** and **D,** Two affected boys. Note the increased head circumference with prominent forehead, prognathism, and big ears. (**A, B,** and **D,** Courtesy of Dr. Lynne M. Bird, Children's Hospital, San Diego.)

SOTOS SYNDROME
(CEREBRAL GIGANTISM SYNDROME)

Large Size, Large Hands and Feet, Poor Coordination

Sotos and colleagues described five such patients in 1964, and more than 300 cases have subsequently been reported.

ABNORMALITIES

Performance. Variable mental deficiency; IQs of 40 to 129, with a mean of 78; poor coordination; hypotonia; hyperreflexia; delayed gross motor function; significant behavioral abnormalities.

Growth. Prenatal onset of excessive size; at birth, length more likely to be increased than weight; mean full-term birth length 55.2 cm and birth weight 3.9 kg; length increases rapidly, remains at or above 97th percentile throughout childhood and early adolescence, and is more significantly increased than weight; final height often within normal range; relatively large span; large hands and feet (greater than 50th percentile even when plotted for height age); advanced osseous maturation in childhood (84%).

Craniofacial. Macrocephaly of prenatal onset in 50% and by 1 year of age in 100%; mild dilatation of the cerebral ventricles; prominent forehead (dolichocephalic); sparse hair in frontoparietal region; downslanting palpebral fissures; apparent hypertelorism not always confirmed by measurement; prominent jaw; high, narrow palate with prominent lateral palatine ridges; facial flushing frequently of nose but also cheeks and perioral region; premature eruption of teeth.

Other. Orthopedic problems (60%) primarily including pes planus and genu valgus; thin, brittle fingernails.

OCCASIONAL ABNORMALITIES.
Seizures, electroencephalograph abnormalities, strabismus, nystagmus, optic disc pallor and retinal atrophy, cataracts, iris hypoplasia, glaucoma, cardiac defects, kyphoscoliosis, abnormal glucose tolerance test (14%), malignancy (2.2%) including Wilms tumor (two patients), vaginal carcinoma (one), hepatocarcinoma (one), cavernous hemangioma (one), mixed parotid tumor (one), osteochondroma (one), neuroectodermal tumor (one), small cell lung carcinoma (one), neuroblastoma (one), acute lymphocytic leukemia (two), non-Hodgkin lymphoma (one).

NATURAL HISTORY. Neonatal problems have been frequent, including difficulties with respiration and feeding. Thereafter, appetite and fluid intake are frequently noted to be increased over normal and constipation is often a problem. An increased incidence of otitis media has been noted with conductive hearing loss and associated complications. Early developmental milestones are delayed. The median age of individuals at first sitting has been 9 months; walking, 17 months; and saying a few words, 25 months. However, these early assessments, which rely heavily on specific motor and verbal skills that are particularly delayed in Sotos syndrome, may well be poor predictors of ultimate intellectual performance. Even in those patients with normal intelligence, delay of expressive language and motor development is characteristically present in infancy. Behavior problems are significant. Excessive size, with poor coordination, leads to problems of social adjustment, often with undue aggressiveness and temper tantrums. Immaturity persisting into adulthood adds to the difficulties with socialization. A propensity to fracture with minimal trauma has been documented. A slightly increased risk for malignancy appears to exist. However, because the sites and types vary greatly, no routine screening with the exception of periodic clinical evaluation seems appropriate.

ETIOLOGY. This disorder has an autosomal dominant inheritance pattern. Although parent-to-child transmission has occurred, the majority of cases are sporadic. Mutations of NSD1 (nuclear receptor SET-domain-containing protein) located at 5q35 are responsible for most cases. However, NSD1 deletions are also seen and are associated with more severe mental retardation.

COMMENT. Typical abnormalities have been noted on brain magnetic resonance imaging that can be helpful relative to diagnosis. Abnormalities of the cerebral ventricles include prominence of the trigone, prominence of the occipital horns, and ventriculomegaly. Midline defects include abnormalities of the corpus callosum with complete or partial agenesis or hypoplasia. The supratentorial extracerebral fluid spaces and the fluid spaces in the posterior fossa are increased in 70% of cases.

References

Sotos JF et al: Cerebral gigantism in childhood: A syndrome of excessively rapid growth with acromegalic features and a nonprogressive neurologic disorder. N Engl J Med 271:109, 1964.

Jaecken J, van der Schueren-Lodeweyckx, Eekels R: Cerebral gigantism syndrome. Z Kinderheilkd 112:332, 1972.

Dodge PR, Holmes SJ, Sotos JF: Cerebral gigantism. Dev Med Child Neurol 25:248, 1983.

Rutter SC, Cole TRP: Psychological characteristics of Sotos syndrome. Dev Med Child Neurol 33:898, 1991.

Hersh JH et al: Risk of malignancy in Sotos syndrome. J Pediatr 120:572, 1992.

Cole TRP, Hughes HE: Sotos syndrome: A study of the diagnostic criteria and natural history. J Med Genet 31:20, 1994.

Schaefer GB et al: The neuroimaging findings in Sotos syndrome. Am J Med Genet 68:462, 1997.

Opitz JM et al: The syndromes of Sotos and Weaver: Reports and review. Am J Med Genet 79:294, 1998.

Douglas J et al: NSD1 mutations are the major cause of Sotos syndrome and occur in some cases of Weaver syndrome but are rare in other overgrowth phenotypes. Am J Hum Genet 72:132, 2003.

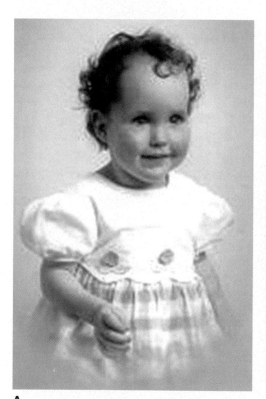

A

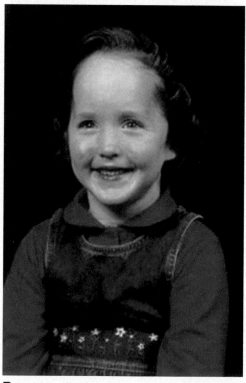

B

Continued

FIGURE 1. Sotos syndrome. **A–D,** Affected girl from childhood to adolescence. (Courtesy of Dr. Angela Lin, Brigham and Women's Hospital, Boston.)

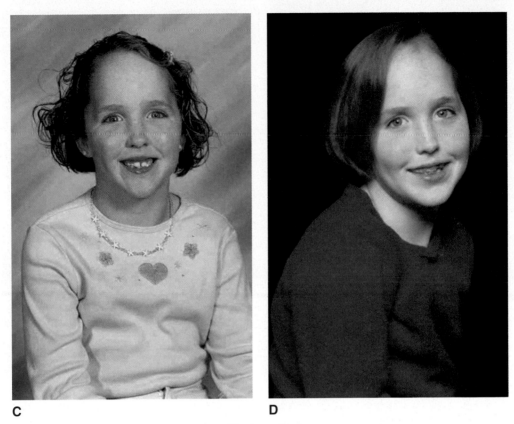

C   D

Fig. 1, cont'd.

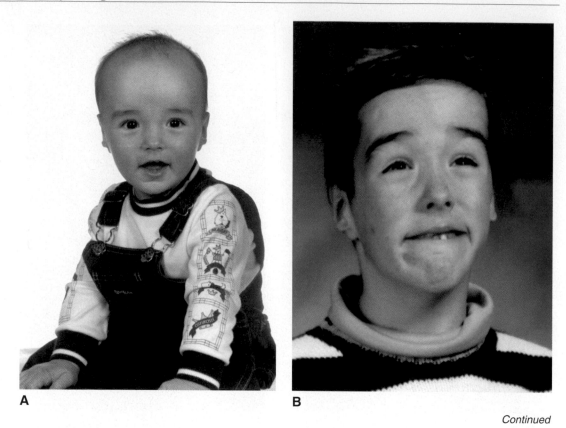

A

B

Continued

FIGURE 2. **A–D,** Affected boy from 9 months through 14 years. (Courtesy of Dr. Angela Lin, Brigham and Women's Hospital, Boston.)

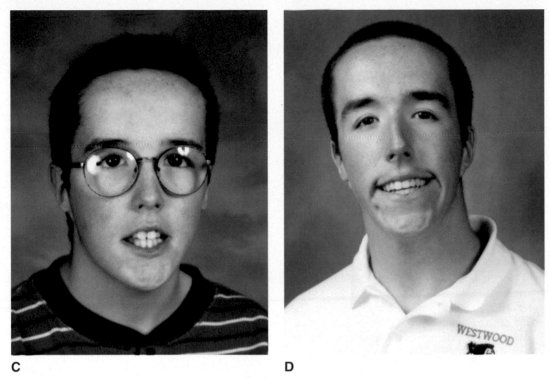

C　　　　　　　　　　　　　　　**D**

Fig. 2, cont'd.

WEAVER SYNDROME

Macrosomia, Accelerated Skeletal Maturation, Camptodactyly, Unusual Facies

Weaver and colleagues reported two strikingly similar boys with this pattern of overgrowth. Documentation of a number of additional cases indicates that this is a distinct disorder separate from Marshall-Smith or Sotos syndromes.

ABNORMALITIES

Growth. Accelerated growth and maturation, of prenatal onset; weight is more significantly increased than height.

Performance. Developmental delay or mental retardation, usually mild (81%); mild hypertonia, developmental lag, coarse low-pitched voice with slurred or dysarthric speech that is delayed in onset; progressive spasticity; strabismus.

Craniofacial. Macrocephaly (83%), large bifrontal diameter, flat occiput, ocular hypertelorism, epicanthal folds, depressed nasal bridge, downslanting palpebral fissures, large ears, long philtrum, relative micrognathia.

Limbs. Camptodactyly, broad thumbs, thin deepset nails, prominent fingertip pads, limited elbow and knee extension, clinodactyly leading to overriding of toes, flared metaphyses, especially distal femora and humeri, foot deformities including talipes equinovarus, calcaneovalgus, and metatarsus adductus.

Other. Relatively loose skin, inverted nipples, thin hair, umbilical hernia, inguinal hernia, cryptorchidism, scoliosis, kyphosis.

OCCASIONAL ABNORMALITIES.

Cardiac defects, cleft palate, atretic ear canal, postaxial polydactyly, diaphragmatic eventration, short ribs, short fourth metatarsals, hypotonia, instability of the upper cervical spine, seizures, cyst in the septum pellucidum, cerebral atrophy, enlarged vessels and hypervascularization in the areas of the middle and left posterior cerebral arteries, neuroblastoma, endodermal sinus, tumor of ovary, and sacrococcygeal teratoma.

NATURAL HISTORY. These children are usually large at birth and show accelerated growth and markedly advanced skeletal maturation during infancy, with carpal centers more advanced than phalangeal centers. In a minority of patients, overgrowth does not develop until a few months of age. Final height 194.2 cm in males and 176.3 cm in females with occipito-frontal circumference of 61 cm and 59.5 cm in males and females, respectively. Although initially development is delayed, with advancing age, few are described as mentally retarded. Attention deficit and hyperactivity occur occasionally.

ETIOLOGY. This disorder has an autosomal dominant inheritance pattern. Although parent-to-child transmission has occurred in at least five instances, the majority of cases are sporadic. It has been suggested that some cases are due to mutations of NSD1, which is the major cause of Sotos syndrome. However, other studies have shown this not to be the case.

References

Weaver DD et al: A new overgrowth syndrome with accelerated skeletal maturation, unusual facies, and camptodactyly. J Pediatr 84:547, 1974.

Fitch N: The syndromes of Marshall and Weaver. J Med Genet 17:174, 1980.

Fitch N: Letter to the editor: Update on the Marshall-Smith-Weaver controversy. Am J Med Genet 20: 559, 1985.

Ardinger HH et al: Further delineation of Weaver syndrome. J Pediatr 108:229, 1986.

Ramos-Arroyo MA et al: Weaver syndrome: A case without early overgrowth and review of the literature. Pediatrics 88:1106, 1991.

Cole TRP et al: Weaver syndrome. J Med Genet 29:332, 1992.

Opitz JM et al: The syndromes of Sotos and Weaver: Reports and review. Am J Med Genet 79:294, 1998.

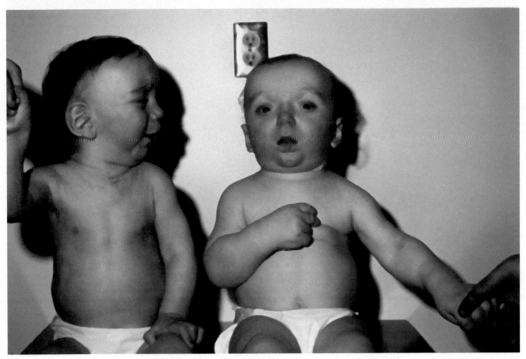

FIGURE 1. Unrelated affected boys at 18 months and 11 months of age, respectively. (From Weaver DD et al: J Pediatr 84:547, 1974, with permission.)

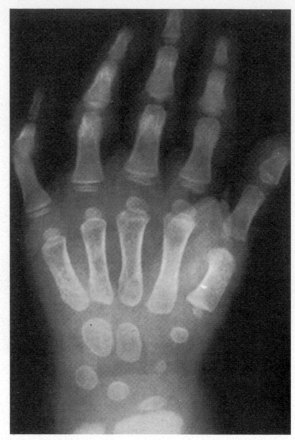

Continued

FIGURE 2. Radiographs showing accelerated osseous maturation and broad distal splaying of femurs. (From Weaver DD et al: J Pediatr 84:547, 1974, with permission.)

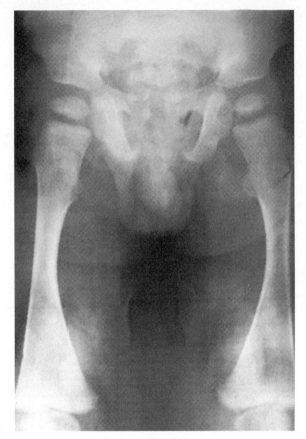

Fig. 2, cont'd.

MARSHALL-SMITH SYNDROME

Accelerated Growth and Maturation, Shallow Orbits, Broad Middle Phalanges

Initially described by Marshall and Smith in 1977, at least 19 patients with this disorder have been reported. Although categorized as an overgrowth syndrome, recent evidence suggests that this disorder involves an intrinsic structural or biochemical defect of cartilage, bone, or connective tissue, rather than generalized or localized cellular hyperplasia.

ABNORMALITIES

Growth. Accelerated linear growth and markedly accelerated skeletal maturation of prenatal onset, underweight for length with failure to thrive in weight.

Performance. Motor and mental deficiency, average IQ of 50, hypotonia.

Craniofacial. Long cranium with prominent forehead, shallow orbits with prominent eyes, bluish sclerae, upturned nose, low nasal bridge, small mandibular ramus.

Limbs. Broad proximal and middle phalanges with narrow distal phalanges.

Other. Hypertrichosis, umbilical hernia.

OCCASIONAL ABNORMALITIES.
Choanal atresia or stenosis or both; abnormal larynx/laryngomalacia; dysplastic teeth; deafness and ear anomalies; brain abnormalities including macrogyria, cerebral atrophy, and absent corpus callosum; instability of the craniocervical junction with severe spinal stenoses; short sternum; scoliosis; hypersegmented sacrococcyx; rudimentary epiglottis; omphalocele; deep crease between hallux and second toe; immunologic defect.

NATURAL HISTORY.
These patients have failed to thrive in terms of weight. They have persistent respiratory difficulties manifested by stridor, hyperextension of the neck, and obstructing tongue. Although the majority die by 20 months with pneumonia, atelectasis, aspiration, or pulmonary hypertension, two children, 7 and 8 years of age, respectively, are being followed by Hoyme and colleagues. Although neither can speak and both have a mild to moderate, conductive hearing loss, overall intellectual performance is in the lower range of normal. Aggressive management of respiratory difficulties is extremely important with respect to ultimate prognosis. The accelerated osseous maturation, of unknown cause, is of prenatal onset, as indicated by a wrist "bone age" of 3 to 4 years in one patient at 2 weeks of life.

ETIOLOGY.
The etiology of this disorder is unknown. Each case has been a sporadic occurrence in the family.

COMMENT.
Changes in the lower medulla secondary to the craniocervical instability may contribute to the respiratory distress leading to sudden early death in this disorder.

References

Marshall RE et al: Syndrome of accelerated skeletal maturation and relative failure to thrive: A newly recognized clinical growth disorder. J Pediatr 78:95, 1971.

Visveshware N, Rudolph N, Dragutsky D: Syndrome of accelerated skeletal maturation in infancy, peculiar facies and multiple congenital anomalies—an additional case. J Pediatr 84:553, 1974.

Fitch N: The syndromes of Marshall and Weaver. J Med Genet 17:174, 1980.

Johnson JP et al: Marshall-Smith syndrome: Two case reports and a review of pulmonary manifestations. Pediatrics 77:219, 1983.

Fitch N: Letter to the editor: Update on the Marshall-Smith-Weaver controversy. Am J Med Genet 20:559, 1985.

Eich GF et al: Marshall-Smith syndrome: New radiographic clinical and pathological observations. Radiology 181:183, 1991.

Hoyme HE et al: The Marshall-Smith syndrome: Further evidence of osteochondrodysplasia in long term survivors. Proc Greenwood Genet Clin 72:70, 1993.

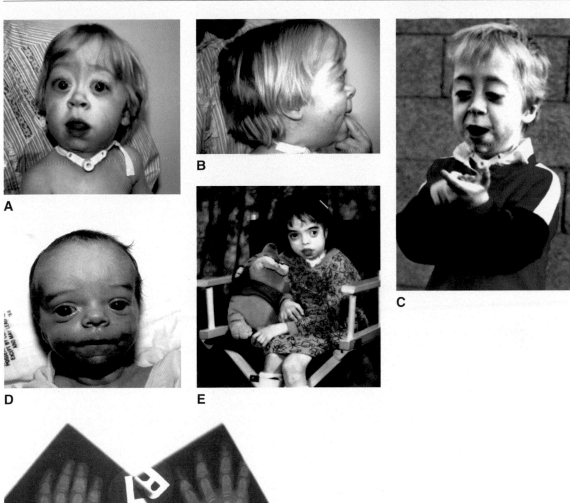

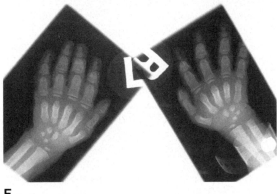

FIGURE 1. Marshall-Smith syndrome. Affected boy as a neonate and at 7 years (**A–C**) and affected girl as a neonate and at 8 years (**D** and **E**). **A–F,** Note the prominent forehead, shallow orbits with prominent eyes, blue sclera, low nasal bridge, and the hand of one showing an accelerated carpal bone age and broad phalanges. (Courtesy of H. Eugene Hoyme, Stanford University, Palo Alto.)

BECKWITH-WIEDEMANN SYNDROME
(Exomphalos-Macroglossia-Gigantism Syndrome)

Macroglossia, Omphalocele, Macrosomia, Ear Creases

Beckwith and Wiedemann first reported this distinct clinical entity, and more than 200 cases have subsequently been reported.

ABNORMALITIES

Performance. Unknown incidence of mild to moderate mental retardation; may be normal.

Growth. Macrosomia with large muscle mass and thick subcutaneous tissue, accelerated osseous maturation, metaphyseal flaring with over-constriction of diaphyses, diminished tubulation of proximal humerus.

Craniofacial. Macroglossia; prominent eyes with *relative* infraorbital hypoplasia; capillary nevus flammeus, central forehead and eyelids; metopic ridge; large fontanels; prominent occiput; malocclusion with tendency toward mandibular prognathism and maxillary underdevelopment; unusual linear fissures in lobule of external ear; indentations on posterior rim of helix.

Hyperplasia and Dysplasia. Large kidneys with renal medullary dysplasia; pancreatic hyperplasia, including excess of islets; fetal adrenocortical cytomegaly—a *consistent feature*; interstitial cell hyperplasia, gonads; pituitary amphophil hyperplasia.

Other. Neonatal polycythemia, hypoglycemia in early infancy (about one third to one half of cases), omphalocele or other umbilical anomaly, diastasis recti, posterior diaphragmatic eventration, cryptorchidism, cardiovascular defects including isolated cardiomegaly.

OCCASIONAL ABNORMALITIES.
Hepatomegaly, mild microcephaly, hemihypertrophy, adrenal carcinoma, Wilms tumor, gonadoblastoma, hepatoblastoma, clitoromegaly, large ovaries, hyperplastic uterus and bladder, bicornuate uterus, hypospadias, immunodeficiency, cardiac hamartoma, focal cardiomyopathy, hypercalciuria.

NATURAL HISTORY. Hydramnios and a relatively high incidence of prematurity provide further indication of the rather profound prenatal alterations. Birth weight has averaged 4 kg, and length, 52.6 cm. Thereafter, length parallels the normal curve at or above the 95th percentile through adolescence. After 9 years of age, mean weight remains between the 75th and 95th percentile. Advanced bone age, most pronounced during the first 4 years, only rarely persists until maturity. Spontaneous pubertal development occurs at a normal time. Severe problems of neonatal adaptation may occur, with apnea, cyanosis, and seizures as symptoms. The large tongue may partially occlude the respiratory tract and lead to feeding difficulties. Placing the baby on the side or face down may help respiration, and a large, soft nipple may facilitate feeding. Infant mortality rate is estimated to be as high as 21%. Detection and treatment of hypoglycemia in any neonate with features of this syndrome are critical. The hypoglycemia is responsive to hydrocortisone analogue therapy, which is usually required for only 1 to 4 months. Polycythemia might only merit therapeutic intervention during the early neonatal period. The frequency of tumor in this disorder is suggested to be 6.5%. Obtaining renal ultrasounds and measuring serum alpha-fetoprotein (AFP) to rule out Wilms tumor and hepatoblastoma, respectively, are warranted. An increased risk of malignancy seems to be associated with those children who have hemihypertrophy. Serum alpha-fetoprotein concentration is greater in Beckwith-Wiedemann syndrome (BWS) and declines at a slower rate than normal in the neonatal period. Affected individuals who survive infancy generally are healthy. Growth may allow adequate oral room for the large tongue. Partial glossectomy has been performed successfully in a number of cases. Evidence suggests the prognathia and dental malocclusion are secondary to the large tongue.

ETIOLOGY. Although usually sporadic, autosomal dominant inheritance with preferential maternal transmission has occurred in approximately 10% to 15% of cases. BWS is caused by perturbations of the normal dosage balance of a number of genes clustered at 11p15, a highly imprinted region in the genome. Both genetic

(factors that change the structure of the gene) and epigenetic (factors that influence the function/expression of a gene without changing its structure) play a role. Genes at 11p15 are organized in two separately controlled imprinted domains.

Domain 1 contains paternally expressed insulin-like growth factor 2 (IGF2) as well as a number of genes and transcripts that control expression of insulin-like growth factor 2. Mechanisms that increase expression of insulin-like growth factor 2, including maternally derived translocations and inversions of chromosome 11p15, duplications of the paternal chromosome 11p15, paternal uniparental disomy (20% of cases of BWS) and imprinting anomalies, all lead to BWS.

Domain 2 contains several imprinted genes including CDKNIC (10% of sporadic cases have a mutation of this gene and 40% of the dominant cases are due to this mutation), and KCNQ1OT1 (LIT1), a paternally expressed transcript that regulates the expression of other genes in domain 2. (Loss of imprint in LIT1 accounts for 40% to 50% of cases of BWS.)

Currently, clinical testing is available for roughly 70% of mechanisms that produce BWS. BWS has occurred discordantly in a number of monozygotic twins (mostly females). The mechanism behind this discordance is currently unclear. BWS may occur more frequently in pregnancies conceived with assisted reproductive technology, although the absolute risk is low.

References

Wiedemann HR: Complexe malformatif familial avec hernie ombilicale et macroglossie—un "syndrome nouveau"? J Genet Hum 13:223, 1964.

Beckwith JB: Macroglossia, omphalocele, adrenal cytomegaly, gigantism, and hyperplastic visceromegaly. Birth Defects 5(2):188, 1969.

Pettenati MJ et al: Wiedemann-Beckwith syndrome: Presentation of clinical and cytogenetic data on 22 new cases and review of the literature. Hum Genet 74:143, 1986.

Sippell WG et al: Growth, bone maturation and pubertal development in children with the EMG syndrome. Clin Genet 35:20, 1989.

Normal AM et al: Recurrent Wiedmann-Beckwith syndrome with inversion of chromosome (11) (p11.2p15.5). Am J Med Genet 42:638, 1992.

Weksburg R et al: Disruption of insulin-like growth factor 2 imprinting in Beckwith-Wiedemann syndrome. Nat Genet 5:143, 1993.

Weksburg R et al: Molecular characterization of cytogenetic alterations associated with the Beckwith-Wiedemann syndrome (BWS) phenotype refines the localization and suggests the gene for BWS is imprinted. Hum Mol Genet 2:549, 1993.

Everman DB et al: Serum alpha-fetoprotein levels in Beckwith-Wiedemann syndrome. J Pediatr 137:123, 2000.

DeBaun MR et al: Association of in vitro fertilization with Beckwith-Wiedemann syndrome and epigenetic alterations of LIT1 and H19. Am J Hum Genet 72:156, 2003.

Weksberg R et al: Beckwith-Wiedemann syndrome demonstrates a role for epigenetic control of normal development. Hum Mol Genet 12: R61, 2003.

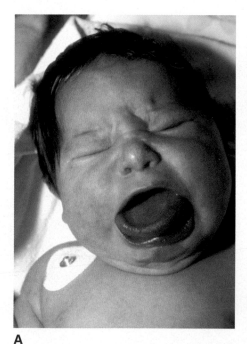
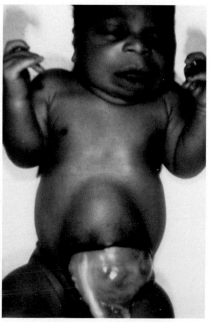

A   **B**

FIGURE 1. Beckwith-Wiedemann syndrome. **A** and **B,** Newborn infants. (Courtesy of Dr. Michael Cohen, Dalhousie University, Halifax, Nova Scotia.)

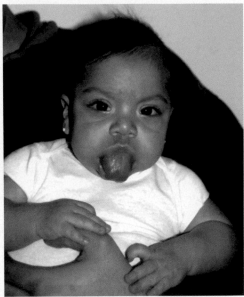

A

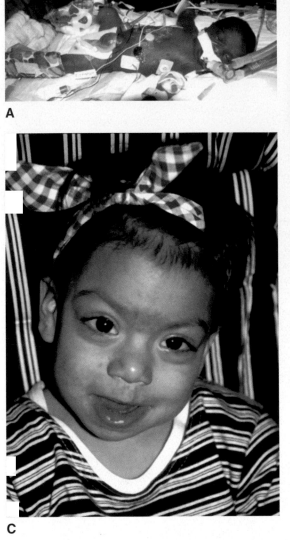

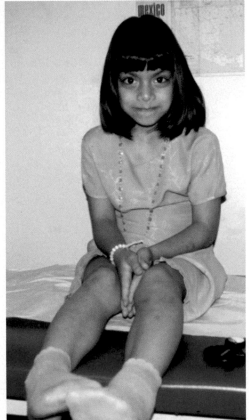

B

C

D

FIGURE 2. **A–D,** Affected child from birth through 5 years of age. Partial glossectomy was performed at 18 months (see **C**). (Courtesy of Dr. Lynne M. Bird, Children's Hospital, San Diego.)

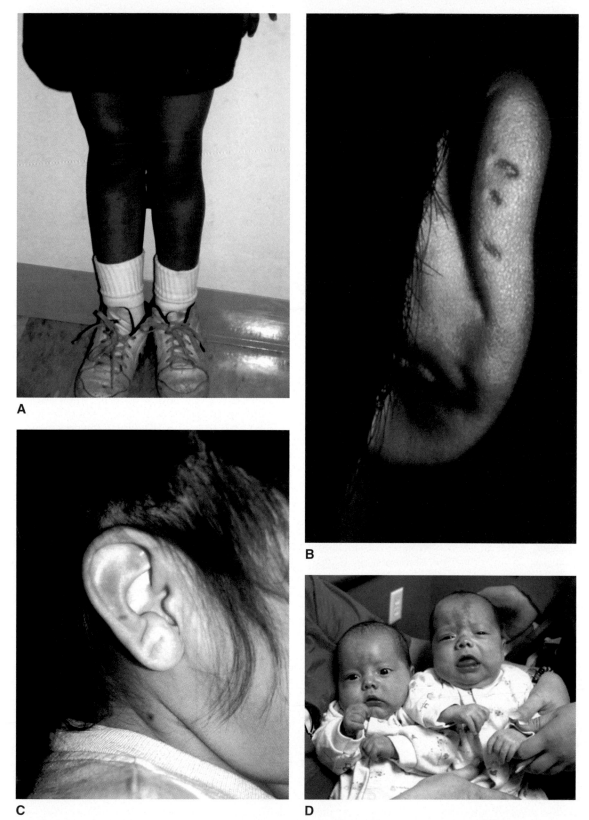

FIGURE 3. **A,** Asymmetry of legs. (Courtesy of Dr. Lynne M. Bird, Children's Hospital, San Diego.) **B,** Indentations on the posterior rim of the helix. **C,** Linear crease on the ear lobe. **D,** Newborn monozygotic twins discordant for BWS. (**D,** Courtesy of Dr. Cynthia Curry, University of California, San Francisco.)

SIMPSON-GOLABI-BEHMEL SYNDROME

Neri and colleagues and Opitz and colleagues recognized in 1988 that the disorder initially reported by Simpson and colleagues in 1975 was the same as that described in 1984 by both Behmel and colleagues and by Golabi and Rosen. Marked inter- and intrafamilial variability in expression has been documented in this X-linked recessive disorder. Carrier females sometimes have mild manifestations.

ABNORMALITIES

Performance. Intelligence has varied from severely retarded to normal, average IQ is approximately 1 SD below the mean, hypotonia.

Growth. Prenatal onset of overgrowth; birth weight as high as 5.9 kg; in seven of eight affected adults, height was greater than the 97th percentile and ranged from 188 cm to 210 cm; bone age, initially increased, becomes normal.

Craniofacial. Macrocephaly, present at birth, continues in childhood; coarse facies; down-slanting palpebral fissures; ocular hypertelorism; epicanthal folds; broad flat nasal bridge with short nose; macrostomia; macroglossia; midline groove of lower lip; broad secondary alveolar ridge; low-set posteriorly rotated ears.

Limbs. Postaxial polydactyly of hands, syndactyly of second and third fingers and toes, nail hypoplasia (particularly of index finger), broad thumbs and great toes.

Skeletal. Vertebral segmentation defects including fusion of posterior elements of C2/C3, cervical ribs, six lumbar vertebrae, and sacral and coccygeal defects; pectus excavatum.

Other. Short webbed neck, cardiac conduction defects; supernumerary nipples; cryptorchidism; spotty perioral or palatal pigmentation; thickened or dark skin; umbilical or inguinal hernias.

OCCASIONAL ABNORMALITIES.

Cleft lip, cleft palate, or both; indentations on posterior rim of helix; preauricular pits and tags; coloboma of optic disk; scoliosis; cleft of xiphisternum; preaxial polydactyly of feet; brachydactyly; camptodactyly; clinodactyly; broad thumbs; pectus excavatum; scoliosis; congenital hip dislocation; clubfeet; short limbs; vertebral anomalies; gastrointestinal anomalies including intestinal malrotation, pyloric ring, polysplenia, hepatosplenomegaly, and increased number of islets of Langerhans; genitourinary anomalies including large kidneys, cystic kidneys, duplication of renal pelvis, mild hydronephrosis with lobular cystic kidneys, and hypospadias; cardiac defects including ventricular septal defect, pulmonic stenosis, transposition of great vessels, and patent ductus arteriosus; choledochal cyst; central nervous system abnormalities including agenesis of corpus callosum, hypoplasia of cerebellar vermis, and hydrocephalus; embryonal tumors; diaphragmatic hernias; diffuse neonatal hemangiomatosis.

NATURAL HISTORY. Both a severe neonatal form in which babies often die in utero or in the neonatal period from cor pulmonale, heart failure, congenital heart defects or conduction defects, diaphragmatic hernias, overwhelming sepsis, or hypoglycemia from increased insulin production and a less severe form in which affected individuals live into adulthood have been described. An increased risk exists for development of Wilms tumor, neuroblastoma, hepatocellular carcinoma, and testicular gonadoblastoma.

ETIOLOGY. This disorder has an X-linked recessive inheritance pattern. Most cases have been attributed to mutations in the glypican-3 gene (GPC3) located at Xq26. Glypican 3 is thought to play an important role in growth control in embryonic mesodermal tissue. A severe form has been mapped to Xp22. Female carriers have a milder phenotype.

References

Simpson JL et al: A previously unrecognized X-linked syndrome of dysmorphia. Birth Defects 11:18, 1975.

Behmel A et al: A new X-linked dysplasia gigantism syndrome: Identical with the Simpson dysplasia syndrome? Hum Genet 67:409, 1984.

Golabi M, Rosen L: A new X-linked mental retardation–overgrowth syndrome. Am J Med Genet 17:345, 1984.

Neri G et al: Simpson-Golabi-Behmel syndrome: An X-linked encephalo-tropho-schisis syndrome. Am J Med Genet 30:287, 1988.

Gargunta CL, Bodurtha JN: Report of another family with Simpson-Golabi-Behmel syndrome and a review of the literature. Am J Med Genet 44:129, 1992.

Hughes-Benzie RM et al: Simpson-Golabi-Behmel syndrome associated with renal dysplasia and embryonal tumor: Localization of the gene to Xqcen-q21. Am J Med Genet 43:428, 1992.

Pilia G et al: Mutations in GPC3, a glypican gene, cause the Simpson-Golabi-Behmel overgrowth syndrome. Nat Genet 12:1, 1996.

Brzustowicz LM et al: Mapping of a new SGBS locus to chromosome Xp22 in a family with a severe form of Simpson-Golabi-Behmel syndrome. Am J Hum Genet 65:779, 1999.

DeBaun MR et al: Simpson-Golabi-Behmel syndrome: Progress toward understanding the molecular basis for overgrowth, malformation, and cancer predisposition. Mol Genet Metab 72:279, 2001.

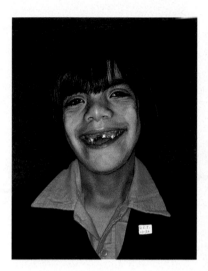
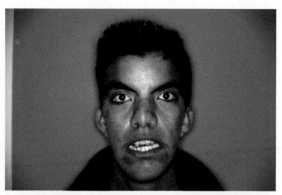
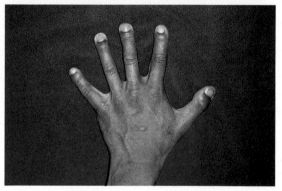

FIGURE 1. Simpson-Golabi-Behmel syndrome. Affected boy at 7 and 16 years of age. Note the ocular hypertelorism, broad flat nose, 2–3 syndactyly, and nail hypoplasia. (From Golabi M, Rosen L: Am J Med Genet 17:345, 1984, with permission. Copyright © 1984. Reprinted with permission of Wiley-Liss, Inc., a subsidiary of John Wiley & Sons, Inc.)

F Unusual Brain and/or Neuromuscular Findings with Associated Defects

AMYOPLASIA CONGENITA DISRUPTIVE SEQUENCE

Arms Extended with Flexion of Hands and Wrists, Shoulders Internally Rotated with Decreased Muscle Mass, Bilateral Equinovarus, Variable Contractures of Other Major Joints

ABNORMALITIES

Facies. Round face with micrognathia, small upturned nose, midline capillary hemangioma.

Shoulders. Rounded and sloping with decreased muscle mass, internally rotated.

Upper Limbs. Elbows usually in extension with wrists and hands flexed ("policeman tip" position). Severe flexion contractures at metacarpophalangeal joints with mild contractures at interphalangeal joints.

Lower Limbs. Hips, usually flexed, dislocated, adducted, or abducted; knees, flexed or extended; feet, usually equinovarus positioning bilaterally; many combinations of hip and knee positions observed.

Other. Stiff, straight spine.

OCCASIONAL ABNORMALITIES.

Cord wrapping of limb, amniotic bands, smashed digits, cryptorchidism, hypoplastic labia, dimples at contracture sites, torticollis, scoliosis, hernias, gastroschisis, nonduodenal intestinal atresia, defects of muscular layer of trunk and abdominal musculature, Poland sequence, Moebius anomaly, hypoplasia of deltoids and biceps.

NATURAL HISTORY.

There is decreased movement in utero. Delivery is often difficult and breech presentation is common. Fractures of the limbs secondary to traumatic delivery occur. Intelligence is usually normal unless birth trauma because of stiff joints has occurred. There is decreased bone growth of involved limbs, and there may be increased flexion and pterygium at large joints with time. By 5 years of age, the majority of patients (85%) become ambulatory with good physical therapy. It is important to begin physical therapy and occupational therapy early to mobilize any muscle tissue present (particularly intrinsic muscles). Splinting and casting are used to maintain and improve range of joint mobility. More than two thirds will require orthopedic surgery, an average of 5.7 procedures per child. All four limbs are involved in 92% of patients; the legs alone in 7% and the arms alone in 1%. Most will attend regular classrooms at appropriate grade levels and most will be independent in their activities of daily living.

ETIOLOGY.

This disorder is sporadic. There is a higher incidence than expected in identical twins, with only one affected. Based on the fact that many of the associated abnormalities have been shown to be caused by an intrauterine vascular accident, it is most likely that hypotension in the developing fetal spinal cord at a time when anterior horn cells are susceptible to insults is the mechanism responsible for the unique arthrogrypotic changes seen in this disorder. Prenatal diagnosis with use of serial real-time ultrasonography, looking for abnormal movement, could be used to allay parental anxiety.

References

Howard R: A case of congenital defect of the muscular system and its association with congenital talipes equinovarus. Proc Soc Med 1:157, 1907.

Hall JG, Reed SD, Driscoll EP: Part I. Amyoplasia: A common sporadic condition with congenital contractures. Am J Med Genet 15:571, 1983.

Hall JG et al: Part II: Amyoplasia—a specific type of arthrogryposis with an apparent excess of discordantly affected identical twins. Am J Med Genet 15:591, 1983.

Reid COMV et al: Association of amyoplasia with gastroschisis, bowel atresia and defects of the muscular layer of the trunk. Am J Med Genet 24:701, 1986.

Robertson WL et al: Further evidence that arthrogryposis multiple congenita in the human sometimes is caused by an intrauterine vascular accident. Teratology 45:345, 1992.

Sells JM et al: Amyoplasia, the most common type of arthrogryposis: The potential for good outcome. Pediatrics 97:225, 1996.

DISTAL ARTHROGRYPOSIS SYNDROME, TYPE 1

Distal Congenital Contractures, Clenched Hands with Medial Overlapping of the Fingers at Birth, Opening of Clenched Hands with Ulnar Deviation

In 1932, Lundblom described a mother and her son with congenital ulnar deviation and flexion of the fingers. In addition, the son had a calcaneovalgus positioning of the feet. Hall recognized this condition as an entity in 1982 in her report of 37 patients with congenital contractures of the distal joints. Two groups of patients were recognized: type I (typical) and type II (atypical), based on the association of other specific anomalies. Bamshad and colleagues have revised and extended the classification to include type 1 (formerly DA type I) through type 9.

ABNORMALITIES

Hands. Neonate's hands are clenched tightly in a fist, with thumb adduction and medially overlapping fingers; hypoplastic/absent flexion creases; ulnar deviation and camptodactyly.

Feet. Position deformities (88%): bilateral calcaneovalgus (33%), bilateral equinovarus (25%), combinations (30%).

Hips. Hip involvement (38%): congenital dislocations, decreased abduction, mild flexion, contracture deformities.

Knees. Mild flexion contractures (30%).

Shoulders. Stiff at birth (17%).

OCCASIONAL ABNORMALITIES.

Trismus, mild scoliosis, limited range of motion of proximal joints, small calves, dimples, cryptorchidism, hernias.

NATURAL HISTORY. "Trisomy 18 position" of hand at birth in vast majority. Variable talipes involvement. The hands eventually unclench and may have residual camptodactyly and ulnar deviation. Twenty percent of adults have straight and fully functional fingers. Both neurologic examinations and intelligence are normal. There is remarkably good response to treatment in all joints.

ETIOLOGY. This disorder has an autosomal dominant inheritance pattern with extensive intrafamilial and interfamilial variability. The parent of an affected child might possibly express the gene through mild hand contractures only. This disorder is now divided into Distal Arthrogryposis 1 (DA1A) and DA1B based on whether the disease allele segregating in the family maps to the DA1A locus on chromosome 9. DA1 families in which the gene is not mapped to chromosome 9 are designated DA1B.

COMMENT. Eight additional disorders, all autosomal dominant, have been designated as Distal Arthrogryposis (DA) syndromes and are listed subsequently.

DA2A. Freeman-Sheldon syndrome (see page 242).

DA2B. Less severe than DA2A, but more severe than DA1. Affected individuals have vertical talus, ulnar deviation, severe camptodactyly, and a distinctive facies including a triangular shape, prominent nasolabial folds, downslanting palpebral fissures, small mouth, and a prominent chin. Inheritance is autosomal dominant. A gene for DA2B has been mapped to chromosome 11p15.5.

DA3. Gordon syndrome — Distal arthrogryposis in association with short stature, cleft palate, submucous cleft palate or bifid uvula, ptosis, epicanthal folds, mild facial asymmetry, and short neck (see Hall et al., 1982).

DA4. Distal arthrogryposis in association with scoliosis (see Hall et al., 1982).

DA5. Distal arthrogryposis in association with short stature, short neck, ptosis, immobility of face with or without keratoconus and decreased ocular range of movement, and smooth, shiny, tapering fingers with mild camptodactyly (see Hall et al., 1982).

DA6. Distal arthrogryposis in association with sensorineural hearing loss (see Stewart and Bergstrom, 1971).

DA7. Hecht syndrome (see page 256).

DA8. Autosomal dominant multiple pterygium syndrome (see McKowen and Harris, 1982).

DA9. Beals congenital contractural arachnodactyly (see page 552).

References

Lundblom A: On congenital ulnar deviation of the fingers of familial occurrence. Acta Orthop Scand 8:393, 1932.

Stewart JM, Bergstrom L: Familial hand abnormality and sensorineural deafness: A new syndrome. J Pediatr 78:102, 1971.

Hall JG, Reed SD, Greene D: The distal arthrogryposes: Delineation of new entities—review and nosologic discussion. Am J Med Genet 11:185, 1982.

McKeown CME, Harris R: An autosomal dominant multiple pterygium syndrome. J Med Genet 25:96, 1982.

Bamshad M et al: A gene for distal arthrogryposis type I maps to the pericentromeric region of chromosome 9. Am J Hum Genet 55:1153, 1994.

Bamshad M et al: A revised and extended classification of the distal arthrogryposis. Am J Med Genet 65:277, 1996.

Krakowiak PA: Clinical analysis of a variant of Freeman-Sheldon syndrome (DA2B). Am J Med Genet 76:93, 1998.

NEU-LAXOVA SYNDROME

Microcephaly/Lissencephaly, Canine Facies with Exophthalmos, Syndactyly with Subcutaneous Edema

Neu and colleagues reported three siblings with microcephaly and multiple congenital abnormalities in 1971. An additional family with three affected siblings from a first-cousin mating was reported by Laxova and colleagues in 1972. At least 40 cases have been reported subsequently.

ABNORMALITIES

Growth. Prenatal onset of marked growth deficiency (100%).

Central Nervous System. Microcephaly (84%); lissencephaly (40%); absence of corpus callosum (53%); hypoplasia of cerebellum (53%), pons; absence of olfactory bulbs.

Facies. Sloping forehead (100%); ocular hypertelorism (94%); protruding eyes with absent lids (40%); flattened nose; round, gaping mouth and thick everted lips; micrognathia (97%); large ears; short neck.

Skin. Yellow subcutaneous tissue covered by thin, transparent, scaling skin and edema (85%); ichthyosis (50%).

Limbs. Short limbs, syndactyly of fingers and toes (60%), extreme puffiness of hands and feet, overlapping of digits, calcaneovalgus, vertical talus, flexion contractures of major joints with pterygia (79%), poorly mineralized bones.

Other. Cataracts (25%), microphthalmia, persistence of some embryonic structures of eye, absent eyelashes and head hair, muscular atrophy with hypertrophy of fatty tissue, hypoplastic or atelectatic lungs, hypoplastic genitalia (50%), polyhydramnios, short umbilical cord, small placenta.

OCCASIONAL ABNORMALITIES.

Hydranencephaly, spina bifida, Dandy-Walker malformation, choroid plexus cysts, hypodontia, patent foramen ovale and ductus arteriosus, atrial septal defect, ventricular septal detect, transposition of great vessels, cleft lip, cleft palate, renal agenesis, bifid uterus, cryptorchidism.

NATURAL HISTORY.

Most patients were stillborn or died in the immediate neonatal period. Three infants survived 7 weeks, 2 months, and 6 months, respectively.

ETIOLOGY.

This disorder has an autosomal recessive inheritance pattern.

References

Neu RL et al: A lethal syndrome of microcephaly with multiple congenital anomalies in three siblings. Pediatrics 47:610, 1971.

Laxova R, Ohdra PT, Timothy JAD: A further example of a lethal autosomal recessive condition in siblings. J Ment Def Res 16:139, 1972.

Curry CJR: Letter to the editor: Further comments on the Neu-Laxova syndrome. Am J Med Genet 13:441, 1982.

Shved IA, Lazjuk GI, Cherstovoy ED: Elaboration of the phenotypic changes of the upper limbs in the Neu-Laxova syndrome. Am J Med Genet 20:1, 1985.

Ostrovskaya TI, Lazjuk GI: Cerebral abnormalities in the Neu-Laxova syndrome. Am J Med Genet 30:747, 1988.

Shapiro I et al: Neu-Laxova syndrome: Prenatal ultrasonographic diagnosis, clinical and pathological studies, and new manifestations. Am J Med Genet 43:602, 1992.

King JAC et al: Neu-Laxova syndrome: Pathological evaluation of a fetus and review of the literature. Pediatr Pathol Lab Med 15:57, 1995.

Carder KR et al: What syndrome is this? Pediatr Dermatol 20:78, 2003.

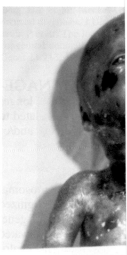

A

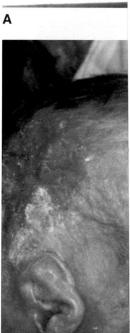

C

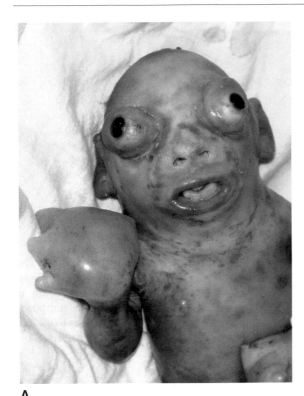

A

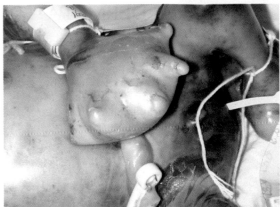

B

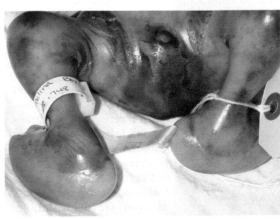

C

FIGURE 1. Neu-Laxova syndrome. **A–C,** Newborn with microcephaly, sloping forehead, protruding eyes with absent lids, flat nose, gaping mouth and thick lips, scaling skin with edema, extreme puffiness of hands and feet, syndactyly, and joint contractures. (From Manning M et al: Am J Med Genet 125:240, 2004, with permission.)

RESTRICTI

Initially described
colleagues in 198:
reported in appro
the features are c
restricted in utero
defective skin.

ABNORMALI

Growth. Intrauteri
Craniofacial. Enla
    entropion, sm
    with ankylos
    joints, microg
Skin. Tightly adher
    prominent ve:
    fissures often
    nails may be
    eyebrows, and
    head hair may
    is hyperkerato
    pilosebaceous
    and absence
    subcutaneous
    dermis is thin
    in parallel w
    absence of the
Skeletal. Multiple
    bottom feet; tl
    cles, ribbon-l
    bones of the a
    skull are prese
Other. Polyhydram
    short umbilic
    posterior diai
    hypoplasia.

X-LINKED HYDROCEPHALUS SPECTRUM
(X-Linked Hydrocephalus Syndrome, MASA Syndrome)

Hydrocephalus, Short Flexed Thumbs, Mental Deficiency

In 1949, Bickers and Adams first described X-linked recessive hydrocephalus associated with aqueductal stenosis. In 1974, Bianchine and Lewis delineated an X-linked recessive disorder referred to as MASA syndrome, an acronym for *m*ental retardation, *a*dducted thumbs, *s*huffling gait, and *a*phasia. Based on the similarities of their clinical phenotype as well as molecular studies that have placed the locus for both disorders, as well as X-linked corpus callosal agenesis, at Xq28, it seems clear that the three conditions are phenotypic variations of mutations in the same gene.

ABNORMALITIES

Performance. Mental retardation and spasticity, especially of lower extremities.
Brain. Aqueductal stenosis with hydrocephalus.
Hands. Thumb flexed over palm (cortical thumb) in approximately 50%.

OCCASIONAL ABNORMALITIES.
Asymmetry of somewhat coarse facies; brain defects such as absence of the pyramidal tract, fusion of thalamic fornices, agenesis/dysgenesis of corpus callosum, small brainstem, porencephalic cyst.

NATURAL HISTORY.
Prenatal hydrocephalus may be severe enough to impede delivery. However, many of the affected males have no hydrocephalus. Such individuals often have a narrow scaphocephalic cranium with an IQ in the range of 30 and tend to have spasticity, a shuffling gait, and aphasia.

ETIOLOGY.
This disorder has an X-linked recessive inheritance pattern. A number of different mutations in the gene encoding for the neural cell adhesion molecule L1CAM located at Xq28 have been reported in X-linked hydrocephalus families, in families with MASA syndrome, and in families with X-linked agenesis of the corpus callosum. The carrier female is usually normal but may have dull intelligence and/or adducted thumbs.

COMMENT.
Prenatal diagnosis is not always reliable in that ventriculomegaly usually starts after 20 weeks' gestation. Ultrasonographic studies should be performed every 2 to 4 weeks from 16 through 28 weeks' gestation. However, it should be recognized that hydrocephalus might develop postnatally or might never occur.

References
Bickers DS, Adams RD: Hereditary stenosis of the aqueduct of Sylvius as a cause of congenital hydrocephalus. Brain 72:246, 1949.
Edwards JH: The syndrome of sex-linked hydrocephalus. Arch Dis Child 36:486, 1961.
Holmes LB et al: X-linked aqueductal stenosis. Pediatrics 51:697, 1973.
Bianchine JW, Lewis RC Jr: The MASA syndrome: A new heritable mental retardation syndrome. Clin Genet 5:298, 1974.
Fryns JP et al: X-linked complicated spastic paraplegia, MASA syndrome, and X-linked hydrocephalus owing to congenital stenosis of the aqueduct of Sylvius: Variable expression of the same mutation at Xq28. J Med Genet 28:429, 1991.
Van Camp G et al: A duplication in the L1CAM gene associated with X-linked hydrocephalus. Nat Genet 4:421, 1993.
Schrander-Stumpel C et al: The spectrum of complicated spastic paraplegia, MASA syndrome and X-linked hydrocephalus: Contribution of DNA linkage analysis in genetic counseling of individual families. Genet Couns 5:1, 1994.
Schrander-Stumpel C, Fryns J-P: Congenital hydrocephalus: Nosology and guidelines for clinical approach and genetic counselling. Eur J Pediatr 157:355, 1998.
Weller S, Gartner J: Genetic and clinical aspects X-linked hydrocephalus (L1 disease): Mutations in the L1CAM gene. Hum Mutat 18:1, 2001.

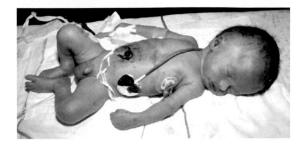

FIGURE 1. X-linked hydrocephalus spectrum. A male infant, who later died, was shown to have aqueductal stenosis as the cause for hydrocephalus. (Courtesy of Dr. Marilyn C. Jones, Children's Hospital, San Diego.)

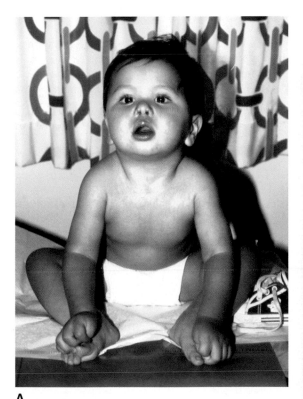

A

B

FIGURE 2. **A** and **B,** Boy with MASA syndrome. He has mental retardation, adducted thumb, shuffling gait, and aphasia. (Courtesy of Dr. Marilyn C. Jones, Children's Hospital, San Diego.)

HYDROLETHALUS SYNDROME

Hydrocephalus, Micrognathia, Polydactyly

This disorder was described initially by Salonen and colleagues in 1981. Hydrolethalus refers to hydramnios, hydrocephalus, and lethality, three of the most common features of this condition. Of the approximately 80 cases reported, the vast majority have been from Finland.

ABNORMALITIES

Central Nervous System. Severe prenatal onset of hydrocephalus, absent corpus callosum and septum pellucidum, abnormal gyrations, colobomatous dysplasia and hypoplasia of the optic nerve, cleft in the base of the skull. The resulting defect made up of the foramen magnum and the bony cleft extending posterior from it form a "keyhole-shaped" opening in the base of the skull.

Craniofacial. Micrognathia, cleft palate, cleft lip that is lateral or midline, broad nose especially at the root, microphthalmia, broad neck relative to the shoulders, malformed low-set ears.

Limbs. Postaxial polydactyly of hands, preaxial polydactyly of feet, clubfeet.

Cardiac. Defects in 50%, most commonly a large ventricular septal defect combined with an atrial septal defect to form an atrio-ventricular canal.

Respiratory. Defective lung lobation, malformed or hypoplastic larynx, trachea and/or bronchi are stenotic or rarely dilated.

Genitourinary. Duplicated uterus, hypospadias, malformations of vagina.

OCCASIONAL ABNORMALITIES.

Absent pituitary, arrhinencephaly, anencephaly, clefts in the lower lip, bifid nose, agenesis of tongue, hydronephrosis, urethral atresia, short arms, syndactyly, agenesis of the diaphragm, omphalocele.

NATURAL HISTORY.

The gestation of most affected patients is complicated by polyhydramnios. Intrauterine growth deficiency is the rule. Seventy percent of cases are stillborn. Liveborn infants survive for only a few minutes to a few hours.

ETIOLOGY.

This disorder has an autosomal recessive inheritance pattern. The hydrolethalus syndrome locus has been assigned to chromosome 11q23-25.

References

Salonen R et al: The hydrolethalus syndrome: Delineation of a "new" lethal malformation syndrome based on 28 patients. Clin Genet 19:321, 1981.

Toriello H, Bauserman SC: Bilateral pulmonary agenesis: Association with the hydrolethalus syndrome and review of the literature from a developmental field perspective. Am J Med Genet 21:93, 1985.

Salonen R, Herva R: Hydrolethalus syndrome. J Med Genet 27:756, 1990.

Visapaa I et al: Assignment of the locus for hydrolethalus syndrome to a highly restricted region on 11q23-25. Am J Hum Genet 65:1086, 1999.

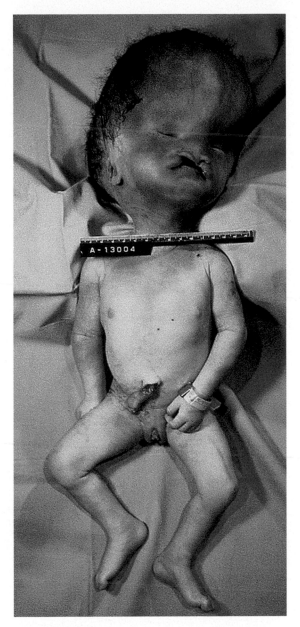

FIGURE 1. Hydrolethalus syndrome. Newborn infant.
Note the broad nasal root, cleft lip, and macrocephaly,
which is due to hydrocephalus. (From Toriello HV,
Bauserman SC: Am J Med Genet 21:93, 1985. Copyright
© 1985. Reprinted with permission of Wiley-Liss, Inc., a
subsidiary of John Wiley & Sons, Inc.)

WALKER-WARBURG SYNDROME
(Hard ± E Syndrome, Warburg Syndrome)

Initially described by Walker in 1942, this disorder was first suggested as a distinct entity by Warburg in 1971. The first familial cases were reported by Chemke and colleagues, and the full spectrum of associated defects was outlined by Pagon and colleagues and by Whitley and colleagues.

ABNORMALITIES

Brain. Type II lissencephaly (100%) manifest by widespread argyria with scattered areas of macrogyria and/or polymicrogyria; abnormally thick cortex with absent white matter interdigitations; absent or hypoplastic septum pellucidum and corpus callosum; cerebellar malformation (100%) including a polymicrogyric or smooth surface and hypoplasia of vermis; occipital encephalocele, which may be small (24%); Dandy-Walker malformation (53%); hydrocephalus usually from mechanical obstruction in the posterior fossa (53%); ventriculomegaly even in the absence of increased intracranial pressure (95%).

Eye. Anterior chamber malformation (91%) including cataract, corneal clouding usually secondary to Peters anomaly, and narrow iridocorneal angle with or without glaucoma; retinal malformations (100%) retrolental masses caused by hyperplastic primary vitreous, coloboma (24%), retinal detachment secondary to retinal dysplasia; microphthalmia (53%).

Other. Congenital muscular dystrophy (100%), genital anomalies in males (65%).

OCCASIONAL ABNORMALITIES.
Cleft lip with or without cleft palate (14%), microcephaly (16%), slit-like ventricles (5%), mild renal dysplasia, imperforate anus, congenital contractures (43%), megalocornea, microtia and absent auditory canals, gonadoblastoid testicular dysplasia.

NATURAL HISTORY. The majority of
affected children die within the first year of life secondary to the severe defect in brain development. Of those who survive, the majority have had profound mental retardation. Five percent to 10%, especially those with less severe retardation, survive longer than 5 years. For them rolling over and sitting should be expected to commence between 1 and 3 years. Seizures are common with increasing age.

ETIOLOGY. This disorder has an autosomal
recessive inheritance pattern. In some patients with Walker-Warburg syndrome, the disorder is due to mutations in the POMT1 gene, which encodes O-mannosyltransferase 1, the enzyme that reportedly catalyzes the first step in O-mannosyl glycan synthesis. Prenatal diagnosis at 20 weeks' gestation has been made on an affected fetus based on the presence of hydrocephalus.

COMMENT. Because of the wide spectrum of
brain and eye defects, the diagnosis is frequently not considered. Postmortem examination of the brain and eyes is often necessary. Elevation of the serum creatine kinase and "myopathic" changes on electromyography can be helpful in documenting the presence of congenital muscular dystrophy, which is present in virtually all affected patients.

References

Warburg M: The heterogenicity of microphthalmia in the mentally retarded. Birth Defects 7:136, 1971.

Chemke J et al: A familial syndrome of central nervous system and ocular malformations. Clin Genet 7:1, 1975.

Pagon RA et al: Autosomal recessive eye and brain anomalies: Warburg syndrome. J Pediatr 102:542, 1983.

Whitley CB et al: Warburg syndrome: Lethal neurodysplasia with autosomal recessive inheritance. J Pediatr 102:547, 1983.

Dobyns WB et al: Diagnostic criteria for Walker-Warburg syndrome. Am J Med Genet 32:195, 1989.

Rodgers BL et al: Walker-Warburg syndrome: Report of three affected sibs. Am J Med Genet 49:198, 1994.

Monteagudo A et al: Walker-Warburg syndrome: Case report and review of the literature. J Ultrasound Med 20:419, 2001.

Beltran-Valero de Bernabe D et al: Mutations in the O-mannosyltransferase gene POMT1 give rise to the severe neuronal migration disorder Walker-Warburg syndrome. Am J Hum Genet 71:1033, 2002.

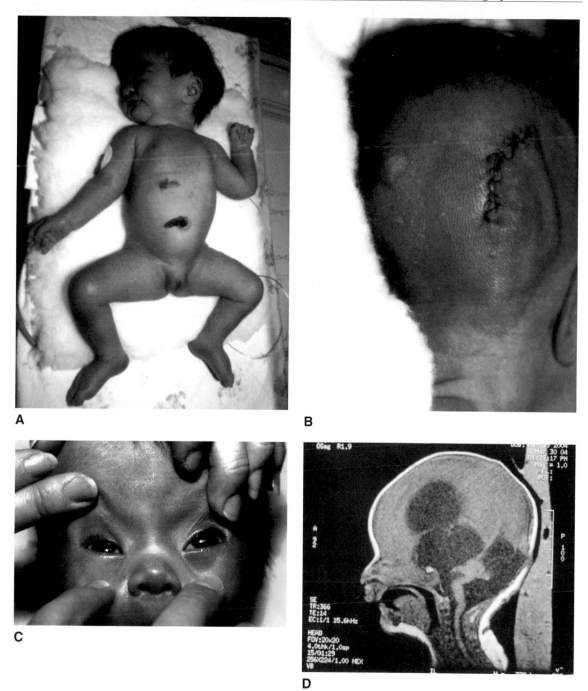

FIGURE 1. Walker-Warburg syndrome. **A,** Newborn female infant with hydrocephalus. Note the small occipital encephalocele (**B**), the unilateral microphthalmic eye (**C**), the encephalocele, and the magnetic resonance image showing an occipital defect (**D**). (Courtesy of Dr. Marilyn C. Jones, Children's Hospital, San Diego.)

MILLER-DIEKER SYNDROME
(LISSENCEPHALY SYNDROME)

Miller in 1963 and later Dieker and colleagues described a specific pattern of malformation, one feature of which was lissencephaly (smooth brain). Jones and colleagues expanded the clinical phenotype and introduced the term Miller-Dieker syndrome to distinguish this disorder from other conditions associated with lissencephaly.

ABNORMALITIES

Brain and Performance. Incomplete development of brain, often with a smooth surface, although areas of pachygyria are often seen inferiorly; heterotopias; both frontal and temporal opercula fail to develop, leaving a wide-open Sylvian fossa and a figure-eight appearance on computed tomography; absent or hypoplastic corpus callosum (74%) and large cavum septi pellucidi (77%); small midline calcifications in the region of third ventricle (45%); brainstem and cerebellum appear grossly normal; severe mental deficiency with initial hypotonia, opisthotonos, spasticity, failure to thrive, seizures, occasionally hypsarrhythmia on electroencephalography.

Craniofacial. Microcephaly with bitemporal narrowing; variable high forehead, vertical ridging and furrowing in central forehead, especially when crying; small nose with anteverted nostrils, upslant to palpebral fissures, protuberant upper lip, thin vermilion border of upper lip, and micrognathia; appearance of "low-set" and/or posteriorly angulated auricles; wide secondary alveolar ridge; late eruption of primary teeth.

Other. Cryptorchidism, pilonidal sinus, fifth finger clinodactyly, transverse palmar crease, polyhydramnios.

OCCASIONAL ABNORMALITIES.
Cardiac defect (tetralogy of Fallot, ventricular septal defect, valvular pulmonic stenosis), intrauterine growth retardation, decreased fetal activity, omphalocele, pelvic kidney, cystic dysplasia of kidney, lipomeningocele with tethered cord, sacral tail, cleft palate, cataract.

NATURAL HISTORY. Postnatal failure to thrive; gastrostomy because of feeding problems, poor nutrition, and repeated aspiration pneumonia; brief visual fixation, smiling, and nonspecific motor responses to stimulation are the only developmental skills usually acquired, although a few patients have rolled over occasionally; death usually occurs before 2 years and often within the first 3 months; one child lived to 9 years of age.

ETIOLOGY. A deletion at 17p13.3 has been documented in the majority of patients with this disorder. This defect has been found in association with ring chromosome 17, terminal deletion 17, unbalanced translocation inherited from a balanced reciprocal translocation carrier and a recombinant chromosome 17 because of crossover in a pericentric inversion carrier. For de novo abnormalities such as ring 17 or terminal deletions, the recurrence risk is negligible. In families with balanced rearrangements, the recurrence risk might be high. However, prenatal diagnosis is possible. In patients with highly suggestive phenotypes in which high-resolution chromosomal analysis is normal, the diagnosis can sometimes be established with fluorescent in situ hybridization using probes specific for the lissencephaly critical region on 17p. The LIS1 gene that has been cloned from the lissencephaly critical region at 17p13.3 encodes a protein referred to as PAFAH1B1, which is required for optimal neuronal migration. The major facial features of Miller-Dieker syndrome are thought to be due to deletion of additional genes in the critical region.

References

Miller JQ: Lissencephaly in two siblings. Neurology 13:841, 1963.

Dieker H et al: The Lissencephaly syndrome. Birth Defects 5:53, 1969.

Jones KL et al: The Miller-Dieker syndrome. Pediatrics 66:277, 1980.

Dobyns WB et al: Miller-Dieker syndrome. Lissencephaly and monosomy 17p. J Pediatr 102:552, 1983.

Dobyns WB, Stratton RF, Greenberg F: Syndromes with lissencephaly. I: Miller-Dieker and Norman-Roberts syndrome and isolated lissencephaly syndromes. Am J Med Genet 22:197, 1984.

Dobyns WB et al: Clinical and molecular diagnosis of Miller-Dieker syndrome. Am J Hum Genet 48:584, 1991.

Hattori M et al: Miller-Dieker syndrome gene encodes a subunit of brain platelet activating factor. Nature 370:216, 1994.

Dobyns WB et al: Differences in the gyral pattern distinguish chromosome 17-linked and X-linked lissencephaly. Neurology 53:270, 1999.

Pollin TI et al: Risk of abnormal pregnancy outcome in carriers of balanced reciprocal translocations involving the Miller-Dieker syndrome (MDS) critical region in chromosome 17p13.3. Am J Med Genet 85:369, 1999.

Cardoso C et al: The location and type of mutation predict malformation severity in isolated lissencephaly caused by abnormalities within the LIS1 gene. Hum Mol Genet 9:3019, 2000.

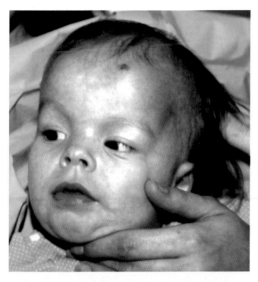

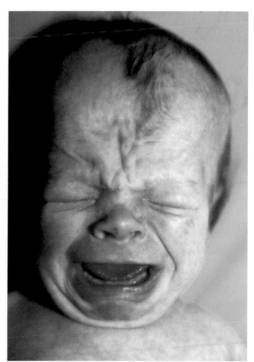

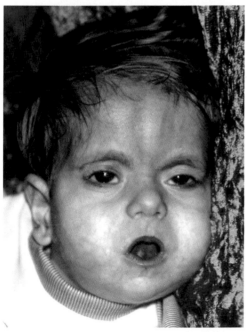

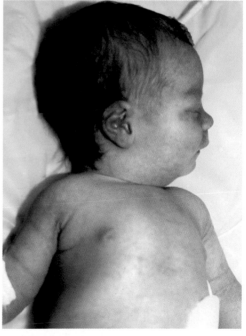

FIGURE 1. Facies of an infant with Miller-Dieker syndrome, showing high forehead with vertical soft tissue ridging and furrowing when crying, and small, anteverted nose.

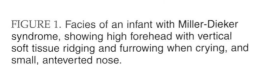

SMITH-MAGENIS SYNDROME

Broad, Flat Midface with Brachycephaly, Brachydactyly, Speech Delay

Initially described in 1982 by Smith and colleagues, the clinical phenotype including characteristic behavioral abnormalities have been more completely delineated by Stratton and colleagues and Greenberg and colleagues. Over 100 cases have been described. The minimum birth prevalence may be as high as 1/25,000.

ABNORMALITIES

Growth. Failure to thrive in infancy, postnatal growth deficiency.

Performance. Infantile hypotonia; intelligence quotients range from 20 to 78 with most falling between 40 and 54; speech delay with expressive language more delayed than receptive; hoarse, deep voice; self-destructive behavior including head banging, wrist biting, onychotillomania (pulling out fingernails and toenails) and polyembolokoilamania (insertion of foreign objects into body orifices); sleep disorders.

Craniofacial. Brachycephaly with flat midface, prominent forehead, broad nasal bridge, synophrys, downturned upper lip with protruding premaxilla, prognathia, low-set ears and/or other ear anomalies.

Limbs. Short broad hands and short fingers (brachydactyly), decreased range of motion at elbows, pes planus/varus.

Other. Cardiac defects; renal anomalies especially duplication of collecting system, brain anomalies (primarily ventriculomegaly); eye abnormalities including strabismus, myopia, microcornea, and iris dysplasia; hearing loss (both conductive and sensorineural); scoliosis; insensitivity to pain.

OCCASIONAL ABNORMALITIES.

Microcephaly, craniosynostosis, upslanting palpebral fissures, micrognathia (in infancy), Brushfield spots, cleft lip ± palate, cleft palate, iris coloboma, velopharyngeal incompetence, laryngeal abnormalities (polyps, nodules, edema, and paralysis), bifid rib, hemivertebrae, fifth finger clinodactyly, prominent finger tip pads, lymphedema of hands and feet, short or bowed ulna, cryptorchidism, borderline hypothyroidism, decreased immunoglobulins, jejunal atresia, bladder exstrophy.

NATURAL HISTORY. The clinical phenotype is rarely evident before late childhood or early adolescence. With increasing age, the frontal prominence; prognathism; brachydactyly; hoarse, deep voice; and coarsening of facial features become apparent. Although onychotillomania, most likely the result of insensitivity to pain, is uncommon in children younger than 5 to 6 years of age, head banging and wrist biting have been documented as early as the second year of life. Severe sleep disturbances are common. Usual bedtime is early (8:00 or 8:30 PM); one to three arousals throughout the night are common; and affected individuals frequently awaken between 4 and 6 AM. Exhaustion during morning hours, naps throughout the day, and inability to remain awake during the early evening are associated with tantrums.

ETIOLOGY. This disorder involves an interstitial deletion of chromosome band 17p11.2. The deletion can be difficult to detect at resolution levels of less than 500 bands. Although the vast majority of cases have been sporadic, transmission from a mosaic mother has occurred on one occasion, suggesting that parental chromosomes should be examined in all cases.

COMMENT. Individuals with Smith-Magenis syndrome have a phase shift of their circadian rhythm of melatonin with a paradoxical diurnal secretion of the hormone. It has been hypothesized that some of the hyperactivity and other behavioral problems may occur as the child struggles to remain awake during the day at the time of paradoxical increase in melatonin levels.

References

Smith ACM et al: Deletion of the 17 short arm in the two patients with facial clefts. Am J Hum Genet 34(Suppl):A410, 1982.

Smith ACM et al: Interstitial deletion of (17) (p11.2p11.2) in nine patients. Am J Med Genet 24:383, 1986.

Stratton RF et al: Interstitial deletion of (17) (p11.2p11.2): Report of six additional patients with a new chromosome deletion syndrome. Am J Med Genet 24:421, 1986.

Greenberg F et al: Molecular analysis of the Smith-Magenis syndrome: A possible contiguous gene syndrome associated with del (17) (p11.2). Am J Hum Genet 49:1207, 1991.

Greenberg F et al: Multi-disciplinary clinical study of Smith-Magenis syndrome (Deletion 17p11.2). Am J Med Genet 62:247, 1996.

De leersynder H et al: Inversion of the circadian rhythm of melatonin in the Smith-Magenis syndrome. J Pediatr 139:111, 2001.

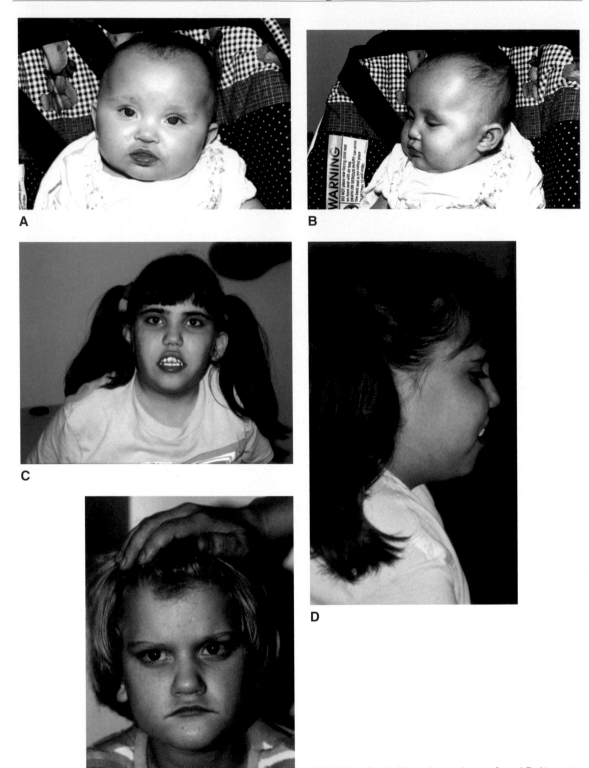

FIGURE 1. Smith-Magenis syndrome. **A** and **B,** Neonate showing brachycephaly, flat face, and prominent forehead. Note the similarity of this child's face to that of the Down syndrome. (Courtesy of Dr. Marilyn C. Jones, Children's Hospital, San Diego.) **C–E,** Note the downturned upper lip and protruding premaxilla.

ATAXIA-TELANGIECTASIA SYNDROME
(Louis-Bar Syndrome)

Ataxia, Telangiectasia, Lymphopenia, Immune Deficit

This disease was initially described by Louis-Bar in 1941. More recently it has received broader recognition, with many cases having been reported and its broader implications documented.

ABNORMALITIES

Growth. Deficiency, variable in age of onset.

Central Nervous System. Progressive ataxia and other evidence of degeneration of central nervous system (CNS) function, particularly in the cerebellum.

Skin and Conjunctivae. Telangiectasia in bulbar conjunctivae and later over bridge of nose, auricles, and elsewhere.

Respiratory. Inflammation of mucous membranes, frequent respiratory infections, bronchiectasis.

Immune System. Deficiency in cellular immunity with thymic hypoplasia, hypoplasia of tonsil and adenoid lymphoid tissue, lymphopenia, low to absent serum and secretory IgA and serum IgE, and the presence of a low-molecular-weight IgM.

OCCASIONAL FEATURES

Skin and Hair. Areas of altered skin or hair pigmentation, including café au lait spots; sclerodermatous changes.

Lymphoreticular System. Malignancy, including leukemia, sarcoma, and Hodgkin's disease, in approximately 10% of patients.

Gonads. Hypogonadism with absent or hypoplastic ovaries, ovarian dysgerminoma or hypoplasia, infertility.

Other. Endocrine abnormalities including hyperinsulinism, insulin resistance, and hyperglycemia; hepatic abnormalities with increased alpha-fetoprotein; hypersensitivity of fibroblasts and lymphocytes to ionizing radiation; primary carcinomas of stomach, liver, ovary, salivary glands, oral cavity, breast, and pancreas have been reported infrequently.

NATURAL HISTORY. Growth deficiency, although it may be prenatal in onset, more commonly becomes evident in later infancy or in childhood. Progressive ataxia usually develops during infancy and is commonly accompanied by features of choreoathetosis and by dysrhythmic speech, drooling, aberrant ocular movements such as fixation nystagmus, stooped posture plus dull sad facies, and occasionally seizures. Instability, suggesting vestibular deficit, often becomes so severe that ambulation is no longer possible in later childhood. These children are usually affable and pleasant despite their progressive handicap. Mental deficiency, although difficult to access, becomes evident in some cases in later stages of this fatal disease. Telangiectasias usually appear between 2 and 8 years. The immune deficiency probably contributes to the frequent respiratory infections and bronchiectasis that become prominent after 3 years of age. The persistent inflammation and progressive generalized bronchiectasis are relatively unresponsive to antibiotic management, and there may be a basic problem in the mucous membranes besides the cellular immune deficit. Death is usually a consequence of lung infection, neurologic deficit, or malignancy. Patients seldom survive later childhood. The oldest survivor was 37 years old, and the disease had been quiescent for 20 years.

ETIOLOGY. This disorder has an autosomal recessive inheritance pattern. The gene, ATM, has been localized to chromosomal region 11q23. Although it is located primarily in the nucleus of cultured human cells, consistent with its proposed role in cellular response to DNA repair, ATM is also present in the cytoplasm. In addition to patients who are homozygous for ataxia-telangiectasia, it has been suggested that individuals who are heterozygous have an increased cancer risk, in particular breast cancer in women. Prenatal detection of an affected fetus has been performed successfully.

References

Louis-Bar D: Sur un syndrome progressif comprenant des télangiectasies capillaires cutanées et conjonctivales, à disposition naevoide et des troubles cérébelleux. Confin Neurol 4:32, 1941.

McFarlin DW, Strober W, Waldmann TA: Ataxia telangiectasia. Medicine 51:281, 1972.

Shaham M et al: Prenatal diagnosis of ataxia-telangiectasia. J Pediatr 100:134, 1982.

Swift M et al: Breast and other cancers in families with ataxia-telangiectasia. N Engl J Med 316:1289, 1987.

Gatti RA et al: Localization of an ataxia-telangiectasia gene to chromosome 11q22-23. Nature 336:577, 1988.

Swift M et al: Incidence of cancer in 161 families affected by ataxia-telangiectasia. N Engl J Med 325:1831, 1991.

FitzGerald MG et al: Heterozygous ATM mutations do not contribute to early onset of breast cancer. Nat Genet 15:307, 1997.

Brown KD et al: Multiple ATM-dependent pathways: An explanation for pleiotropy. Am J Hum Genet 64:46, 1999.

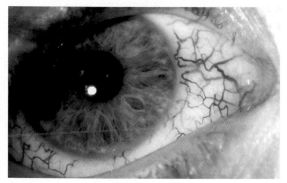

B

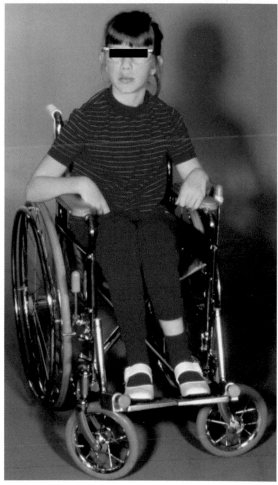

A

FIGURE 1. Ataxia-telangiectasia syndrome. **A,** Affected female. **B,** Bulbar conjunctiva. (**A** and **B,** Courtesy of Dr. Hans Ochs, University of Washington, Seattle.)

MENKES SYNDROME
(MENKES KINKY HAIR SYNDROME)

Progressive Cerebral Deterioration with Seizures, Twisted and Fractured Hair

Menkes and colleagues described five related male infants with this disease in 1962, and Danks and colleagues subsequently indicated that all features of the disorder are the result of copper deficiency.

ABNORMALITIES

Growth. Deficiency, sometimes small at birth.

Central Nervous System. Severe degenerative process in cerebral cortex with gliosis and atrophy; profound and progressive neurologic deficit beginning at 1 to 2 months of age with hypertonia, irritability, seizures, intracranial hemorrhage, hypothermia, and feeding difficulties.

Facies. Lack of expressive movement, pudgy cheeks.

Hair. Sparse, stubby, and lightly pigmented; shows twisting and partial breakage by magnified inspection.

Skin. Occasionally thick and relatively dry; unequal skin pigmentation at birth, particularly in darkly pigmented patients.

Skeletal. Wormian bones; metaphyseal widening, particularly of ribs and femur, with formation of lateral spurs that frequently fracture.

Other. Ocular findings including very poor visual acuity, myopia, and strabismus; gingival enlargement and delayed eruption of primary teeth; gastric polyps associated with gastrointestinal bleeding; pyloric stenosis; sliding hiatal hernia; bladder diverticuli; widespread arterial elongation and tortuousity noted on arteriograms and at autopsy most likely caused by deficiency of copper dependent cross-linking in the internal elastic membrane of the arterial wall.

NATURAL HISTORY. Progressive deterioration beginning in early infancy, with death usually by 3 years, although in one child as late as 13 years. Hair is normal at birth but by 6 weeks begins to lose pigmentation.

ETIOLOGY. This disorder has an X-linked recessive inheritance pattern. The gene responsible for this disorder encodes a copper transporting ATPase and is located at Xq13.3. Manifestations in the carrier female include hair that is lighter than would be expected for the family, pili torti (180-degree twist of hair shaft), and increased fragility and breakage of hair. Prenatal diagnosis can be made by gene analysis and by demonstrating excessive copper uptake in cultured amniotic fluid cells. The disease results from an abnormality in copper transport so that low levels of serum copper and ceruloplasmin are found in all patients studied. The basic defect at least partially involves reduced ability to incorporate copper into certain enzymes that need it as a cofactor. The clinical phenotype is due to a deficiency of these enzymes. For example, hypopigmentation due to tyrosinase deficiency; vascular tortuousity and bladder diverticuli due to lysyl oxidase deficiency. Subcutaneous therapy with copper-histidine may be an effective treatment if started early.

COMMENT. A child with Menkes syndrome presenting with subdural hematomas with a nontraumatic origin has been mistakenly diagnosed as having been the victim of child abuse.

References

Menkes JH et al: A sex-linked recessive disorder with retardation of growth, peculiar hair, and focal cerebral and cerebellar degeneration. Pediatrics 29:764, 1962.

Danks DM et al: Menkes' kinky hair syndrome. An inherited defect in copper absorption with wide-spread effects. Pediatrics 50:188, 1972.

Danks DM et al: Menkes' kinky hair syndrome. Lancet 1:1100, 1972.

Horn N: Menkes X-linked disease: Prenatal diagnosis of hemizygous males and heterozygous females. Prenat Diagn 1:121, 1981.

Kaler SG et al: Gastrointestinal hemorrhage associated with gastric polyps in Menkes disease. J Pediatr 122:93, 1993.

Sarkar B et al: Copper-histidine therapy for Menkes disease. J Pediatr 123:828, 1993.

Vulpe C et al: Isolation of a candidate gene for Menkes disease and evidence that it encodes a copper-transporting ATPase. Nat Genet 3:7, 1993.

Bankier A: Menkes disease. J Med Genet 32:213, 1995.

Gasch AT et al: Menkes syndrome: Ophthalmic findings. Ophthalmology 109:1477, 2002.

Nassogne MC et al: Massive subdural haematomas in Menkes disease mimicking shaken baby syndrome. Childs Nerv Syst 18:729, 2002.

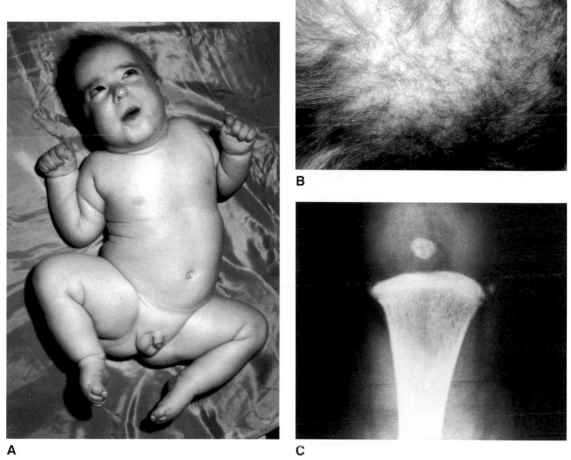

A

B

C

FIGURE 1. Menkes syndrome. **A–C,** Note the sparse, stubby hair and on radiograph the metaphyseal widening with lateral spur that has fractured.

22q13 DELETION SYNDROME
(PHELAN-MCDERMID SYNDROME)

Initially identified as a recognizable pattern of malformation in 1994, this disorder was more completely characterized by Phelan and colleagues in 2001. More than 50 cases have been published. The nonspecificity of the phenotype in newborns suggests that it is far more common than presently recognized.

ABNORMALITIES

Growth. Normal to accelerated.

Performance. Mental retardation, severe to profound in majority of cases; absent or severely delayed speech; hypotonia; frequent mouthing/chewing of objects.

Craniofacial. Dolichocephaly; prominent, dysplastic ears; pointed chin.

Limbs. Relatively large, fleshy hands; abnormal, dysplastic toenails.

OCCASIONAL ABNORMALITIES.
Microcephaly; seizures; CNS abnormalities including ventricular dilatation, delayed myelination, decreased periventricular white matter and arachnoid cyst; sensorineural hearing loss; ptosis; epicanthal folds; fifth finger clinodactyly; 2-3 toe syndactyly; cardiac defects, primarily patent ductus arteriosus and ventricular septal defects; vesicoureteral reflux and polycystic kidney; puffy, swollen feet.

NATURAL HISTORY. Hypotonia is common in infancy and is associated with poor oral intake, dehydration, and failure to thrive. Early developmental milestones are often delayed. Although lack of expressive speech is the rule, the ability of affected children to understand language is far more advanced. In one third of cases, a significant regression of skills has been observed.

ETIOLOGY. This disorder is caused by loss of genetic material near the terminal end of the long arm of one chromosome 22 at 22q13. It may result from a simple deletion, an unbalanced translocation, or formation of a ring. Although most cases occur de novo, can be identified with FISH analysis for 22q13, and have no increased risk for recurrence, 10% of cases result from the inheritance of an unbalanced translocation. In those cases, an increased recurrence risk exists. The gene SHANK3, which codes for a structural protein found in the postsynaptic density, is thought to be a major factor in development of the associated neurological features.

COMMENT. FISH analysis for 22q13 should be considered in all infants presenting with normal growth and hypotonia in the absence of a neurologic cause.

References

Nesslinger NJ et al: Clinical, cytogenetic, and molecular characterization of seven patients with deletion of chromosome 22q13.3. Am J Hum Genet 54:464, 1994.

Phelan MC et al: 22q13 deletion syndrome. Am J Med Genet 101:91, 2001.

Wilson HL et al: Molecular characterization of the 22q13 deletion syndrome supports the role of haploinsufficiency of SHANK3/PROSAP2 in the major neurological symptoms. J Med Genet 40:575, 2003.

Havens JM et al: 22q13 deletion syndrome: An update and review for the primary pediatrician. Clin Pediatr 43:43, 2004.

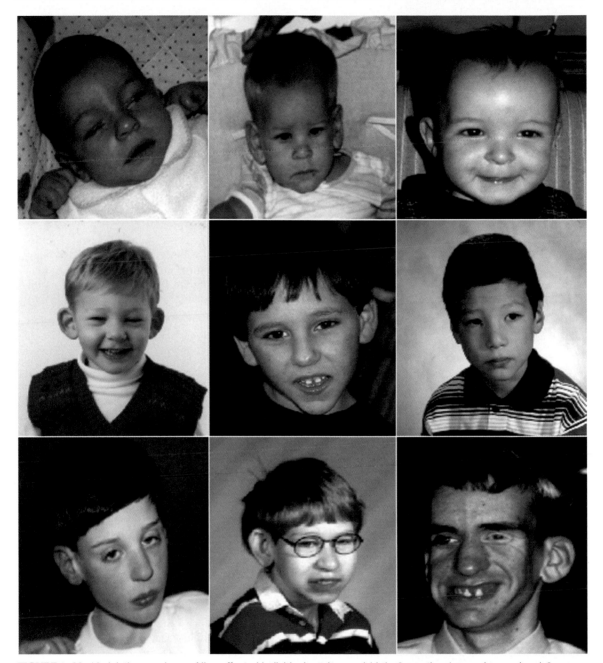

FIGURE 1. 22q13 deletion syndrome. Nine affected individuals at (*top row*) birth, 6 months, 1 year; (*second row*) 3 years, 5 years, 7 years; (*third row*) 9 years, 13 years, and 24 years. (From Phelan MC et al: Am J Med Genet 101:91, 2001, with permission.)

ANGELMAN SYNDROME
(Happy Puppet Syndrome)

"Puppet-Like" Gait, Paroxysms of Laughter, Characteristic Facies

This disorder, initially described in 1965 by Angelman in three unrelated children with severe mental deficiency, abnormal puppet-like gait, characteristic facies, and frequent paroxysms of laughter, has been more completely delineated by Williams and Frias, who have documented the natural history of this disorder and suggested that the term "happy puppet" is inappropriate.

ABNORMALITIES

Performance. Severe mental retardation with marked delay in attainment of motor milestones (100%), paroxysms of inappropriate laughter, absent speech or fewer than six words (100%).

Craniofacial. Microbrachycephaly; blond hair (65%); ocular anomalies, including decreased pigmentation of the choroid and iris, the latter resulting in pale blue eyes (88%); maxillary hypoplasia, deep-set eyes, a large mouth with tongue protrusion and widely spaced teeth; prognathia.

Neurologic. Ataxia and jerky arm movements resembling a puppet gait (100%); characteristic position of arms, which are upheld with flexion at wrists and elbows; seizures varying from major motor to akinetic, beginning usually between 18 and 24 months (86%); electroencephalographic abnormalities consisting of high-amplitude spike and slow waves at 2 to 3 Hz, posterior, large-amplitude slow waves mixed with spikes facilitated by eye closure, and generalized large-amplitude intermediate slow activity persisting for most of the record (92%); hypotonia and occasionally hyperreflexia; computed tomography shows cerebral atrophy (33%); left hand preference.

OCCASIONAL ABNORMALITIES.
Scoliosis; hypopigmentation (39%); strabismus (42%); myopia and hypermetropia; nystagmus.

NATURAL HISTORY.
The mental deficiency, although nonprogressive, is severe. Seizure activity most severe around 4 years, may stop by 10 years of age. The laughter is not apparently associated with happiness but rather is suggestive of a defect at the brainstem level. Decreased need for sleep particularly between 2 and 6 years.

Although severe problems exist with speech, the vast majority communicate in other ways, such as sign language. Receptive ability may be sufficient to understand simple commands. Most individuals become toilet-trained by day and some by night. None were capable of an independent living situation.

ETIOLOGY.
There are several known genetic abnormalities resulting in this disorder, all involving the chromosome 15q11-q13 region: a de novo interstitial deletion of maternal 15q11-q13 in 70% to 75% of cases; paternal uniparental disomy (UPD) of chromosome 15 in 2%; an imprinting center mutation in 2%; a mutation in the E3 ubiquitin protein ligase gene (UBE3A) in 5% to 10%; and an unidentified mechanism. Whereas the parental origin of the deleted chromosome 15 is paternal in Prader-Willi syndrome, it is always maternal in Angelman syndrome. The fact that the parent of origin of the deleted chromosome impacts the phenotype implies that genes located at 15q11-q13 on the maternally inherited chromosome are expressed differently from those at the same locus on the paternally inherited chromosome, a phenomenon known as genomic imprinting.

The vast majority occur sporadically except in the following situations: a chromosomal rearrangement or unbalanced translocation in which the same rearrangement occurs in the mother and an inherited imprinting center mutation.

COMMENT.
Patients with chromosome 15 deletions are more severely affected with a higher incidence of seizures, microcephaly, and hypopigmentation. A response to the standard physician issue tuning fork held close to their ear, including a wide smile, laughter, and a tendency to lean toward the vibrating tuning fork, has been documented and can be used as an adjunct test for this disorder in children as young as 12 months of age.

References

Angelman H: "Puppet" children: A report on three cases. Dev Med Child Neurol 7:681, 1965.

Williams CA, Frias JL: The Angelman ("happy puppet") syndrome. Am J Med Genet 11:453, 1982.

Boyd SG et al: The EEG in early diagnosis of the Angelman (happy puppet) syndrome. Eur J Pediatr 147:508, 1988.

Clayton-Smith J: Clinical research on Angelman syndrome in the United Kingdom: Observations on 82 affected individuals. Am J Med Genet 46:12, 1993.

Knoll JHM et al: Cytogenetic and molecular studies in the Prader-Willi and Angelman syndromes. Am J Med Genet 46:2, 1993.

Nicholls RD: Genomic imprinting and uniparental disomy in Angelman and Prader-Willi syndromes: A review. Am J Med Genet 46:16, 1993.

Hall BD: Adjunct diagnostic test for Angelman syndrome: The tuning fork response. Am J Med Genet 109:238, 2002.

Clayton-Smith J, Loan L: Angelman syndrome: A review of the clinical and genetic aspects. J Med Genet 40:87, 2003.

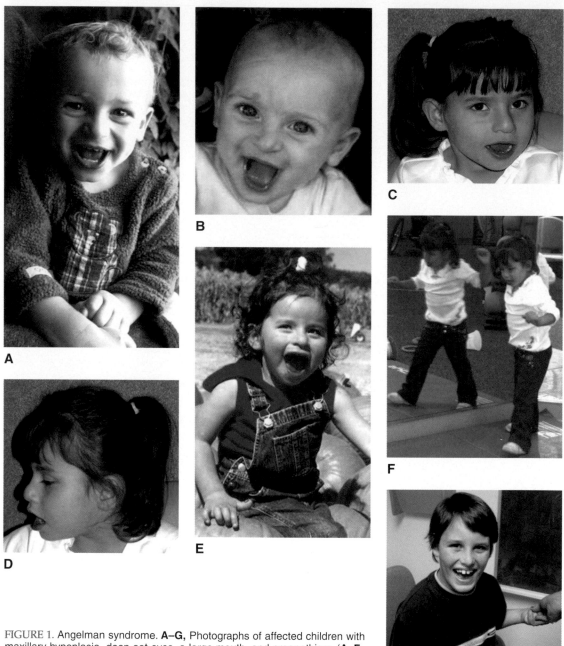

FIGURE 1. Angelman syndrome. **A–G,** Photographs of affected children with maxillary hypoplasia, deep-set eyes, a large mouth, and prognathism. (**A–F,** Courtesy of Dr. Lynne M. Bird, Children's Hospital, San Diego.)

PRADER-WILLI SYNDROME
Hypotonia, Obesity, Small Hands and Feet

Charles Dickens, in *The Pickwick Papers*, described "a fat and red-faced boy in a state of somnolency." The boy was subsequently addressed as "young dropsy," "young opium eater," and "boa constrictor," no doubt in reference to his obesity, somnolence, and excessive appetite, respectively. This may have been the first reported instance of Prader-Willi syndrome.

Prader and colleagues reported this pattern of abnormality in nine children in 1956. The prevalence is estimated to be 1 in 15,000.

ABNORMALITIES. Variability in the extent and severity of features based particularly on age.

Growth. Normal birth length with deceleration in the first 2 months of life, steady linear growth rate during childhood, and decrease in adolescence; mean adult height in males is 155 cm and in females is 147 cm.

Obesity. Onset from 6 months to 6 years.

Craniofacial. Almond-shaped appearance to palpebral fissures, which may be upslanting; narrow bifrontal diameter; strabismus; thin upper lip.

Hair, Eyes, and Skin. Blond to light brown hair with blue eyes and fair skin that is sunsensitive; picks excessively at sores.

Performance. Mental retardation is mild in 63%, moderate in 31%, and severe in the remainder; almost three fourths of affected individuals receive special education and function at a sixth-grade level or below in reading and third-grade level or below in math; food-related behavior problems including excessive appetite, absent sense of satiation, obsession with eating; speech articulation problems, particularly hypernasal speech; hypotonia, severe in early infancy.

Hands and Feet. Small; slowing in growth of hands and/or feet, usually becoming evident in midchildhood, one patient wore size 3 shoes at 23 years of age; narrow hands with straight ulnar border.

Genitalia. Small penis and cryptorchidism, hypoplastic labia minora and clitoris, frequent hypogonadism secondary to hypogonadotropism.

Other. Scoliosis, osteoporosis, temperature instability, high pain threshold, skill with jigsaw puzzles, decreased vomiting, growth hormone deficiency.

OCCASIONAL ABNORMALITIES. Poor fine and gross motor coordination; upsweep of frontal scalp hair; microcephaly, seizures, clinodactyly, syndactyly, hypoplasia of auricular cartilage; kyphosis; early dental caries; diabetes mellitus; early adrenarche; precocious puberty.

NATURAL HISTORY. The mother may have noted feeble fetal activity, and the baby is often born in the breech position. The hypotonia is most severe in early infancy, when there may be respiratory tract and feeding problems, not uncommonly necessitating tube feeding. The degree of mental deficiency may appear to be greater in infancy than at a later age because of the severity of the hypotonia hindering developmental performance. Regarding behavior, these patients have been noted to be cheerful and good-natured. However, behavioral problems, including stubbornness and rage-type responses, tend to become more frequent in later childhood. Verbal perseverance on favorite topics is common. Failure to thrive is frequent in early infancy, with obesity presenting between 6 months and 6 years of age, especially over the lower abdomen, buttocks, and thighs. The obesity, which is due to excess intake and reduced activity, paradoxically develops at a time when the hypotonia is improving. Bizarre and binge-type eating are common. The presence of a diabetic type of glucose tolerance curve relates to the severity of the obesity, and only an occasional patient develops diabetes mellitus during childhood. Therapy with growth hormone results in significant improvement of body composition (decreased fat mass, increased lean body mass, and increased linear growth) and physical function (strength and agility). However, a significant concern has been raised regarding a small risk of death in severely obese, respiratory-compromised individuals with Prader-Willi syndrome within 3 to 7 months of the start of treatment.

Reduced life expectancy appears to relate to complications of morbid obesity. In addition, the decline of IQ with age is obviated with weight control. Early short-term testosterone therapy has resulted in enlargement of the penis to normal size for age. Any boy who is doing reasonably well at the age of adolescence should be considered for full testosterone replacement therapy, because his testosterone production is usually inadequate. Sixty percent of females have amenorrhea and the remaining begin to menstruate between 10 and 28 years with an average of 17 years.

ETIOLOGY. Approximately 75% of affected individuals have a deletion of the long arm of chromosome 15 at q11-q13. In all cases studied, the paternally derived chromosome has been deleted. Maternal UPD (i.e., two maternal copies and no paternal copies of 15q) accounts for a further 20%. The remaining 5% are due to a mutation of the imprinting center or to a chromosomal translocation involving proximal 15q. Methylation analysis detects all three molecular defects. If the methylation pattern is abnormal, fluorescent in situ hybridization (FISH) can be used to document a deletion, and microsatellite probes can be used to confirm maternal disomy. An abnormal methylation analysis and normal FISH and UPD studies indicate an imprinting defect. Recurrence risk is negligible except for cases involving a chromosome translocation, or for those in which there is an imprinting center mutation.

COMMENT. Compared to those with deletion 15q, individuals with UPD 15 are less likely to be hypopigmented or to have the typical facial features as well as to show skin picking, skill with jigsaw puzzles, and high pain threshold. However, they are more likely to have psychotic illness.

References

Prader A, Labhart A, Willi H: Ein Syndrom von Adipositas, Kleinwuchs, Kryptorchismus und Oligophrenie nach myatonieartigem Zustand im Neugeborenenalter. Schweiz Med Wochenschr 86:1260, 1956.

Hall BD, Smith DW: Prader-Willi syndrome. J Pediatr 81:286, 1972.

Clarren SK, Smith DW: Prader-Willi syndrome. Am J Dis Child 131:798, 1977.

Ledbetter DH et al: Deletion of chromosome 15 as a cause of the Prader-Willi syndrome. N Engl J Med 304:325, 1981.

Creel DJ et al: Abnormalities of the central visual pathways in the Prader-Willi syndrome associated with hypopigmentation. N Engl J Med 314:1606, 1986.

Butler MG et al: Prader-Willi syndrome: Current understanding of cause and diagnosis. Am J Med Genet 35:319, 1990.

Holm VA et al: Prader-Willi syndrome: Consensus diagnostic criteria. Pediatrics 91:398, 1993.

Donaldson MDC et al: The Prader-Willi syndrome. Arch Dis Child 70:58, 1994.

Cassidy SB et al: Comparison of phenotype between patients with Prader-Willi syndrome due to deletion 15q and uniparental disomy 15. Am J Med Genet 68:433, 1997.

McEntagart ME et al: Familial Prader-Willi syndrome; case report and a literature review. Clin Genet 58:216, 2000.

Gunay-Aygun M et al: The changing purpose of Prader-Willi syndrome clinical diagnostic criteria and proposed revised criteria. Pediatrics 108(5), 2001. Available at: http://www.pediatrics.org/cgi/content/full/108/5/e92.

Boer H et al: Psychotic illness in people with Prader-Willi syndrome due to chromosome 15 maternal uniparental disomy. Lancet 359:135, 2002.

Carrel AL et al: Benefits of long-term GH therapy in Prader-Willi syndrome: A 4-year study. J Clin Endocrinol Metab 87:1581, 2002.

Cassidy SB: Prader-Willi syndrome: Is growth hormone replacement risky? Twenty-fifth Annual David W. Smith Workshop on Malformations and Morphogenesis. August 18–21, 2004.

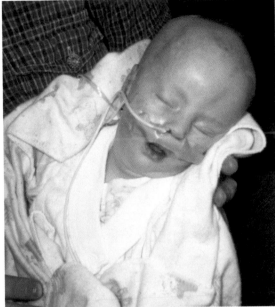

A

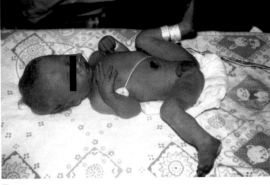

B

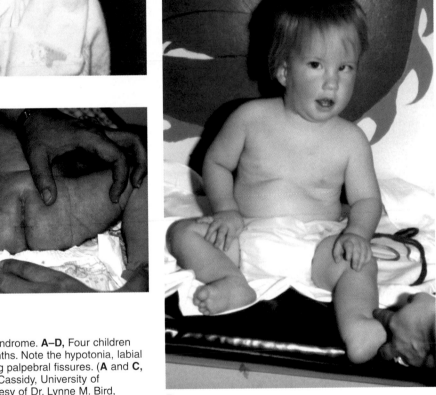

C

D

FIGURE 1. Prader-Willi syndrome. **A–D,** Four children from birth through 14 months. Note the hypotonia, labial hypoplasia, and upslanting palpebral fissures. (**A** and **C,** Courtesy of Dr. Suzanne Cassidy, University of California, Irvine; **B,** courtesy of Dr. Lynne M. Bird, Children's Hospital, San Diego.)

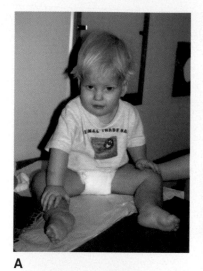

A

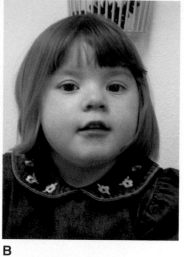

B

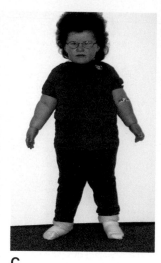

C

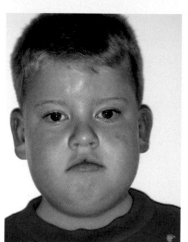

D

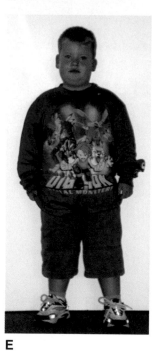

E

FIGURE 2. **A–E,** Note the almond-shaped eyes, narrow bifrontal diameter, and small hands and feet. (**A** and **B,** Courtesy of Dr. Lynne M. Bird, Children's Hospital, San Diego; **C–E,** courtesy of Dr. Suzanne Cassidy, University of California, Irvine.)

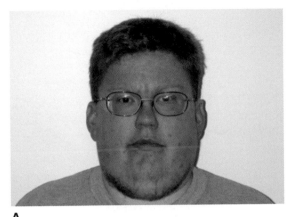

A

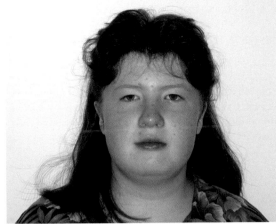

B

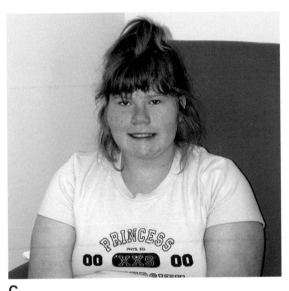

C

FIGURE 3. **A–C,** Affected young adults. (Courtesy of Dr. Suzanne Cassidy, University of California, Irvine.)

COHEN SYNDROME

Hypotonia, Obesity, Prominent Incisors

This disorder was recognized in 1973 in two affected siblings and one isolated case by Cohen and colleagues. In excess of 80 cases have subsequently been described.

ABNORMALITIES

Growth. Truncal obesity of midchildhood onset, low birth weight, postnatal growth deficiency.

Performance. Persisting hypotonia and weakness, mental retardation (22% profound, 61% severe, 6% moderate, and 11% mild), clumsiness.

Craniofacial. Microcephaly, high nasal bridge, maxillary hypoplasia with mild downslant to palpebral fissures, high-arched or wave-shaped eyelids, long/thick eyelashes, thick eyebrows, short philtrum, open mouth with prominent maxillary central incisors, high narrow palate, mild micrognathia, large ears.

Eyes. Decreased visual acuity, strabismus, defective vision in bright light, constricted visual fields, retinochoroidal dystrophy with bull's-eye–like maculae, pigmentary deposits, and optic atrophy.

Limbs. Narrow hands and feet with mild shortening of metacarpals and metatarsals, simian creases, hyperextensible joints, genu valgus, cubitus valgus, pes planovalgus.

Spine. Lumbar lordosis with mild scoliosis.

Other. Delayed puberty, cryptorchidism, granulocytopenia, thick hair, low hairline.

OCCASIONAL ABNORMALITIES.

Cardiac defects; microphthalmia, colobomata, enlarged corpus callosum, mild cutaneous syndactyly, seizures, growth hormone deficiency, ureteropelvic obstruction, tall stature, mitral valve prolapse.

NATURAL HISTORY. Neonatal feeding difficulties; weakness and hypotonia persist beyond infancy, and obesity of moderate degree has developed in midchildhood; motor milestones are delayed; all have developed speech, although to variable extent; a high-pitched voice is common; despite their moderate to severe degree of mental deficiency, the majority have a cheerful disposition; vision begins to deteriorate early but slowly; progressive myopia and retinochoroidal dystrophy in all patients older than 5 years of age; decreased left ventricular cardiac function occurs with advancing age.

ETIOLOGY. This disorder has an autosomal recessive inheritance pattern. Mutations in COH1, a gene located on chromosome 8q22 that encodes a transmembrane protein with a presumed role in vesicle-mediated sorting and intracellular protein transport, is responsible for this disorder.

References

Cohen MM Jr et al.: A new syndrome with hypotonia, obesity, mental deficiency, and facial, oral, ocular, and limb anomalies. J Pediatr 83:280, 1973.

Carey JC, Hall BD: Confirmation of the Cohen syndrome. J Pediatr 93:239, 1978.

Kousseff BG: Cohen syndrome: Further delineation and inheritance. Am J Med Genet 9:25, 1981.

Norio R, Christina R, Lindahl E: Further delineation of the Cohen syndrome: Report on chorioretinal dystrophy, leukopenia, and consanguinity. Clin Genet 25:1, 1984.

North C et al: The clinical features of the Cohen syndrome. J Med Genet 22:131, 1985.

Young ID, Moore JR: Intrafamilial variation in Cohen syndrome. J Med Genet 24:488, 1987.

Massa G et al: Growth hormone deficiency in a girl with the Cohen syndrome. J Med Genet 28:48, 1991.

Kivitie-Kallio S et al: Cohen syndrome: Essential features, natural history, and heterogeneity. Am J Med Genet 102:125, 2001.

Kolehmainen J et al: Cohen syndrome is caused by mutations in a novel gene, COH1, encoding a transmembrane protein with a presumed role in vesicle-mediated sorting and intracellular protein transport. Am J Hum Genet 72:1359, 2003.

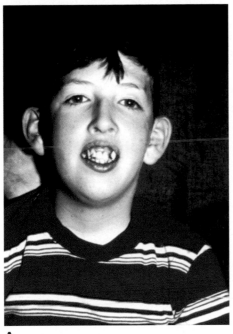
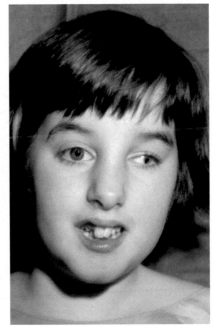

A

B

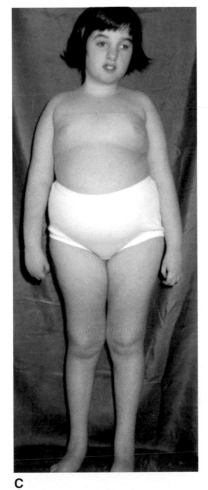

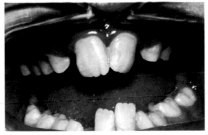

D

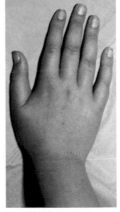

E

C

FIGURE 1. Cohen syndrome. **A** and **B,** Brother and sister at 11 and 14 years of age, respectively. **C,** An 8-year-old child in whom obesity developed at 5 to 6 years. **D** and **E,** Prominent central incisors and narrow hands with slim fingers. (**A–E,** From Cohen MM Jr: J Pediatr 83:280, 1973, with permission.)

KILLIAN/TESCHLER-NICOLA SYNDROME
(PALLISTER MOSAIC SYNDROME, TETRASOMY 12P)

Teschler-Nicola and Killian described a 3-year-old girl with this disorder in 1981. A second case was reported by Schroer and Stevenson in 1983. It was subsequently recognized that two adults with a similar phenotype and mosaicism for a marker chromosome reported by Pallister and colleagues in 1976 had the same condition. Tetrasomy 12p, either mosaic or total, has been documented in skin fibroblasts from affected individuals, but not in peripheral blood.

ABNORMALITIES

Growth. Normal or increased birth length, weight, and head circumference, with postnatal deceleration of length and head circumference; obesity frequently develops.

Performance. Profound mental deficiency with only minimal speech development, seizures, hypotonia with contractures developing with advancing age.

Craniofacial. Sparse anterior scalp hair particularly in temporal areas in infancy, with sparse eyebrows and eyelashes; prominent forehead; coarsening of face over time. Upslanting palpebral fissures; ocular hypertelorism; ptosis; strabismus; epicanthal folds; flat, broad nasal root and short nose with anteverted nostrils; chubby cheeks; long philtrum with thin upper lip and distinct cupid-bow shape; protruding lower lip; delayed dental eruption; large ears with thick protruding lobules; short neck.

Other. Streaks of hyperpigmentation and hypopigmentation, broad hands with short digits, accessory nipples, disproportionate shortening of arms and legs.

OCCASIONAL ABNORMALITIES.
Microcephaly; polymicrogyria; cataracts; stenosis of external auditory canal; hearing loss; mild mental retardation; hypopigmentation of fundus; macroglossia; prominent lateral palatine ridges; cleft palate; bifid uvula; micrognathia; umbilical and inguinal hernias; hypermobile joints; kyphoscoliosis; hemihypertrophy; fifth finger clinodactyly; distal digital hypoplasia; postaxial polydactyly of hands and feet; congenital hip dislocation; simian crease; sweating abnormalities; lymphedema; cardiac defect; pericardial agenesis; diaphragmatic hernia; persistence of urogenital sinus/cloaca; intestinal malrotation; imperforate anus; hypospadias; sacral appendage; renal defect; omphalocele.

NATURAL HISTORY. A significant number of affected patients are stillborn or die in the neonatal period. Seizures usually begin in infancy. Survivors are frequently bedridden. Most will never talk. Physical characteristics change with age. Initially sparse, anterior scalp hair grows in by 2 to 5 years; a normal-size tongue becomes macroglossic; initial micrognathia progresses to prognathism, and contractures develop between 5 and 10 years after initial hypotonia. The face of adolescents and adults is coarse with thick lips, an everted lower lip, a broad nasal root, and high forehead. The oldest reported patient is a profoundly retarded, nonambulatory 45-year-old man with multiple joint contractures.

ETIOLOGY. Tetrasomy 12p, either mosaic or total, in skin fibroblasts. An older maternal age affect has been suggested. Although most patients tested have had normal karyotype in peripheral lymphocytes, at least five patients have had lymphocyte mosaicism for an isochromosome of 12p. Fluorescent in situ hybridization (FISH) using chromosome 12–specific DNA probes has been successfully used to detect the isochromosome 12p in fibroblasts. Prenatal diagnosis is possible by amniocentesis and chorionic villus sampling.

References

Pallister PD et al: The Pallister mosaic syndrome. Birth Defects 5XIII(3B):103, 1976.

Teschler-Nicola M, Killian W: Case report 72: Mental retardation, unusual facial appearance, abnormal hair. Synd Ident 7(1):6, 1981.

Buyse ML, Korf BR: Killian syndrome, Pallister mosaic syndrome, or mosaic tetrasomy 12p? An analysis. J Clin Dysmorphol 1(3):2, 1983.

Hall BD: Teschler-Nicola/Killian syndrome: A sporadic case in an 11 year old male. J Clin Dysmorphol 1(3):14, 1983.

Schroer RJ, Stevenson RE: Further clinical delineation of the syndrome of unusual facial appearance, abnormal hair and mental retardation reported by Teschler-Nicola and Killian. Proc Greenwood Genet Cntr 2:3, 1983.

Reynolds JF et al: Isochromosome 12p mosaicism (Pallister mosaic aneuploidy or Pallister-Killian syndrome): Report of 11 cases. Am J Med Genet 27:257, 1987.

Schinzel A: Tetrasomy 12p (Pallister-Killian syndrome). J Med Genet 28:122, 1991.

Bernert J et al: Prenatal diagnosis of the Pallister-Killian mosaic aneuploidy syndrome by CVS. Am J Med Genet 42:747, 1992.

Bielanska MA et al.: Pallister-Killian syndrome: A mild case diagnosed by fluorescence in situ hybridization: Review of the literature and expansion of the phenotype. Am J Med Genet 65:104, 1996.

Adachi M et al: Pallister-Hall syndrome and neuronal migration disorder. Brain Devel 25:357, 2003.

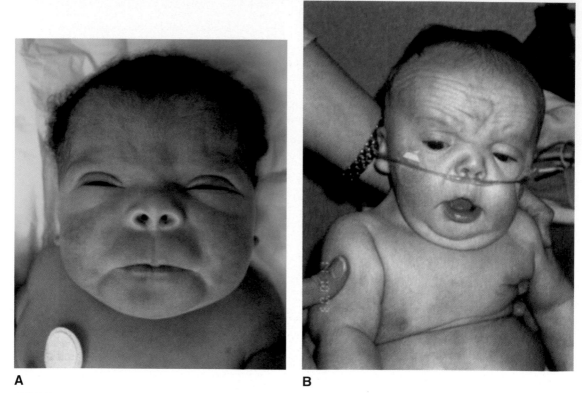

A   B

FIGURE 1. Killian/Teschler-Nicola syndrome. **A** and **B,** Affected newborn. (**B,** Courtesy of Dr. Stephen Braddock, University of Missouri, Columbia.)

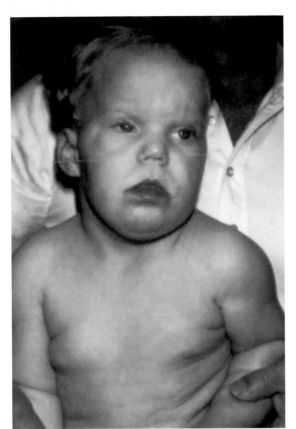

A

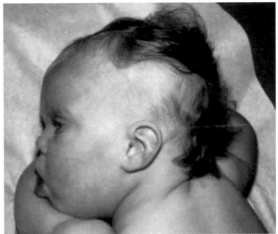

B

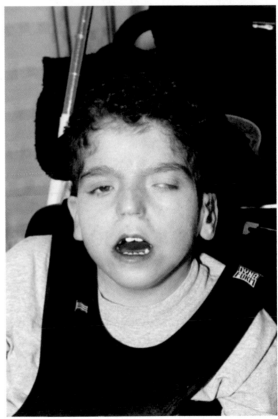

C

FIGURE 2. **A** and **B,** A 2-year-old affected child with sparse anterior scalp hair, eyebrows, and eyelashes. Note the prominent forehead, long philtrum with thin upper lip, and distinct cupid-bow configuration. (Courtesy of Dr. Robert Saul, Dr. Richard Schroer, and Dr. Roger Stevenson, Greenwood Genetic Center, Greenwood, SC.) **C,** An affected 10-year-old girl. Note that the hair, initially sparse anteriorly, has grown in and that the initial micrognathia has progressed to prognathism. (**C,** Courtesy of Dr. Marilyn C. Jones, Children's Hospital, San Diego.)

1P36 DELETION SYNDROME

Large Anterior Fontanel, Deep-Set Eyes, Pointed Chin

First delineated in 1997 as a recognizable pattern of malformation, monosomy 1p36 is the most commonly observed terminal deletion in the human population with an estimated prevalence of 1 in 5000.

ABNORMALITIES

Growth. Postnatal onset of growth deficiency, obesity.

Performance. Mental retardation, severe in the majority of cases; speech more severely affected than motor development; hypotonia; seizures.

Craniofacial. Microcephaly; brachycephaly; large, late-closing anterior fontanel; prominent forehead; deep-set eyes; flat nose and nasal bridge; thickened ear helices; pointed chin.

Cardiac. Structural defects in 43%, including patent ductus arteriosus, ventricular septal defect, atrial septal defect, bicommisural aortic valve, Ebstein anomaly; dilated cardiomyopathy in infancy (23%).

Other. Hypermetropia, hearing loss, short fifth finger.

OCCASIONAL ABNORMALITIES.

Cortical atrophy; ventricular asymmetry and enlargement; hydrocephalus; posteriorly rotated, low-set asymmetric ears; visual inattentiveness; strabismus; myopia; nystagmus; sixth nerve palsies; cataracts; colobomas; moderate optic atrophy; cleft lip with or without palate; bifid uvula; long philtrum; facial asymmetry; fifth finger clinodactyly; camptodactyly; small hands and feet; hypothyroidism; kyphoscoliosis; hip dysplasia; congenital spinal stenosis; metatarsus adductus; 11 pairs of ribs; bifid rib; polydactyly; cryptorchidism shawl scrotum; imperforate anus; abnormal pulmonary lobation.

NATURAL HISTORY.

Hypotonia occurs in the majority of neonates. Feeding problems including poor suck and swallowing, reflux, and vomiting are common in infancy. Hearing impairment, primarily sensorineural, is common and visual disturbances have been observed frequently. Full scale IQ scores are generally less than 60 and IQ less than 20 has been described. Seizures beginning in infancy, cease in the first few years in some children but persist, requiring long-term therapy, in others. Disturbed behaviors including temper tantrums, aggressivity, and self-injurious behavior are common. Survival into adulthood is the rule.

ETIOLOGY.

Terminal deletions of the short arm of chromosome 1 from 1p36.13 to 1p36.33, with the majority in band lp36.2. Although in some cases the deletion can be detected by high resolution karyotype, confirmation by FISH analysis is required in most. The breakpoints are variable leading to a variety of deletion sizes. This raises the possibility that differences in the clinical phenotype may be due to certain genes that map to certain deletion intervals suggesting that this condition is a contiguous gene syndrome.

References

Shapira SK et al: Chromosome 1p36 deletions: The clinical phenotype and molecular characterization of a common newly delineated syndrome. Am J Hum Genet 61:642, 1997.

Riegel M et al: Terminal deletion, del (1) (p36.3), detected through screening for terminal deletions in patients with unclassified malformation syndromes. Am J Med Genet 82:249, 1999.

Slavotinek A et al: Monosomy 1p36. J Med Genet 36:657, 1999.

Heilstedt HA et al: Physical map of 1p36, placement of breakpoints in monosomy 1p36, and clinical characterization of the syndrome. Am J Hum Genet 72:1200, 2003.

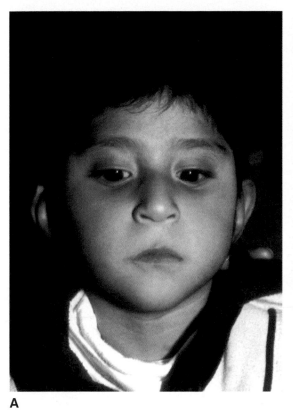

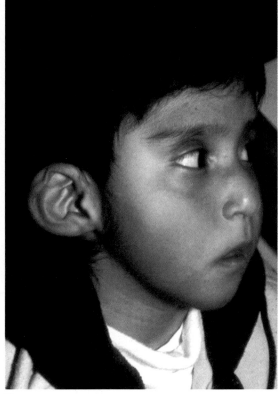

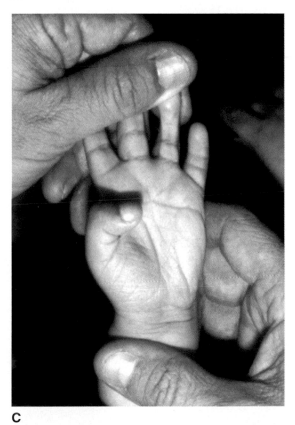

FIGURE 1. 1p36 deletion syndrome. **A–C,** Affected child with thickened ear helices, pointed chin, and missing distal crease on fourth finger with contracture (camptodactyly). (Courtesy of Dr. Marilyn C. Jones, Children's Hospital, San Diego.)

FRYNS SYNDROME

Diaphragmatic Abnormalities, Coarse Facies, Distal Digital Hypoplasia

This disorder was initially described in 1979 by Fryns and colleagues in two female siblings. Subsequently, 50 affected individuals have been reported.

ABNORMALITIES

Craniofacial. "Coarse" face (100%), abnormal ear shape (85%), cleft lip and/or palate (70%), large mouth (92%), microretrognathia (92%), broad nasal bridge (69%), anteverted nares (69%).

Thorax. Diaphragmatic defects (89%), abnormal lung lobations (60%).

Limbs. Distal digital hypoplasia (100%), usually represented by hypoplastic to absent nails and short terminal phalanges.

Genitourinary. Anomalies of genital tract in 86% including bicornuate uterus, uterus and vagina duplex, and/or uterine and cervical atresia in females; cryptorchidism, hypospadias, scrotalization of the phallus, and/or bifid scrotum in males; cystic dysplasia of kidneys (54%).

Central Nervous System. Malformation in 50%, including Dandy-Walker malformation, hypoplasia of optic or olfactory tracts, arrhinencephaly, and agenesis of corpus callosum.

Other. Intestinal malrotation and nonfixation, ventricular septal defects, broad medial ends of clavicles.

OCCASIONAL ABNORMALITIES.

Large for gestational age, microphthalmia, cloudy corneas, bowman irregularities, retinal dysplasia, thickened posterior lens capsule, camptodactyly, prominent fingertip pads, axial deviation of fingers, single transverse palmar crease, digitalization, proximal placement, wide or club-shaped and/or small thumbs, omphalocele, Meckel diverticulum, multiple accessory spleens, duodenal atresia, ectopic pancreatic tissue, anterior or posterior placement and/or imperforate anus, aganglionosis of colon and ureters.

NATURAL HISTORY. Cystic hygroma of the neck is common prenatally. The vast majority of affected individuals have been stillborn or have died in the early neonatal period. The survivors, one of whom did not have a diaphragmatic hernia and the other who was maintained on extracorporeal membrane oxygenation therapy for 5 days followed by high-frequency oscillatory ventilation for 1 month, both have significant mental retardation. A third, also with severe mental retardation, died in status epilepticus at 15 years of age.

ETIOLOGY. This disorder has an autosomal recessive inheritance pattern.

References

Fryns JP et al: A new lethal syndrome with cloudy corneae, diaphragmatic defects and distal limb deformities. Hum Genet 50:65, 1979.

Bamforth JS et al: Congenital diaphragmatic hernia, coarse facies, and acral hypoplasia: Fryns syndrome. Am J Med Genet 32:93, 1989.

Cunniff C et al: Fryns syndrome: An autosomal recessive disorder associated with craniofacial anomalies, diaphragmatic hernia and distal digital hypoplasia. Pediatrics 85:499, 1990.

Kershisnik MM et al: Osteochondrodysplasia in Fryns syndrome. Am J Dis Child 145: 656, 1991.

Dingens M, Fryns JP: Hematometra and sudden death in an adolescent female with Fryns syndrome. Genet Couns 10:329, 1999.

Cursiefen C et al: Ocular findings in Fryns syndrome. Acta Opthalmol Scand 78:710, 2000.

Ramsing M et al: Variability in the phenotypic expression of Fryns syndrome: A report of two siblings. Am J Med Genet 95:415, 2000.

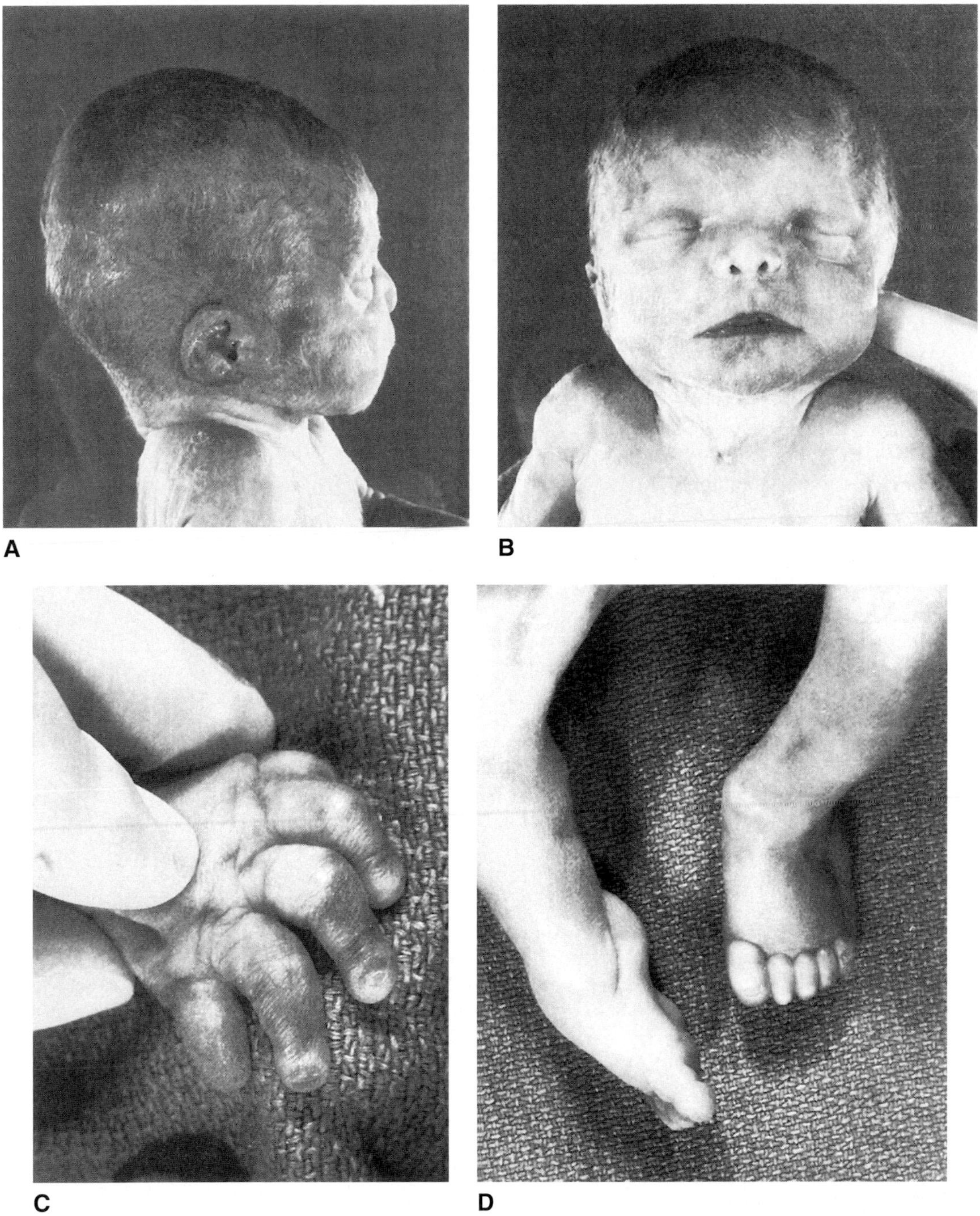

FIGURE 1. Fryns syndrome. **A–D,** Postmortem photograph of newborn infant. Note the broad, depressed nasal bridge; anteverted nares; poorly formed auricles; and hypoplastic nails. (From Cunniff C et al: Pediatrics 85:499, 1990, with permission.)

ZELLWEGER SYNDROME
(Cerebro-Hepato-Renal Syndrome)

Hypotonia, High Forehead with Flat Facies, Hepatomegaly

Bowen and colleagues and Smith and colleagues independently reported siblings with this pattern of malformation in 1964 and 1965. In 1973, Goldfischer and colleagues reported that peroxisomes, subcellular organelles that are present in all human cells except for the mature erythrocyte and have been shown to play a role in the production and degradation of hydrogen peroxide as well as in lipid metabolism, were absent in the liver and kidneys of two affected children. Multiple biochemical markers of peroxisomal dysfunction have subsequently been demonstrated.

ABNORMALITIES

Growth. Postnatal growth deficiency; mean birth weight, 2740 g.

Performance. Hypotonia, seizures, poor suck, severe mental retardation in survivors, deafness.

Brain. Gross defects of early brain development including pachymicrogyria, heterotopias/abnormal migration, subependymal cysts, astrocytosis and gliosis, hypoplastic corpus callosum, hypoplastic olfactory lobes.

Craniofacial. Large fontanels, flat occiput, high forehead with shallow supraorbital ridges and flat facies, anteverted nares, minor ear anomaly, inner epicanthal folds, Brushfield spots, mild micrognathia, redundant skin of neck.

Eyes. Congenital cataracts; pallid, hypoplastic optic disk; retinal pigmentary changes.

Liver. Hepatomegaly with dysgenesis, including cirrhotic changes.

Kidneys. Albuminuria; small cysts, chiefly of glomeruli.

Adrenals. Decreased weight, striated adrenocortical cells.

Cardiac. Patent ductus arteriosus, septal defect.

Limbs. Variable contractures with camptodactyly, limited extension of knee, equinovarus deformity; simian crease; radiographic stippling of patellae, greater trochanters, and/or triradiate cartilages.

Other. Variable elevated serum iron level and evidence of excess iron storage, pipecolic acidemia (not always diagnostic in first weeks of life), abnormal bile acids, accumulation of very long-chain fatty acids, and absent liver peroxisomes.

OCCASIONAL ABNORMALITIES. Prenatal growth deficiency, glaucoma, nystagmus, cubitus valgus, ulnar deviation of hands, deep sacral dimple, hypospadias, cryptorchidism, hypertrophied pylorus, single umbilical artery, breech presentation.

NATURAL HISTORY. Most of these babies were born from the breech presentation and failed to thrive. Some developed icterus and some had bloody stools, possibly related to hypoprothrombinemia. The vast majority die within the first year of life. Survivors have severe mental retardation and seizures.

ETIOLOGY. This disorder has an autosomal recessive inheritance pattern. Zellweger syndrome is one of a number of peroxisome biogenesis disorders (PBDs) that are manifest by absence or reduced numbers of peroxisomes in tissues as well as multiple enzyme abnormalities. All are caused by defects in a number of PEX genes, which encode peroxins, proteins necessary for peroxisome biosynthesis and import of peroxisomal proteins.

COMMENT. Zellweger syndrome (most severe), neonatal adrenoleukodystrophy (intermediate), and infantile Refsum disease (least severe) represent variants of the same disorder with a decreasing continuum of severity of the phenotype. They are associated with nine distinct defects in PEX genes.

References
Bowen P et al: A familial syndrome of multiple congenital defects. Bull Johns Hopkins Hosp 114:402, 1964.

Smith DW, Opitz JM, Inhorn SL: A syndrome of multiple developmental defects including polycystic kidneys and intrahepatic biliary dysgenesis in two siblings. J Pediatr 67:617, 1965.

Opitz JM et al: The Zellweger syndrome. Birth Defects 5:144, 1969.

Goldfischer S et al: Peroxisomal and mitochondrial defects in the cerebro-hepato-renal syndrome. Science 182:62, 1973.

Kelley RI: Review: The cerebrohepatorenal syndrome of Zellweger: Morphologic and metabolic aspects. Am J Med Genet 16:503, 1983.

Datta NS, Wilson GN, Hajra AK: Deficiency of enzymes catalyzing the biosynthesis of glycerol ether lipids in Zellweger syndrome. N Engl J Med 311:1080, 1984.

Hajra AK et al: Prenatal diagnosis of Zellweger cerebro-hepatorenal syndrome. N Engl J Med 312:445, 1985.

Solish JI et al: The prenatal diagnosis of the cerebro-hepato-renal syndrome of Zellweger. Prenat Diagn 5:27, 1985.

Wilson GN et al: Zellweger syndrome: Diagnostic assays, syndrome delineation, and potential therapy. Am J Med Genet 24:69, 1986.

Moser HW: Genotype-phenotype correlations in disorders of peroxisome biogenesis. Mol Genet Metab 68:316, 1999.

Steinberg SJ et al: Peroxisomal disorders: Clinical and biochemical studies in 15 children and prenatal diagnosis in seven families. Am J Med Genet 85:502, 1999.

Suzuki Y et al: Genetic and molecular bases of peroxisome biogenesis disorders. Gen Med 3:372, 2001.

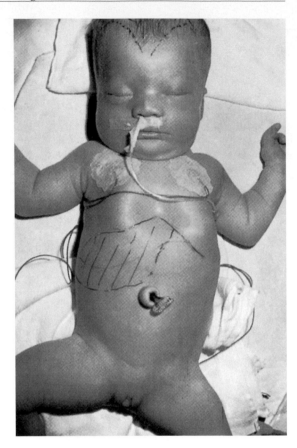

FIGURE 1. Zellweger syndrome. Affected infant showing hypotonia, enlarged fontanel, and enlarged liver.

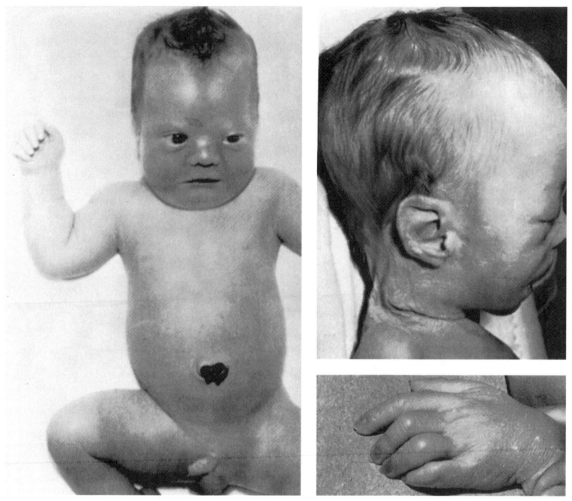

FIGURE 2. Affected siblings at 1 day of age (*left*) and postmortem at 10 weeks of age (*right*). Note camptodactyly of third, fourth, and fifth fingers. (From Smith DW et al: J Pediatr 67:617, 1965, with permission.)

FREEMAN-SHELDON SYNDROME
(WHISTLING FACE SYNDROME)

Mask-Like "Whistling" Facies, Hypoplastic Alae Nasi, Talipes Equinovarus

This disorder was described by Freeman and Sheldon in 1938 and at least 60 cases have been reported.

ABNORMALITIES

Most of the features are secondary to increased muscle tone.

Facies. Full forehead and mask-like facies with small mouth giving a "whistling" appearance (100%), deep-set eyes, broad nasal bridge, telecanthus, epicanthal folds, strabismus, blepharophimosis, small nose, hypoplastic alae nasi with coloboma, long philtrum, H-shaped cutaneous dimpling on chin, high palate, small tongue, limited palatal movement with nasal speech.

Joints and Skeletal. Ulnar deviation of hands (91%), cortical thumbs, flexion of fingers (88%), thick skin over flexor surface of proximal phalanges, equinovarus with contracted toes (59%), vertical talus, kyphoscoliosis (84%), contracture of hips and/or knees (73%), contractures of shoulders, steeply inclined anterior cranial fossa on radiographs.

Other. Postnatal growth deficiency (62%), inguinal hernia, incomplete descent of testes.

OCCASIONAL ABNORMALITIES.

Microcephaly (44%), mental deficiency (31%), seizures (19%), flat face, ptosis, upper airway narrowing, subcutaneous ridge across lower forehead, short neck, low birth weight, dislocation of hip, spina bifida occulta, cerebellar and brainstem atrophy, absent brainstem auditory evoked response, prominent mental protuberance on radiographs of facial bones.

NATURAL HISTORY. These patients are not uncommonly born in the breech position, and/or their delivery may be difficult. Vomiting and dysphagia may lead to failure to thrive in infancy. There may be early mortality, often related to aspiration. Difficulties with speech, oral hygiene, and dental treatment secondary to the small mouth can be a problem. Eventual intelligence is in the normal range in the majority of patients. Obstructive sleep apnea/hypopnea exclusively during REM sleep has been described. Muscle rigidity following halothane anesthesia has been reported, which gives credence to the theory that this disorder is the result of an underlying myopathy.

ETIOLOGY. This disorder has an autosomal dominant inheritance pattern. A clinically indistinguishable autosomal recessive type has been reported in three separate families.

References

Freeman EA, Sheldon JH: Craniocarpotarsal dystrophy: An undescribed congenital malformation. Arch Dis Child 13:277, 1938.

Burian F: The "whistling face" characteristic in a compound cranio-facio-corporal syndrome. Br J Plast Surg 16:140, 1963.

Antley RM et al.: Diagnostic criteria for the whistling face syndrome. Birth Defects 11:161, 1975.

O'Connell DJ, Hall CM: Cranio-carpotarsal dysplasia: A report of seven cases. Radiology 123:719, 1977.

Kousseff BG, McConnachie P, Hadro TA: Autosomal recessive type of whistling face syndrome in twins. Pediatrics 69:328, 1982.

Vanek J et al: Freeman-Sheldon syndrome: A disorder of congenital myopathic origin? J Med Genet 23:231, 1986.

Millner MM et al: Whistling face syndrome: A case report and literature review. Acta Paediatr Hung 31:279, 1991.

Jones R, Dolcourt JL: Muscle rigidity following halothane anesthesia in two patients with Freeman-Sheldon syndrome. Anesthesiology 77:599, 1992.

Kohyama J et al: Sleep disordered breathing during REM sleep in Freeman-Sheldon syndrome. Acta Neurol Scand 102:395, 2000.

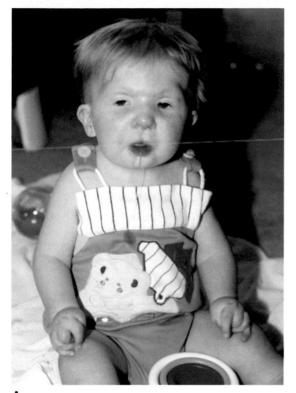

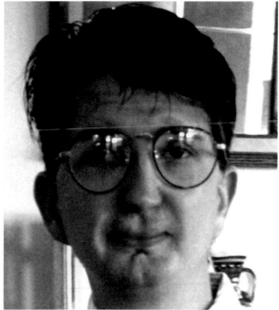

B

A

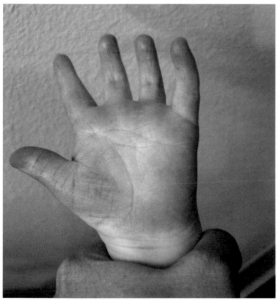

C

FIGURE 1. Freeman-Sheldon syndrome. **A–C,** Affected boy and his father. Note the crease pattern on chin, deep-set eyes, hypoplastic ala nasi, and camptodactyly. (Courtesy of Dr. Michael Bamshad, University of Utah, Salt Lake City.)

MYOTONIC DYSTROPHY SYNDROME
(MYOTONIC DYSTROPHY TYPE 1, STEINERT SYNDROME, DYSTROPHIA MYOTONICA)

Myotonia with Muscle Atrophy, Cataract, Hypogonadism

The text by Caughey and Myrianthopoulos presents the manifold abnormalities that may occur as features of this single mutant gene. Approximately 1 in 8000 individuals are affected.

ABNORMALITIES

Muscle Degeneration. Myotonia (difficulty in relaxing a contracted muscle), often best appreciated in the hand or jaw or by tapping the tongue; degeneration of swollen muscle cells giving way to thin and atrophic muscle fibers with weakness; ptosis of the eyelids is frequent; myopathic facies.
Eyes. Cataract, often evident only as "myotonic dust" by slit lamp inspection.
Gonadal Insufficiency. Testicular atrophy (80%) in males. Amenorrhea, dysmenorrhea, ovarian cyst in females.
Scalp. Premature frontal hair recession, especially in males.
Cardiac. Conduction defects with arrhythmias.

OCCASIONAL ABNORMALITIES.
Hypotonia in infancy, mental deficiency, microcephaly, brain abnormalities especially the anterior temporal and frontal lobes, talipes, clinodactyly, hernia, cryptorchidism, kyphoscoliosis, hyperostotic cranial bones, atrophic thin skin, macular abnormality, blepharitis, keratitis sicca, goiter, thyroid adenomata, diabetes mellitus.

NATURAL HISTORY.
The age of onset is from prenatal life to the sixth or seventh decade, with the average being between 20 and 25 years of age. Lens opacification is usually evident by slit lamp examination in the 20s. Initial signs of the disease are variable. Myotonia may be so mild as to be detected only when specifically tested for. Muscle wasting and weakness, occasionally asymmetric, most often involving the facial and temporal muscles, yielding the expressionless "myopathic facies." The most consistent evident weakness is in

the orbicularis oculi muscles. Other involved muscles are the anterior cervical and those of the arms, thighs, and anterior lower leg, with progression from proximal to distal. Ptosis of the eyelids is frequent, and pseudo-hypertrophy is an occasional feature. One of the most sensitive early indicators of muscle dysfunction is the radiologic evidence of partial retention of radiopaque material in the pharynx after swallowing. Mental deterioration may also be a feature. There is increasing debility, with death, usually by the fifth or sixth decade, as a consequence of pneumonia, cardiac failure, or intercurrent illness.

Congenital myotonic dystrophy is associated with polyhydramnios and decreased fetal activity. Severe hypotonia, difficulty in swallowing and sucking, a tented upper lip, talipes equinovarus (in some cases multiple joint contractures), cerebral ventricular enlargement, edema, and hematomas of the skin are all frequently present in the newborn period. Myotonia, muscle wasting, and cataracts are not seen initially. An infant mortality rate of approximately 25% has been documented, the majority of deaths occurring in the neonatal period because of respiratory failure. For those that survive, the symptoms diminish. However, at adolescence, typical features of the adult variant develop. Although the vast majority of affected children walk by 3 years of age, psychomotor retardation is present in all survivors. With the exception of five known cases of paternal transmission, congenital myotonic dystrophy has occurred only in the offspring of mothers who have myotonic dystrophy.

ETIOLOGY.
This disorder has an autosomal dominant inheritance pattern with variability in expression. The disorder is caused by an unstable trinucleotide repeat expansion containing cytosine-thymidine-guanosine (CTG) in the DM1 gene located at chromosome region 19q13.3. With transmission of the disorder to family members in subsequent generations, the severity of clinical symptoms increases and their onset occurs earlier. This phenomenon, known as anticipation, is due to expansion of the repeat, which is estimated to have

a 93% chance of occurring when the altered allele is passed from parent to child. It is generally thought that the size of the triplet expansion correlates with the severity of the disease and the age of onset. Thus, newborns presenting with congenital myotonic dystrophy have on the average the largest repeat sizes.

COMMENT. DNA based testing is indicated for evaluation of neonates with hypotonia and severe feeding problems, for confirmation of a clinical diagnosis, and for evaluation of at-risk asymptomatic individuals with a confirmed family history of myotonic dystrophy.

References

Caughey JE, Myrianthopoulos ND: Dystrophia Myotonica and Related Disorders. Springfield, Ill: Charles C Thomas, 1963.

Pruzanski W: Myotonic dystrophy—a multisystem disease: Report of 67 cases and a review of the literature. Psychiatr Neurol Med Pyschol (Leipz) 149:302, 1965.

Calderon R: Myotonic dystrophy: A neglected cause of mental retardation. J Pediatr 68:423, 1966.

Pruzanski W: Variants of myotonic dystrophy in preadolescent life (the syndrome of myotonic dysembryoplasia). Brain 89:563, 1966.

Bell DB, Smith DW: Myotonic dystrophy in the neonate. J Pediatr 81:83, 1972.

Brook JD et al: Molecular basis of myotonic dystrophy: Expansion of a trinucleotide (CTG) repeat at the 3' end of a transcript encoding a protein kinase family member. Cell 68:799, 1992.

Fu YH et al: An unstable repeat in a gene related to myotonic dystrophy. Science 255:1256, 1992.

Mahadevan M et al: Myotonic dystrophy mutation: An unstable CTG repeat in the 3' untranslated region of the gene. Science 255:1253, 1992.

Reardon W et al: The natural history of congenital myotonic dystrophy: Mortality and long term clinical aspects. Arch Dis Child 68:177, 1993.

Wieringa B: Commentary: Myotonic dystrophy reviewed: Back to the future? Hum Mol Genet 3:1, 1994.

Keller C et al: Congenital myotonic dystrophy requiring prolonged endotracheal and noninvasive assisted ventilation: Not a uniformly fatal condition. Pediatrics 101:704, 1998.

Meola G: Clinical and genetic heterogeneity in myotonic dystrophies. Muscle Nerve 23:1789, 2000.

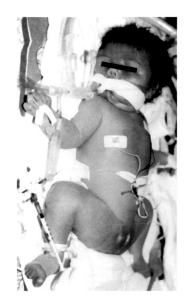

	FETAL-NEONATAL INFANCY	CHILDHOOD	ADULTHOOD
CNS	Mental deficiency ----------------------→		
OCULAR	Cataracts -----------------------→ Ptosis -----------------------→		
SKELETAL	Clubfeet	Scoliosis/lordosis ------→ Cranial hyperostosis ------→	
RESPIRATORY	Neonatal distress Recurrent infection ---------------→		Chronic insufficiency
NEURO – MUSCULAR	Hypotonia/"floppy" Facial diplegia Weakness/atrophy ----------------→ Variable myotonia ----------------→	Dysarthria -----------→	
GI	Poor feeding Impaired deglutition ---------------→		
GONADAL	Cryptorchidism ------------------→		Hypogonadism
CARDIAC		Disturbed conduction -------→	
MISC.		Frontal baldness -------→ Decreased IgG and IgM -------→	

FIGURE 1. *Above left,* Severely affected, almost immobile newborn baby of mother with myotonic dystrophy. (Courtesy of David Weaver, Indiana University, Indianapolis.) *Above right,* Correlation of protean features of myotonic dystrophy with age of onset, beginning with earliest age reported.

SCHWARTZ-JAMPEL SYNDROME
(CHONDRODYSTROPHIA MYOTONIA)

Myotonia, Blepharophimosis, Joint Limitation

Although Pinto and de Sousa were the first to report this disorder, this fact was only recently appreciated. Schwartz and Jampel described a brother and sister with this condition in 1962, and later Aberfeld and colleagues reported further observations on the same patients. At least 50 cases have been reported. Many, if not most, of the features appear to be secondary to a primary muscle disorder with myotonia. Based on the severity and age of onset of symptoms, three different types have been delineated. Type 1A is described subsequently. Types 1B and 2 are summarized in the comment section.

ABNORMALITIES

Growth. Small stature, usually of postnatal onset.

Muscle. Myotonia with sad, fixed facies, pursed lips, and narrowed palpebral fissures; small mandible; muscular hypertrophy in one half of patients; hyporeflexia.

Joints. Limitation in hips, wrists, fingers, toes, and spine.

Other Skeletal. Vertical shortness of vertebrae (platyspondyly) with short neck, enlarged epiphysis at the knees, progressive dysplasia of femoral heads, diaphyses of leg bones bowed anteriorly, hip dysplasia with acetabular flattening, narrow pelvis, coxa valga/vara, wide metaphyses, osteoporosis, pectus carinatum.

Larynx. Small and high-pitched voice.

Eyes. Blepharophimosis, myopia, medial displacement of outer canthi, long eyelashes in irregular rows.

Other. Low hairline, flat facies, small mouth, low-set ears, small testicles, umbilical and inguinal hernias.

OCCASIONAL ABNORMALITIES.

Mental deficiency (25%), intrauterine growth deficiency, delayed bone age, equinovarus foot deformation, hip dislocation, cataract, microcornea.

NATURAL HISTORY. Diagnosis of type 1A is usually made in midchildhood when the

myotonic face is recognized. Progressive myotonia, muscle wasting, and orthopedic problems, with slow linear growth occur. Myotonia, which usually reaches a plateau in midchildhood, is almost always recorded on electromyography, even when not present clinically. Light and electron microscopic and histochemical examinations of muscles show inconsistent myopathic abnormalities. Contractures are most severe by midadolescence and then remain static. Anesthesia may constitute a serious risk because of difficulties with intubation and malignant hyperthermia. There is slowing of growth, and there are problems of motor function. Affected patients frequently have a waddling gait and crouched stance. Tiredness results from stiffness of joints. Intelligence is usually considered normal. However, myotonia may result in drooling and indistinct speech. Normal pubertal development occurs.

ETIOLOGY. This disorder has an autosomal recessive inheritance pattern. Mutations of the gene encoding perlecan (HSPG2) located at chromosome 1p34-p36.1 are responsible for types 1A and 1B. Type 2 (the neonatal type) does not map to 1p34-p36.1.

COMMENT. Two additional types have been delineated. Findings in type 1B are more marked than those in type 1A. Bone dysplasia is present at birth. Long bones are shortened, femurs are dumbbell-shaped in infancy, and epiphyses of long bones are large during childhood. There is flattening of vertebral bodies and coronal clefts. Flared iliac wings, supra-acetabular lateral notches, and a wide ischium are characteristic. Type 2 is more severe with onset in neonatal period. At birth, short-limbed dysplasia is present with bowed long bones. Early death is frequent. In survivors, there is undertubulation of the metaphyses, marked osteoporosis, but only minimal vertebral involvement.

References

Pinto LM, de Sousa JS: Um caso de "doenca muscular" de dificil classificacao. Rev Port Pediatr Pueric 6:1, 1961.

Schwartz O, Jampel RS: Congenital blepharophimosis associated with a unique generalized myopathy. Arch Ophthalmol 68:52, 1962.

Aberfeld DC, Hinterbuchner LP, Schneider M: Myotonia, dwarfism, diffuse bone disease and unusual ocular and facial abnormalities (a new syndrome). Brain 88:313, 1965.

Horan F, Beighton P: Orthopedic aspects of Schwartz syndrome. J Bone Joint Surg 57:542, 1975.

Edward WC, Root AW: Chondrodystrophic myotonia (Schwartz-Jampel syndrome): Report of a new case and follow-up of patients initially reported in 1969. Am J Med Genet 13:51, 1982.

Viljoen D, Beighton P: Schwartz-Jampel syndrome (chondrodystrophic myotonia). J Med Genet 29:58, 1992.

Al Gazali LI: The Schwartz-Jampel syndrome. Clin Dysmorph 2:47, 1993.

Giedion A: Heterogeneity in Schwartz-Jampel chondrodysplasia myotonia. Eur J Pediatr 156:214, 1997.

Nicole S et al: Perlecan, the major proteoglycan of basement membranes, is altered in patients with Schwartz-Jampel syndrome (chondrodystrophic myotonia). Nat Genet 26:480, 2000.

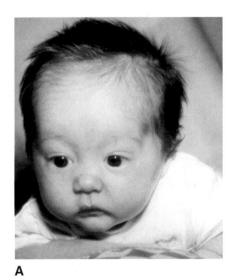

A

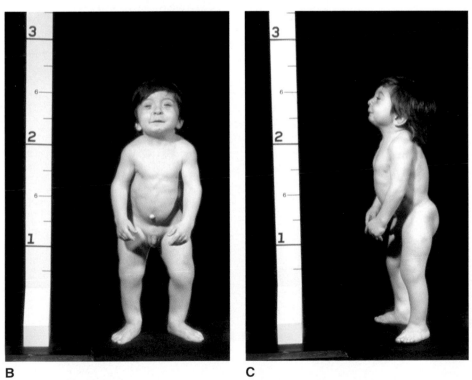

B   **C**

FIGURE 1. Schwartz-Jampel syndrome. **A–C,** Affected child at 2 months and 12 years. Note the myotonia and sad, fixed face, blepharophimosis, and micrognathia.

MARDEN-WALKER SYNDROME

Blepharophimosis, Joint Contractures, Immobile Facies

This disorder was reported initially in 1966 by Marden and Walker, who described a female infant who died at 3 months of age. Subsequently, approximately 30 affected individuals have been reported.

ABNORMALITIES

Growth. Prenatal (35%) and severe postnatal (88%) growth deficiency.

Performance. Moderate to severe mental retardation (89%), hypotonia (86%), strabismus (69%).

Craniofacies. Microcephaly (56%), large anterior fontanel, fixed facial expression (100%), blepharophimosis (100%), cleft palate (38%), high-arched palate (88%), micrognathia (100%), small mouth (63%).

Musculoskeletal. Multiple joint contractures present at birth (100%), camptodactyly (69%), arachnodactyly (71%), talipes equinovarus (63%), scoliosis/kyphosis (71%), pectus excavatum/carinatum (75%), decreased muscle mass (92%).

OCCASIONAL ABNORMALITIES.

Seizures, electroencephalographic abnormalities, microphthalmia, ventricular dilatation, agenesis of corpus callosum, hypoplasia of cerebellum and inferior vermis, hypoplastic brainstem, Dandy-Walker malformation with vertebral anomalies, short neck, cardiac defect, hypospadias, cryptorchidism, micropenis, microcystic or hypoplastic kidneys, inguinal hernia, radioulnar synostosis, Zollinger-Ellison syndrome, pyloric stenosis and duodenal bands, absent clavicle, hypoplastic lung, patent omphalomesenteric duct.

NATURAL HISTORY. Death has occurred at approximately 3 months of age because of aspiration, sepsis, and/or cardiac failure in 19%. The joint contractures become less severe with age and physical therapy. The vast majority of survivors have been significantly mentally retarded.

ETIOLOGY. This disorder has an autosomal recessive inheritance pattern. The primary abnormality is most likely related to a major defect in CNS development. Muscle biopsy specimens obtained from some affected individuals have revealed nonspecific changes that are most likely secondary to the primary CNS process.

References

Marden PM, Walker WA: A new generalized connective tissue syndrome. Am J Dis Child 112:225, 1966.

Ramer JC et al: Marden-Walker phenotype: Spectrum of variability in three infants. Am J Med Genet 45:285, 1993.

Schrander-Stumple C et al: Marden-Walker syndrome: Case report, literature review and nosologic discussion. Clin Genet 43:303, 1993.

Williams MS et al: Marden-Walker syndrome: A case report and a critical review of the literature. Clin Dysmorph 2:211, 1993.

Orrico A et al: Additional case of Marden-Walker syndrome: Support for the autosomal recessive inheritance and refinement of phenotype in a surviving patient. J Clin Neurol 16:150, 2001.

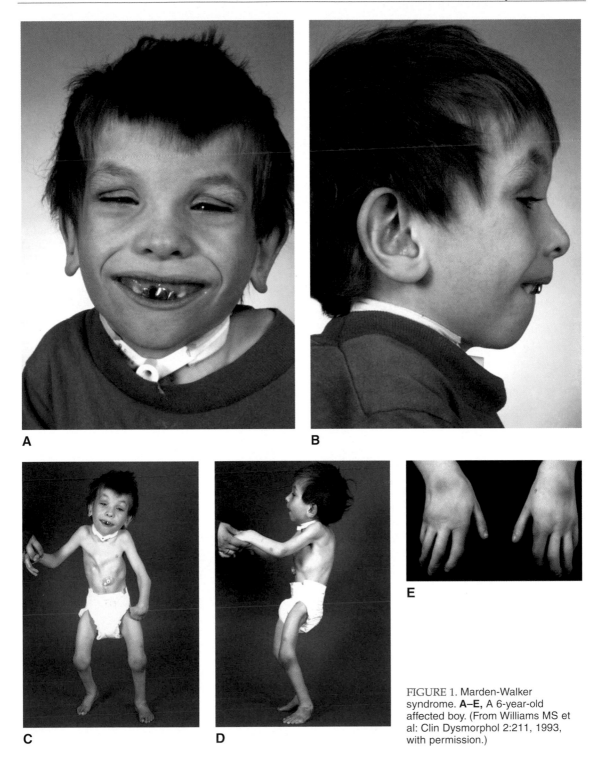

FIGURE 1. Marden-Walker syndrome. **A–E,** A 6-year-old affected boy. (From Williams MS et al: Clin Dysmorphol 2:211, 1993, with permission.)

SCHINZEL-GIEDION SYNDROME

A brother and sister with this disorder were described in 1978 by Schinzel and Giedion. Approximately 30 cases have been reported.

ABNORMALITIES

Growth. Postnatal growth deficiency.

Performance. Profound mental deficiency, seizures, opisthotonus, spasticity, hypsarrhythmia, ventriculomegaly secondary to cerebral atrophy and thinning of the corpus callosum.

Craniofacial. Coarse face; widely patent fontanels and sutures (100%) with metopic suture extending anteriorly to nasal root; high, protruding forehead (100%); short nose with low nasal bridge and anteverted nares (83%); shallow orbits with apparent proptosis (100%); ocular hypertelorism; midface hypoplasia (100%); choanal stenosis (45%); attached helix with protruding lobules of low-set ear (91%).

Limbs. Moderate shortening of forearms and legs (70%), talipes equinovarus, hyperconvex nails (75%), hypoplastic dermal ridges (100%), simian crease (70%).

Genital. Anomalies in 100% including hypospadias, short penis, hypoplastic scrotum in males; deep interlabial sulcus, hypoplasia of labia majora or minora, hymenal atresia, and a short perineum in females.

Renal. Anomalies in 92%, including hydronephrosis, vesicoureteric junction dysplasia, ureteric stenosis, hydroureter, and megacalyces.

Radiologic. Steep short base of skull (60%), sclerotic skull base (80%), wide occipital synchondrosis (60%), multiple wormian bones (63%), hypoplastic first ribs, broad ribs (90%), long clavicles, hypoplastic/aplastic pubic bones (36%), hypoplasia of distal phalanges (78%), short metacarpals of thumbs (56%), broad cortex and increased density of long bones, widening of distal femurs, tibial bowing, mesomelic brachymelia.

Other. Hypertrichosis (91%), short neck with redundant skin, hypoplastic nipples.

OCCASIONAL ABNORMALITIES.

Macroglossia, facial hemangiomata (27%), type I Arnold-Chiari malformation, alacrima (absence of reflex tearing) and corneal hypoesthesia, hearing loss with tuning-fork malformation of the stapes, visual impairment, postaxial polydactyly, syndactyly, fifth toe overlapping fourth, cardiac defect (30%), short sternum, bicornuate uterus, embryonal tumors (14%), including a hepatoblastoma and a malignant sacrococcygeal teratoma.

NATURAL HISTORY. Severe postnatal growth deficiency and profound mental retardation and seizures as well as visual and hearing problems have occurred in all patients who have survived. Death before 2 years of age in 55% of cases. Although no specific cause of death has been determined, it is most likely related to the severe alteration in CNS function. There is some evidence that this disorder is associated with a severe neurodegenerative process with progressive cerebral and brainstem atrophy.

ETIOLOGY. This disorder has an autosomal recessive inheritance pattern.

References

Schinzel A, Giedion A: A syndrome of severe midface retraction, multiple skull anomalies, clubfeet, and cardiac and renal malformations in siblings. Am J Med Genet 1:361, 1978.

Donnai D, Harris R: A further case of a new syndrome including midface retraction, hypertrichosis and skeletal anomalies. J Med Genet 16:483, 1979.

Kelley RI, Zackai EH, Charney EG: Congenital hydronephrosis, skeletal dysplasia, and severe developmental retardation: The Schinzel-Giedion syndrome. J Pediatr 100:943, 1982.

Al-Gazali LI et al: The Schinzel-Giedion syndrome. J Med Genet 27:42, 1990.

Robin NH et al: New findings of Schinzel-Giedion syndrome: A case with a malignant sacrococcygeal teratoma. Am J Med Genet 47:852, 1993.

Labrune P et al: Three new cases of Schinzel-Giedion syndrome and review of the literature. Am J Med Genet 50:90, 1994.

Elliott A et al: Schinzel-Giedion syndrome: Further delineation of the phenotype. Clin Dysmorph 5:135, 1996.

Shah AM et al: Schienzel-Giedion syndrome: Evidence for a neurodegenerative process. Am J Med Genet 82:344, 1999.

Minn D et al: Further clinical and sensorial delineation of Schinzel-Giedion syndrome: Report of two cases. Am J Med Genet 109:211, 2002.

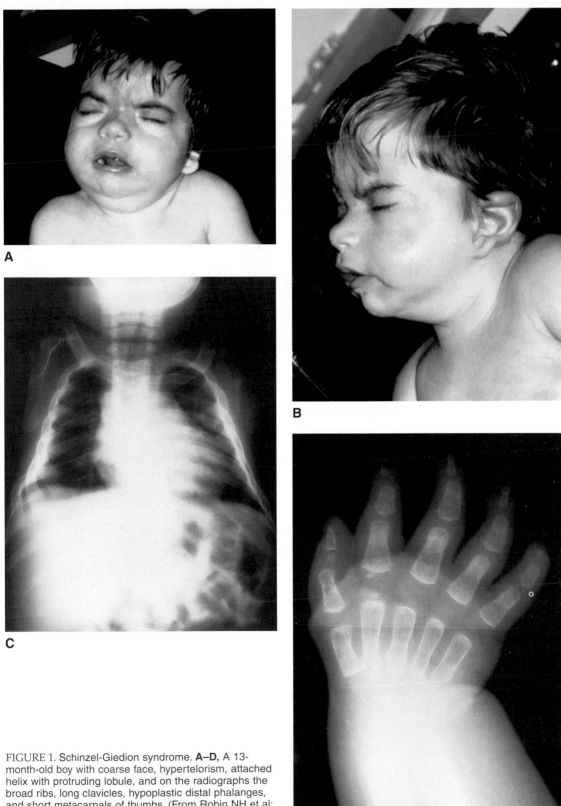

FIGURE 1. Schinzel-Giedion syndrome. **A–D,** A 13-month-old boy with coarse face, hypertelorism, attached helix with protruding lobule, and on the radiographs the broad ribs, long clavicles, hypoplastic distal phalanges, and short metacarpals of thumbs. (From Robin NH et al: Am J Med Genet 47:852, 1993. Copyright © 1993. Reprinted with permission of Wiley-Liss, Inc., a subsidiary of John Wiley & Sons, Inc.)

ACROCALLOSAL SYNDROME

Hypoplastic or Absent Corpus Callosum, Postaxial Polydactyly of Hands and Feet, Hallux Duplication

Since the initial description of this disorder by Schinzel in 1979, approximately 26 cases have been reported.

ABNORMALITIES

Neurologic. Hypoplastic or absent corpus callosum; intracranial cysts; other brain anomalies in 20%, including polymicrogyria, cerebral atrophy, hypothalamic dysfunction, hypoplastic pons, medulla oblongata, cerebellar hemispheres, small cerebellum, agenesis or hypoplasia of cerebellar vermis; severe mental retardation (80%); seizures (33%); strabismus; hypotonia.

Craniofacial. Macrocephaly, prominent forehead, large anterior fontanel, hypertelorism, epicanthal folds, downslanting palpebral fissures, small nose with broad nasal bridge and antiverted nares, malformed ears, short philtrum.

Limbs. Postaxial polydactyly of hands and feet, preaxial polydactyly of feet, mild syndactyly of hands and feet, tapered fingers, fifth finger clinodactyly.

Other. Eye findings including optic atrophy, and decreased retinal pigmentation; cardiac defects, primarily septal defects and abnormalities of the pulmonary valves; umbilical hernia.

OCCASIONAL ABNORMALITIES.

Mild mental retardation, prominent occiput, hyperreflexia, nystagmus, cleft lip, cleft palate, anterior displaced glottis, laryngomalacia, mixed hearing loss, supernumerary nipples, rib hypoplasia, preaxial polydactyly of hands, syndactyly of feet, simian crease, cryptorchidism, hypospadias, prenatal overgrowth, postnatal growth deficiency, intestinal malrotation.

NATURAL HISTORY. Marked retardation in the attainment of developmental milestones. Neonatal respiratory distress and intercurrent infection leading to early death occur in approximately 15% of patients. Family data documenting an increased incidence of spontaneous abortion suggests an apparent increased lethality of the gene.

ETIOLOGY. This disorder has an autosomal recessive inheritance pattern. Although one patient has been reported with a mutation of GLI3, mutations of which cause Grieg cephalopolysyndactyly syndrome, GLI3 has been excluded in other individuals with this disorder.

COMMENT. Three affected children have had siblings with anencephaly, two of which had polydactyly, suggesting that anencephaly may be the severe end of the spectrum of brain defects in the acrocallosal syndrome.

References

Schinzel A: Postaxial polydactyly, hallux duplication, absence of the corpus callosum, macrencephaly and severe mental retardation: A new syndrome? Helv Paediatr Acta 34:141, 1979.

Schinzel A, Schmid W: Hallux duplication, postaxial polydactyly, absence of the corpus callosum, severe mental retardation, and additional anomalies in two unrelated patients: A new syndrome. Am J Med Genet 6:241, 1980.

Schinzel A: The acrocallosal syndrome in first cousins: Widening of the spectrum of clinical features and further support for autosomal recessive inheritance. J Med Genet 25:332, 1988.

Casamassima AC et al: Acrocallosal syndrome: Additional manifestations. Am J Med Genet 32:311, 1989.

Lurie IW et al: The acrocallosal syndrome: Expansion of the phenotypic spectrum. Clin Dysmorphol 3:31, 1994.

Elson E et al: De novo GLI3 mutation in acrocallosal syndrome: broadening the phenotypic spectrum of GLI3 defects and overlap with murine models. J Med Genet 39:804, 2002.

Koenig R et al: Spectrum of the acrocallosal syndrome. Am J Med Genet 108:7, 2002.

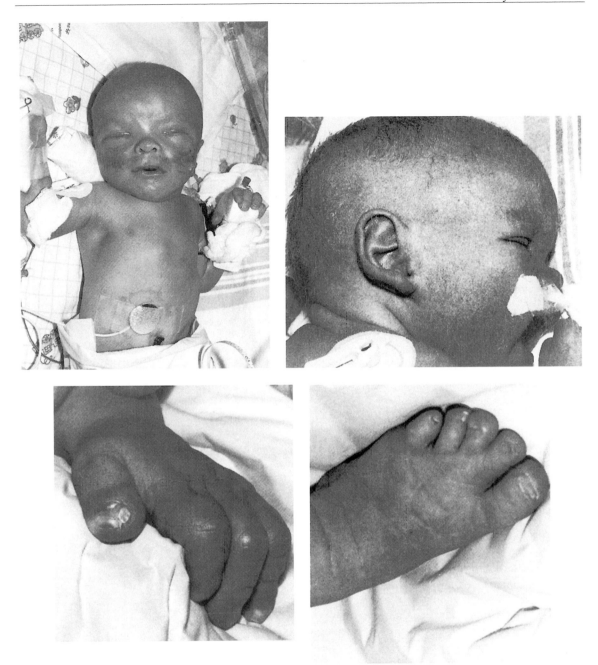

FIGURE 1. Acrocallosal syndrome. Newborn boy with broad forehead, hypertelorism, broad nose with anteverted nares, abnormal auricles, and redundant nuchal skin. In addition, note the broad thumbs and great toes with partial duplication of the thumb, nail hypoplasia, and syndactyly of the feet. (From Casamassima AC et al: Am J Med Genet 32:11, 1989. Copyright © 1989. Reprinted with permission of Wiley-Liss, Inc., a subsidiary of John Wiley & Sons, Inc.)

3C SYNDROME
(RITSCHER-SCHINZEL SYNDROME)

In 1987, Ritscher and colleagues reported two sisters with similar craniofacial anomalies, one of which had a complete common atrioventricular canal and Dandy-Walker variant while the other had a partial atrioventricular canal and a Dandy-Walker malformation. Subsequently Verloes and colleagues reported a third child with this disorder, which they referred to as 3C (craniofacial, cerebellar, cardiac) syndrome.

ABNORMALITIES

Growth. Postnatal growth deficiency with respect to both length and weight.

Performance. Hypotonia, gross motor delay, speech delay.

Craniofacial. Prominent forehead, large anterior fontanel, ocular hypertelorism, depressed nasal bridge, downslanting palpebral fissures.

Central Nervous System. Variable degrees of Dandy-Walker malformation/variant including cerebellar vermis hypoplasia, enlarged fourth ventricle, enlarged cisterna magna, and hydrocephalus.

Cardiac. Complete/partial atrioventricular canal defects, tetralogy of Fallot, double outlet right ventricle, atrial septal defect, ventricular septal defect.

OCCASIONAL ABNORMALITIES.
Macrocephaly, prominent occiput, mental retardation, coloboma, glaucoma, cleft palate, bifid uvula, hemivertebrae, absent/hypoplastic ribs, short neck, syndactyly, brachydactyly, proximally-placed thumb, hypospadias, growth hormone deficiency, bowel malrotation, anal atresia, sensorineural hearing loss, single umbilical artery, hydronephrosis, immunodeficiency.

NATURAL HISTORY.
Death before 4 years of age, primarily related to the severity of the cardiovascular malformation, has occurred in one half of reported cases. Shunting for hydrocephalus was required infrequently. Limited information is available regarding intellectual performance. A 6-year-old girl performed at the 4½- to 5-year-old level and a 13-year-old child had "mild mental retardation." The degree to which the growth deficiency is related to growth hormone deficiency is unknown.

ETIOLOGY.
This disorder has an autosomal recessive inheritance pattern. Some data are available indicating that the gene is located at chromosome 22q11.2.

References

Ritscher D et al: Dandy-Walker (like) malformation, atrioventricular septal defect and a similar pattern of minor anomalies in two sisters: A new syndrome? Am J Med Genet 26:481–491, 1987.

Verloes H et al: 3C syndrome: Third occurrence of cranio-cerebello-cardiac dysplasia (Ritscher-Schinzel syndrome). Clin Genet 35:205–208, 1989.

Kosaki K et al: Ritscher-Schinzel (3C) syndrome: Documentation of the phenotype. Am J Med Genet 68:421–427, 1997.

Leonardi ML et al: Ritscher-Schinzel cranio-cerebello-cardiac (3C) syndrome: Report of four new cases and review. Am J Med Genet 102:237–242, 2001.

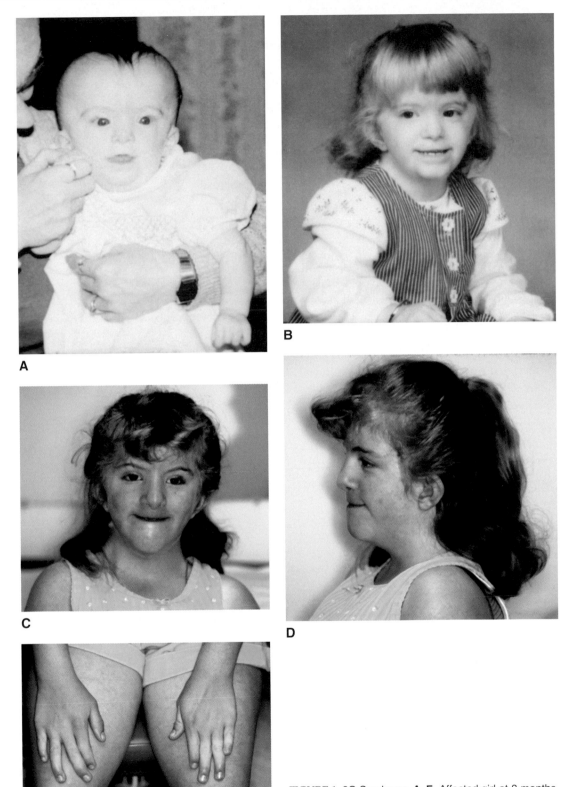

FIGURE 1. 3C Syndrome. **A–E,** Affected girl at 8 months, 4 years, and 13 years of age. Note the high forehead, low-set ears, mild maxillary hypoplasia, short fifth fingers, and DIP contractures. (From Wheeler PG et al : Am J Med Genet 87:61, 1999, with permission.)

HECHT SYNDROME
(Trismus Pseudocamptodactyly Syndrome)

This disorder of muscle development and function was first described by Hecht and Beals and by Wilson and colleagues in 1968. It was more recently well delineated by Mabry and colleagues in a huge kindred in which the initial United States case was a young Dutch girl who arrived in this country with "crooked hands and a small mouth."

ABNORMALITIES. Abnormalities appear to be based on short muscles and especially tendons.

Muscles and Tendons. Limited opening of mouth, sometimes with an enlarged coronoid process; short flexor tendons, so that when the hand is dorsiflexed, the fingers are partially flexed; occasionally short flexor muscles to the feet cause such problems as downturning toes, talipes equinovarus, calcaneovalgus, and metatarsus adductus; short hamstrings and gastrocnemius muscles.

NATURAL HISTORY. The newborn baby may have tightly fisted hands and later usually crawls on the knuckles. These patients may have feeding problems because of the small mouth, and they tend to eat slowly. Tonsillectomy and/or intubation may present serious problems. There can be occupational handicaps relative to the military service, typing, or other situations requiring high levels of hand dexterity. Surgical correction of the trismus has been reported in one case.

ETIOLOGY. This disorder has an autosomal dominant inheritance pattern, with an unexplained 2:1 excess of affected females.

References

Hecht F, Beals RK: Inability to open the mouth fully. In Bergsma D (ed): Birth Defects Original Article Series. Part III: Limb Malformation, vol. V. New York: National Foundation March of Dimes, 1968, p 96.

Wilson RV et al: Autosomal dominant inheritance of shortening of flexor profundus muscle tendon. In Bergsma D (ed): Birth Defects Original Article Series. Part III: Limb Malformation, vol. V. New York: National Foundation March of Dimes, 1968, p 99.

Mabry CC et al: Trismus camptomelic syndrome. J Pediatr 85:503, 1974.

Lefaivre J-F et al: Surgical correction of trismus in a child with Hecht syndrome. Ann Plast Surg 50:310, 2003.

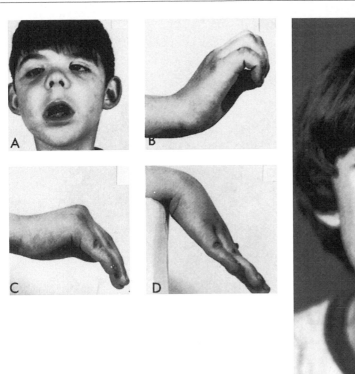

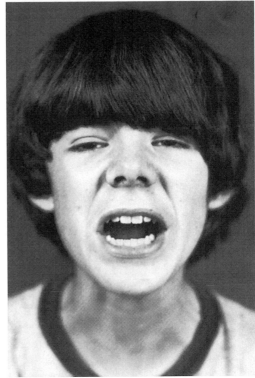

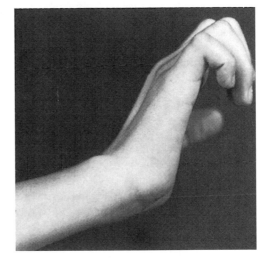

FIGURE 1. Hecht syndrome. *Above,* Boy with maximal opening of mouth (**A**), dorsiflexed hand showing flexion of fingers (**B**), extended hand with some flexion of fingers (**C**), but volar flexed hand with no finger flexion (**D**). *Right,* A 13-year-old boy with maximal mouth opening and flexed fingers following hand flexion. (*Above* and *right,* Courtesy of Dr. C. Charlton Mabry, University of Kentucky Medical School, Lexington.)

G Facial Defects as Major Feature

MOEBIUS SEQUENCE
Sixth and Seventh Nerve Palsy

The basic features of Moebius sequence are mask-like facies with sixth and seventh cranial nerve palsy, usually bilaterally. The necropsy cases implicate at least four modes of developmental pathology in the genesis of the problem. These are (1) hypoplasia to absence of the central brain nuclei, (2) destructive degeneration of the central brain nuclei (most common type), (3) peripheral nerve involvement, and (4) a myopathy. Thus, the Moebius sequence is but a sign and is quite nonspecific. Micrognathia, a frequent feature, may be interpreted as secondary to a neuromuscular deficit in early movement of the mandible. It leads to a U-shaped cleft palate or cleft uvula in one third of cases. Some patients have more extensive cranial nerve involvement, including the third, fourth, fifth, ninth, tenth, and twelfth cranial nerves. In cases where there is more extensive cranial nerve involvement, the tongue may be limited in mobility and/or small. There may be ocular ptosis and/or a protruding auricle. Abnormal tearing, the result of aberrant innervation of the lacrimal gland and limited involvement of both abduction and adduction are common. Hearing loss, most frequently the result of chronic otitis media, is frequent. Approximately one third of patients have talipes equinovarus, which is most likely the consequence of neurologic deficiency relative to early foot movement. Autism occurs in approximately 25% of cases, and approximately 30% of patients have mental retardation, the majority of which are severe, as a more obvious indication that in some cases the central nervous system (CNS) defect involves more than the cranial nerve nuclei alone. All individuals with severe mental retardation show severe autistic symptoms. Impaired speech occurs in the majority of cases. Feeding difficulties and problems of aspiration often lead to failure to thrive during infancy. The expressionless facies and speech impediments create problems in acceptance and social adaptation. Associated non–CNS-related defects have included hypodontia, limb reduction defects, syndactyly, the Poland sequence, and occasionally the Klippel-Feil anomaly.

The Moebius sequence is most commonly a sporadic occurrence in an otherwise normal family. In the majority of those cases, insufficient blood supply to structures supplied by the developing primitive subclavian artery lead to the variable features seen in this disorder. Evidence that a number of affected individuals have been born to women who experienced events during pregnancy that could cause transient ischemic/hypoxic insults to the fetus suggests that this disorder may be due to any event that interferes with the uterine/fetal circulation.

The association of seventh cranial nerve palsy with or without sixth cranial nerve palsy but without limb reduction defects may be familial with an autosomal dominant mode of inheritance in some cases.

References

Moebius PJ: Ueber engeborene doppelseitige Abducens-Facialis-Laehmung. Munch Med Wochenschr 35:91, 1888.

Henderson JL: The congenital facial diplegia syndrome: Clinical features, pathology, and aetiology: A review of sixty-one cases. Brain 62:381, 1939.

Sugarman GI, Stark HH: Möbius anomaly with Poland's anomaly. J Med Genet 10:192, 1973.

Baraitser M: Genetics of Möbius syndrome. J Med Genet 14:415, 1977.

Meyerson MD, Foushee DR: Speech, language and hearing in Moebius syndrome. Dev Med Child Neurol 20:357, 1978.

Bouwes-Bavinck JN, Weaver DD: Subclavian artery supply disruption sequence: Hypothesis of a vascular etiology for Poland, Klippel-Feil, and Mobius anomalies. Am J Med Genet 23:903, 1986.

Lipson AH et al: Moebius syndrome: Animal model–human correlations and evidence for a brainstem vascular etiology. Teratology 40:339, 1989.

Kumar D: Moebius syndrome. J Med Genet 27:122, 1990.

St. Charles S et al: Mobius sequence: Further in vivo support for the subclavian artery supply disruption sequence. Am J Med Genet 47:289, 1993.

Stromland K et al.: Mobius sequence—a Swedish multi-discipline study. Eur J Pediat Neurol 6:35, 2002.

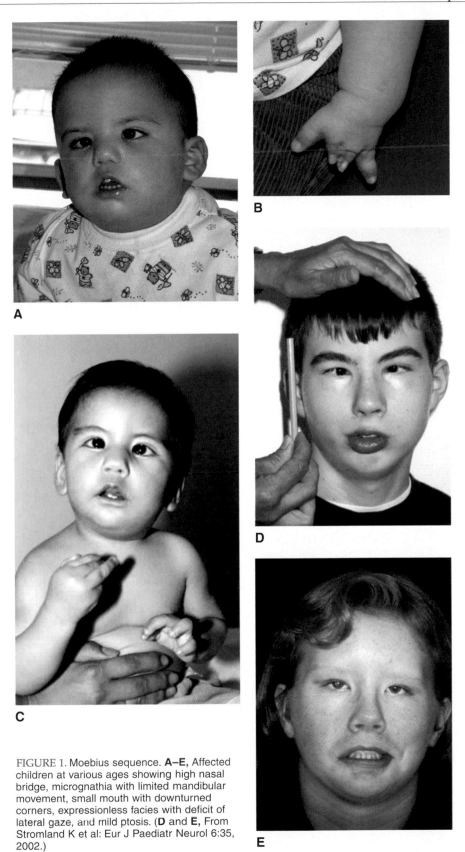

FIGURE 1. Moebius sequence. **A–E,** Affected children at various ages showing high nasal bridge, micrognathia with limited mandibular movement, small mouth with downturned corners, expressionless facies with deficit of lateral gaze, and mild ptosis. (**D** and **E,** From Stromland K et al: Eur J Paediatr Neurol 6:35, 2002.)

BLEPHAROPHIMOSIS-PTOSIS-EPICANTHUS INVERSUS SYNDROME
(Familial Blepharophimosis Syndrome)

Inner Canthal Fold, Lateral Displacement of Inner Canthi, Ptosis

This entity, predominantly a dysplasia of the eyelids, was described by Vignes in 1889, and more than 200 families have been reported. The existence of two types has been suggested: type I, associated with infertility in affected females; and type II, transmitted by both males and females.

ABNORMALITIES

Eyes. Inverted inner canthal fold between upper and lower lid, short palpebral fissures with lateral displacement of inner canthi, low nasal bridge and ptosis of eyelids, hypoplasia, fibrosis of the levator palpebrae muscle, strabismus, amblyopia, eyebrows are increased in their vertical height and are arched.

Ears. Incomplete development, cupping.

Endocrine. Females with type I have menstrual irregularities or amenorrhea, infertility, and elevated gonadotropin levels.

Other. Variable hypotonia in early life.

OCCASIONAL ABNORMALITIES.

Mental deficiency; cardiac defect; ocular abnormalities including microphthalmia, microcornea, hypermetropia, trichiasis, colobomas of the optic disk, trabecular dysgenesis, congenital optic nerve hypoplasia, nystagmus; endometrial carcinoma; granulosa cell tumor.

NATURAL HISTORY.

Plastic surgery is indicated both for cosmetic reasons and for improvement of ocular function. Amblyopia, which occurs in greater than one half of patients, is most frequently associated with asymmetrical ptosis, although it also occurs when the ptosis is bilateral. Although most women with type I have a normal menarche and may initially be fertile, they soon develop ovarian resistance to gonadotropins or true premature ovarian failure. In at least one case, primary ovarian failure has been documented in early childhood.

ETIOLOGY.

There is an autosomal dominant inheritance pattern for both type I and type II. Mutations in the forkhead transcription factor gene 2 (FOXL2) located at 3q22.3-q23 have been documented in 67% of cases and are responsible for both types. Type I is caused by truncating mutations leading to haploinsufficiency, while type II is caused by mutations that generate elongated protein products. The importance of distinguishing between the types relates to reproductive capabilities and menstrual irregularities, including amenorrhea in females with type I. With the exception of infertility in females, the two types are indistinguishable clinically. Unfortunately female fertility cannot be definitely predicted based on the FOXL2 molecular defect. Therefore, separating the two types can be accomplished only through a combination of molecular testing and careful family history. If the affected individual, either male or female, is a member of a family in which the disorder has been transmitted only through males, it is most likely type I, whereas if transmission has occurred through both males and females, it is type II.

References

Vignes A: Epicanthus héréditaire. Rev Gen Ophthalmol (Paris) 8:438, 1889.

Sacrez R et al: Le blépharophimosis compliqué familial: Étude des membres de la famille Blé. Ann Pediatr (Paris) 10:493, 1963.

Kohn R, Romano PE: Blepharoptosis, blepharophimosis, epicanthus inversus, and telecanthus—a syndrome with no name. Am J Ophthalmol 72:625, 1972.

Zlotogora J, Sagi M, Cohen T: The blepharophimosis, ptosis and epicanthus inversus syndrome: Delineation of two types. Am J Hum Genet 35:1020, 1983.

Jones CA, Collin JRD: Blepharophimosis and its association with female infertility. Br J Ophthalmol 68:533, 1984.

Oley C, Baraister M: Blepharophimosis, ptosis, epicanthus inversus syndrome (BPES syndrome). J Med Genet 25:47, 1988.

Beaconsfield M et al: Visual development in the blepharophimosis syndrome. Br J Ophthalmol 75:746, 1991.

DeBaere E et al: Spectrum of FOXL2 gene mutations in blepharophimosis-ptosis-epicanthus inversus (BPES) families demonstrates a genotype-phenotype correlation. Hum Mol Genet 10:1591, 2001.

Fokstuen S et al: FOXL2-Mutations in blepharophimosis-ptosis-epicanthus inversus syndrome (BPES): Challenges for genetic counseling in female patients. Am J Med Genet 117:143, 2003.

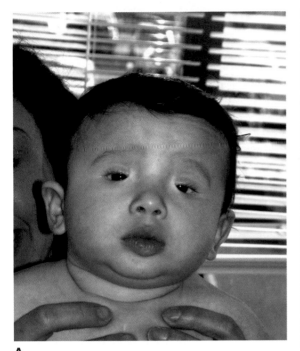

A

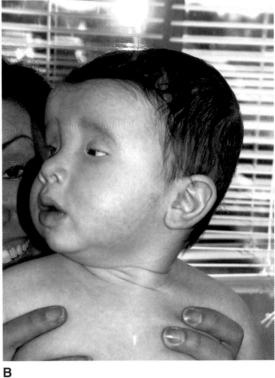

B

C

FIGURE 1. Blepharophimosis syndrome. **A–C,** Mother and infant son. (Courtesy of Dr. Lynne M. Bird, Children's Hospital, San Diego.)

ROBIN SEQUENCE
(PIERRE ROBIN SYNDROME)

Micrognathia, Glossoptosis, Cleft Soft Palate; Primary Defect—Early Mandibular Hypoplasia

The single initiating defect of this disorder may be hypoplasia of the mandibular area before 9 weeks in utero, allowing the tongue to be posteriorly located and thereby impairing the closure of the posterior palatal shelves that must "grow over" the tongue to meet the midline. The mode of pathogenesis is depicted to the right. The rounded contour of the "cleft" palate in some of these patients (see illustration) is compatible with this mode of developmental pathology and differs from the usual inverted V shape of most palatal clefts. Latham's study of a 17-week-old fetus with the Robin sequence led him to the same conclusion: that early mandibular retrognathia is the primary anomaly. The posterior airway obstruction may require in order of increasing invasiveness prone positioning, nasal pharyngeal airway, nasal esophageal intubation, lip-tongue adhesion, mandibular distraction, and tracheostomy. Airway obstruction can lead to hypoxia, cor pulmonale, failure to thrive, and cerebral impairment. Mortality rates as high as 30% have been reported. Significant airway obstruction may develop over the first 1 to 4 weeks of life. Therefore, affected children should be monitored carefully during that period, focusing on the obstruction pathogenesis of the apnea and airway concerns in the condition. In that significant hypoxia may occur without obvious clinical signs of obstruction, serial polysomnography may be helpful over the first month to identify infants at

significant risk. Feeding problems requiring nasogastric tube feeding are common and are related in many cases to lower esophageal sphincter hypertonia, failure of lower esophageal sphincter relaxation at deglutition, and esophageal dyskinesis. Although the Robin sequence often occurs in otherwise normal individuals, in whom the prognosis is very good if they survive the early period of respiratory obstruction, this disorder commonly occurs as one feature in a multiple malformation syndrome, such as the trisomy 18 syndrome, the Stickler syndrome, or a number of other disorders. It may also be a result of early in utero mechanical constraint, with the chin compressed in such a manner as to limit its growth before palatine closure.

References

Dennison WM: The Pierre Robin syndrome. Pediatrics 36:336, 1965.

Latham RA: The pathogenesis of cleft palate associated with the Pierre Robin syndrome. Br J Plast Surg 19:205, 1966.

Hanson JW, Smith DW: U-shaped palatal defect in the Robin anomalad: Developmental and clinical relevance. J Pediatr 87:30, 1975.

Bull MJ et al: Improved outcome in Pierre Robin sequence: Effect of multidisciplinary evaluation and management. Pediatrics 86:294, 1990.

Baujat G et al: Oroesophageal motor disorders in Pierre Robin syndrome. J Pediatr Gastroenterol Nutr 32:297, 2001.

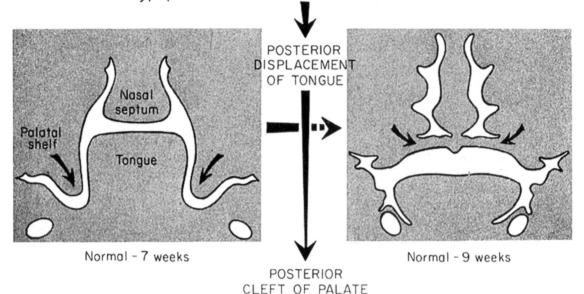

PIERRE ROBIN SYNDROME
A Primary Anomaly in Mandibular Development
Hypoplasia of Mandible Prior to 9 Weeks

POSTERIOR DISPLACEMENT OF TONGUE

Nasal septum

Palatal shelf

Tongue

Normal – 7 weeks

Normal – 9 weeks

POSTERIOR CLEFT OF PALATE

A

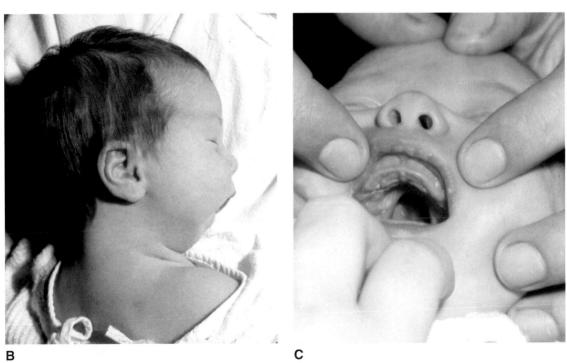

B

C

FIGURE 1. **A,** Mode of pathogenesis of the Robin sequence. **B,** Note the severe micrognathia. **C,** Note the unusual rounded shape to palatal "cleft" in a patient with the Robin sequence compatible with the incomplete closure of the palate having been secondary to the posterior displacement of the tongue.

CLEFT LIP SEQUENCE
Primary Defect—Closure of Lip

By 35 days of uterine age, the lip is normally fused, as illustrated in Figure 1. A failure of lip fusion, as shown, may impair the subsequent closure of the palatal shelves, which do not completely fuse until the eighth to ninth week. Thus, cleft palate is a frequent association with cleft lip. Other secondary anomalies include defects of tooth development in the area of the cleft lip and incomplete growth of the ala nasi on the side of the cleft. There may be mild ocular hypertelorism, the precise reason for which is undetermined. Tertiary abnormalities can include poor speech and multiple episodes of otitis media as a consequence of palatal incompetence and conductive hearing loss.

ETIOLOGY AND RECURRENCE RISK COUNSELING.
The cause of this disorder is usually unknown. It is more likely to occur in the male. The more severe the defect, the higher the recurrence risk for future siblings. For a unilateral defect, the recurrence risk is 2.7%; for bilateral defect, it is 5.4%. The following are the general risk figures: unaffected parents with one affected child, 4% for future siblings; unaffected parents with two affected children, 10% for future siblings. If either the mother or father is affected, the risk for offspring is 4%. An affected parent with one affected child has a 14% risk for future offspring.

COMMENT.
As many as 15% of infants surviving the newborn period with cleft lip, with or without cleft palate, and 42% of those with cleft palate alone have the defect as part of a broader pattern of altered morphogenesis. One should identify such individuals before using the above figures for recurrence risk counseling. In addition, the underlying diagnosis may well have an impact on prognosis.

References
Bixler D: Heritability of clefts of the lip and palate. J Prosthet Dent 33:100, 1975.

Carter CO et al: A three generations family study of cleft lip with or without cleft palate. J Med Genet 19:246, 1982.

Shprintzen RJ et al: Anomalies associated with cleft lip, cleft palate, or both. Am J Med Genet 20:585, 1985.

Jones MC: Facial clefting: Etiology and developmental pathogenesis. Clin Plast Surg 20:599, 1993.

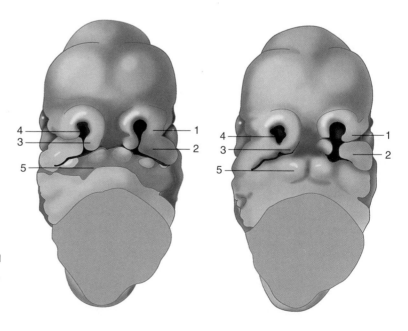

FIGURE 1. Cleft lip sequence. *Left,* Normal embryo of 35 days. *Right,* Spontaneously aborted 35-day embryo with hypoplasia of the left lateral nasal swelling and, therefore, a cleft lip. *1,* Lateral nasal swelling; *2,* maxillary swelling; *3,* medial nasal swelling; *4,* nares; *5,* mandibular swelling. (*Left* and *right,* Courtesy of Professor G. Töndury, University of Zurich.)

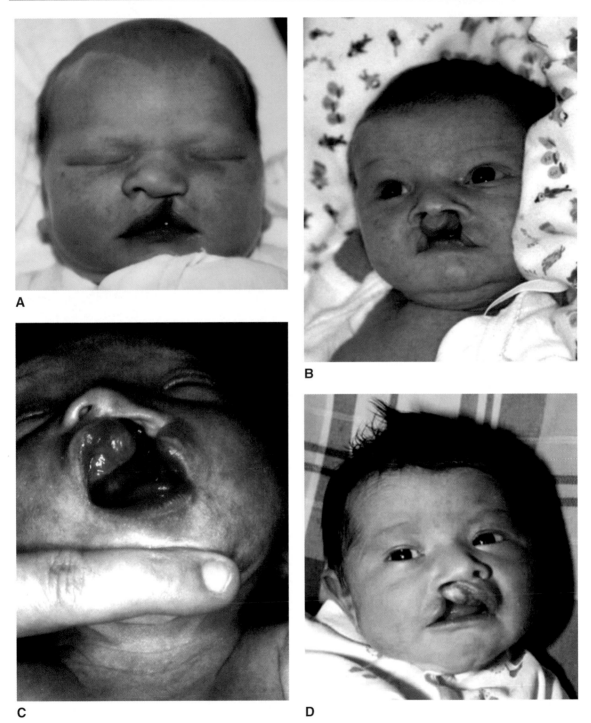

FIGURE 2. **A–D,** All gradations of cleft lip and its consequences occur, from an isolated unilateral cleft lip to a widely open cleft with secondary consequences of cleft palate, flared ala nasi, and mild ocular hypertelorism. (Courtesy of Dr. Marilyn C. Jones, Children's Hospital, San Diego.)

VAN DER WOUDE SYNDROME
(Lip Pit–Cleft Lip Syndrome)

Lower Lip Pit(s), with or without Cleft Lip, with or without Missing Second Premolars

Originally reported by Van der Woude in 1954, this disorder is the most common multiple malformation syndrome associated with cleft lip with or without cleft palate.

ABNORMALITIES

Oral. Lower lip pits (80%); hypodontia, missing central and lateral incisors, canines, or bicuspids; cleft lip with or without cleft palate, cleft palate alone, cleft uvula.

NATURAL HISTORY. Surgical removal of the fistulas, which represent small accessory salivary glands, is recommended because they may produce a watery mucoid discharge that can be embarrassing for the individual.

ETIOLOGY. This disorder has an autosomal dominant inheritance pattern. The gene responsible in the vast majority of cases of this disorder, interferon inhibiting factor 6 (IRF6) has been mapped to the long arm of chromosome 1 at q32-41. Mutations in IRF6 lead not only to Van der Woude syndrome, but to the popliteal pterygium syndrome. Interestingly, both of these disorders have been observed in the same family.

References

Van der Woude A: Fistula labii inferioris congenita and its association with cleft lip and palate. Am J Hum Genet 6:244, 1954.

Cervenka J, Gorlin RJ, Anderson VE: The syndrome of pits of the lower lip and cleft lip or cleft palate: Genetic considerations. Am J Hum Genet 19:416, 1967.

Janku P et al: The Van der Woude syndrome in a large kindred: Variability, penetrance, genetic risks. Am J Med Genet 5:117, 1980.

Sander A et al: Evidence for a microdeletion in 1q32-41 involving the gene responsible for Van der Woude syndrome. Hum Mol Genet 3:575, 1994.

Kondo S et al: Mutations in IRF6 causes Van der Woude and popliteal pterygium syndromes. Nat Genet 32:285, 2002.

Muenke M: The pit, the cleft and the web. Nat Genet 32:219, 2002.

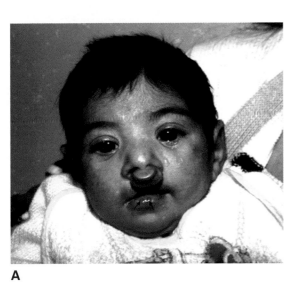 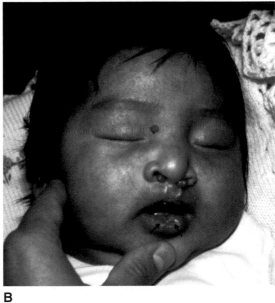

A　　　　　　　　　　　　　　　　　　　**B**

FIGURE 1. Van der Woude syndrome. **A** and **B,** Two affected children. Note the lip pits in both. Bilateral cleft palate has been repaired in **B.** (**B,** Courtesy of Dr. Marilyn C. Jones, Children's Hospital, San Diego.)

FRONTONASAL DYSPLASIA SEQUENCE
(MEDIAN CLEFT FACE SYNDROME)

Unknown Primary Defect in Midfacial Development with Incomplete Anterior Appositional Alignment of Eyes

DeMyer recognized the transitional gradations in severity of this presumed single primary localized defect in 33 cases and called this pattern of anomaly the median cleft face syndrome. Sedano and colleagues subsequently extended these observations and recommended frontonasal dysplasia as a more appropriate designation for this defect. The accompanying figure sets forth a crude interpretation of the developmental pathogenesis and gradations of the sequence.

ABNORMALITIES. Defects that may occur in the more severe cases; the milder cases may have only a few of the defects.

Eyes. Ocular hypertelorism, lateral displacement of inner canthi.

Forehead. Widow's peak, deficit in midline frontal bone (cranium bifidum occultum).

Nose. Variability from notched broad nasal tip to completely divided nostrils with hypoplasia to absence of the prolabium and premaxilla with a median cleft lip, variable notching of alae nasi, broad nasal root, lack of formation of nasal tip.

OCCASIONAL ABNORMALITIES.

Accessory nasal tags; microphthalmia; preauricular tags, low-set ears, conductive deafness; mental retardation; frontal cutaneous lipoma or lipoma of corpus callosum; agenesis of the corpus callosum; tetralogy of Fallot.

NATURAL HISTORY. Depending on the severity of the defect, radical cosmetic surgery is usually merited. The majority of affected individuals are of normal intelligence. DeMyer noted 8% severe mental retardation and 12% mild impairment of intelligence.

ETIOLOGY. The cause of this disorder is unknown, with a sporadic occurrence; it may occasionally be familial.

COMMENT. Frontonasal dysplasia in association with defects of the CNS and limb anomalies including tibial hypoplasia/aplasia, talipes equinovarus, and preaxial polydactyly of the feet has been seen in 13 individuals and is referred to as acromelic frontonasal dysostosis. A number of the affected children were the offspring of consanguineous marriages, raising the possibility of autosomal recessive inheritance.

Frontonasal dysplasia associated with optic disk anomalies, basal encephalocele, absent corpus callosum, diabetes insipidus, and pituitary deficiency appears to be another distinct subgroup within the spectrum of frontonasal dysplasia. All cases have been sporadic.

References

DeMyer W: The median cleft face syndrome: Differential diagnosis of cranium bifidum occultum, hypertelorism, and median cleft nose, lip, and palate. Neurology [Minn] 17:961, 1967.

Sedano HO et al: Frontonasal dysplasia. J Pediatr 76:906, 1970.

Pascual-Castroviejo I, Pascual-Pascual SI, Perez-Hiqueras A: Fronto-nasal dysplasia and lipoma of the corpus callosum. Eur J Pediatr 144:66, 1985.

Sedano HO, Gorlin RJ: Frontonasal malformation as a field defect and in syndromic associations. Oral Surg Oral Med Oral Pathol 65:704, 1988.

Grubben C et al: Anterior basal encephalocele in the median cleft face syndrome: Comments on nosology and treatment. Genet Couns 38:103, 1990.

Lees MM et al: Frontonasal dysplasia with optic disc anomalies and other midline craniofacial defects: A report of six cases. Clin Dysmorphol 7:157, 1998.

Slaney S et al: Acromelic frontonasal dysostosis. Am J Med Genet 83:109, 1999.

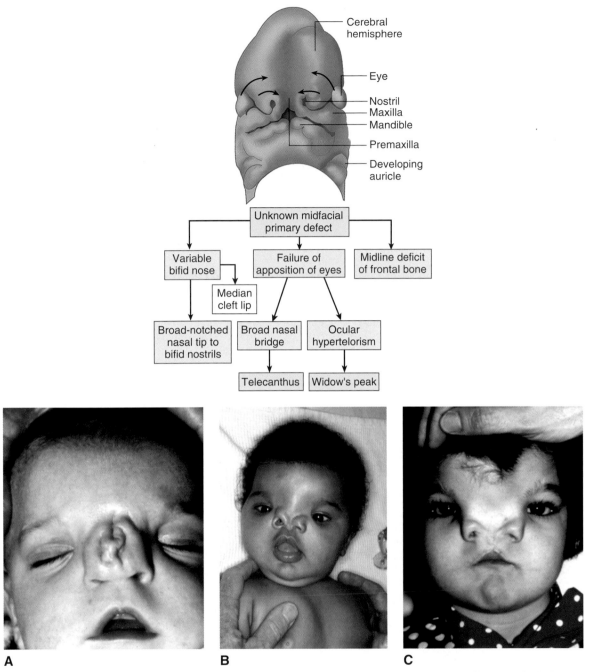

FIGURE 1. *Top*, Developmental pathogenesis of the frontonasal dysplasia sequence. *Bottom*, Affected individuals.

FRASER SYNDROME
(Cryptophthalmos Syndrome)

Cryptophthalmos,* Defect of Auricle, Genital Anomaly

The association of other multiple malformations in patients with the rare anomaly of cryptophthalmos had been appreciated before 1962, when a rather distinctive syndrome found in two sets of siblings was set forth by Fraser. More than 100 patients have been reported. Since cryptophthalmos is not an obligate feature of this disorder, it is more appropriately termed Fraser syndrome.

ABNORMALITIES

Facial. Cryptophthalmos (93%), usually bilateral and frequently with defect of eye; hair growth on lateral forehead extending to lateral eyebrow (34%), often associated with a depression of underlying frontal bone; hypoplastic notched nares; broad nose with depressed bridge; ear anomalies (44%), most commonly atresia of external auditory canal and cupped ears.

Performance. Mental deficiency in approximately 50% of survivors.

Limbs. Partial cutaneous syndactyly (57%).

Genitalia. Incomplete development (49%); male: hypospadias, cryptorchidism; female: bicornuate uterus, vaginal atresia, clitoromegaly.

Other. Laryngeal stenosis or atresia (21%), renal hypoplasia or agenesis (37%).

OCCASIONAL ABNORMALITIES.

Microcephaly, hydrocephalus, encephalocele, abnormal gyral pattern, meningomyelocele, midline groove toward nasal tip, unilateral absence of a nostril, choanal atresia or stenosis, subglottic stenosis, cleft lip, with or without cleft palate (4%), and cleft palate (3%), tongue tie (6%), dental malocclusion and crowding, bony skull defects, hypertelorism, lacrimal duct defect (9%), coloboma of upper lid (6%), absent eyebrows or eyelashes, microphthalmia, anophthalmia, corneal opacification, partial midfacial cleft, defect of middle ear,

fusion of superior helix to scalp, microtia, low-set ears, widely spaced nipples, pulmonary hyperplasia, abnormalities of ureters or bladder, low-set umbilicus, anal atresia, malformation of small bowel, cardiac defects, thymic aplasia/hypoplasia, diastasis of symphysis pubis, partial absence of sternum, absent phalanges, hypoplastic or absent thumb.

NATURAL HISTORY. This disorder should be considered in stillborn babies with renal agenesis. Because the defect of eyelid development is frequently accompanied by ocular anomaly, the likelihood of achieving adequate visual perception is small, although early surgical intervention was of value in one case. Hearing is usually normal. Twenty-five percent of affected individuals are stillborn and an additional 20% die before 1 year of age. Death is related primarily to the renal or laryngeal defects. No affected individual has been reported to have reproduced.

ETIOLOGY. This disorder has an autosomal recessive inheritance pattern. There is etiologic heterogeneity for the cryptophthalmos anomaly. A number of individuals with isolated cryptophthalmos who do not have the Fraser syndrome have been reported.

References

Fraser CR: Our genetical "load": A review of some aspects of genetical variation. Ann Hum Genet 25:387, 1962.

Gupta SP, Saxena RC: Cryptophthalmos. Br J Ophthalmol 46:629, 1962.

Azvedo ES, Biondi J, Ramaldo LM: Cryptophthalmos in two families. J Med Genet 10:389, 1973.

Mortimer G, McEwen HP, Yates JRW: Fraser syndrome presenting as monozygous twins with bilateral renal agenesis. J Med Genet 22:76, 1985.

Thomas IT et al: Isolated and syndromic cryptophthalmos. Am J Med Genet 25:85, 1986.

Gattuso J et al: The clinical spectrum of the Fraser syndrome: Report of three new cases and review. J Med Genet 24:549, 1987.

Ford GR et al: ENT manifestations of Fraser syndrome. J Laryngol Otol 106:1, 1992.

Slavotinek AM, Tifft CJ: Fraser syndrome and cryptophthalmos: Review of the diagnostic criteria and evidence for phenotypic modules in complex malformation syndromes. J Med Genet 39:623, 2002.

---

*Cryptophthalmos (hidden eye) fundamentally means absence of the palpebral fissure but usually includes varying absence of eyelashes and eyebrows and defects of the eye, especially the anterior part.

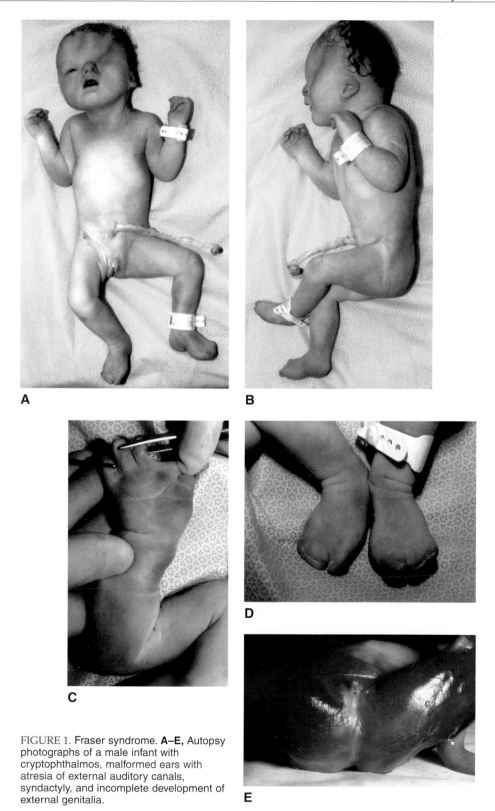

FIGURE 1. Fraser syndrome. **A–E,** Autopsy photographs of a male infant with cryptophthalmos, malformed ears with atresia of external auditory canals, syndactyly, and incomplete development of external genitalia.

MELNICK-FRASER SYNDROME
(Branchio-Oto-Renal Syndrome)

The association of branchial arch anomalies (preauricular pits, branchial fistulas), hearing loss, and renal hypoplasia constitutes the branchio-oto-renal (BOR) syndrome first described by Melnick and colleagues in 1975 and further delineated by Fraser and colleagues. The prevalence is roughly 1 in 40,000. The syndrome occurs in approximately 2% of profoundly deaf children.

ABNORMALITIES

Hearing loss	90%
Preauricular pits	80%
Branchial fistulas or cysts	50%
Anomalous pinna	35%
External auditory canal stenosis	30%
Malformed middle or inner ear	—
Lacrimal duct stenosis/aplasia	10%
Renal dysplasia	65%

OCCASIONAL ABNORMALITIES.
Long, narrow face, preauricular tag, congenital cholesteatoma, anomalies of the facial nerve, "constricted palate," deep overbite, microdontia of permanent teeth, cleft palate, bifid uvula, facial paralysis, gustatory lacrimation (the shedding of tears during eating because of misdirected growth of seventh cranial nerve fibers), congenital hip dislocation, nonrotation of bowel, pancreatic duplication cyst, euthyroid goiter, benign intracranial tumor.

NATURAL HISTORY. The ear pits or branchial clefts may go unnoticed until the hearing loss appears, or they may become infected and require surgery. The hearing loss may be sensorineural (25%), conductive (25%), or mixed (50%) and ranges from mild to severe. Age of onset can be from early childhood to young adulthood, and hearing loss is occasionally precipitous. In some families, it has been progressive. There may be malformations of the middle ear, vestibular system, and cochlea, including displaced, malformed, or fused ossicles and the Mondini malformation of the cochlea. Defects of the external ear range from severe microtia to minor anomalies of the pinna, which is variously described as cup- or loop-shaped, flattened, or hypoplastic. The external canal can be narrow, slanted upward, or malformed, making otoscopic examination difficult.

The renal anomalies range from minor dysplasia (sharply tapered superior poles, blunting of calyces, duplication of the collecting system) to bilateral renal agenesis with renal failure in approximately 6% of patients.

ETIOLOGY. This disorder is caused by an autosomal dominant gene with variable expression. Mutations in the human homologue of the Drosophila eyes absent gene (eya) called EYA1 localized to chromosome 8q13.3 are responsible for approximately 50% of cases. It has been hypothesized that the lack of confirmed mutations in the remainder reflects a failure to screen for complex disease-causing genomic rearrangements using Southern blot analysis or that mutations in another gene in the same region could cause a similar phenotype.

COMMENT. Mutations of the EYA1 gene occur in the majority of individuals with the branchio-otic syndrome, which manifests the same clinical features as branchio-oto-renal syndrome with the exception of renal anomalies. This, in addition to their marked phenotypic overlap, indicates that they are phenotypic variants of the same disorder or allelic defects of the EYA1 gene.

References
Melnick M et al.: Autosomal dominant branchio-otorenal dysplasia. Birth Defects 11(5):121, 1975.

Melnick M et al: Familial branchio-oto-renal dysplasia: A new addition to the branchial arch syndromes. Clin Genet 9:25, 1976.

Fraser FC et al: Genetic aspects of the BOR syndrome—branchial fistulas, ear pits, hearing loss, and renal anomalies. Am J Med Genet 2:241, 1978.

Fraser FC, Sproule JR, Halal F: Frequency of the branchio-oto-renal (BOR) syndrome in children with profound hearing loss. Am J Med Genet 7:341, 1980.

Heimler A, Lieber E: Branchio-oto-renal syndrome: Reduced penetrance and variable expressivity in four generations of a large kindred. Am J Med Genet 25:15, 1986.

Smith RJH, Schwartz C: Branchio-oto-renal syndrome. J Commun Disord 31:411, 1998.

Vervoort VS et al: Genomic rearrangements of EYA1 account for a large fraction of families with BOR syndrome. Eur J Hum Genet 10:757, 2002.

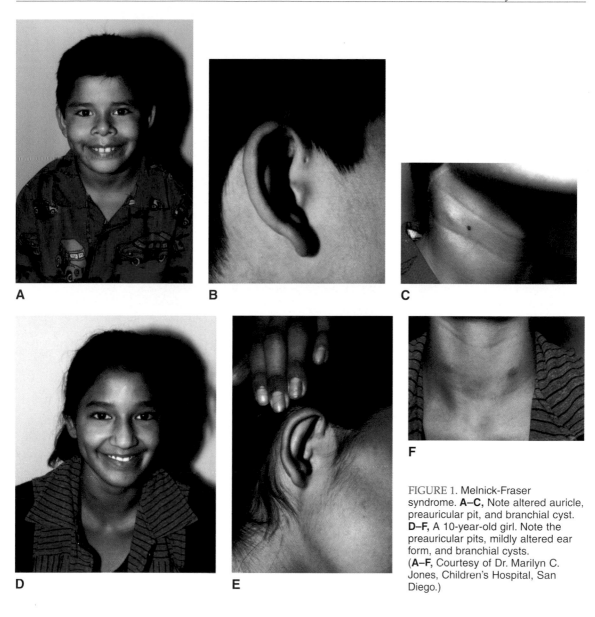

FIGURE 1. Melnick-Fraser syndrome. **A–C,** Note altered auricle, preauricular pit, and branchial cyst. **D–F,** A 10-year-old girl. Note the preauricular pits, mildly altered ear form, and branchial cysts. (**A–F,** Courtesy of Dr. Marilyn C. Jones, Children's Hospital, San Diego.)

BRANCHIO-OCULO-FACIAL SYNDROME

Branchial Defects, Lacrimal Duct Obstruction, Pseudocleft of Upper Lip

Individuals with this disorder were initially described in 1982 by Lee and colleagues and in 1983 by Hall and colleagues. The designation branchio-oculo-facial syndrome was introduced by Fujimoto and colleagues. More than 30 cases have been described.

ABNORMALITIES

Performance. Mental retardation (25%) in most cases mild.

Growth. Prenatal growth deficiency (27%), postnatal growth deficiency (50%).

Branchial. Sinus/fistulous tract (45%), atrophic skin lesion/aplasia cutis congenita/scarring (57%), hemangiomatous lesion (36%).

Ocular. Lacrimal duct obstruction (78%), colobomata (47%), microphthalmia/anophthalmia (44%), upslanting palpebral fissures (48%), telecanthus (58%), myopia (46%).

Auricular. Low-set, posteriorly rotated, overfolded or malformed ears (85%); hypoplastic superior helix (43%); conductive hearing loss (71%); supra-auricular sinuses (15%).

Oral. Abnormal upper lip (90%), which includes pseudocleft (appearance of repaired cleft lip), incomplete or complete cleft lip; dental abnormalities (56%); micrognathia (50%).

Other. Premature graying of hair (67%).

OCCASIONAL ABNORMALITIES.

Microcephaly; white forelock; ptosis; orbital cyst; facial nerve paralysis; cataract; strabismus; preauricular pit; posterior auricular pit; microtia; sensorineural hearing loss; cleft palate; lip pits; ectopic dermal thymus in cervical region; broad or divided nasal tip; subcutaneous cysts of the scalp; renal agenesis; hand anomalies including polydactyly, clinodactyly, preaxial polydactyly, and a single transverse palmar crease; agenesis of cerebellar vermis.

NATURAL HISTORY. Hypernasal speech with conductive hearing loss is common. Premature graying of scalp hair normally begins around 18 years but has been seen as early as 10 years. Intelligence is usually normal. Reduced reproductive fitness in both males and females has been suggested.

ETIOLOGY. This disorder has an autosomal dominant inheritance pattern.

References

Lee WK et al: Bilateral branchial cleft sinuses associated with intrauterine and postnatal growth retardation, premature aging, and unusual facial appearance: A new syndrome with dominant transmission. Am J Med Genet 11:345, 1982.

Hall BD et al: A new syndrome of hemangiomatous branchial clefts, lip pseudoclefts, and unusual facial appearance. Am J Med Genet 14:135, 1983.

Fujimoto A et al: New autosomal dominant branchio-oculofacial syndrome. Am J Med Genet 27:943, 1987.

McCool M, Weaver D: Branchio-oculo-facial syndrome: Broadening the spectrum. Am J Med Genet 49:414, 1994.

Raveh E et al: Branchio-oculo-facial syndrome. Int J Pediatr Otorhinolaryngol 53:149, 2000.

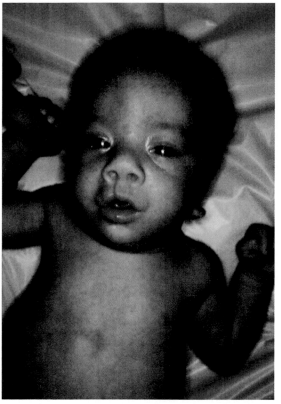

A

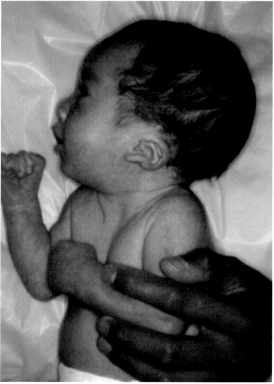

B

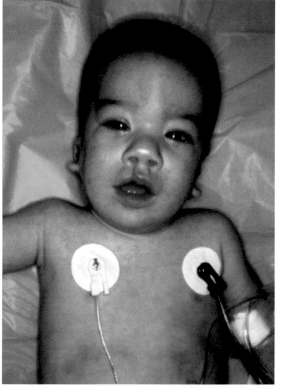

C

FIGURE 1. Branchio-oculo-facial syndrome. **A–C,** Male infant at 3 days and at 8 months of age. Note the pseudocleft of the lip and the low-set, posteriorly rotated ears with hypoplastic superior helix. (From Fujimoto A et al: Am J Med Genet 27:943, 1987. Copyright © 1987. Reprinted with permission of Wiley-Liss, Inc., a subsidiary of John Wiley & Sons, Inc.)

CHARGE SYNDROME

This disorder, initially referred to as an association, was first summarized by Hall, and many similar anomalies have been observed in patients ascertained for ocular coloboma. The spectrum was broadened by Pagon and colleagues to include *c*oloboma, *h*eart disease, *a*tresia choanae, *r*etarded growth and development and/or CNS anomalies, *g*enital anomalies and hypogonadism, and *e*ar anomalies and deafness. Based on the specificity of the pattern of malformation, it has been suggested that this condition represents a recognizable syndrome. A genetic etiology has recently been identified that gives support to that concept.

ABNORMALITIES

Colobomatous malformation sequence (ranging from isolated iris coloboma without visual impairment to clinical anophthalmos; retinal coloboma most common)	80%–90%
Heart defect (tetralogy of Fallot, patent ductus arteriosus, double-outlet right ventricle with an atrioventricular canal, ventricular septal defect, atrial septal defect, right-sided aortic arch)	75%–80%
Atresia choanae (membranous or bony)	58%
Growth deficiency (usually postnatal)	70%
Mental deficiency (ranging from mild to profound with several patients at autopsy demonstrating arrhinencephaly variants and several adults demonstrating hypogonadotropic hypogonadism reminiscent of Kallmann syndrome)	100%
Genital hypoplasia (in males)	75%
Ear anomalies or deafness (ranging from small ears without malformation of the pinna to cup-shaped, lop ears; either sensorineural or mixed sensorineural and conductive deafness, ranging from mild to profound)	90%

OCCASIONAL ABNORMALITIES. Micrognathia, including Robin malformation sequence; cleft lip; cleft palate; multiple cranial nerve abnormalities (I, VII, VIII, IX, and/or X); feeding difficulties resulting from poor suck and velopharyngeal incompetence; DiGeorge sequence; renal anomalies; omphalocele; tracheoesophageal fistula; rib anomalies; scoliosis; hemivertebrae; hand anomalies including polydactyly, ectrodactyly, thumb hypoplasia, and altered palmar creases; webbed neck; sloping shoulders; nipple anomalies; ptosis; ocular hypertelorism; microcephaly; anal atresia or stenosis; growth hormone deficiency.

NATURAL HISTORY. In some instances, the severity of these defects has been such that death has occurred during the perinatal period, the result of either respiratory insufficiency, intractable hypocalcemia, or congenital heart disease. Although prenatal growth deficiency has been present in some cases, most patients have been the appropriate size for gestational age, with linear growth shifting down to or below the third percentile during the first 6 months of life, which in some cases has been due to growth hormone deficiency. Most patients have shown some degree of mental deficiency or CNS defects, and visual or auditory handicaps may further compromise cognitive function. Multiple cranial nerve abnormalities may be more common than previously appreciated and may be responsible for the facial palsy, feeding difficulties, and sensorineural hearing loss.

ETIOLOGY. Mutations in the gene CDH7, a member of the chromodomain helicase DNA-binding (CHD) gene family, are responsible. This class of proteins is thought to be important in early embryologic development by affecting chromatin structure and gene expression.

References

Hall BD: Choanal atresia and associated multiple anomalies. J Pediatr 95:395, 1979.

Hittner HM et al: Colobomatous microphthalmia, heart disease, hearing loss, and mental retardation—a syndrome. J Pediatr Ophthalmol Strabismus 16:122, 1979.

Pagon RA et al: Coloboma, congenital heart disease, and

choanal atresia with multiple anomalies: CHARGE association. J Pediatr 99:223,1981.

August JP et al: Hypopituitarism and the CHARGE association. J Pediatr 103:424, 1983.

Davenport SLH et al: The spectrum of clinical features in CHARGE association. Clin Genet 29:298, 1986.

Byerly KA, Pauli RM: Cranial nerve abnormalities in CHARGE association. Am J Med Genet 45:751, 1993.

Derenoncourt A et al: CHARGE association and growth hormone deficiency. Clin Res 42:51A, 1994.

Blake KD et al: CHARGE association: An update and review for the primary pediatrician. Clin Pediatr 37:159, 1998.

Vissers LELM et al: Mutations in a new member of the chromodomain gene family cause CHARGE syndrome. Nat Genet, August 8, 2004. Available at: http://www. nature.com/ naturegenetics/.

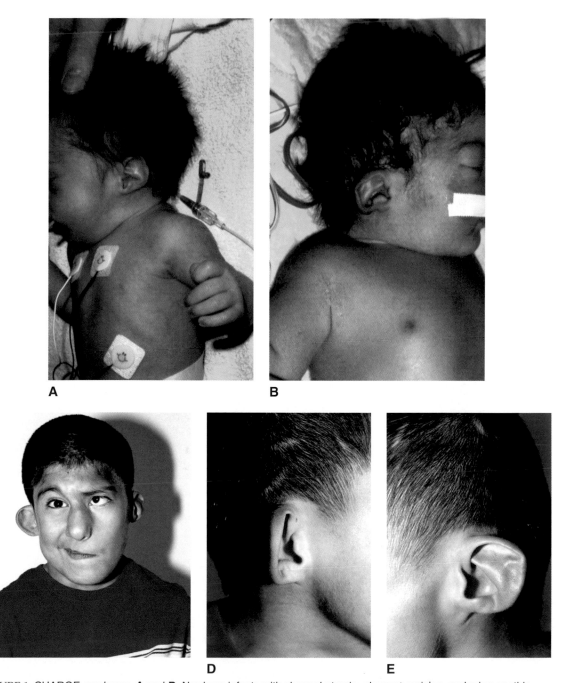

FIGURE 1. CHARGE syndrome. **A** and **B,** Newborn infants with choanal atresia, aberrant auricles, and micrognathia. The infant in **A** had a cardiac defect, and the infant in **B** had colobomata. Note the typical ear anomalies. **C–E,** A 10-year-old boy with mental retardation. Note the unilateral microphthalmia, the facial palsy, and the ear anomalies. (**C–E,** Courtesy of Dr. Marilyn C. Jones, Children's Hospital, San Diego.)

WAARDENBURG SYNDROME, TYPES I AND II

Lateral Displacement of Medial Canthi, Partial Albinism, Deafness

Waardenburg set forth this pattern of malformation in 1951. He found this syndrome in 1.4% of congenitally deaf children and from these data estimated the incidence to be approximately 1 in 42,000 in Holland. Four types have been described: type I is associated with lateral displacement of the medial canthi; type II is characterized by normally placed medial canthi; type III (Klein-Waardenburg syndrome) the principal features of which are upper limb defects including hypoplasia of muscles and bones, flexion contractures and syndactyly, in addition to the oculoauditory and pigmentary abnormalities characteristic of type I; and type IV (Shah-Waardenburg syndrome), which includes Hirschsprung disease combined with features of type II.

ABNORMALITIES. Lateral displacement of inner canthi with short palpebral fissures; broad and high nasal bridge with hypoplastic alae nasi; medial flare of bushy eyebrows, which may meet in midline; partial albinism manifest by hypopigmented ocular fundus, white eyelashes, eyebrows and forelock, premature graying, hypopigmented skin lesions, hypochromic iridis; deafness; aplasia of the posterior semicircular canal is commonly noted on tomography or computed tomography scan; broad mandible.

OCCASIONAL ABNORMALITIES. Patent metopic suture, strabismus, rounded tip of nose, full lips with accentuated "Cupid's bow" to upper lip, smooth philtrum, cleft lip and palate, anisocoria, cardiac anomaly (ventricular septal defect), upper limb defect; Hirschsprung aganglionosis, esophageal atresia, and anal atresia; Sprengel anomaly, supernumerary vertebrae and ribs, neural tube closure defect, scoliosis; multicystic dysplastic kidney; absence of vagina and adnexa uteri.

NATURAL HISTORY. The partial albinism is most commonly expressed as a white forelock and/or isochromic beautiful pale blue eyes with hypoplastic iridic stroma; however, it may be present as heterochromia of the iris, areas of vitiligo on the skin, patches of white hair other than the forelock, and/or mottled peripheral pigmentation of the retina. The white forelock may be present at birth only to become pigmented early in life; the hair may become prematurely gray or white.

Deafness, the most serious feature, is sensorineural, congenital, and usually nonprogressive. It can be unilateral or bilateral and varies from slight to profound, although usually the latter. The defect appears to be in the organ of Corti, with atrophic changes in the spiral ganglion and nerve. Deafness is a feature in 25% of type I cases (with lateral displacement of inner canthi) and in about 50% of type II cases.

ETIOLOGY. This disorder has an autosomal dominant inheritance pattern for types I, II, III, and some cases of type IV. Type I and type III are caused by mutations in the PAX3 gene located at 2q35. Approximately 15% of type II cases are caused by mutations in the human microphthalmia (MITF) gene at 3p12.3-p14.1. Mutations in the endothelin-B receptor gene (EDNRP), the gene for its ligand endothelin-3 (EDN3), and the SOX10 gene are all responsibe for type IV. Type IV is inherited as an autosomal recessive disorder when caused by mutations in EDNRP and EDN3, and as an autosomal dominant disorder when the result of mutations in SOX10.

References

Waardenburg PJ: A new syndrome combining developmental anomalies of the eyelids, eyebrows and nose root with pigmentary defects of the iris and head hair and with congenital deafness. Am J Hum Genet 3:195, 1951.

DiGeorge AM, Olmsted RW, Harley RD: Waardenburg's syndrome. J Pediatr 57:649, 1960.

Hageman MJ, Delleman JW: Heterogeneity in Waardenburg syndrome. Am J Hum Genet 29:468, 1977.

Klein D: Historical background and evidence for dominant inheritance of the Klein-Waardenburg syndrome (type III). Am J Med Genet 14:231, 1983.

Tassabehji M et al: Waardenburg's syndrome patients have

mutations in the human homologue of the PAX-3 paired box gene. Nature 355:635, 1992.

Hoth CF et al: Mutations in the paired domain of the human PAX3 gene cause Klein-Waardenburg syndrome (WS-III) as well as Waardenburg syndrome type I (WS-I). Am J Hum Genet 52:455, 1993.

Tassabehji M et al: Waardenburg syndrome type II caused by mutations in the human microphthalmia (MITF) gene. Nat Genet 8:251, 1994.

Read AP, Newton VP: Waardenburg syndrome. J Med Genet 34:656, 1997.

Touraine RL et al: Neurological phenotype in Waardenburg syndrome type 4 correlates with novel SOX10 truncating mutations and expression in developing brain. Am J Hum Genet 66:1496, 2000.

Pardono E et al: Waardenburg syndrome: Clinical differentiation between types I and II. Am J Med Genet 117:223, 2003.

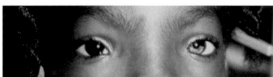

B

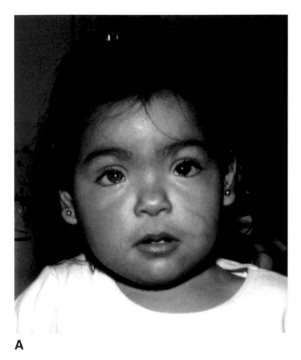

A

FIGURE 1. Waardenburg syndrome. **A** and **B,** Note the lateral displacement of the medial canthi, the broad nasal bridge with hypoplastic ala nasi, medial eyebrow flare, and hypochromic iridis.

TREACHER COLLINS SYNDROME
(MANDIBULOFACIAL DYSOSTOSIS,
FRANCESCHETTI-KLEIN SYNDROME)

Malar Hypoplasia with Downslanting Palpebral Fissures, Defect of Lower Lid, Malformation of External Ear

Although Thomson reported the first case in 1846, the syndrome has been associated with Treacher Collins, who described two cases in 1900. Franceschetti and Klein made extensive reports on this condition and called it mandibulofacial dysostosis (1940s).

ABNORMALITIES

Antimongoloid slanting palpebral fissures	89%
Malar hypoplasia, with or without cleft in zygomatic bone	81%
Mandibular hypoplasia	78%
Lower lid coloboma	69%
Partial to total absence of lower eyelashes	53%
Malformation of auricles	77%
External ear canal defect	36%
Conductive deafness	40%
Visual loss	37%
Cleft palate	28%
Incompetent soft palate	32%
Projection of scalp hair onto lateral cheek	26%

OCCASIONAL ABNORMALITIES.
Pharyngeal hypoplasia, coloboma of the upper lid, dacryostenosis, microphthalmia, strabismus, ptosis, macrostomia, microstomia, choanal atresia, blind fistulas and skin tags between auricle and angle of the mouth, absence of the parotid gland, congenital heart defect, cryptorchidism, mental retardation has been reported in only 5% of the cases.

NATURAL HISTORY.
Early respiratory problems can develop as a result of having a narrow airway and may occasionally require temporary tracheostomy. The narrow airway may make intubation difficult. As the great majority of these patients are of normal intelligence, the early recognition of deafness and its correction with hearing aids or surgery (when possible) are of great importance for development. Amblyopia secondary to refractive errors, anisometropia, strabismus, and/or ptosis is the most common cause of visual loss and should be carefully sought for in all cases. The growth of the facial bones during infancy and childhood results in some cosmetic improvement that may be enhanced by plastic surgery.

ETIOLOGY.
This disorder has an autosomal dominant inheritance pattern. Mutations in a gene, TCOF1, which maps to 5q31.3-32, are responsible for this disorder. TCOF1 encodes a protein named treacle, the function of which is unknown. There is wide variability in expression.

COMMENT.
Despite the marked variability in expression, a careful clinical and radiologic examination to rule out such subtle features as hypoplasia of the zygomatic arch on the occipitomental radiographs are usually diagnostic even in the most mildly affected individual.

References
Thomson A: Notice of several cases of malformation of the external ear, together with experiments on the state of hearing in such persons. Month J Med Sci 7:420, 1846.
Treacher Collins E: Case with symmetrical congenital notches in the outer part of each lower lid and defective development of the malar bones. Trans Ophthalmol Soc UK 20:90, 1900.
Franceschetti A, Klein D: The Mandibulofacial Dysostosis: A New Hereditary Syndrome. Copenhagen: E. Munksgaard, 1949.
Peterson-Falzone S, Pruzansky S: Cleft palate and congenital palatopharyngeal incompetency in mandibulofacial dysostosis. Cleft Palate J 13:354, 1976.
Shprintzen RJ, Berkman MD: Pharyngeal hypoplasia in Treacher Collins syndrome. Arch Otolaryngol 105:127, 1979.
Dixon MJ et al: Narrowing the position of the Treacher Collins syndrome locus to a small interval between three new microsatellite markers at 5q32-33.1. Am J Hum Genet 52:907, 1993.

Hertle RW et al: Ophthalmic features and visual prognosis in the Treacher Collins syndrome. Br J Ophthalmol 77:642, 1993.

Dixon MJ et al: Treacher Collins syndrome: Correlation between clinical and genetic linkage studies. Clin Dysmorph 3:96, 1994.

The Treacher Collins Syndrome Collaborative Group: Positional cloning of a gene involved in the pathogenesis of Treacher Collins syndrome. Nat Genet 12:130, 1996.

Posnick JC, Ruiz RL: Treacher Collins syndrome: Current evaluation, treatment, and future directions. Cleft Palate Craniofac J 37:434, 2000.

Ellis PE et al: Mutation testing in Treacher Collins syndrome. J Orthodontia 29:293, 2002.

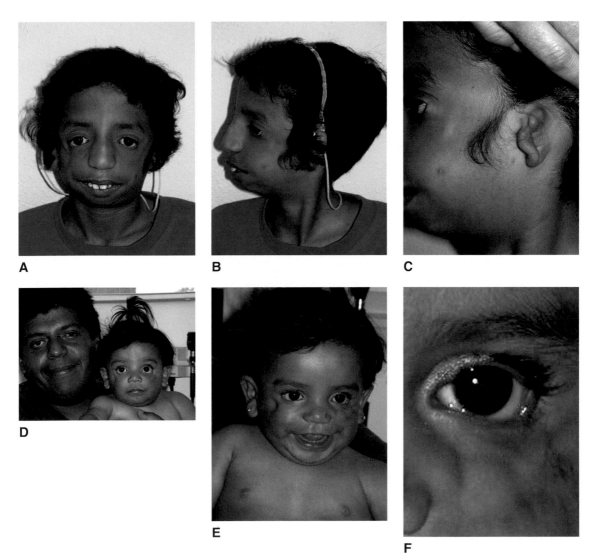

FIGURE 1. Treacher-Collins syndrome. **A–C,** An adolescent boy. Note the hair extending onto the lateral cheek, downslanting palpebral fissures, malar hypoplasia, malformed ears, and micrognathia. **D,** An affected father and his affected daughter. **E** and **F,** Note evidence of a cleft of the zygomatic bone and the coloboma of both the upper and lower lids. (**A–F,** Courtesy of Dr. Lynne M. Bird, Children's Hospital, San Diego.)

MARSHALL SYNDROME

In 1958, Marshall described seven family members in three generations with a disorder characterized by cataracts, sensorineural deafness, and an extremely short nose with a flat bridge.

ABNORMALITIES

Growth. Short stature.

Facies. Short depressed nose with flat nasal bridge and anteverted nares; appearance of large eyes; flat midface; prominent, protruding upper incisors; thick lips.

Eyes. Ocular hypertelorism, myopia, cataracts, esotropia.

Hearing. Sensorineural or mixed loss, primarily affects high frequencies and usually is progressive.

Skeletal. Calvarial thickening; absent frontal sinuses; falx, tentorial, and meningeal calcifications; spondyloepiphyseal abnormalities, including mild platyspondyly, slightly small and irregular distal femoral and proximal tibial epiphyses, outward bowing of radius and ulna, and wide tufts of distal phalanges.

Other. Brachycephaly; sparse scalp hair, eyebrows, and eyelashes.

OCCASIONAL ABNORMALITIES.

Mental retardation, glaucoma, retinal detachment, spontaneous rupture of lens capsule, cleft palate, asymptomatic dysfunction of central and peripheral vestibular system, cryptorchidism, fifth finger clinodactyly.

NATURAL HISTORY. The cataracts may spontaneously resorb. Hearing loss has been noted in early childhood and often progresses to moderate or severe by adulthood.

ETIOLOGY. This disorder has an autosomal dominant inheritance pattern. Mutations in the gene encoding the α1 chain of type XI collagen (COL11A1), mapped to chromosome 1p21, are responsible. Some cases of Stickler syndrome are also due to mutations in COL11A1.

References

Marshall D: Ectodermal dysplasia: Report of a kindred with ocular abnormalities and hearing defect. Am J Ophthalmol 45:143, 1958.

Zellweger H, Smith JK, Grützner P: The Marshall syndrome: Report of a new family. J Pediatr 84:868, 1974.

O'Donnell JJ, Sirkin S, Hall BD: Generalized osseous abnormalities in the Marshall syndrome. Birth Defects 12(5):299, 1976.

Aymé S, Preus M: The Marshall and Stickler syndromes: Objective rejection of lumping. J Med Genet 21:34, 1984.

Shanske AL et al: The Marshall syndrome: Report of a new family and review of the literature. Am J Med Genet 70:52, 1997.

Griffith AJ et al: Marshall syndrome associated with a splicing defect at the COL11A1 locus. Am J Hum Genet 62:816, 1998.

Griffith AJ et al: Audiovestibular phenotype associated with a COL11A1 mutation in Marshall syndrome. Arch Otolaryngol Head Neck Surg 126:891, 2000.

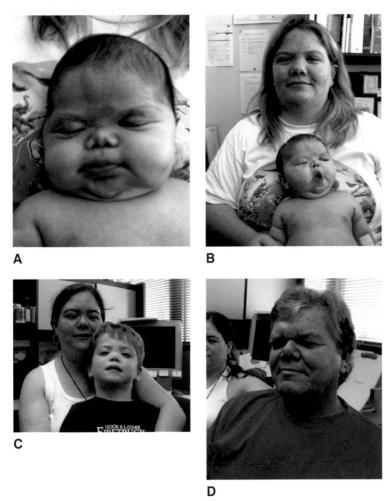

FIGURE 1. Marshall syndrome. **A–D,** Three-generation family including a father, his two daughters, and two of his grandchildren. Note the short depressed nose, flat nasal bridge, anteverted nares, and appearance of large eyes.

CERVICO-OCULO-ACOUSTIC SYNDROME
(WILDERVANCK SYNDROME)

Klippel-Feil Anomaly, Abducens Paralysis with Retracted Globes, Sensorineural Deafness

Initially described by Wildervanck in 1952, this disorder was further characterized by the same investigator, who summarized the clinical features of 62 affected patients in 1978.

ABNORMALITIES

Craniofacial. Asymmetry with a short neck and low hairline, preauricular skin tags and pits.

Eyes. Duane anomaly (abducens paralysis with retraction of the globe and narrowing of the palpebral fissure of the affected eye on adduction), epibulbar dermoids.

Hearing. Sensorineural, conductive, or mixed loss; a malformed vestibular labyrinth is usually present; the cochlea is sometimes altered.

Skeletal. Klippel-Feil anomaly (fusion of two or more cervical and sometimes thoracic vertebrae), torticollis, scoliosis, Sprengel deformity.

OCCASIONAL ABNORMALITIES.
Mental retardation; growth deficiency; occipital meningocele; cerebellar and brainstem hypoplasia, primarily involving the pons and medulla; cervical diastematomyelia; pseudopapilledema; tearing during oral feeding; hydrocephalus; cleft palate; ear anomalies; cardiac defects; cervical ribs; absent kidney; cholelithiasis.

NATURAL HISTORY. Severe deformations of the craniofacial area can progress in cases with significant degrees of torticollis. Intelligence in the vast majority of cases is normal. Computed tomography should be performed to document any abnormality of the inner ear. Magnetic resonance imaging for craniospinal abnormalities should be considered.

ETIOLOGY. The cause of this disorder is unknown; all cases have been sporadic. The majority of affected individuals have been females.

References

Wildervanck LS: The cervico-oculo-acusticus syndrome. In Vinken PJ, Bruyn GW (eds): Handbook of Clinical Neurology: Congenital Malformations of the Spine and Spinal Cord, vol. 32. Amsterdam, NY: Elsevier/North-Holland Biomedical, 1978.

West PDB et al: Wildervanck's syndrome: Unilateral Mondini dysplasia identified by computed tomography. J Laryngol Otol 103:408, 1989.

Gupte G et al: Wildervanck syndrome (cervico-oculo-acoustic syndrome). J Postgrad Med 38:180, 1992.

Brodsky MC et al: Brainstem hypoplasia in the Wildervanck (cervico-oculo-acoustic) syndrome. Arch Ophthalmol 116:383, 1998.

Balci S et al: Cervical diastematomyelia in the cervico-oculo-acoustic (Wildervanck) syndrome: MRI findings. Clin Dysmorphol 11:125, 2002.

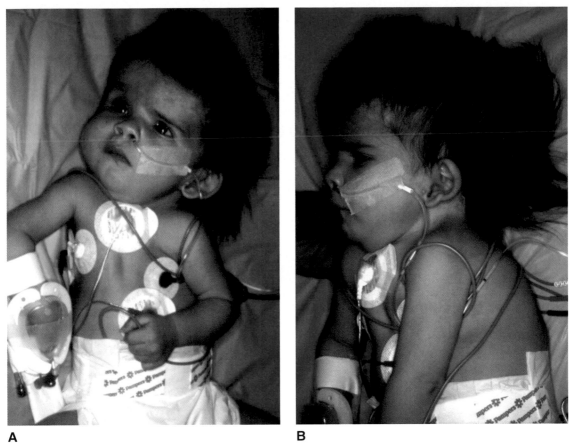

A   **B**

FIGURE 1. Cervico-oculo-acoustic syndrome. **A** and **B,** Note the short neck with low hairline, preauricular skin tag, and ear anomalies.

H Facial-Limb Defects as Major Feature

MILLER SYNDROME
(Postaxial Acrofacial Dysostosis Syndrome)

Treacher Collins–Like Facies; Limb Deficiency, Especially Postaxial

In 1979, Miller and colleagues brought together six cases, four of which were from the literature, and recognized this disorder as a concise entity. The facial appearance is similar to that of Treacher Collins syndrome and, in combination with limb defects, resembles Nager syndrome. The severity of the postaxial deficiencies distinguishes it from the latter syndrome.

ABNORMALITIES

Craniofacial. Malar hypoplasia, sometimes with radiologic evidence of a vertical bony cleft, with downslanting palpebral fissures; colobomata of eyelids and ectropion; micrognathia; cleft lip and/or cleft palate; hypoplastic, cup-shaped ears.

Limbs. Absence of fifth digits of all four limbs with or without shortening and in-curving of forearms with ulnar and radial hypoplasia; syndactyly.

Other. Accessory nipple(s).

OCCASIONAL ABNORMALITIES.
Postnatal growth deficiency, choanal atresia, conductive hearing loss, thumb hypoplasia, low-arch dermal pattern, pectus excavatum, radioulnar synostosis, supernumerary vertebrae, rib defects, congenital hip dislocation, heart defects, absence of hemidiaphragm, pyloric stenosis, renal anomalies, cryptorchidism, midgut malrotation.

NATURAL HISTORY. These individuals are usually of normal intelligence. Hearing evaluation is indicated in all cases. The craniofacial appearance sometimes changes with increasing age with a progressively greater degree of ectropion and facial asymmetry as well as a more triangular facial appearance with thin lips.

ETIOLOGY. This disorder has an autosomal recessive inheritance pattern.

References

Genée E: Une forme extensive de dysostose mandibulofaciale. J Genet Hum 17:45, 1969.

Smith DW, Pashayan H, Wildervanck LS: Case report 28. Syndrome Identification 3(1):7, 1975.

Miller M, Fineman R, Smith DW: Postaxial acrofacial dysostosis syndrome. J Pediatr 95:970, 1979.

Ogilvy-Stuart AL, Parsons AC: Miller syndrome (postaxial acrofacial dysostosis): Further evidence for autosomal recessive inheritance and expansion of the phenotype. J Med Genet 28:695, 1991.

Chrzanowska K, Fryns JP: Miller postaxial acrofacial dysostosis: The phenotypic changes with age. Genet Couns 4:131, 1993.

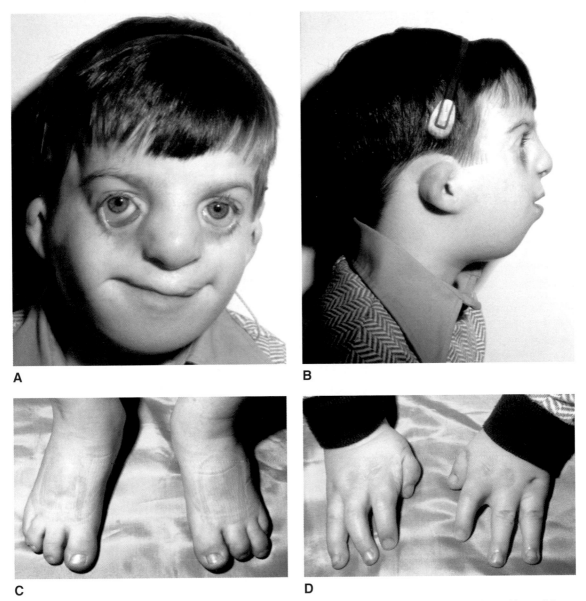

A

B

C

D

FIGURE 1. Miller syndrome. **A–D,** Affected individual showing striking malar and maxillary hypoplasia and lower lid defects. Note the hearing aid, required for middle ear deafness. The deficiency in the hands and feet is complete for the fifth ray and incomplete for the other digits. (From Miller M et al: J Pediatr 95:970, 1979, with permission.)

NAGER SYNDROME
(NAGER ACROFACIAL DYSOSTOSIS SYNDROME)

Radial Limb Hypoplasia, Malar Hypoplasia, Ear Defects

Nager and deReynier described a Treacher Collins syndrome–like patient with radial limb defects in 1948, and subsequently more than 75 cases have been recognized.

ABNORMALITIES

Performance. Intelligence normal, conductive deafness usually bilateral and problems with articulation.

Craniofacial. Malar hypoplasia with downslanting palpebral fissures; high nasal bridge; micrognathia; partial to total absence of lower eyelashes; low-set, posteriorly rotated ears; preauricular tags; atresia of external ear canal; cleft palate.

Limbs. Hypoplasia to aplasia of thumb, with or without radius; proximal radioulnar synostosis and limitation of elbow extension; short forearms.

OCCASIONAL ABNORMALITIES.

Mental retardation; microcephaly; hydrocephalus secondary to aqueductal stenosis; polymicrogyria; postnatal growth deficiency; lower lid coloboma; projection of scalp hair onto lateral cheek; cleft lip; velopharyngeal insufficiency; hypoplasia of larynx or epiglottis; temporomandibular joint fibrosis and ankylosis; syndactyly, clinodactyly, or camptodactyly of hands; duplicated and triphalangeal thumbs; missing or hypoplastic toes; overlapping toes; syndactyly of toes; posteriorly placed hypoplastic halluces, hallux valgus, broad hallux; absent distal flexion creases on toes; limb reduction defects; hip dislocation; clubfeet; hypoplastic first rib; scoliosis; cervical vertebral and spine anomalies; cardiac defects; genitourinary anomalies; Hirschsprung disease; urticaria pigmentosa.

NATURAL HISTORY. The recommendations for early detection of deafness, hearing aid

augmentation, and plastic surgery are similar to those for Treacher Collins syndrome. Anesthetic complications should be considered seriously. Delays in speech and language development are related primarily to hearing loss. Early respiratory and feeding problems frequently occur. Gastrostomy or gavage feeding is often necessary. The incidence of prematurity is high. Perinatal mortality is approximately 20% and is related to respiratory distress secondary to micrognathia and palatal anomalies. Management should be the same as that for the Robin sequence.

ETIOLOGY. Most cases have been sporadic.
However, seven cases of parent-to-child transmission have been documented, suggesting autosomal dominant inheritance for some cases; and six families in which unaffected parents have given birth to more than one affected child have been reported, suggesting autosomal recessive inheritance for others.

References
Nager FR, deReynier JP: Das Gehörogan bei den angeborenen Kopfmissbildungen. Pract Otorhinolaryngol (Basal) 10(Suppl 2):1, 1948.
Bowen P, Harley F: Mandibulofacial dysostosis with limb malformations (Nager's acrofacial dysostosis). Birth Defects 10(5):109, 1974.
Walker F: Apparent autosomal recessive inheritance of Treacher-Collins syndrome. Birth Defects 10(8):135, 1974.
Meyerson MD et al: Nager acrofacial dysostosis: Early invention and long-term planning. Cleft Palate J 14:35, 1977.
Halal F et al: Differential diagnosis of Nager acrofacial dysostosis syndrome: Report of four patients with Nager syndrome and discussion of other related syndromes. Am J Med Genet 14:209, 1983.
Krauss CM, Hassell LA, Gang DL: Brief clinical report: Anomalies in an infant with Nager acrofacial dysostosis. Am J Med Genet 21:761, 1985.
Aylsworth AL et al: Nager acrofacial dysostosis: Male-to-male transmission in 2 families. Am J Med Genet 41:83, 1991.
McDonald MT, Gorski JL: Nager acrofacial dysostosis. J Med Genet 30:779, 1993.
Groeper K et al: Anaesthetic implications of Nager syndrome. Paediatr Anaesth 12:365. 2002.

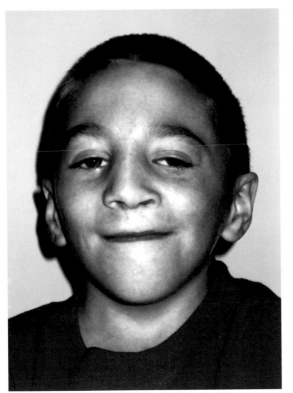 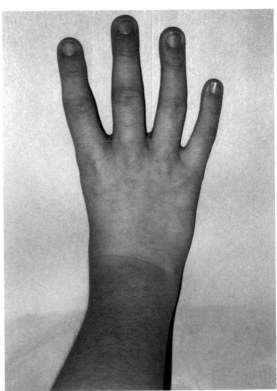

A B

FIGURE 1. Nager syndrome. **A** and **B,** Note the malar hypoplasia, downslanting palpebral fissures, high nasal bridge, micrognathia, and thumb aplasia. (Courtesy of Dr. Stephen Braddock, University of Missouri, Columbia.)

TOWNES-BROCKS SYNDROME

Thumb Anomalies, Auricular Anomalies, Anal Anomalies

Townes and Brocks first described this disorder in 1972, and at least 65 affected individuals have been reported.

ABNORMALITIES

Craniofacial. Auricular anomalies, including overfolding of the superior helix and small, sometimes cupped ears; variable features of hemifacial microsomia, especially preauricular tags.

Hearing. Sensorineural loss, ranging from mild to profound; a small conductive component is often present.

Limbs. Hand anomalies including broad, bifid, or triphalangeal thumb; preaxial polydactyly; distal ulnar deviation of thumb; pseudoepiphysis of second metacarpals; fusion of triquetrum and hamate; absence of triquetrum and navicular bones; fusion or short metatarsals; prominence of distal ends of lateral metatarsals; absent or hypoplastic third toe; clinodactyly of fifth toe.

Anus. Imperforate anus, anterior placement, and stenosis; rectovaginal or rectoperineal fistula.

Genitourinary. Unilateral or bilateral hypoplastic or dysplastic kidneys, renal agenesis, multicystic kidney, posterior urethral valves, vesicoureteral reflux, meatal stenosis.

OCCASIONAL ABNORMALITIES.

Mental retardation; microcephaly; microtia; preauricular pit; structural middle ear anomalies; cardiac defect; duodenal atresia; cystic ovary; prominent perineal raphe; bifid scrotum; hypospadias; 2-3 and 3-4 syndactyly of fingers; abnormalities of toes, including fifth toe clinodactyly, absence or hypoplasia of third toe, 3-4 syndactyly of toes, overlapping second, third, and fourth toes; scoliosis.

NATURAL HISTORY. Hearing loss can be progressive and is worse in the high frequencies. Renal failure or impaired renal function occurs in some cases. Lifelong monitoring of renal function is indicated.

ETIOLOGY. This disorder has an autosomal dominant inheritance pattern with marked variability in the severity of expression for each feature. Mutations in SALL1, which is expressed in all organs affected in this disorder and is located at 16q12.1, are responsible.

COMMENT. This single gene disorder encompasses many of the features of both the VATERR association and the facio-auriculo-vertebral malformation sequence.

References

Townes PL, Brocks ER: Hereditary syndrome of imperforate anus with hand, foot and ear anomalies. J Pediatr 81:321, 1972.

Reid IS, Turner G: Familial anal abnormality. J Pediatr 88:992, 1976.

Kurnit DM et al: Autosomal dominant transmission of a syndrome of anal, ear, renal and radial congenital malformations. J Pediatr 93:270, 1978.

Walpole IR, Hockey A: Syndrome of imperforate anus, abnormalities of hands and feet, satyr ears, and sensorineural deafness. J Pediatr 100:250, 1982.

Monteiro de Pino-Neto J: Phenotypic variability in Townes-Brocks syndrome. Am J Med Genet 18:147, 1984.

O'Callaghan M, Young ID: The Townes-Brocks syndrome. J Med Genet 27:457, 1990.

Cameron TH et al.: Townes-Brocks syndrome in two mentally retarded youngsters. Am J Med Genet 41:1, 1991.

Kohlhase J et al: Molecular analysis of SALL1 mutations in Townes-Brocks syndrome. Am J Hum Genet 64:435, 1999.

Powell CM, Michaelis RC: Townes-Brocks syndrome. J Med Genet 36:89, 1999.

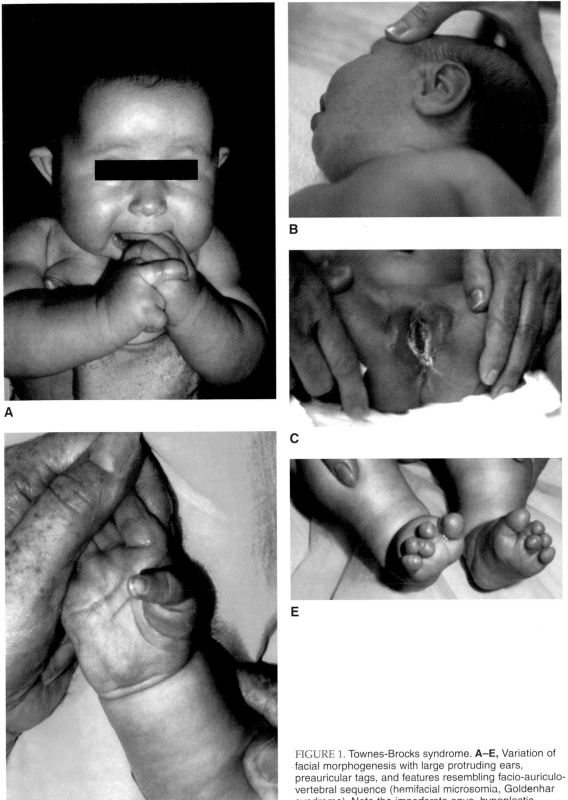

FIGURE 1. Townes-Brocks syndrome. **A–E,** Variation of facial morphogenesis with large protruding ears, preauricular tags, and features resembling facio-auriculo-vertebral sequence (hemifacial microsomia, Goldenhar syndrome). Note the imperforate anus, hypoplastic thenar eminence and thumb, and hypoplastic third toe.

ORAL-FACIAL-DIGITAL SYNDROME
(OFD SYNDROME, TYPE I)

Oral Frenula and Clefts, Hypoplasia of Alae Nasi, Digital Asymmetry

Papillon-Léage and Psaume set forth this condition as a clinical entity in 1954. More than 160 cases have been reported. Nine different oral-facial-digital syndromes have been delineated. Only types I and II have been set forth in detail in this text.

ABNORMALITIES

Oral. Multiple and/or hyperplastic frenuli between the buccal mucous membrane and alveolar ridge, median cleft lip, lobated/bifid tongue with nodules, cleft of alveolar ridge (at area of lateral incisors, which may be missing), cleft palate, dental caries and anomalous anterior teeth.

Facial. Hypoplasia of alar cartilages, lateral placement of inner canthi; milia of ears and upper face in infancy.

Digital. Asymmetric shortening of digits with clinodactyly, syndactyly, or brachydactyly of hands and unilateral polydactyly of feet.

Scalp. Dry, rough, sparse hair, dry scalp.

Central Nervous System. Variable mental deficiency in approximately 57%, with average IQ of 70; brain malformation (20%) including absence of corpus callosum, intracerebral cyst, porencephaly, hydrocephalus, vermis hypoplasia, focal polymicrogyria, cortical, periventricular, subarachnoid heterotopia, and Dandy-Walker malformation.

Cranium. Increased naso-sella-basion angle at base of cranium.

Renal. Adult polycystic kidney disease; histologically, there is a predominance of glomerular cysts.

OCCASIONAL ABNORMALITIES.
Enamel hypoplasia, supernumerary teeth, hamartoma of tongue, fistula in lower lip, choanal atresia, frontal bossing, hypoplastic mandibular ramus and zygoma, nonprogressive metaphyseal rarefaction, alopecia, granular seborrheic skin.

NATURAL HISTORY. Patients may do poorly in early infancy; as many as one third die during this period. Management is directed toward plastic surgical correction of oral clefts and dental care, including dentures when indicated. Psychometric evaluation is merited because about one half of the reported patients have mental retardation. Renal function should be monitored.

ETIOLOGY. This disorder has an X-linked dominant inheritance pattern with lethality in the vast majority of affected males. Mutations in OFD1 (formerly named Cxorf5), mapped to Xp22, are responsible for type I.

COMMENT. Toriello has set forth the major features that distinguish types III through IX. With the exception of type V, all have similar oral, facial, and digital abnormalities. Significant overlap exists between the nine types, making it difficult to provide appropriate counseling relative to prognosis.

Type III (Sugarman syndrome), an autosomal recessive disorder, is distinguished clinically by polydactyly that is only postaxial, a bulbous nose, extra, small teeth, and macular red spots associated with see-saw winking of eyelids or myoclonic jerks.

Type IV (Burn-Baraister syndrome), an autosomal recessive disorder, is distinguished by short tibiae, pre- or postaxial polydactyly of hands and feet, syndactyly of hands, clubfeet, wide metaphyses, and deafness.

Type V (Thurston syndrome), an autosomal recessive condition, includes midline cleft lip, duplicated frenulum, and postaxial polydactyly of hands and feet.

Type VI (Varadi syndrome), an autosomal recessive condition, is distinguished by preaxial polysyndactyly of toes and postaxial polydactyly of fingers, Y-shaped metacarpal with central polydactyly, cerebellar anomalies (vermis hypoplasia/aplasia or Dandy-Walker anomaly). Occasional features include growth hormone deficiency, hypogonadotrophic hypogonadism, and a hypothalamic hamartoma.

Type VII (Whelan syndrome) has been reported in a mother-daughter pair. Features that distinguish this condition include congenital hydronephrosis, coarse hair, facial asymmetry, facial weakness, and preauricular tags.

Type VIII is an X-linked recessive disorder distinguished from type I by pre- and postaxial polydactyly of hands and bilateral duplication of halluces, shortness of long bones, abnormal tibiae, short stature, laryngeal anomalies, absent/abnormal central incisors, broad/bifid nasal tip, and metacarpal forking.

Type IX is an autosomal recessive disorder. The features that distinguish this condition are retinal abnormalities consisting of atrophic areas of colobomatous origin, hamartoma, and detachment.

References

Papillon-Léage Mme, Psaume J: Une malformation héréditaire de la muqueuse buccale: Brides et freins anormaux. Rev Stomatol (Paris) 55:209, 1954.

Gorlin RJ, Psaume J: Orodigitofacial dysostosis—a new syndrome. J Pediatr 61:520, 1962.

Doege TC et al: Studies of a family with the oral-facial-digital syndrome. N Engl J Med 271:1073, 1964.

Majewski F et al: Das oro-facio-digitale Syndrom: Symptome und Prognose. Z Kinderheilkd 112:89, 1972.

Donnai D et al: Familial orofaciodigital syndrome type I presenting as adult polycystic kidney disease. J Med Genet 24:84, 1987.

Toriello HV: Oral-facial-digital syndromes, 1992. Clin Dysmorphol 2:95, 1993.

Toriello HV et al: Six patients with oral-facial-digital syndrome IV: The case for heterogeneity. Am J Med Genet 69:250, 1997.

Doss BJ et al: Neuropathologic findings in a case of OFDS type VI (Varadi syndrome). Am J Med Genet 77:38, 1998.

Ferrante MI et al: Identification of the gene for oral-facial-digital type I syndrome. Am J Hum Genet 68:569, 2001.

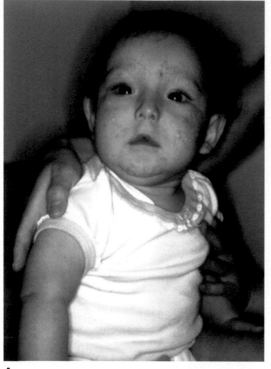

A

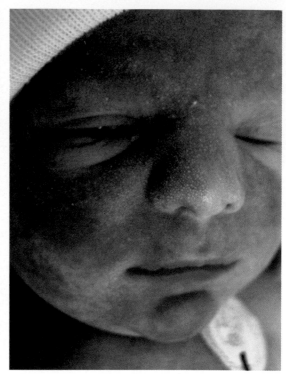

B

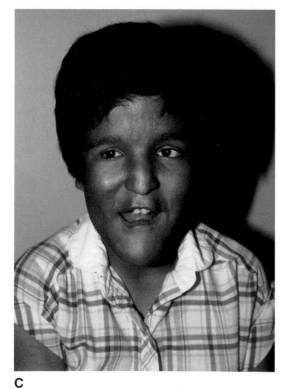

C

FIGURE 1. Oral-facial-digital syndrome, type I. **A–C,** Note the milia of the ears and upper face in infancy, the median cleft lip, and the hypoplastic ala nasi. (**A–G,** Courtesy of Dr. Marilyn C. Jones, Children's Hospital, San Diego.)

Continued

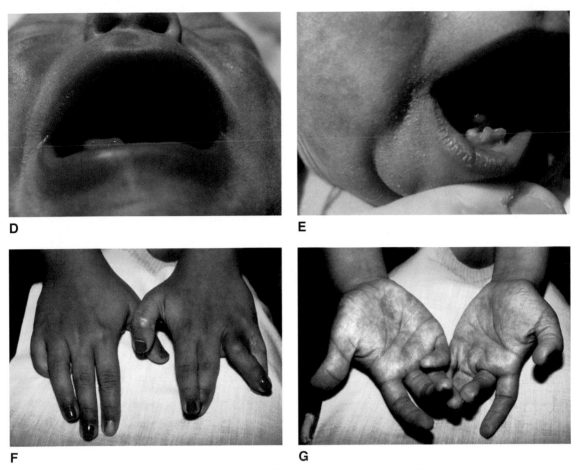

Fig. 1, cont'd. **D** and **E,** Note the clefts of the alveolar ridge, cleft palate, and lobulated tongue. **F** and **G,** Note the asymmetric shortening of digits with syndactyly and clinodactyly.

MOHR SYNDROME
(OFD Syndrome, Type II)

Cleft Tongue, Conductive Deafness, Partial Reduplication of Hallux

Mohr described this pattern in several male siblings in 1941. More than 30 cases have been reported.

ABNORMALITIES

General. Mild shortness of stature, conductive deafness due apparently to defect of incus.

Facies and Mouth. Low nasal bridge with lateral displacement of inner canthi; broad nasal tip, sometimes slightly bifid; midline partial cleft of lip; hypertrophy of usual frenula; midline cleft of tongue, nodules on tongue; flare to alveolar ridge; hypoplasia of zygomatic arch, maxilla, and body of mandible.

Limbs. Partial reduplication of hallux and first metatarsal, cuneiform and cuboid bones; relatively short hands with clinodactyly of fifth finger; bilateral postaxial polydactyly of hands; bilateral preaxial polysyndactyly of feet (occasionally only unilateral); metaphyseal flaring and irregularity.

OCCASIONAL ABNORMALITIES.
Wormian cranial bones, missing central incisors, cleft palate, multiple frenula, pectus excavatum, scoliosis.

NATURAL HISTORY. These patients apparently have normal intelligence, and plastic surgery is indicated for the clefts, frenula, and partial reduplication of the hallux.

ETIOLOGY. This disorder has an autosomal recessive inheritance pattern.

References

Mohr OL: A hereditary sublethal syndrome in man. Skr Norske Vidensk Akad I Mat Naturv Klasse 14:3, 1941.

Rimoin DL, Edgerton MT: Genetic and clinical heterogeneity in the oral-facial-digital syndromes. J Pediatr 71:94, 1967.

Pfeiffer RA, Majewski F, Mannkopf H: Das syndrome von Mohr und Classen. Klin Paediatr 184:224, 1972.

Levy EP, Fletcher BD, Fraser FC: Mohr syndrome with subclinical expression of the bifid great toe. Am J Dis Child 128:531, 1974.

Baraitser M: The orofacial digital (OFD) syndromes. J Med Genet 23:116, 1986.

Hosalkar HS et al: Mohr syndrome: A rare case and distinction from orofacial digital syndrome I. J Postgrad Med 45:123, 1999.

Sakai N et al: Oral-facial-digital syndrome type II (Mohr syndrome): Clinical and genetic manifestations. J Craniofac Surg 13:321, 2002.

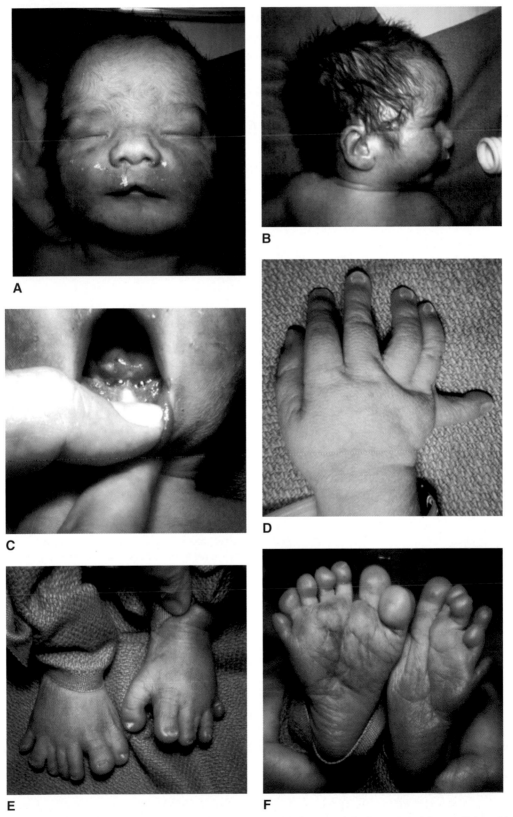

FIGURE 1. Mohr syndrome. **A–C,** Note the midline cleft of the upper lip, lateral displacement of the medial canthi, broad nasal tip, and tongue nodules. **D–F,** Note the postaxial polydactyly of hands and feet and preaxial polydactyly of feet.

DELETION 22q11.2 SYNDROME
(Velo-Cardio-Facial Syndrome, DiGeorge
Syndrome, Shprintzen Syndrome)

In 1965, DiGeorge described a patient with hypo-parathyroidism and cellular immune deficiency secondary to thymic hypoplasia. The pattern of malformation expanded rapidly to include other defects of the third and fourth branchial arches as well as dysmorphic facial features. In 1978, Shprintzen and colleagues reported a group of children with cleft palate or velopharyngeal incompetence, cardiac defects, and a prominent nose (Velo-Cardio-Facial syndrome). It was subsequently determined that individuals with velo-cardio-facial syndrome and the majority of those with the condition described by DiGeorge have a deletion of chromosome 22q11.2. It is now known that the two disorders represent different manifestations of the same genetic defect.

ABNORMALITIES

Performance. Normal development or mild learning problems (62%); moderate or severe learning problems (18%); IQ generally ranges from 70 to 90, with some slightly higher; psychiatric disorders in approximately 10% of cases.

Growth. Postnatal onset of short stature (36%).

Ears and Hearing. Conductive hearing loss secondary to cleft palate; minor auricular anomalies.

Craniofacial. Cleft of the secondary palate, either overt or submucous; velopharyngeal incompetence; small or absent adenoids; prominent nose with squared nasal root and narrow alar base; narrow palpebral fissures; abundant scalp hair; deficient malar area; vertical maxillary excess with long face; retruded mandible with chin deficiency; microcephaly (40% to 50%).

Limbs. Slender and hypotonic with hyperextensible hands and fingers (63%).

Cardiac. Defects present in 85%, the most common being ventricular septal defect (62%); right aortic arch (52%); tetralogy of Fallot (21%); aberrant left subclavian artery.

OCCASIONAL ABNORMALITIES.
Robin malformation sequence; cleft lip; asymmetric crying facies; facial nerve palsy; nasal dimple; enlargement, medial displacement, tortuosity or other abnormalities of internal carotid arteries (25%); umbilical or inguinal hernias; structural brain defects including cerebral atrophy, cerebellar hypoplasia, cerebral vascular defect, septum pellucidum cyst, hydrocephalus, hypoplastic corpus callosum and enlarged ventricles; meningomyelocele; absent, dysplastic, or multicystic kidneys; obstructive uropathy; vesicoureteral reflux; cryptorchidism; hypospadias; anal anomalies; laryngeal web; tortuousity of retinal vessels (30%); small optic disks; ocular coloboma; cataracts; holoprosencephaly; neural tube closure defect; hypothyroidism; Graves' disease; abnormal T cell function and absent thymic tissue; pre- and postaxial polydactyly; talipes equinovarus; scoliosis; abnormal vertebrae; arthritis.

NATURAL HISTORY. Death, due almost exclusively to cardiac defects, has occurred in 8% of cases, over one half in the first month of life and the majority before 6 months. Hypotonia in infancy is frequent (70% to 80%). Transient neonatal hypocalcemia occurs in 60% of cases. Seizures (21%), usually the result of hypocalcemia. Speech development is often delayed, and language is impaired. Speech is almost always hypernasal, with the pharyngeal musculature being hypotonic. Socialization skills may surpass intellectual skills. Personality may tend toward perseverative behavior, with concrete thinking secondary to intellectual impairment or learning disorders. Approximately 10% of affected individuals have developed psychiatric disorders, primarily chronic schizophrenia and paranoid delusions, with onset varying between 10 and 21 years of age. Obstructive sleep apnea has been noted following pharyngeal surgery to improve speech in several patients. The abnormalities of the internal carotid arteries can be diagnosed by the demonstration of visible pulsations in the posterior pharyngeal wall musculature using fiberoptic nasopharyngoscopy and with magnetic resonance imaging (MRI) of the pharynx. Clinically significant immunologic problems are not common.

ETIOLOGY. This disorder has an autosomal dominant inheritance pattern. Affected individuals have an interstitial deletion of chromosome

22q11.2, which is detectable using fluorescent in situ hybridization (FISH). Because of the marked variability of expression, both parents of an affected child should be tested to determine if they carry the deletion.

References

Shprintzen RJ et al.: A new syndrome involving cleft palate, cardiac anomalies, typical facies, and learning disabilities: Velo-cardio-facial syndrome. Cleft Palate J 15:56, 1978.

Young D, Shprintzen RJ, Goldberg RB: Cardiac malformations in the velo-cardio-facial syndrome. Am J Cardiol 46:643, 1980.

Shprintzen RJ et al: The velo-cardio-facial syndrome: A clinical and genetic analysis. Pediatrics 67:167, 1981.

Fitch N: Velo-cardio-facial syndrome and eye abnormality. Am J Med Genet 15:699, 1983.

Williams MA, Shprintzen RJ, Goldberg RB: Male-to-male transmission of the velo-cardio-facial syndrome: A case report and review of 60 cases. J Craniofac Genet Dev Biol 5:175, 1985.

Driscoll DA et al: Deletions and microdeletions of 22q11.2 in velo-cardio-facial syndrome. Am J Med Genet 44:261, 1992.

Scrambler PJ et al: The velo-cardio-facial syndrome is associated with chromosome 22 deletions which encompass the DiGeorge syndrome locus, Lancet 339:1138, 1992.

Goldberg R et al: Velo-cardio-facial: A review of 120 patients. Am J Med Genet 45:313, 1993.

Ryan AK et al: Spectrum of clinical features associated with interstitial chromosome 22q11 deletions: A European collaborative study. J Med Genet 34:798, 1997.

Wooden M et al: Neuropsychological profile of children and adolescents with the 22q11.2 microdeletion. Genet Med 3:34, 2001.

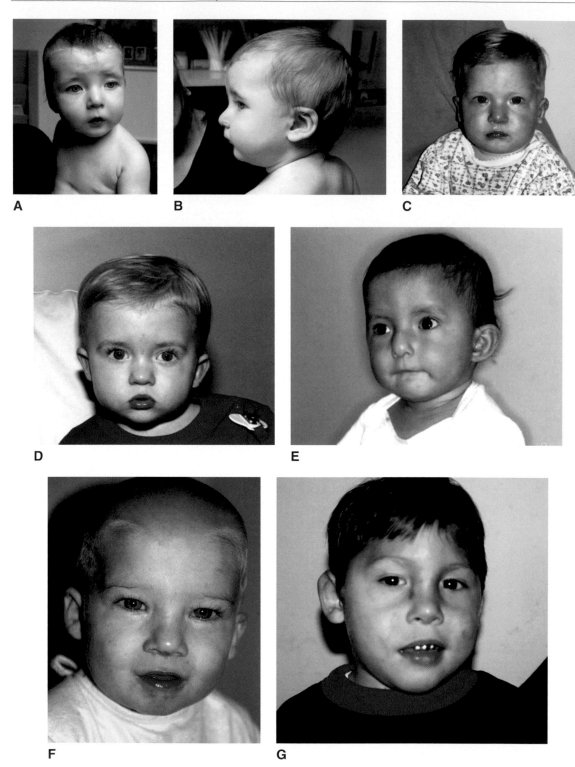

FIGURE 1. Deletion 22q11.2 syndrome. **A–G,** Phenotype in children from 8 months to 3 years of age. Note the narrow nose with squared nasal root and narrow ala nasi; the short palpebral fissures; and the somewhat smooth philtrum. (**C, F,** and **G,** Courtesy of Dr. Lynne M. Bird, Children's Hospital, San Diego; **D** and **E,** courtesy of Dr. Marilyn C. Jones, Children's Hospital, San Diego.)

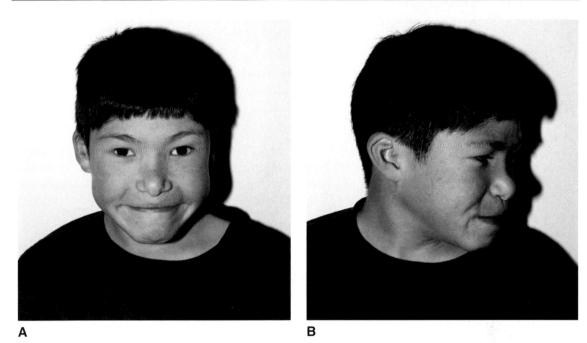

A **B**

FIGURE 2. **A** and **B,** Photograph of 12-year-old boy. Facial features emphasizing the nasal configuration. (Courtesy of Dr. Marilyn C. Jones, Children's Hospital, San Diego.)

OCULODENTODIGITAL SYNDROME
(OCULODENTODIGITAL DYSPLASIA)

Microphthalmos, Enamel Hypoplasia, Camptodactyly of Fifth Fingers

Originally described in 1920 by Lohmann, this pattern was more fully characterized by Gorlin, Meskin, and St. Geme in 1963.

ABNORMALITIES

Eyes. Microphthalmos, microcornea, fine porous iris; short palpebral fissures and epicanthal folds.

Nose. Thin, hypoplastic alae nasi with small nares.

Teeth. Enamel hypoplasia.

Hands and Feet. Syndactyly of fourth and fifth fingers, third and fourth toes; camptodactyly of fifth fingers; midphalangeal hypoplasia or aplasia of one or more fingers or toes.

Hair. Fine, dry, or sparse and slow growing.

Neurologic. Dysarthria, neurogenic bladder, spastic paraparesis, ataxia, nystagmus, anterior tibial muscle weakness, paresthesias, and seizures.

Other Skeletal. Broad tubular bones and mandible with wide alveolar ridge.

OCCASIONAL ABNORMALITIES.

Mental retardation, microcephaly, glaucoma, cataract, hearing loss, bony orbital hypotelorism with normal inner canthal distance, partial anodontia, microdontia, premature loss of teeth, cleft lip and palate, conductive hearing impairment, cubitus valgus, hip dislocation, osteopetrosis, poor posture, skull and vertebral hyperostosis, abnormal CNS white matter on MRI, calcification of basal ganglia.

NATURAL HISTORY. Intellectual performance is usually normal. Progressive neurologic dysfunction is frequent, usually presenting with spastic bladder or gait disturbances, often by the second decade. Demonstration on MRI of diffuse bilateral abnormalities in the subcortical cerebral white matter can be indicative of a slowly progressive leukodystrophy. Facial features become more obvious after the first 3 to 4 years of life. Because open angle glaucoma has been reported as a late complication, periodic ophthalmic evaluation is recommended.

ETIOLOGY. This disorder has an autosomal dominant inheritance pattern with variable expression; many cases represent fresh mutations. Mutations in the connexin 43 gene, or GJA1, located at chromosome 6q22-q23, are responsible for this disorder.

References
Lohmann W: Beitrag zur Kenntnis des reinen Mikrophthalmus. Arch Augenh 86:136, 1920.

Gorlin RJ, Meskin LH, St. Geme JW: Oculodentodigital dysplasia. J Pediatr 63:69, 1963.

Eidelman E, Chosack A, Wagner ML: Orodigitofacial dysostosis and oculodentodigital dysplasia: Two distinct syndromes with some similarities. Oral Surg 23:311, 1967.

Judisch GF et al: Oculodentodigital dysplasia. Arch Ophthalmol 97:878, 1979.

Loddenkemper T et al: Neurological manifestations of the oculodentodigital dysplasia syndrome. J Neurol 249:584, 2002.

Paznekas WA et al: Connexin 43 (GJA1) mutations cause the pleiotropic phenotype of oculodentodigital dysplasia. Am J Hum Genet 72:408, 2003.

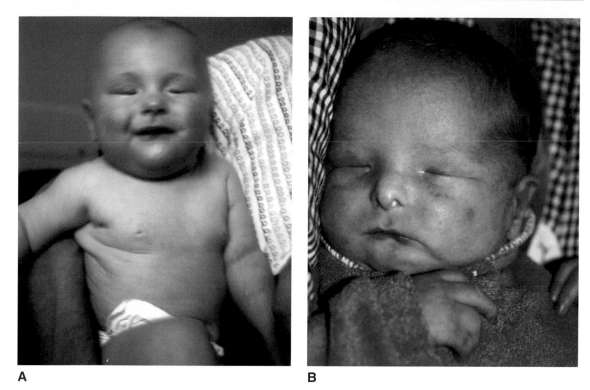

A

B

FIGURE 1. **A** and **B,** Infants with oculodentodigital syndrome. Note the small alae nasi, small mandible, and 4-5 cutaneous syndactyly. (**B,** Courtesy of Dr. Marilyn C. Jones, Children's Hospital, San Diego.)

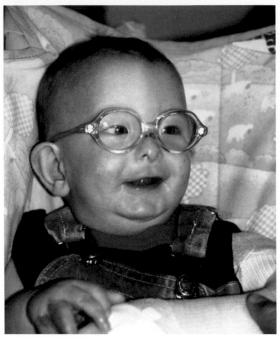

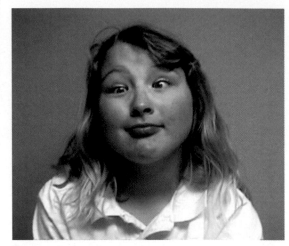

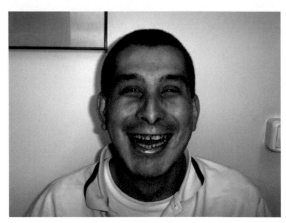

FIGURE 2. **A–C,** Note the microcornea; short palpebral fissures; thin, hypoplastic alae nasi; and enamel hypoplasia. (**A,** Courtesy of Dr. Marilyn C. Jones, Children's Hospital, San Diego; **C,** courtesy of Dr. Blanca Gener Querol, Universitat Pompeu Fabra, Barcelona.)

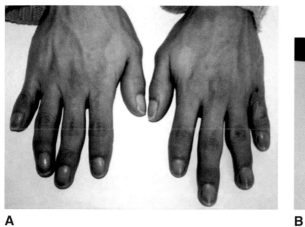
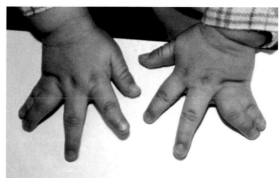

A

B

FIGURE 3. **A** and **B,** Syndactyly of fingers 4 and 5, which has been surgically corrected in **A**. (Courtesy of Dr. Blanca Gener Querol, Universitat Pompeu Fabra, Barcelona.)

LENZ MICROPHTHALMIA SYNDROME

Microphthalmia, Growth Retardation, Ear Abnormalities

Initially described in 1955 by Lenz, more than 20 cases of this disorder have been reported.

ABNORMALITIES

Performance. Delayed motor development, hypotonia, moderate to severe mental retardation.

Growth. Postnatal onset of growth retardation with respect to height and weight.

Craniofacial. Microcephaly. Prominent, protuberant ears lacking cartilage; high-arched palate; widely spaced teeth with missing upper incisors.

Ocular. Colobomatous or noncolobomatous microphthalmia, usually bilateral and symmetric, ranging from mild to complete anophthalmia; ptosis.

Hands and Feet. Fifth finger clinodactyly, syndactyly, fetal finger tip pads.

Other. Cylindrical thorax, sloping shoulders, kyphoscoliosis, thinning of lateral one third of clavicle, lordosis, hypospadias.

OCCASIONAL ABNORMALITIES.

Retinal detachment; peg-like or crowed teeth; cleft palate; preauricular tag; hearing loss; web neck; camptodactyly; hypoplastic, duplicated or broad thumbs; pseudoclubbing; mitral valve prolapse; bicuspid aortic valve; mild coarctation of aorta; renal aplasia/hypoplasia; duplicated renal system; imperforate anus; sacral pit; dysgenesis of corpus callosum and dilatation of lateral ventricles.

ETIOLOGY. This disorder has an X-linked recessive inheritance pattern. Linkage studies have indicated that the gene is located on chromosome region Xq27-Xq28. Obligate carrier females may manifest recurrent spontaneous abortion, short stature, and 2-3 syndactyly of the feet.

References

Lenz W: Recessivqeschlechtsqebundene Microphalmie mit multiplen missbildungen. Z Kinderheilkd 77:384–390, 1955.

Hermann J, Opitz JM: The Lenz microphthalmia syndrome. Birth Defects Orig Artic Ser V:138–143, 1969.

Traboulisi EI et al: The Lenz microphthalmia syndrome. Am J Ophthalmol 105:40–45, 1988.

Forrester S et al: Manifestations in four males with an obligate carrier of the Lenz microphthalmia syndrome. Am J Med Genet 98:92–100, 2001.

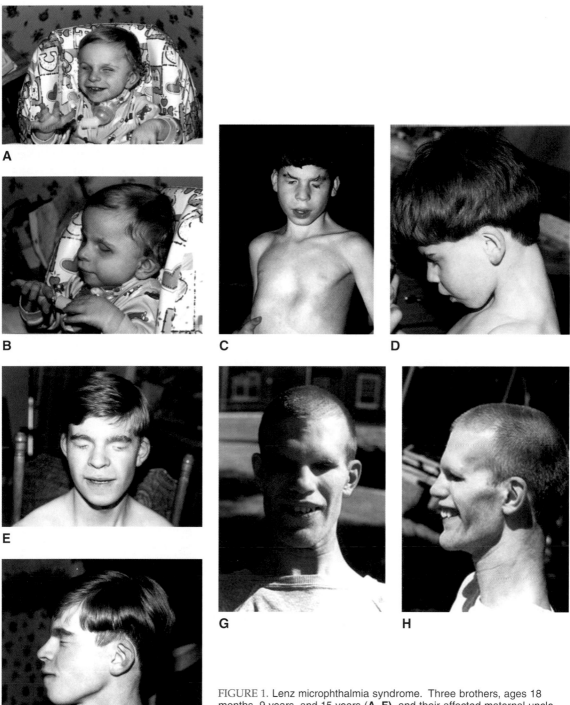

FIGURE 1. Lenz microphthalmia syndrome. Three brothers, ages 18 months, 9 years, and 15 years (**A–F**), and their affected maternal uncle, age 27 years (**G** and **H**). Note the prominent ears, microphthalmos, narrow thorax, and sloping shoulders. (**A–H,** From Forrester S et al: Am J Med Genet 98:92, 2001, with permission.)

OTO-PALATO-DIGITAL SYNDROME, TYPE I
(TAYBI SYNDROME)

Deafness, Cleft Palate, Broad Distal Digits with Short Nails

Initially described by Taybi in 1962, many cases have been recognized subsequently.

ABNORMALITIES

Performance. Mild mental retardation; IQs of 75 to 90.

Growth. Small stature, below 10th percentile for age.

Hearing. Conductive, sensorineural, or mixed loss; severity varies and is almost always bilateral; ossicular anomalies.

Cranium. Frontal and occipital prominence with thick frontal bone and thick base of skull, having a steep naso-basal angulation; absence of frontal and sphenoid sinuses.

Facies. Facial bone hypoplasia and ocular hypertelorism with small nose and mouth but lateral fullness of the supraorbital ridges, broad nasal bridge, midface hypoplasia, downslanting palpebral fissures.

Mouth. Partial anodontia, impacted teeth, or both; cleft soft palate, small tonsils.

Midskeletal. Small trunk, pectus excavatum, failure of neural arch fusion, small iliac crests.

Limbs. Limited elbow extension; inward-bowing tibiae; short, broad distal phalanges of thumbs and great toes, to a lesser extent for other digits, with short nails; fifth finger clinodactyly; relatively short third, fourth, fifth metacarpals; fusion of hamate and capitate bones; accessory ossification center at the base of the second metatarsal; widely spaced toes.

OCCASIONAL ABNORMALITIES.

Delayed closure of anterior fontanel, hip dislocation, limited knee flexion, syndactyly of toes, hallucal nail dystrophy, scoliosis, hypoplasia of transverse sinus with enlarged occipital sinuses.

NATURAL HISTORY. Speech development is retarded on the basis of hearing impairment, mental retardation, or both. The sensorineural component of the hearing loss is progressive.

ETIOLOGY. This disorder has an X-linked transmission pattern with intermediate expression in females and complete expression in males. Mutations in FLNA, a gene that encodes filamin A, a protein that regulates reorganization of the cytoskeleton, are responsible. FLNA has been mapped to Xq28. Features in females include fullness of the lateral supraorbital ridges, short nails, clinodactyly of toes, and radiologic abnormalities in limbs and skull.

COMMENT. Oto-palato-digital syndrome, types I and II, frontometaphyseal dysplasia, and Melnick-Needles syndrome are allelic conditions, all caused by mutations in FLNA.

References

Taybi H: Generalized skeletal dysplasia with multiple anomalies. Am J Roentgenol Radium Ther Nucl Med 88:450, 1962.

Dudding BA, Gorlin RJ, Langer LO: The oto-palato-digital syndrome: A new symptom-complex consisting of deafness, dwarfism, cleft palate, characteristic facies, and a generalized bone dysplasia. Am J Dis Child 113:214, 1967.

Gorlin RJ, Poznanski AK, Hendon I: The oto-palato-digital (OPD) syndrome in females. Oral Surg 35:218, 1973.

Biancalana V et al: Oto-palato-digital syndrome type I: Further evidence for assignment of the locus to Xq28. Hum Genet 88:228, 1991.

Zaytoun GM et al: The oto-palatal-digital syndrome: Variable clinical expressions. Otolaryngol Head Neck Surg 126:129, 2002.

Robertson SP et al: Localized mutations in the gene encoding the cytoskeletal protein filamin A cause diverse malformations in humans. Nat Genet 33:487, 2003.

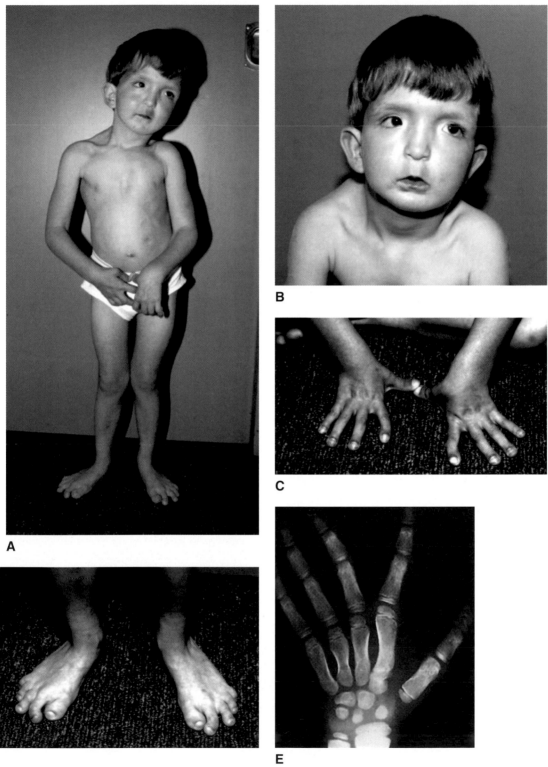

FIGURE 1. Oto-palato-digital syndrome, type I. **A–E,** Note the frontal prominence of the skull; small trunk and pectus excavatum; limited elbow extension; and irregular length and form of distal phalanges, especially thumb and great toe. (**A–D,** Courtesy of Dr. Marilyn C. Jones, Children's Hospital, San Diego; **E,** radiograph from Dudding BA, Gorlin RJ, Langer LO: Am J Dis Child 113:214, 1967, with permission. Copyright 1967, American Medical Association.)

OTO-PALATO-DIGITAL SYNDROME, TYPE II

Fitch and colleagues and later Kozlowski and colleagues each described this pattern of malformation in two half brothers. Approximately 20 cases have been reported.

ABNORMALITIES

Growth. Postnatal growth deficiency in survivors.

Craniofacial. Late closure of large anterior fontanel; wide sutures; prominent forehead; low-set malformed ears; ocular hypertelorism; antimongoloid slant to palpebral fissures; flat nasal bridge; small mouth; micrognathia; cleft palate; radiographic evidence of dense fontanels, supraorbital ridge, and skull base with undermineralization of cranial vault; small mandible with obtuse angle.

Limbs. Flexed, overlapping fingers; short broad thumbs and great toes; polydactyly; variable syndactyly of hands and feet; clinodactyly of second finger; bowing of radius, ulna, femur, and tibia; small to absent fibula; hypoplastic, irregular metacarpals; nonossified fifth metatarsal; short, absent, or poorly ossified phalanges of fingers and toes; subluxed elbows, wrists, and knees; congenital hip dislocation; rocker-bottom feet.

Other. Conductive hearing loss, pectus excavatum, a narrow chest with thin, wavy clavicles and ribs, flattened vertebral bodies, hypoplastic ilia, widened lumbosacral canal, mental retardation, microcephaly, posterior fossa brain anomalies.

OCCASIONAL ABNORMALITIES.

Dental abnormalities, transverse capitate bone, clinodactyly of second finger, retarded carpal bone age and advanced phalangeal bone age, absent halluces, omphalocele, cryptorchidism, hypospadias, absent adrenal glands.

NATURAL HISTORY. The majority of

affected individuals have been stillborn or died before 5 months of age because, in most cases, of respiratory difficulties. The incidence of mental retardation in survivors is unknown. Although significant developmental delay has been documented, one 18-month-old and one 6-year-old affected boy are developmentally normal. The facial appearance as well as the bone curvatures tend to normalize with age. Both membranous ossification and bone remodeling appear to be defective.

ETIOLOGY. This disorder is X-linked, with

mild manifestations such as broad face, antimongoloid slant of palpebral fissures, and cleft palate or bifid uvula in heterozygote females. Mutations in FLNA, which has been mapped to Xq28, are responsible.

COMMENT. Oto-palato-digital syndrome,

types I and II, frontometaphyseal dysplasia, and Melnick-Needles syndrome are allelic conditions, all caused by mutations in FLNA.

References

Fitch N, Jequier S, Papageorgiou A: A familial syndrome of cranial, facial, oral and limb anomalies. Clin Genet 10:226, 1976.

Kozlowski K et al: Oto-palato-digital syndrome with severe x-ray changes in two half brothers. Pediatr Radiol 6:97, 1977.

Fitch N, Jequier S, Gorlin R: The oto-palato-digital syndrome, proposed type II. Am J Med Genet 15:655, 1983.

Brewster TG et al: Oto-palato-digital syndrome, type II—an X-linked skeletal dysplasia. Am J Med Genet 20:249, 1985.

Blanchet P et al: Multiple congenital anomalies associated with an oto-palatal-digital syndrome type II. Genet Couns 4:289, 1993.

Holder SE, Winter RM: Otopalatodigital syndrome type II. J Med Genet 30:310, 1993.

Preis S et al: Oto-palato-digital syndrome type II in two unrelated boys. Clin Genet 45:154, 1994.

Savarirayan R et al: Oto-palato-digital syndrome, type II: Report of three cases with further delineation of the chondro-osseous morphology. Am J Med Genet 95:193, 2000.

Robertson SP et al: Localized mutations in the gene encoding the cytoskeletal protein filamin A cause of diverse malformations in humans. Nat Genet 33:487, 2003.

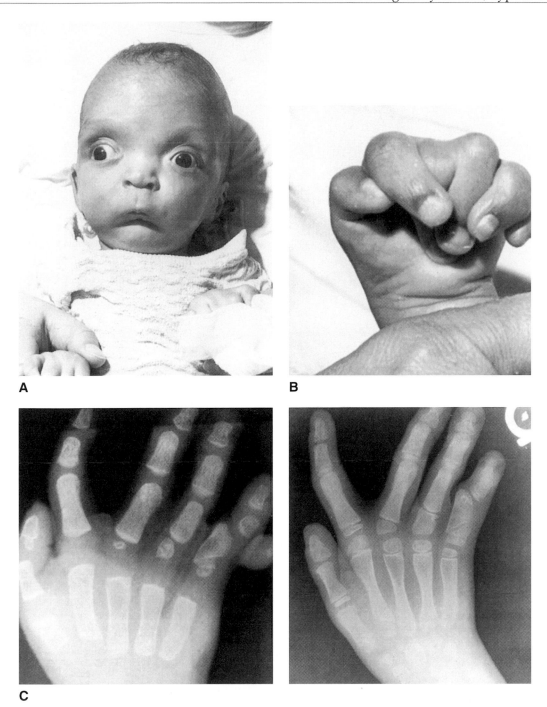

FIGURE 1. **A** and **B,** Neonate with oto-palato-digital syndrome, type II. Note the prominent forehead, ocular hypertelorism, flat nasal bridge, small mouth, micrognathia, and the flexed overlapping fingers. **C,** Radiographs of the hand at 1 and 5 years of age reveal hypoplastic irregular metacarpals, abnormal epiphyses of proximal phalanges 4 and 5, and postaxial polydactyly. (**A–C,** From Fitch N et al: Am J Med Genet 15:655, 1983, with permission.)

COFFIN-LOWRY SYNDROME

Downslanting Palpebral Fissures, Bulbous Nose, Tapering Fingers

Coffin and colleagues in 1966 and Lowry and colleagues in 1971 independently described a mental retardation syndrome associated with coarse facies, short stature, and thick, soft hands with tapering fingers. Temtamy recognized the similarity between the two and referred to the disorder as the Coffin-Lowry syndrome. The facies may appear similar to that of the Williams syndrome.

ABNORMALITIES

Growth. Mild to moderate growth deficiency, apparently of postnatal onset; delayed bone age.
Performance. Mental retardation, usually severe; relative weakness; hypotonia.
Facies. Coarse appearance, with downslanting palpebral fissures and maxillary hypoplasia, mild hypertelorism, prominent brow, and short, broad nose with thick alae nasi and septum, and anteverted nares; large open mouth with thick, everted lower lip; prominent ears.
Dental. Hypodontia, malocclusion, wide-spaced teeth, and large medial incisors.
Thorax. Short bifid sternum with pectus carinatum, and excavatum.
Spine. Anterior superior marginal vertebral defects, thoracolumbar scoliosis, and kyphosis.
Limbs. Broad, soft hands with stubby, tapering, limp fingers that are wide at the base and narrow distally; tufted drumstick appearance to distal phalanges on roentgenogram; small fingernails; accessory transverse hypothenar crease; fullness of the forearms due to increased subcutaneous fat; flat feet; lax ligaments.

OCCASIONAL ABNORMALITIES.

Microcephaly; thick calvarium; dilated lateral ventricles; seizures; cardiomyopathy; mitral valve prolapse; radiographically, there are hypoplastic sinuses and mastoids, delayed closure of anterior fontanel, narrowing of the foramen magnum, and in the thoracolumbar vertebrae, narrowing of the intervertebral spaces, irregular endplates, and anterior wedging; simian crease; inguinal hernia; rectal prolapse; uterine prolapse; mitral valve insufficiency; sensorineural hearing loss; cataracts; retinal changes; premature loss of primary teeth.

NATURAL HISTORY. In males, the mental retardation is usually of severe degree, leaving the patient without speech. Fullness of the brows and lips become more exaggerated with advancing age. The vertebral dysplasia and kyphoscoliosis generally do not develop until after 6 years. Late eruption and premature loss of teeth are common. Psychotic behavior with onset around 20 years sometimes occurs in affected females, whereas males are usually cheerful, easygoing, and friendly. Drop attacks triggered by unexpected tactile or auditory stimuli or by excitement, in which the patient experiences episodes of falling backward, have their onset from midchildhood to the teens. Life expectancy may be reduced in affected males, related primarily to cardiac, respiratory, neurologic, and kyphoscoliosis-related causes.

ETIOLOGY. This disorder has an X-linked inheritance pattern with striking similarity between the severely affected hemizygous males. Clinical findings in affected females include slight to moderate mental retardation, mild facial changes, tapered fingers, obesity and short stature, although some are completely normal. Mutations in the RSK2 gene, which has been mapped to Xp22.2, are responsible.

References

Coffin GS, Siris E, Wegienka LC: Mental retardation with osteocartilaginous anomalies. Am J Dis Child 112:205, 1966.
Lowry B, Miller JR, Fraser FC: A new dominant gene mental retardation syndrome. Am J Dis Child 121:496, 1971.
Temtamy SA et al: The Coffin-Lowry syndrome: A simply inherited trait comprising mental retardation, facio-digital anomalies and skeletal anomalies. Birth Defects 11(6):133, 1975.
Hunter AGW, Partington MW, Evans JA: The Coffin-Lowry syndrome: Experience from four centres. Clin Genet 21:321, 1982.
Vles JSH et al: Early signs in Coffin-Lowry syndrome. Clin Genet 26:448, 1984.

Gilgenkrautz S et al: Coffin-Lowry syndrome: A multicenter study. Clin Genet 34:230, 1988.

Hartsfield JK et al: Pleiotrophy in Coffin-Lowry syndrome: Sensorineural hearing deficit and premature tooth loss as early manifestations. Am J Med Genet 45:552, 1993.

Hanauer A, Young ID: Coffin-Lowry syndrome: Clinical and molecular features. J Med Genet 39:705, 2002.

Hunter AGW: Coffin-Lowry syndrome: A 20-year follow-up and review of long-term outcomes. Am J Med Genet 111:345, 2002.

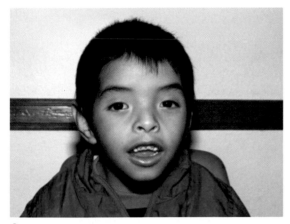

A

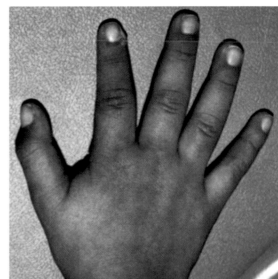

B

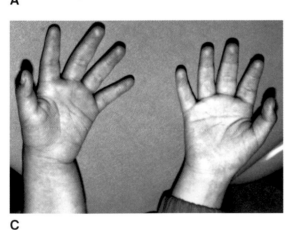

C

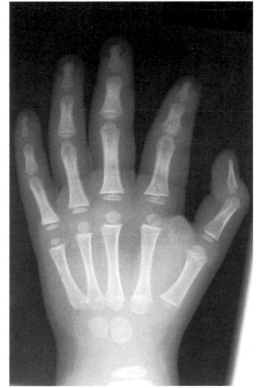

D

FIGURE 1. Coffin-Lowry syndrome. **A–D,** Note the downslanting palpebral fissures; maxillary hypoplasia; prominent brow; large, open mouth with everted lower lip; prominent ears; dental malocclusion; tapering fingers; and tufted drumstick appearance to terminal phalanges on radiograph. (Courtesy of Dr. Marilyn C. Jones, Children's Hospital, San Diego.)

X-LINKED α-THALASSEMIA/MENTAL RETARDATION SYNDROME

Severe Mental Retardation, Characteristic Face, Genital Abnormalities

First described in 1990 by Wilkie and colleagues, this disorder was further characterized by Gibbons and colleagues in 1991. More than 40 affected individuals have been identified.

ABNORMALITIES

Performance. Severe mental retardation, initial hypotonia frequently followed by spasticity, seizures, self-biting/hitting, extreme emotion.

Growth. Postnatal growth deficiency sometimes not evident until adolescence, delayed bone age.

Craniofacial. Microcephaly; telecanthus; epicanthal folds; low nasal bridge; small, triangular nose with anteverted nares; midface hypoplasia; large "carp-like" mouth that is frequently held open; full lips; large, protruding tongue; wide-spaced incisors; small, simple, deformed, low-set, or posteriorly rotated ears.

Limbs. Tapering fingers; fifth finger clinodactyly; overlapping fingers and toes; foot deformities including talipes equinovarus, pes planus, and talipes calcaneovalgus.

Genitalia. Cryptorchidism, testicular dysgenesis, shawl and/or hypoplastic scrotum, small penis, hypospadias.

Hematologic. Mild hypochromic microcytic anemia; mild form of hemoglobin H disease (a type of α-thalassemia); the hemoglobin H that can be detected electrophoretically in this disorder ranges from 0% to 6.7%; in almost all cases, by using 1% brilliant cresyl blue (BCB), hemoglobin H forms inclusions, which can be detected in from 0.01% to 40% of red blood cells.

OCCASIONAL ABNORMALITIES.

Cerebral atrophy, cleft palate, kyphoscoliosis, hemivertebra, missing rib, ovoid vertebral bodies, short sternum, small or drumstick appearing terminal phalanges, absent frontal sinuses, flexion deformity of index finger, umbilical hernia, cardiac defects, renal agenesis, hydronephrosis, male pseudohermaphroditism.

NATURAL HISTORY. Severe mental retardation with lack of expressive speech, limited comprehension, and the development of only partial bladder and bowel control is the rule. Some patients do not walk independently until late teens and some not at all. Apneic and cyanotic episodes as well as cold/blue extremities occur frequently. Regurgitation of food often induced by putting fingers down throat. Excessive salivation, gastroesophageal reflux, and constipation also occur. Recurrent urinary tract and chest infections as well as blepharitis/conjunctivitis are common.

ETIOLOGY. This disorder has an X-linked recessive inheritance pattern. Mutations in the X-linked α−thalassemia/mental retardation (ATR-X) gene, which has been identified and maps to Xq13.3, are responsible for this disorder. Over 70 mutations of the gene have been reported. The function of the X-linked α−thalassemia/mental retardation protein is not yet completely understood. The most sensitive diagnostic test is the demonstration of hemoglobin H inclusions in red blood cells after incubation with BCB. The inability to demonstrate hemoglobin H electrophoretically should not exclude the diagnosis. Carrier females frequently have rare cells containing hemoglobin H in their peripheral blood after incubation with 1% BCB. A faint band of hemoglobin H is sometimes visible on electrophoresis.

References

Wilkie AOM et al: Clinical features and molecular analysis of the α thalassemia/mental retardation syndromes. II. Cases due to deletions involving chromosome band 16p13.3. Am J Hum Genet 46:1112, 1990.

Wilkie AOM et al: Clinical features and molecular analysis of the α thalassemia/mental retardation syndromes. II. Cases without detectable abnormality of the α globin complex. Am J Hum Genet 46:1127, 1990.

Gibbons RJ et al: A newly defined X linked mental retardation syndrome with α thalassemia. J Med Genet 28:729, 1991.

Gibbons RJ et al: X linked α thalassemia/mental retardation (ATR-X) syndrome: Localization to Xq12-q21.31 by X inactivation and linkage analysis. Am J Hum Genet 51:1136, 1992.

Logie LJ et al: Alpha thalassemia mental retardation (ATR-X): A typical family. Arch Dis Child 70:439, 1994.

Gibbons RJ et al: Mutations in a putative global transcriptional regulator cause X-linked mental retardation with α-thalassemia (ATR-X syndrome). Cell 80:837, 1995.

Gibbons RJ et al: Clinical and hematological aspects of the X-linked alpha-thalassemia/mental retardation syndrome (ATR-X). Am J Med Genet 55:288, 1995.

McPherson EW et al: X-linked alpha-thalassemia/mental retardation (ATR-X) syndrome: A new kindred with severe genital anomalies and mild hematological expression. Am J Med Genet 55:302, 1995.

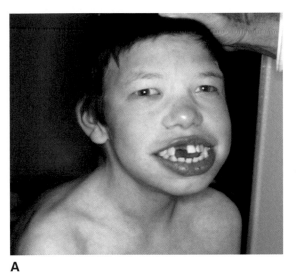

A

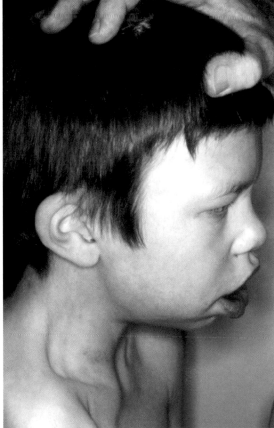

B

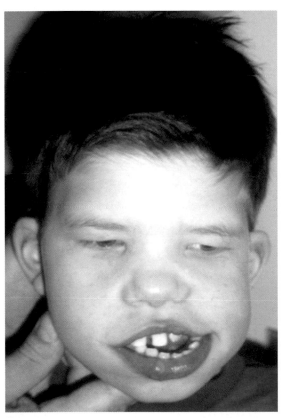

C

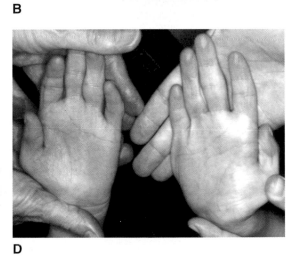

D

FIGURE 1. X-Linked α-thalassemia/mental retardation syndrome. **A** and **B**, Affected boy at 12 years of age. **C**, Same patient at 15 years of age. Note the telecanthus, epicanthal folds, low nasal bridge, and large mouth with thick lips. **D**, Note the tapering fingers and fifth finger clinodactyly.

FG SYNDROME

Imperforate Anus, Hypotonia, Prominent Forehead

Initially described by Opitz and Kaveggia in three brothers and two of their male first cousins, over 50 cases of this X-linked recessive disorder now have been documented.

ABNORMALITIES

Performance. Mental retardation (97%); delayed motor development or hypotonia (90%); electroencephalographic disturbances with seizures (70%); strabismus (52%); hyperactive behavior with short attention span (70%); affable, extroverted personality with occasional temper tantrums in response to frustration (54%).

Growth. Postnatal onset of short stature.

Craniofacies. Postnatal onset of macrocephaly (74%); large anterior fontanel (77%); prominent forehead (95%); frontal hair upsweep (91%); ocular hypertelorism (83%); prominent lower lip (44%); small ears with simple structure (66%); facial skin wrinkling; fine, sparse hair (66%); epicanthal folds; short downslanting palpebral fissures (85%); narrow palate; large-appearing cornea (75%).

Gastrointestinal. Anal anomalies including stenosis, imperforate anus, and anteriorly placed anus (38%); constipation (69%).

Skeletal. Broad thumbs and great toes (81%); clinodactyly (53%); camptodactyly (55%); multiple joint contractures; syndactyly (54%); simian crease (60%); minor vertebral defects (64%); abnormal sternum (69%).

Other. Complete or partial agenesis of the corpus callosum, sacral dimple, cryptorchidism (36%), low total dermal ridge count, persistent fetal fingertip pads (50%).

OCCASIONAL ABNORMALITIES.
Craniosynostosis, cleft palate, cleft lip, choanal atresia, hydrocephalus, stenotic ear canal, short neck, defects of neuronal migration, malrotation of cecum, absence of mesentery, pyloric stenosis, dilatation of urinary tract, hypospadias, cardiac defect, ectrodactyly, sensorineural deafness, high-pitched voice.

NATURAL HISTORY. Death due to pulmonary complications may occur in the first 2 years of life. Constipation, common in infancy, usually resolves in midchildhood. Although mental retardation has been severe in the survivors, their generally affable personality has led to an adequate social adjustment in most cases. The initial hypotonia with lax joints tends to evolve into spasticity with joint contractures and unsteady gait in adults.

ETIOLOGY. This disorder has an X-linked recessive inheritance pattern. At least four different loci on the X chromosome have been identified as causative for this disorder, thus documenting genetic heterogeneity.

References

Opitz JM, Kaveggia EG: Studies of malformation syndromes of man XXXIII: The FG syndrome. An X-linked recessive syndrome of multiple congenital anomalies and mental retardation. Z Kinderhlkd 117:1, 1974.

Romano C et al: A clinical follow-up of British patients with FG syndrome. Clin Dysmorphol 3:104, 1994.

Graham JM et al: FG syndrome: Report of three new families with linkage to Xq12-q22.1. Am J Med Genet 80:145, 1998.

Ozonoff S et al: Behavioral phenotype of FG syndrome: Cognition, personality, and behavior in eleven affected boys. Am J Med Genet 97:112, 2000.

Piluso G et al: Genetic heterogeneity of FG syndrome: A fourth locus (FGS4) maps to Xp11.4-p11.3 in an Italian family. Hum Genet 112:124, 2002.

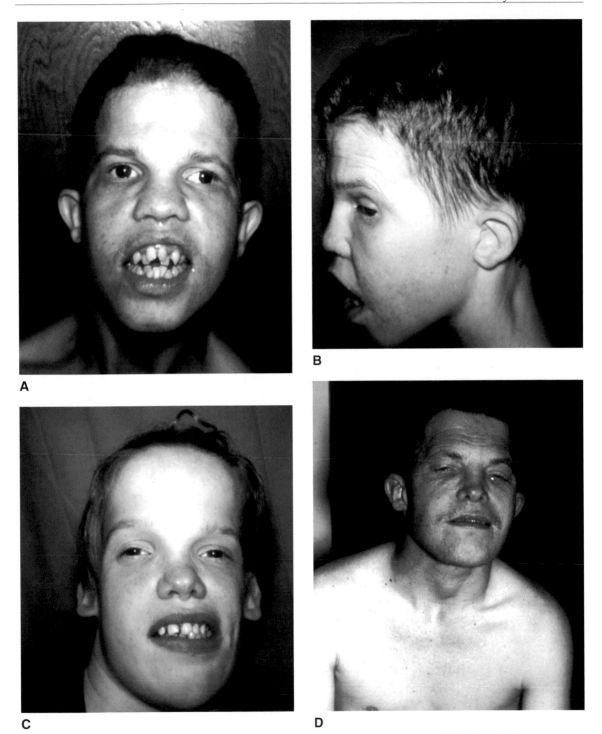

FIGURE 1. FG syndrome. Three affected male siblings, ages 27 (**A** and **B**), 17 (**C**), and 29 (**D**). Note the frontal upsweep, lateral displacement of the medial canthi, and small ears.

STICKLER SYNDROME
(HEREDITARY ARTHRO-OPHTHALMOPATHY)

Flat Facies, Myopia, Spondyloepiphyseal Dysplasia

In 1965, Stickler and colleagues reported the initial observations on affected individuals in five generations of one family; the skeletal aspects have been further documented by Spranger, and the total spectrum of the disorder has been set forth by Herrmann and colleagues.

ABNORMALITIES

Orofacial. Flat facies with depressed nasal bridge, prominent eyes, epicanthal folds, a short nose and anteverted nares; midfacial or mandibular hypoplasia; clefts of hard and/or soft palate and occasionally of uvula, Robin sequence deafness (both sensorineural and conductive); dental anomalies.

Ocular. Myopia, usually present before age 6, which is nonprogressive and of high degree; retinal detachment; cataracts; abnormalities of vitreous formation and gel architecture are manifest in the majority of patients by a vestigial vitreous gel, which occupies the immediate retrolental space, is bordered by a distinct folded membrane, and is referred to as the type 1 phenotype; in the type 2 phenotype, sparse and irregularly thickened bundles of fibres exist throughout the vitreous cavity.

Musculoskeletal. Hypotonia, hyperextensible joints, talipes equinovarus; prominence of large joints may be present at birth; severe arthropathy can occur in childhood; lesser joint pains simulate juvenile rheumatoid arthritis; subluxation of hip; roentgenographic findings beginning in childhood include mild to moderate spondyloepiphyseal dysplasia (i.e., flat vertebrae with anterior wedging, underdevelopment of the distal tibial epiphyses, and flat irregular femoral epiphyses); long bones show disproportionately narrow shafts relative to their metaphyseal width; secondary degeneration of articular surfaces occurs in adulthood.

Other. Mitral valve prolapse.

OCCASIONAL ABNORMALITIES.
Scoliosis, kyphosis, and increased lumbar lordosis; arachnodactyly with marfanoid habitus; pectus excavatum; thoracic disk herniation; thoracic myelopathy; pes planus; genu valgus; mental deficiency; short stature; lens dislocation; glaucoma.

NATURAL HISTORY. Arthritis, if present, most commonly becomes a problem after 30 years of age. Symptoms become more severe with advancing years, leading in some cases to total hip replacement. Spinal abnormalities, which occur almost universally, progress with age and are associated with back pain. Progressive myopia may give rise to retinal detachment and lead to blindness, the most severe complication of this disorder. Although myopia develops in 40% of patients before 10 years of age and 75% by age 20, it does not occur in some patients until after age 50. Retinal detachment can occur in childhood but usually not until after 20 years of age. It is to be hoped that the detachment can be corrected surgically if recognized early. Affected individuals with mitral valve prolapse should be evaluated periodically and should receive antibiotic prophylaxis for certain surgical procedures.

ETIOLOGY. This disorder has an autosomal dominant inheritance pattern. Although highly variable expression of this disorder has been documented, the variability is mostly between families. Within individual families, similarity in the clinical phenotype from patient to patient is the rule. The majority of cases are associated with the type 1 vitreous phenotype and show linkage to the gene encoding type II collagen (COL2AI) located on chromosome 12q13. Some patients with the type 2 vitreous phenotype have mutations in the gene encoding the $\alpha1$ chain of type XI collagen (COL11A1) on chromosome 1p21. Mutations in the gene encoding the $\alpha2$ chain of type XI collagen (COL11A2) on chromosome 6q21.3 have been reported in individuals with Stickler syndrome who lack any ocular abnormality.

COMMENT. The Stickler syndrome should be considered in any neonate with the Robin sequence, particularly in those with a family history of cleft palate and in patients with dominantly inherited myopia, nontraumatic retinal detachment, and/or mild spondyloepiphyseal dysplasia.

References

Stickler GB et al: Hereditary progressive arthroophthalmopathy. Mayo Clin Proc 40:433, 1965.

Stickler GB, Pugh DG: Hereditary progressive arthro-ophthalmopathy. II. Additional observations on vertebral abnormalities, a hearing defect, and a report of a similar case. Mayo Clin Proc 42:495, 1967.

Spranger J: Arthro-ophthalmopathia hereditaria. Ann Radiol (Paris) 11:359, 1968.

Herrmann J et al: The Stickler syndrome (hereditary arthro-ophthalmopathy). Birth Defects 11(2):76, 1975.

Liberfarb RM, Hirose T, Holmes LB: The Wagner-Stickler syndrome: A study of 22 families. J Pediatr 99:394, 1981.

Temple IK: Stickler's syndrome. J Med Genet 26:119, 1989.

Lewkonia RA: The arthropathy of hereditary arthroophthalmopathy (Stickler syndrome). J Rheumatol 19:1271, 1992.

Zlotogora J et al: Variability of Stickler syndrome. Am J Med Genet 42:337, 1992.

Snead MP, Yates JRW: Clinical and molecular genetics of Stickler syndrome. J Med Genet 36:353, 1999.

Rose PS et al: The hip in Stickler syndrome. J Pediatr Orthop 21:657, 2001.

Rose PS et al: Thoracolumbar spinal abnormalities in Stickler syndrome. Spine 26:403, 2001.

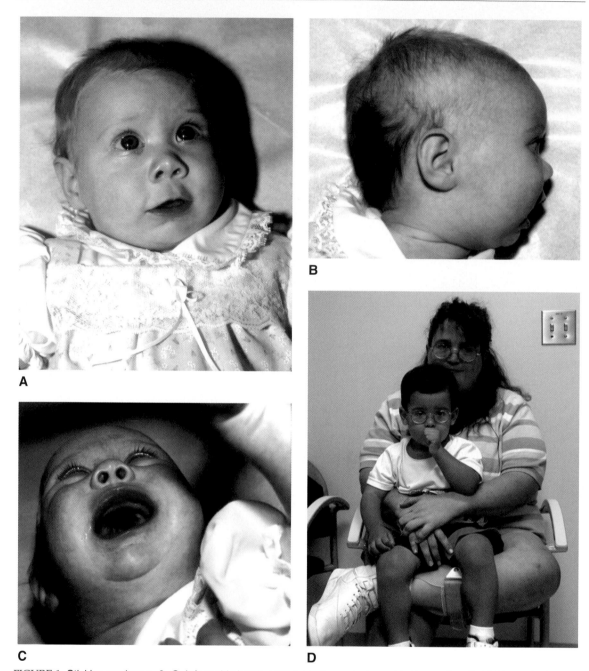

FIGURE 1. Stickler syndrome. **A–C,** Infant girl showing flat face, depressed nasal bridge, epicanthal folds, a short nose with anteverted nares, maxillary hypoplasia, micrognathia, and U-shaped palatal cleft (Robin sequence). **D,** Mother and her affected son.

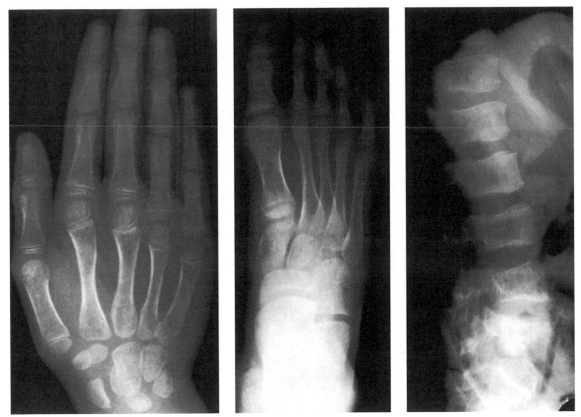

FIGURE 2. Radiographs showing arachnodactyly, fusion of some carpal centers, and mild spondyloepiphyseal dysplasia.

CATEL-MANZKE SYNDROME

Micrognathia, Cleft Palate, Hyperphalangy of Index Finger

First reported by Catel in 1961 in a patient who was reevaluated by Manzke in 1966, more than 20 patients have been described with this condition.

ABNORMALITIES

Growth. Postnatal growth deficiency (75%).

Facies. Cleft palate (78%), micrognathia (72%), malformed ears (33%).

Limbs. Hyperphalangy of index finger in 100% (an accessory bone between proximal phalanges of fingers 2 and 3), fifth finger clinodactyly (39%), single palmar crease (40%).

Other. Cardiac defects (39%), primarily septal defects accompanied by overriding aorta, aortic coarctation, or dextrocardia.

OCCASIONAL ABNORMALITIES.

Developmental delay, seizures, prenatal growth deficiency, short neck, cleft lip, vertebral/rib anomalies, pectus excavatum/carinatum, talipes equinovarus, joint laxity/dislocation, camptodactyly, cryptorchidism, umbilical and inguinal hernias, facial paresis.

NATURAL HISTORY. Careful observation to recognize upper airway obstruction secondary to the Robin sequence should be part of routine care of newborns with this disorder. Failure to thrive is related to respiratory or cardiac problems. The vast majority of cases have normal intelligence. With advancing age, the accessory bone fuses to the proximal phalangeal epiphysis.

ETIOLOGY. The cause of this disorder is unknown. The majority of cases have been sporadic. Although most cases have been males, at least four affected females have been reported.

References

Catel W: Differentialdiagnose von Krankheitsymptomen bei kindern und jugendlichten, vol. 1, ed. 3. Stuttgart: Thieme, 1961.

Manzke VH: Symmetrische hyperphalangie des zweiten fingers durch ein akzessorisches metacarpale. Fortschr Roentgenstr 105:425, 1966.

Skinner SA et al: Catel-Manzke syndrome. Proc Greenwood Genet Center 8:60, 1989.

Wilson GN et al: Index finger hyperphalangy and multiple anomalies: Catel-Manzke syndrome? Am J Med Genet 46:176, 1993.

Kant SG et al: The Catel-Manzke syndrome in a female infant. Genet Couns 9:187, 1998.

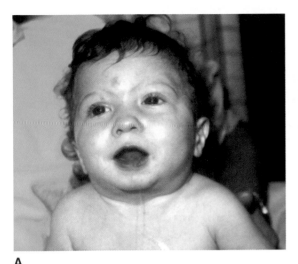

A

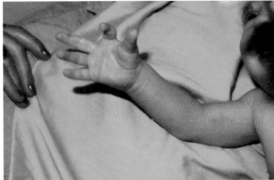

B

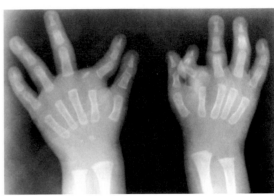

C

FIGURE 1. Catel-Manzke syndrome. **A–C,** A 15-month-old boy. Note the micrognathia and typical hand anomalies with accessory bones at the base of the index finger and hypoplasia of the second metacarpal. (From Stevenson RE et al: J Med Genet 17:238, 1980, with permission.)

LANGER-GIEDION SYNDROME
(TRICHO-RHINO-PHALANGEAL SYNDROME, TYPE II, TRP II)

Multiple Exostoses, Bulbous Nose with Peculiar Facies, Loose Redundant Skin in Infancy

Hall and colleagues in 1974 reported five new cases of this disorder and included two further sporadic cases from the literature. An extensive review of the literature, including data from over 30 patients, has been published by Langer and colleagues. Although the facies of these patients resemble the facies of tricho-rhino-phalangeal syndrome, type I, other features allow for separation of the two syndromes.

ABNORMALITIES

Growth. Postnatal onset of mild growth deficiency.
Performance. Mild to severe mental retardation in 70%, with the remaining patients in the normal to dull-normal range; delayed onset of speech; sensorineural hearing loss.
Cranium. Microcephaly.
Facies. Large laterally protruding ears; heavy eyebrows; deep-set eyes; large bulbous nose with thickened alae nasi and septum, dorsally tented nares, and broad nasal bridge; simple philtrum, which is prominent and elongated; thin upper lip; recessed mandible.
Hair. Sparse scalp hair.
Skin. Redundancy or looseness in infancy, which regresses with age; maculopapular nevi around the scalp, face, neck, upper trunk, and upper limbs.
Hands. Cone-shaped epiphyses, which become radiologically evident at approximately 3 to 4 years of age; lack of normal modeling in metaphyseal regions; poor funnelization at proximal ends of phalanges; metaphyseal hooking over the lateral edges of the cone-shaped epiphyses; exostoses; brittle nails.
Bones. Multiple exostoses of long tubular bones, with onset and distribution similar to the autosomal dominant variety of multiple cartilaginous exostoses; exostoses can involve other areas, such as the ribs, scapulae, and pelvic bones.
Other. Perthes-like changes in capital femoral epiphysis, segmentation defects of vertebrae with scoliosis, narrow posterior ribs; winged scapulae; syndactyly; lax joints; hypotonia; exotropia; recurrent upper respiratory tract infections; malocclusion; dental abnormalities.

OCCASIONAL ABNORMALITIES.
Tendency toward fractures, thin hypomineralized bones, clinobrachydactyly, simian crease, bowed femurs, tibial hemimelia, ocular hypotelorism, ptosis, prominent eyes, epicanthal folds, iris coloboma, abducens palsy, tragal skin tag, cardiac defects, inguinal and umbilical hernia, ureteral reflux, widely spaced nipples, delayed sexual development, small phallus, cryptorchidism, premature thelarche and pubarche, hydrometrocolpos, abnormal electroencephalograph, seizures, conductive hearing loss, hypochromic anemia.

NATURAL HISTORY.
Some of these children have such redundancy or looseness to their skin at birth that they are misdiagnosed as having the Ehlers-Danlos syndrome. The children experience recurrent respiratory tract infections until they are 4 to 5 years old. General health is usually good after that except for a tendency toward fractures and the usual problems of multiple exostoses with their variable effects on bone growth.

ETIOLOGY.
This disorder is caused by a deletion in the region 8q24.11-q24.13. In most cases, the deletion is visible with cytogenetic studies. A few cases of vertical transmission have been described. However, the vast majority have been sporadic. Langer-Giedion syndrome is a contiguous gene syndrome involving the tricho-rhino-phalangeal (TRPS) gene located at 8q24 and the gene involved in multiple exostosis (EXT1). Mental retardation is expected when larger pieces of 8q are deleted.

References
Hall BD et al: Langer-Giedion syndrome. Birth Defects 10(12):147, 1974.

Langer LO et al: The tricho-rhino-phalangeal syndrome with exostosis (or Langer-Giedion syndrome): Four additional patients without mental retardation and review of the literature. Am J Med Genet 19:81, 1984.

Bühler EM et al: A final word on the tricho-rhino-phalangeal syndromes. Clin Genet 31:273, 1987.

Nardmann J et al: The tricho-rhino-phalangeal syndromes: Frequency and parental origin of 8q deletions. Hum Genet 99:638, 1997.

Stevens CA, Moore CA: Tibial hemimelia in Lange-Giedion syndrome—possible gene location for the tibial hemimelia at 8q. Am J Med Genet 85:409, 1999.

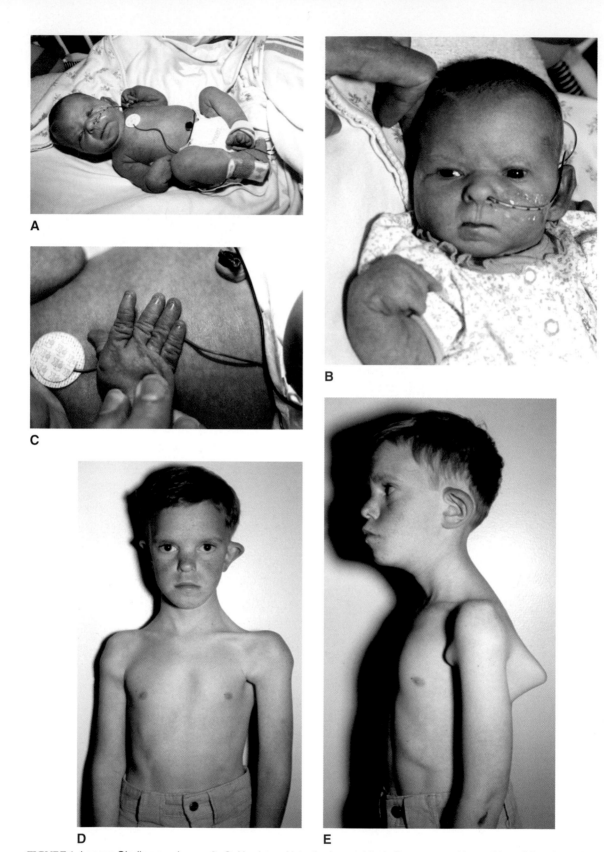

FIGURE 1. Langer-Giedion syndrome. **A–C,** Newborn. Note the loose skin, bulbous nose with notching of the ala nasi, and simple but prominent philtrum. (Courtesy of Dr. Marilyn C. Jones, Children's Hospital, San Diego.) **D** and **E,** A 7-year-old child. Note the sparseness of hair, bulbous nose, simple but prominent philtrum, superiorly tented nares, thin upper lip, prominent ears, and exostoses on the scapula and proximal humerus. (**D** and **E,** Courtesy of Dr. Bryan Hall, University of Kentucky, Lexington.)

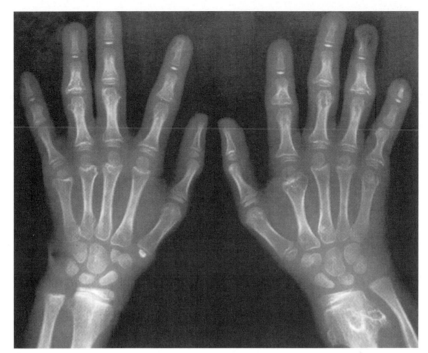

FIGURE 2. An 11½-year-old with exostoses, cone-shaped epiphyses, and metaphyseal hooking at the proximal ends of several of the middle phalanges.

TRICHO-RHINO-PHALANGEAL SYNDROME, TYPE I
(TRP I)

Bulbous Nose, Sparse Hair, Epiphyseal Coning

Klingmuller reported two siblings with this pattern of malformation in 1956. Giedion further established the syndrome and set forth the tricho-rhino-phalangeal designation for it.

ABNORMALITIES

Growth. Mild growth deficiency (3rd to 10th percentiles).

Facial. Pear-shaped nose, prominent and long philtrum, narrow palate, with or without micrognathia, large prominent ears; small, carious teeth with dental malocclusion; horizontal groove on chin.

Hair. Sparse, thin hair with relative hypopigmentation.

Nails. Thin.

Skeletal. Short metacarpals and metatarsals, especially the fourth and fifth; development of broadened middle phalangeal joint with cone-shaped epiphyses, especially the second through fourth fingers and toes; split distal radial epiphyses; winged scapulae.

OCCASIONAL ABNORMALITIES.

Coxa plana and coxa magna, flattening of capital femoral epiphysis, partial syndactyly, pectus carinatum, pes planus, short stature, mental deficiency, craniosynostosis, deep voice, hypotonia during infancy.

NATURAL HISTORY. The hair is usually sparse at birth. Osseous changes such as the cone-shaped epiphyses may develop in early childhood and become worse until adolescent growth is complete. Increased frequency of upper respiratory tract infections has been noted in some cases. A form of degenerative hip disease often develops in young adulthood or later life.

ETIOLOGY. This disorder has an autosomal dominant inheritance pattern. Mutations in TRPS1, a gene encoding a zinc finger transcription factor, have been found in the majority of patients with tricho-rhino-phalangeal syndrome, type I. The gene is located on chromosome band 8q24.1.

COMMENT. In addition to TRPS types I and II, a disorder has been recognized that represents the severe end of the TRPS spectrum, manifest by features of TRPS type I plus severe shortness of all phalanges and metacarpals and short stature. Intelligence is normal, and there are no exostoses. This disorder, referred to as TRPS type III, can be caused by specific mutations in TRPS1.

References

Klingmuller G: Über eigentumliche Konstitutions-anomalien bei 2 Schwestern und ihre Beziehungen zu neueren-entwicklungspathologischen Befunden. Hautarzt 7:105, 1956.

Giedion A: Das tricho-rhino-phalangeale Syndrom. Helv Paediatr Acta 21:475, 1966.

Gorlin RJ, Cohen MM, Wolfson J: Trichorhino-phalangeal syndrome. Am J Dis Child 118:585, 1969.

Fontaine G et al: Le syndrome trichorhinophalangien. Arch Fr Pediatr 27:635, 1970.

Felman AH, Frias JL: The tricho-rhino-phalangeal syndrome: Study of 16 patients in one family. AJR 129:631, 1977.

Goodman RM et al: New clinical observations in the trichorhinophalangeal syndrome. J Craniofac Genet Dev Biol 1:15, 1981.

Buhler EM et al: A final word on the tricho-rhino-phalangeal syndromes. Clin Genet 31:273, 1987.

Momeni P et al: Mutations in a new gene, encoding a zinc-finger protein, cause tricho-rhino-phalangeal syndrome type I. Nat Genet 24:71, 2000.

Ludecke H-J et al: Genotype and phenotype spectrum in the tricho-rhino-phalangeal syndromes types I and III. Am J Hum Genet 68:81, 2001.

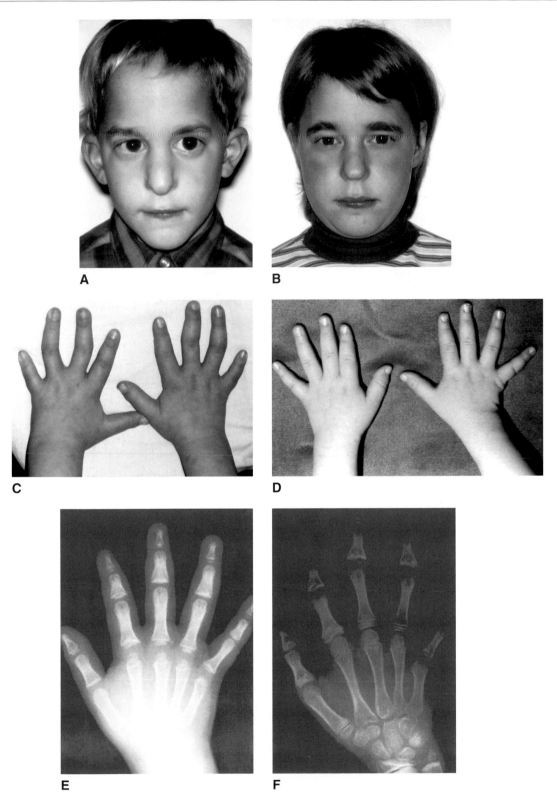

FIGURE 1. Tricho-rhino-phalangeal syndrome. A 6-year-old son (**A**) and 9-year-old daughter (**B**) of an affected father who became bald at 21 years of age. The children have fine, slow-growing hair. Note the tented hypoplastic nares and prominent philtrum. **C–F,** Note too the asymmetric length of fingers related to radiographic evidence of irregular metaphyseal cupping with cone-shaped epiphyses. (**A–F,** Courtesy of D. Weaver, Indiana University, Indianapolis.)

ECTRODACTYLY–ECTODERMAL DYSPLASIA–CLEFTING SYNDROME
(EEC SYNDROME)

Ectrodactyly, Ectodermal Dysplasia, Cleft Lip-Palate

Although the association of ectrodactyly and cleft lip had been noted, it was not until 1970 that Rüdiger and colleagues appreciated that at least some of these patients also had features of ectodermal dysplasia and named the disorder the EEC syndrome. Bixler and colleagues added two additional cases and summarized the past observations. Well over 200 cases have been reported.

ABNORMALITIES. All features are variable.
Skin. Fair and thin, with mild hyperkeratosis; hypoplastic nipples.
Hair. Light-colored, sparse, thin, wiry hair on all hair-bearing areas; distortion of the hair bulb and longitudinal grooving of hair shaft is seen on scanning electron microscopic observation.
Teeth. Partial anodontia, microdontia, caries.
Eyes. Blue irides, photophobia, blepharophimosis, defects of lacrimal duct system (59%), blepharitis, dacryocystitis.
Face. Cleft lip, with or without cleft palate (68%); maxillary hypoplasia; mild malar hypoplasia.
Limbs. Defects in midportion of hands and feet, varying from syndactyly to ectrodactyly (84%); mild nail dysplasia.
Genitourinary. Anomalies in 52% including megaureter, duplicated collecting system, vesicoureteral reflux, ureterocele, bladder diverticuli, renal agenesis/dysplasia, hydronephrosis, micropenis, cryptorchidism, transverse vaginal septum.

OCCASIONAL ABNORMALITIES.
Conductive hearing loss (14%); mental retardation (7%); microcephaly; small or malformed auricles; broad nasal tip; choanal atresia, semilobar holoprosencephaly; polydactyly; clinodactyly; ear dysplasia; telecanthus/hypertelorism; inguinal hernia; anal atresia/rectovaginal fistula; growth hormone deficiency; hypogonadotropic hypogonadism; central diabetes insipidus.

NATURAL HISTORY. These individuals are usually of normal intelligence and adapt

reasonably well with surgical closure of the facial clefts plus (as needed) limb surgery, dentures, and wigs. Chonic/recurrent respiratory infections occur in 6% of cases. Early and continued ophthalmologic evaluation and management for the defective lacrimal duct system are imperative, because chronic dacryocystitis with corneal scarring can be the major debilitating problem in this disorder.

ETIOLOGY. This disorder has an autosomal dominant inheritance with variable expression. No single feature, including ectrodactyly, is obligatory. At least three types and their gene loci have been identified. Type 1 has been assigned to chromosome 7q11.2-q21.3; type 2 to chromosome 19; and type 3 to chromosome 3q27. Mutations of the p63 gene at 3q27 have been identified. Most are amino acid substitutions in the DNA-binding domain. p63 is a homologue of the tumor-suppressor gene p53. At least three reports have documented an association of the EEC syndrome with malignant lymphoma. In one of those reports, mutation analysis was performed and a p63 mutation was documented.

References
Cockayne EA: Cleft palate, hare lip, dacryocystitis and cleft hand and feet. Biometrika 28:60, 1936.
Walker JC, Clodius L: The syndromes of cleft lip, cleft palate and lobster-claw deformities of hands and feet. Plast Reconstr Surg 32:627, 1963.
Rüdiger RA, Haase W, Passarge E: Association of ectrodactyly, ectodermal dysplasia, and cleft lip-palate. Am J Dis Child 120:160, 1970.
Bixler D et al: The ectrodactyly-ectodermal dysplasia-clefting (EEC) syndrome. Clin Genet 3:43, 1972.
Rodini ESO, Richieri-Costa A: EEC syndrome: Report on 20 new patients, clinical and genetic considerations. Am J Med Genet 37:42, 1990.
Roelfsema NM, Cobben JM et al: The EEC syndrome: A literature study. Clin Dysmorphol 5:115, 1996.
Celli J et al: Heterozygous germline mutations in the p53 homolog p63 are the cause of EEC syndrome. Cell 99:143, 1999.
Barrow LL et al: Analysis of p63 gene in the classical EEC syndrome, related syndromes, and non-syndromic orofacial clefts. J Med Genet 39:559, 2002.
Akahoshi K et al: EEC syndrome type 3 with a heterozygous germline mutation in the P63 gene and B cell lymphoma. Am J Med Genet 120:370, 2003.

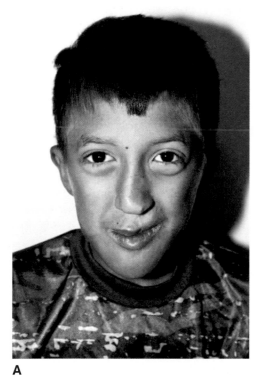

A

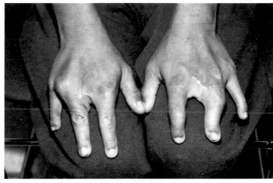

B

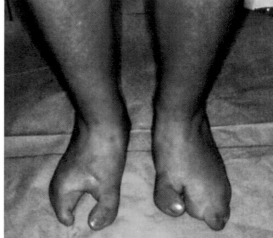

D

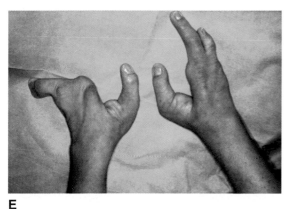

C

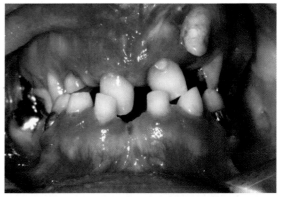

F

E

FIGURE 1. Ectrodactyly–ectodermal dysplasia–clefting syndrome. **A–C,** A 13-year-old boy and adult woman, both with thin, dry, lightly pigmented skin; sparse, fine hair; repaired cleft lip and ectrodactyly. Note the inflammation of the conjunctiva in the adult who has photophobia. (**A** and **B,** Courtesy of Dr. Marilyn C. Jones, Children's Hospital, San Diego; **C,** courtesy of Dr. Michael Bamshad, University of Utah, Salt Lake City.) **D–F,** Note the variability of the ectrodactyly, the partial anodontia, and microdontia.

HAY-WELLS SYNDROME OF ECTODERMAL DYSPLASIA
(Ankyloblepharon–Ectodermal Dysplasia–Clefting Syndrome, AEC Syndrome)

Ankyloblepharon, Ectodermal Dysplasia, Cleft Lip-Palate

In 1976, Hay and Wells described a specific type of ectodermal dysplasia associated with cleft lip or cleft palate and congenital filiform fusion of the eyelids. The association of facial clefting with ankyloblepharon filiforme adnatum had previously been documented in several case reports.

ABNORMALITIES

Craniofacial. Oval face; broadened nasal bridge; maxillary hypoplasia; cleft lip, cleft palate, or both; conical, widely spaced teeth; hypodontia to partial anodontia; ankyloblepharon filiforme adnatum.

Skin. Palmar and plantar keratoderma; peeling erythematous, eroded skin at birth from limited to high percentage of body surface area; hyperkeratosis; patchy, partial deficiency of sweat glands; partial anhidrosis; hyperpigmentation.

Nails. Absent or dystrophic.

Hair. Wiry and sparse to alopecia.

OCCASIONAL ABNORMALITIES.

Deafness; atretic external auditory canal; cup-shaped auricles; lacrimal duct atresia; supernumerary nipples; soft-tissue syndactyly; rarely, ventricular septal defect or patent ductus arteriosus; hypospadias; micropenis; vaginal dryness or erosions; Wilms tumor.

NATURAL HISTORY.
Surgical excision of the ankyloblepharon filiforme adnatum is required during the early neonatal period. Anomalies of the eye are not associated with these tissue bands. However, photophobia is common. Surgical closure of facial clefting and early ophthalmologic evaluation of the lacrimal duct system are required. Otitis media occurs frequently. Severe chronic granulomas of the scalp, which begin as infections, have been a serious problem and in one case have required multiple skin grafts. Although these patients have a partial capacity to produce sweat from fewer glands so that hyperthermia is not a serious threat, heat intolerance is common. Intelligence is normal.

ETIOLOGY.
This disorder has an autosomal dominant inheritance pattern with marked variability of expression. Mutations in the p63 gene, which give rise to amino acid substitutions in the sterile alpha motif (SAM) domain, are responsible for this disorder. The gene is a homologue of the tumor-suppressor gene p53 and is located at 3q27.

COMMENT.
Ankyloblepharon filiforme adnatum is not a simple failure of eyelid separation. The eyelid fusion bands histologically are composed of a central core of vascular connective tissue entirely surrounded by epithelium. Muscle fibers may be observed as well. These bands may represent abnormal proliferation of mesenchymal tissue at certain points on the lid margin or an ectodermal deficit allowing mesodermal union.

References

Duke-Elder S: Textbook of Ophthalmology, vol. 5. London: Kimpton, 1952.

Khanna VN: Ankyloblepharon filiforme adnatum. Am J Ophthalmol 43:774, 1957.

Rogers JW: Ankyloblepharon filiforme adnatum. Arch Ophthalmol 65:114, 1961.

Long JC, Blandford SE: Ankyloblepharon filiforme adnatum with cleft lip and palate. Am J Ophthalmol 53:126, 1962.

Hay RJ, Wells RS: The syndrome of ankyloblepharon, ectodermal defects, and cleft lip and palate: An autosomal dominant condition. Br J Dermatol 94:277, 1976.

Spiegel J, Colton A: AEC syndrome: Ankyloblepharon, ectodermal defects, and cleft lip and palate. J Am Acad Dermatol 12:810, 1985.

Vanderhooft SL et al: Severe skin erosions and scalp infections in AEC syndrome. Pediatr Dermatol 10:334, 1993.

McGrath JA et al: Hay-Wells syndrome is caused by heterozygous missense mutations in the SAM domain of p63. Hum Mol Genet 10:221, 2001.

Fomenkov K et al: p63 Mutations lead to aberrant splicing of the keratinocyte growth factor receptor in the Hay-Wells syndrome. J Biol Chem 278:23906, 2003.

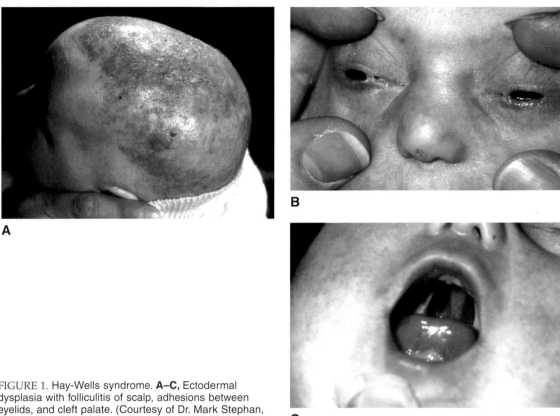

FIGURE 1. Hay-Wells syndrome. **A–C,** Ectodermal dysplasia with folliculitis of scalp, adhesions between eyelids, and cleft palate. (Courtesy of Dr. Mark Stephan, Madigan General Hospital, Tacoma, Wash.)

ROBERTS SYNDROME
(Pseudothalidomide Syndrome,
Hypomelia-Hypotrichosis–Facial
Hemangioma Syndrome)

Hypomelia, Midfacial Defect, Severe Growth Deficiency

This disorder was initially described by Roberts in 1919 and more recently by Appelt and colleagues. Freeman and colleagues reported five cases and reviewed the features in the 17 previously recognized patients. The cases reported by Herrmann and colleagues as "pseudothalidomide or SC syndrome" and the case reported by Hall and Greenberg as "hypomelia-hypotrichosis–facial hemangioma syndrome" are probably examples of this disorder.

ABNORMALITIES

Performance. Microcephaly (80%), severe mental defect in some and borderline to mild mental deficiency in others.

Growth. Profound growth deficiency of prenatal onset, birth weight in full-term infants 1.5 to 2.2 kg (88%) and birth length frequently less than 40 cm, mild or severe postnatal growth deficiency.

Facial. Cleft lip with or without cleft palate and prominent premaxilla, hypertelorism (87%), midfacial capillary hemangioma (78%), thin nares, shallow orbits and prominent eyes (69%), bluish sclerae, corneal clouding (68%), micrognathia, malformed ears with hypoplastic lobules.

Hair. Sparse, often silvery blond in some survivors.

Limbs. Hypomelia, more severe in upper limbs, varying from tetra-amelia to tetraphocomelia to lesser degrees of limb reduction, often including reduction in length or absence of the humerus (77%), radius (98%), or ulna (96%); reduction in numbers or length of fingers (75%), syndactyly (42%), or clinodactyly; reduction or absence of femur (65%), tibia (74%), or fibula (80%); reduction in number of toes (27%); incomplete development of dermal ridges; flexion contractures of knees, ankles, wrists, or elbows.

Genitalia. Cryptorchidism, phallus may *appear* relatively large in relation to body size.

OCCASIONAL ABNORMALITIES.
Frontal encephalocele, hydrocephalus, brachycephaly, craniosynostosis, microphthalmia, cataract, lid coloboma, cranial nerve paralysis, short neck, nuchal cystic-hygroma, cardiac anomaly (atrial septal defect), renal anomaly (polycystic or horseshoe kidney), bicornuate uterus, rudimentary gallbladder, accessory spleen, splenogonadal fusion, polyhydramnios, thrombocytopenia, hypospadias.

NATURAL HISTORY. Most individuals born at term with birth length less than 37 cm and severe defects in midfacial and limb development have been stillborn or have died in early infancy. The survivors have had marked growth deficiency, and some have had severe mental retardation as well. Birth length greater than 37 cm, less severe limb defects, absence of cleft palate, and presence of thin nares have been associated with a better prognosis.

ETIOLOGY. This disorder has an autosomal recessive inheritance pattern with great variability of expression within families.

COMMENT. Approximately 80% of tested individuals have had premature centromere separation, which consists of "puffing" or "repulsion" of the constitutive heterochromatin of many chromosomes. It is best demonstrated using the C-band staining technique.

References

Roberts JB: A child with double cleft of lip and palate, protrusion of the intermaxillary portion of the upper jaw and imperfect development of the bones of the four extremities. Ann Surg 70:252, 1919.

Appelt H, Gerken H, Lenz W: Tetraphokomelie mit Lippen-Kiefer-Gaumenspalte und Clitorishypertrophie—Ein Syndrome. Paediatr Paedol 2:119, 1966.

Herrmann J et al: A familial dysmorphogenetic syndrome of limb deformities, characteristic facial appearance and associated anomalies: The pseudothalidomide or SC-syndrome. Birth Defects 5:81, 1969.

Freeman MVR et al: Roberts syndrome. Clin Genet 5:1, 1974.

Grosse FR, Pandel C, Wiedemann HR: Tetraphocomelia–cleft palate syndrome. Humangenetik 28:353, 1975.

Herrmann J, Opitz JM: The SC phocomelia and the Roberts syndrome: Nosologic aspects. Eur J Pediatr 125:117, 1977.

Waldenmaier C, Aldenhoff P, Klemm T: The Roberts syndrome. Hum Genet 40:345, 1978.

Parry DM et al: SC phocomelia syndrome, premature centromere separation, and congenital cranial nerve paralysis in two sisters, one with malignant melanoma. Am J Med Genet 24:653, 1986.

Holmes-Siedle M et al: A sibship with Roberts/SC phocomelia syndrome. Am J Med Genet 37:18, 1990.

Van Den Berg DJ, Francke U: Roberts syndrome: A review of 100 cases and a new rating syndrome for severity. Am J Med Genet 47:1104, 1993.

Sinha AK et al: Clinical heterogeneity of skeletal dysplasia in Roberts syndrome: A review. Hum Hered 44:121, 1994.

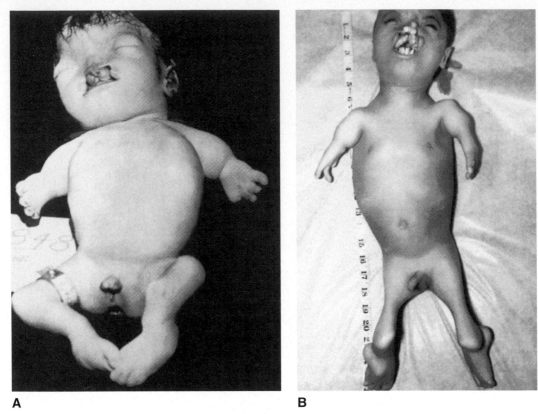

A   **B**

FIGURE 1. Roberts-SC phocomelia. **A,** Severely affected infant girl at autopsy. **B,** Her severely growth-deficient and mentally deficient 10-year-old brother. (**A** and **B,** From Freeman MV et al: Clin Genet 5:1, 1974, with permission.)

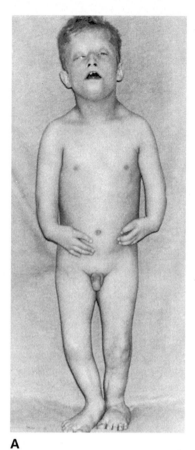

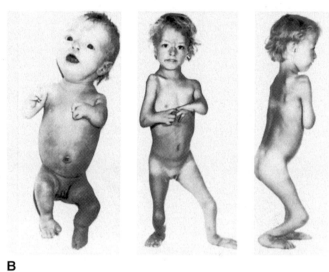

B

FIGURE 2. **A,** An 8-year-old severely mentally deficient boy with silvery blond hair and a height age of 3½ years. (Courtesy of S. Jurenka, St. Amant Wards, Winnipeg, Manitoba.) **B,** Same patient as an infant and at 8 years of age. Note capillary hemangioma on forehead in infancy and sparse scalp hair as a child. (From Hall BD, Greenberg MH: Am J Dis Child 123:602, 1972, with permission.)

A

I Limb Defect as Major Feature

GREBE SYNDROME

Grebe described this disorder in 1952, Quelce-Salgado reported 47 cases in five kindreds in an inbred Brazilian population, and Scott more recently summarized the findings.

ABNORMALITIES

Growth. Disproportionate short stature with short limbs, adult height ranges from 90.5 cm in females to 100.5 cm in males.

Limbs. Arms: Middle segment shorter than proximal, short hands, fingers replaced by globular appendages without apparent articulation at metacarpophalangeal joints, short nails, lack of pronation-supination at elbows, no apparent bony articulation at wrist.

Legs: Middle segment shorter than proximal, bulky muscles that extend to ankles, limited range of motion at knees and ankles, no apparent articulation of toes with foot.

Radiographic. Short radii and ulnae, the latter most severe; rudimentary carpal bones and phalanges; short tibiae, with increased severity from proximal to distal segments; short feet in valgus, with rudimentary phalanges.

OCCASIONAL ABNORMALITIES.
Polydactyly, autoamputation of toes.

NATURAL HISTORY. Affected patients
are of normal intelligence, develop normal secondary sexual characteristics, walk without difficulty, and can develop sophisticated dexterity.

ETIOLOGY. This disorder has an autosomal recessive inheritance pattern. Mutations in the gene encoding cartilage-derived morphogenetic protein-1 (CDMP-1) located on chromosome 20q11.2 are responsible. CDMP-1 is expressed mainly at sites of cartilage differentiation in developing limbs as well as at the position of future joint spaces suggesting a role in the formation of articulation.

COMMENT. Obligate heterozygotes are of normal height, but frequently have minor limb anomalies. Radiographic defects include short tubular bones particularly metacarpals and middle phalanges.

References

Grebe H: Die Achondrogenesis: Ein einfach rezessives Erbmerkmal. Folia Hered Pathol (Milano) 2:23, 1952.

Quelce-Salgado A: A new type of dwarfism with various bone aplasias and hypoplasia of the extremities. Acta Genet 14:63, 1964.

Scott CI: Skeletal dysplasias. Birth Defects 5(3):14, 1969.

Garcio-Castro JM, Pereze-Comas A: Nonlethal achondrogenesis in two Puerto Rican sibships. J Pediatr 87:948, 1975.

Romeo G et al: Heterogeneity of non-lethal severe short-limb dwarfism. J Pediatr 91:918, 1977.

Thomas JT et al: Disruption of human limb morphogenesis by a dominant negative mutation in CDMP-1. Nat Genet 17:58, 1997.

Costa T et al: Grebe syndrome: clinical and radiographic findings in affected individuals and heterozygotic carriers. Am J Med Genet 75:523, 1998.

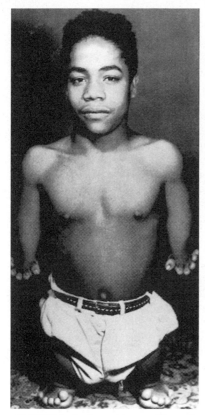 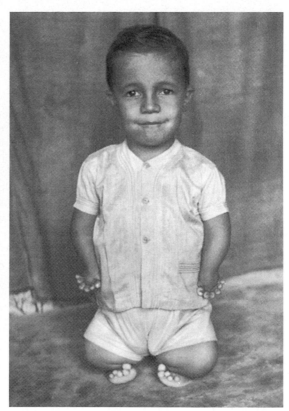

FIGURE 1. Grebe syndrome. (From Quelco-Salgado A: Acta Genet 14:63, 1964, with permission.)

POLAND SEQUENCE

Unilateral Defect of Pectoralis Muscle, Syndactyly of Hand

In 1841, Poland reported unilateral absence of the pectoralis minor and the sternal portion of the pectoralis major muscles in an individual who also had cutaneous syndactyly of the hand on the same side. This unique pattern of defects has subsequently been noted in numerous cases and has an incidence of approximately 1 in 20,000. It has been estimated that 10% of patients with syndactyly of the hand have the Poland sequence.

ABNORMALITIES. Variable *unilateral* features from among the following:

Thorax. Hypoplasia to absence of the pectoralis major muscle, nipple, and areola; rib defects.

Upper Limbs. Hypoplasia distally with varying degrees of syndactyly, brachydactyly, oligodactyly, and occasionally more severe reduction deficiency.

Other. Occasional hemivertebrae, renal anomaly, Sprengel anomaly, isolated dextrocardia without other cardiovascular defects associated with ipsilateral rib defects in left-sided Poland sequence.

NATURAL HISTORY. Generally an otherwise normal individual.

ETIOLOGY. The cause of this disorder is unknown. It is three times as common in the male as in the female and is 75% right-sided. Bouvet and colleagues presented evidence of diminished blood flow to the affected side and suggested that the primary defect may be in the development of the proximal subclavian artery, with early deficit of blood flow to the distal limb and the pectoral region, yielding partial loss of tissue in those regions. Bavinck and Weaver have proposed that early interruption of blood flow in the subclavian artery occurs proximal to the origin of the internal thoracic artery but distal to the origin of the vertebral artery. Credence for a vascular pathogenesis comes from the suggestion that maternal smoking may increase the risk by approximately twofold.

Although the vast majority of cases are sporadic and recurrence risk is negligible, there are several reports of parent-to-child transmission as well as affected siblings born to unaffected parents. Marked variability in expression has been documented including two sibships in which the propositus had the "full" Poland sequence, whereas a sibling in one instance had only absence of the pectoral muscle and, in the other instance, only syndactyly of the hand.

COMMENT. Bavinck and Weaver suggested that the Poland, Klippel-Feil, and Moebius sequences, all of which may occur in various combinations in the same individual, should be grouped together based on a similar developmental pathogenesis into a single category referred to as the subclavian artery disruption sequence. They hypothesized that these conditions are the result of diminished blood flow in the subclavian artery, vertebral artery, or their branches during or around the sixth week of development. The pattern of defects depends on the specific area of diminished blood flow.

References

Poland A: Deficiency of the pectoral muscles. Guy's Hosp Rep 6:191, 1841.

Clarkson P: Poland's syndactyly. Guy's Hosp Rep 111:335, 1962.

David TJ: Nature and etiology of the Poland anomaly. N Engl J Med 287:487, 1972.

Mace JW et al: Poland's syndrome. Clin Pediatr (Phila) 11:98, 1972.

Bouvet J, Maroteaux P, Briard-Guillemot M: Poland's syndrome: Clinical and genetic studies—physiopathology. Nouv Presse Med 5:185, 1976.

Bavinck JNB, Weaver DD: Subclavian artery supply disruption sequence: Hypothesis of a vascular etiology for Poland, Klippel-Feil and Möebius anomalies. Am J Med Genet 23:903, 1986.

Fraser FC et al: Pectoralis major defect and Poland sequence in second cousins: Extension of the Poland sequence spectrum. Am J Med Genet 33:468, 1989.

Fraser FC et al: Poland sequence with dextrocardia: Which comes first? Am J Med Genet 73:194, 1997.

Martinez-Frias ML et al: Smoking during pregnancy and Poland sequence: Results of a population-based registry and case-control registry. Teratology 59:35, 1999.

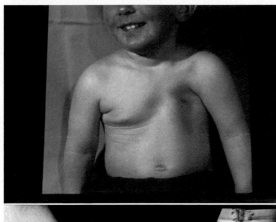
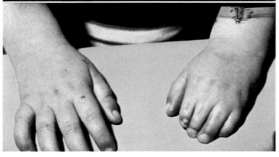

FIGURE 1. Poland sequence. The absence of the pectoralis minor and the sternal portion of the pectoralis major plus the ipsilateral syndactyly of the hand are the more usual features of this complex sequence. The bony thoracic anomaly and the hypoplasia of the hand, as noted in this otherwise normal boy, are more severe expressions of this defect.

ULNAR-MAMMARY SYNDROME

Ulnar Ray Defects, Absence/Hypoplasia of Breast Development, Diminished/Absent Axillary Hair and Perspiration

Originally described in 1882 by Gilly in a woman with mammary hypoplasia, inability to lactate and absence of the third, fourth, and fifth fingers and ulna, this disorder now has been reported in over 50 patients, both males and females. The clinical phenotype as well as the molecular characterization have been most extensively delineated by Bamshad.

ABNORMALITIES

Limb. Hypoplasia of phalanges of fifth digits, partial or complete fifth digit phalangeal fusion with absent interphalangeal creases, postaxial polydactyly, absence of digits 3 to 5, partial ventral duplication of fifth fingernail, aplasia/hypoplasia of ulna, short radius, absent/hypoplasia of metacarpals 3 to 5.

Aprocrine. Diminished/absent axillary hair and perspiration, lack of body odor.

Mammary. Hypopigmentation and hypoplasia of areola, nipple and breast; normal to absent lactation.

Other. Delayed puberty and skeletal maturation in males, genital anomalies including shawl scrotum, micropenis, and cryptorchidism.

Occasional Abnormalities. Absent or ectopic canine teeth, cleft palate, bifid uvula, subglottic stenosis, imperforate hymen, complete absence of forearm and hand, patent ductus arteriorsus, mitral valve prolapse, accessory nipples, carpal bone absence or fusion on ulnar side, hypoplastic flexion creases of first and second digits, short terminal phalanges of toes 4 and 5, hypoplastic humerus, scapula and clavicle, absent/short xiphisternum, obesity, inguinal hernia, renal agenesis, pyloric stenosis, anal atresia/stenosis, gonadotropin deficiency.

NATURAL HISTORY. Males as opposed to females become obese and develop significant delay in growth and skeletal maturation. Puberty and catch-up growth occurs but frequently are 5 to 7 years delayed.

ETIOLOGY. This disorder has an autosomal dominant inheritance pattern. Mutations in TBX3, a member of the T-Box gene family that has been mapped to 12q23-24.1 are responsible for this disorder. This region, in addition, contains a gene (TBX5) for Holt-Oram syndrome.

References

Gilly E: Absence complete des mamelles chez une femme mere: Atrophie du membre superieur droit. Courrier Med 32:27, 1882.

Pallister PD et al: Studies of malformation syndrome in man XXXXII: A pleiotrophic dominant mutation affecting skeletal, sexual and apocrine-mammary development. BD: OAS 12(5):247, 1976.

Schinzel A: Ulnar-Mammary syndrome. J Med Genet 24:778, 1987.

Bamshad M et al: Clinical analysis of a large kindred with the Pallister ulnar mammary syndrome. Am J Med Genet 65:325, 1996.

Bamshad M et al: Mutations in human BX3 alter limb, apocrine and genital development in ulnar-mammary syndrome. Nat Genet 16:311, 1997.

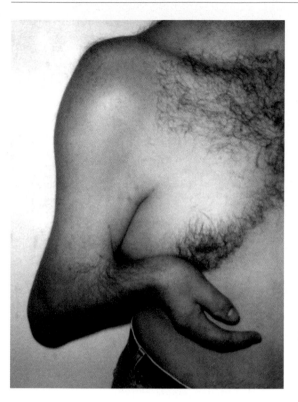

FIGURE 1. Ulnar-mammary syndrome. There is an absent ulna, short radius, absence of metacarpals 3 to 5, diminished axillary hair, and hypoplasia of the breast. (Courtesy of Dr. Michael Bamshad, University of Utah, Salt Lake City.)

POPLITEAL PTERYGIUM SYNDROME
(Facio-Genito-Popliteal Syndrome)

Popliteal Web, Cleft Palate, Lower Lip Pits

This disorder was first reported by Trelat in 1869; greater than 80 cases have been recorded.

ABNORMALITIES

Oral. Cleft palate with or without cleft lip (90%), salivary lower lip pits (46%), intraoral fibrous band connecting maxillary and mandibular alveolar ridges (43%), thin upper lip.

Limbs. Popliteal web, in extreme form from heel to ischium (90%). Toenail dysplasia, pyramidal skinfold extending from base to tip of great toe (33%), syndactyly of toes.

Genitalia. Anomalies in 51% including hypoplastic labia majora, scrotal dysplasia, cryptorchidism.

OCCASIONAL ABNORMALITIES.
Unusual oral frenula, hypodontia, cutaneous webs between eyelids (20%), atresia of external ear canal, intercrural pterygium (9%), syndactyly of fingers most commonly digits 3 to 4, bifid toenail, hypoplasia or aplasia of digits, reduction defect of thumb, fusion of distal interphalangeal joints, valgus deformity of feet, hypoplasia of tibia, bifid or absent patella, posterior dislocation of fibulae, low acetabular angle, spina bifida occulta, other vertebral anomalies, bifid ribs, short sternum, scoliosis, ambiguous external genitalia, penile ectopia or torsion, ectopic testes, underdevelopment of vagina or uterus, inguinal hernia, abnormal scalp hair.

NATURAL HISTORY.
There is usually a dense fibrous cord in the posterior portion of the popliteal pterygium. Magnetic resonance imaging has been successfully used to locate the peroneal nerve and popliteal artery, which often run through the fibrous band, prior to surgical repair. There may be associated defects of muscle in the lower extremities, with limitation of function despite repair of the pterygium. The genital anomalies are most likely due to distortion by intercrural webs that often run from medial thigh to the base of the phallus. Other webbing across the eyelids or in the mouth may require excision. Although a number of cosmetic and orthopedic corrective procedures are frequently required, normal intelligence and good ambulation should be anticipated in the majority of affected individuals.

ETIOLOGY.
An autosomal dominant inheritance pattern is implied, with wide variability in severity. Mutations in the gene encoding Interferon Regulatory Factor 6 (IRF6), located at chromosome 1q32-q41 are responsible for this disorder as well as Van der Woude syndrome, indicating that these two disorders are allelic. The function of IRF6 is at present unknown.

References

Trelat U: Sur un vice conformation trés-rare de la lèvre-inférieure. J Med Chir Prat 40:442, 1869.

Hecht F, Jarvinen JM: Heritable dysmorphic syndrome with normal intelligence. J Pediatr 70:927, 1967.

Escobar V, Weaver D: The facio-genito-popliteal syndrome. Birth Defects 14:185, 1978.

Raithel H, Schweckendiek W, Hillig U: The popliteal pterygium syndrome in three generations. Z Kinderchir 26:56, 1979.

Hall JG et al: Limb pterygium syndromes: A review and report of eleven patients. Am J Med Genet 12:377, 1982.

Froster-Iskenius UG: Popliteal pterygium syndrome. J Med Genet 27:320, 1990.

Hunter A: The popliteal pterygium syndrome: Report of a new family and review of the literature. Am J Med Genet 36:196, 1990.

Lees MM et al: Popliteal pterygium syndrome: A clinical study of three families and report of linkage to the Van der Woude syndrome locus at 1q32. J Med Genet 36:888, 1999.

Donnelly LF et al: MR imaging of popliteal pterygium syndrome in pediatric patients. AJR 178:1281, 2002.

Kondo S et al: Mutations in IRF6 cause Van der Woude and popliteal pterygium syndromes. Nat Genet 32:285, 2002.

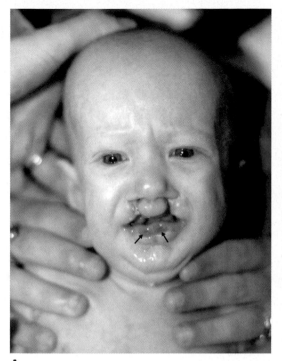

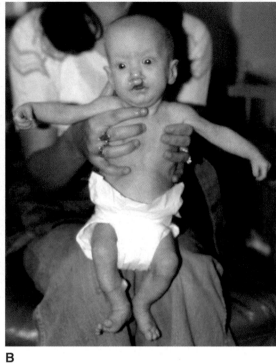

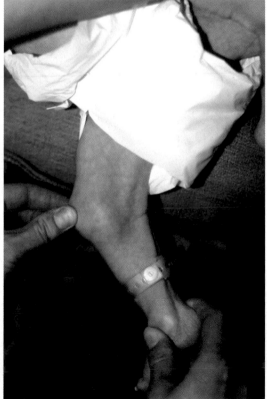

FIGURE 1. Popliteal pterygium syndrome. **A–C,** Infant with bilateral cleft lip, lip pits and popliteal web. Note the rod-like taut core. (Courtesy of Dr. David Weaver, Indiana University, Indianapolis.)

ESCOBAR SYNDROME
(MULTIPLE PTERYGIUM SYNDROME)

Multiple Pterygia, Camptodactyly, Syndactyly

Originally described by Bussiere in 1902, this disorder was fully delineated as a distinct entity by Escobar and colleagues in 1978. Approximately 50 cases have been noted.

ABNORMALITIES

Growth. Small stature.

Facies. Ptosis of eyelids with antimongoloid slant of palpebral fissures; inner canthal folds; hypertelorism; micrognathia with downturning corners of mouth; difficulty opening mouth widely; long philtrum; cleft palate; sad, flat, emotionless face; low-set ears.

Pterygia. Pterygia of neck, axillae, antecubital, popliteal, and intercrural areas.

Limbs. Pterygia plus camptodactyly, syndactyly, equinovarus, or rocker-bottom feet.

Genitalia. Cryptorchidism, absence of labia majora.

Other. Scoliosis, kyphosis, fusion of vertebrae or fused laminae, rib anomalies, absent or dysplastic patella.

OCCASIONAL ABNORMALITIES.

Anterior clefts of vertebral bodies, tall vertebral bodies with decreased anteroposterior diameter, failed fusion of posterior neural arches; rib fusion; long clavicles with lateral hooks; modeled scapulae; dislocated radial head; distal radioulnar separation; muscle atrophy; dislocation of hip; hypoplastic and/or widely spaced nipples; conductive hearing loss; abnormal ossicles; diaphragmatic hernia; hypospadias; cardiac defects.

NATURAL HISTORY. The majority of affected individuals become ambulatory. Intelligence is normal. Respiratory problems including pneumonia plus episodes of dyspnea and apnea presumably secondary to the kyphoscoliosis and small chest size lead to significant morbidity as well as death in the first year of life in approximately 6% of patients.

The pterygia may become more obvious with time, leading to fixed contractures. Early, vigorous physical therapy is indicated to retain the greatest joint mobility. Scoliosis occurs before 5 years of age in the majority of patients and frequently requires surgical fusion. Formal hearing evaluation is indicated in all individuals.

ETIOLOGY. This disorder has an autosomal recessive inheritance pattern.

References

Escobar V et al: Multiple pterygium syndrome. Am J Dis Child 132:609, 1978.

Hall JG et al: Limb pterygium syndromes: A review and report of eleven patients. Am J Med Genet 12:377, 1982.

Thompson EM et al: Multiple pterygium syndrome: Evolution of the phenotype. J Med Genet 24:733, 1987.

Ramer JC et al: Multiple pterygium syndrome: An overview. Am J Dis Child 142:794, 1988.

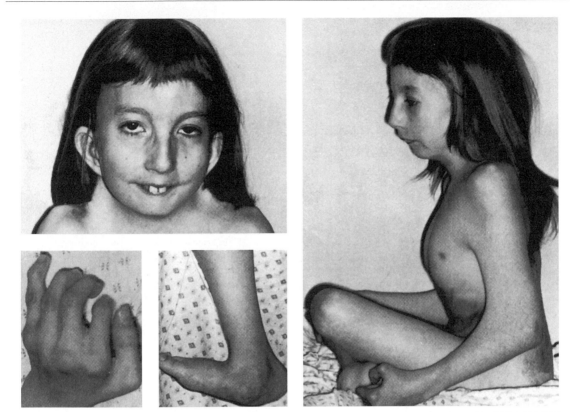

FIGURE 1. A 12-year-old girl showing features of Escobar syndrome. (From Escobar V et al: Am J Dis Child 132:609, 1978, with permission.)

CHILD SYNDROME

Unilateral Hypomelia and Skin Hypoplasia, Cardiac Defect

Falek and colleagues reported two female siblings with this unique pattern of malformation in 1968, and Shear noted a comparable case. The term CHILD is an acronym for *c*ongenital *h*emidysplasia with *i*chthyosiform erythroderma and *l*imb *d*efects.

ABNORMALITIES

Growth. Mild prenatal growth deficiency.

Limbs. Unilateral hypomelia varying from absence of a limb to hypoplasia of some metacarpals and phalanges, webbing at elbows and knees, joint contractures.

Skin. Unilateral ichthyosiform skin lesion, sometimes referred to as an ichthyosiform nevus or inflammatory epidermal nevus, with sharp midline demarcation; small patches of involved skin may occur on opposite side; unilateral alopecia, hyperkeratosis, and nail destruction; histologically, there is a thick parakeratotic stratum corneum overlying a psoriasiform, acanthotic epidermis, often with inflammatory infiltration and lipid-laden histiocytes.

Other Skeletal. Ipsilateral hypoplasia of bones involving any part of the skeleton, including mandible, clavicle, scapula, ribs, and vertebrae; ipsilateral punctate epiphyseal calcifications during infancy.

Other. Cardiac septal defects, single coronary ostium, single ventricle, unilateral renal agenesis.

OCCASIONAL ABNORMALITIES.

Ipsilateral hypoplasia of brain, cranial nerves, spinal cord, lung, thyroid, adrenal gland, ovary, and fallopian tube; mild mental deficiency; mild contralateral anomalies of skin, bone, or viscera; scoliosis; cleft lip; umbilical hernia; hearing loss; meningomyelocele.

NATURAL HISTORY. The skin lesions, usually present at birth, may develop during the first few weeks of life. New areas of involvement may occur as late as 9 years. The face is spared. Early death is due primarily to cardiac defects. When the left side of the body is involved, which occurs far less frequently than the right, severity is far greater. Treatment with etretinate, an aromatic retinoid, has been successful in management of the skin problems in some cases.

ETIOLOGY. This disorder has an X-linked dominant inheritance pattern with lethality in males. Although the majority of cases are sporadic, rare familial cases with mother-daughter transmission have been reported. The majority of cases are caused by mutations in the NSDHL (NADH steroid dehydrogenase-like) gene located at Xq28. However, at least two patients have been reported with a mutation in EBP (Emopamil Binding Protein) located at Xp11.2. Mutations in the latter also are responsible for X-linked dominant chondrodysplasia punctata.

References

Falek A et al: Unilateral limb and skin deformities with congenital heart disease in twin siblings: A lethal syndrome. J Pediatr 73:910, 1968.

Shear CS et al: Syndrome of unilateral ectromelia, psoriasis, and central nervous system anomalies. Birth Defects 7:197, 1971.

Happle R, Koch H, Lenz W: The CHILD syndrome. Eur J Pediatr 134:27, 1980.

Christiansen JR, Petersen HO, Søgaard H: The CHILD syndrome—congenital hemidysplasia with ichthyosiform erythroderma and limb defects: A case report. Acta Dermatol Venereol (Stockh) 64:165, 1984.

Hebert A et al: The CHILD syndrome: Histologic and ultrastructural studies. Arch Dermatol 123:503, 1987.

Emami S et al: Peroxisomal abnormality in fibroblasts from involved skin of CHILD syndrome: Case study and review of peroxisomal disorders in relation to skin disease. Arch Dermatol 128:1213, 1992.

Konig A et al: Mutations in the NSDHL gene, encoding a 3β-hydroxysteroid dehydrogenase, cause CHILD syndrome. Am J Med Genet 90:339, 2000.

Kelley RI et al: Inborn errors of sterol biosynthesis. Annu Rev Genomics Hum Genet 2:299, 2001.

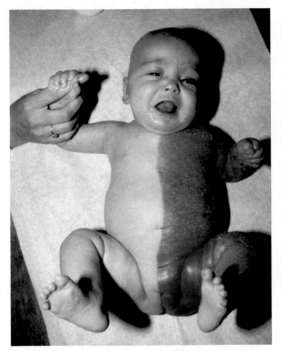
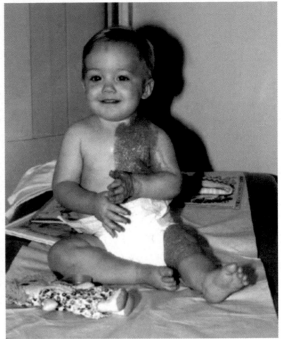
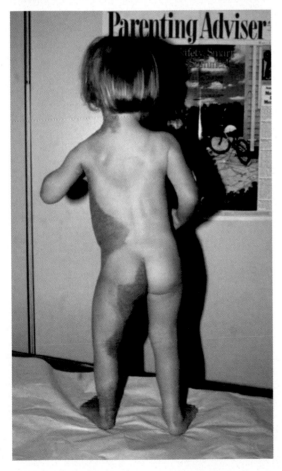

FIGURE 1. CHILD syndrome. Affected child at 3 months, 13 months, and 23 months of age. Note the unilateral erythema and scaling with ipsilateral hypoplasia. (Courtesy of Dr. Marilyn C. Jones, Children's Hospital, San Diego.)

FEMORAL HYPOPLASIA–UNUSUAL FACIES SYNDROME

Femoral Hypoplasia, Short Nose, Cleft Palate

Following single case reports in 1961 and 1965 by Franz and O'Rahilly and by Kucera and colleagues, Daentl and colleagues recognized four additional patients and set forth this unique syndrome in 1975.

ABNORMALITIES

Growth. Small stature, predominantly the result of short lower limbs.

Facial. Short nose with hypoplastic alae nasi, long philtrum, and thin upper lip; micrognathia, cleft palate; upslanting palpebral fissures; low-set, poorly formed pinnae.

Limbs. Bilateral, usually asymmetric involvement; hypoplastic to absent femora and variable asymmetric involvement of fibula and tibia; variable hypoplasia of humeri with restricted elbow movement, including radioulnar and radiohumeral synostosis and limited shoulder movement; Sprengel deformity; talipes equinovarus.

Pelvis. Hypoplastic acetabulae, constricted iliac base with vertical ischial axis, and large obturator foramina.

Spine. Dysplastic sacrum, missing vertebrae or hemivertebrae, sacralization of lumbar vertebrae, scoliosis.

Genitourinary. Cryptorchidism; inguinal hernia; small penis, testes, or labia majora; polycystic kidneys, absent kidneys, abnormal collecting system.

OCCASIONAL ABNORMALITIES.

Astigmatism; esotropia; short third, fourth, and fifth metatarsals; preaxial polydactyly of feet; tapered, fused, or missing ribs; inguinal hernia; cardiac defects including ventricular septal defect, pulmonary stenosis, and truncus arteriosus; craniosynostosis.

NATURAL HISTORY.

Although there may be problems in speech development, the patients have been of normal intelligence; most of them have been ambulatory.

ETIOLOGY.

The cause of this disorder is unknown. Although the vast majority of cases are sporadic, an affected male whose daughter is similarly affected raises the possibility of autosomal dominant inheritance. Maternal diabetes has been documented frequently.

References

Franz CH, O'Rahilly R: Congenital skeletal limb deficiencies. J Bone Joint Surg [Am] 43:1202, 1961.

Kucera VJ, Lenz W, Maier W: Missbildungen der Beine und der Kaudalen Wirbelsaeule bei Kindern diabetischer Muetter. Dtsch Med Wochenschr 90:901, 1965.

Daentl DL et al: Femoral hypoplasia–unusual facies syndrome. J Pediatr 86:107, 1975.

Lampert RP: Dominant inheritance of femoral hypoplasia–unusual facies syndrome. Clin Genet 17:255, 1980.

Johnson JP et al: Femoral hypoplasia–unusual facies syndrome in infants of diabetic mothers. J Pediatr 102:866, 1983.

Baraitser M et al: Femoral hypoplasia unusual facies syndrome with preaxial polydactyly. Clin Dysmorphol 3:40, 1994.

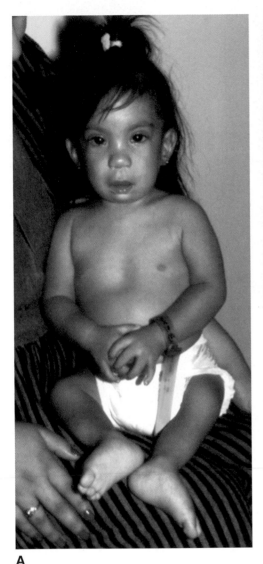

A

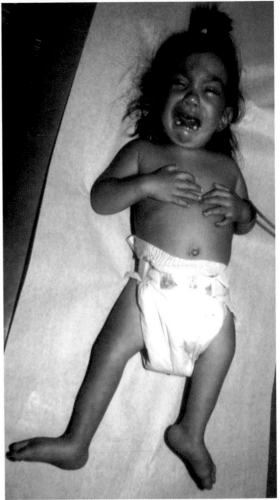

B

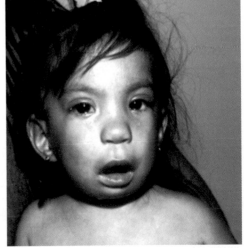

C

FIGURE 1. Femoral hypoplasia–unusual facies syndrome. **A–C,** Photograph of a 21-month-old girl. Note the short nose, small mandible, variable and asymmetric hypoplasia of the femurs and humeri, and inability to extend the elbow fully. (Courtesy of Dr. Marilyn C. Jones, Children's Hospital, San Diego.)

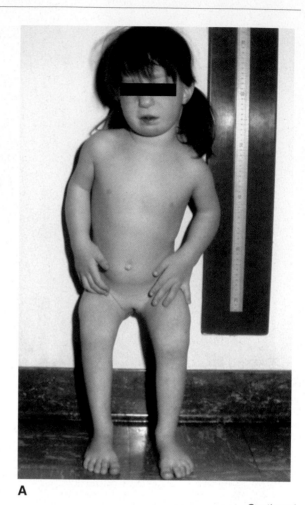

FIGURE 2. **A** and **B,** Girl showing short humeri with
synostosis at the elbow, in addition to femoral shortness.   **A**

Continued

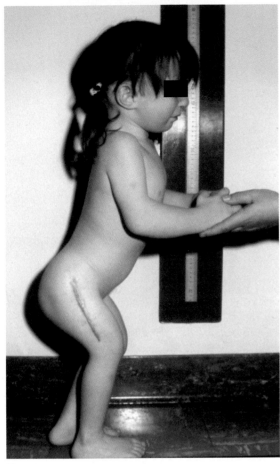

B

Fig. 2, cont'd.

TIBIAL APLASIA–ECTRODACTYLY SYNDROME

Split-Hand/Split-Foot, Absence of Long Bones of Arms and Legs

A single patient with this pattern of malformation was described in 1575 by Ambroise Paré. Subsequently, more than 100 affected individuals have been reported. The complete spectrum of this condition has been set forth by Majewski and colleagues and by Hoyme and colleagues.

ABNORMALITIES

Hands. Abnormalities in 68%, most commonly ectrodactyly (split hand); absence of multiple fingers.

Feet. Abnormalities in 64%, most commonly variable absence of tarsals, metatarsals, and toes.

Limbs. Absence of long bone of legs in 55%, most commonly tibial aplasia; tibial hypoplasia; fibular hypoplasia or aplasia.

OCCASIONAL ABNORMALITIES.

Cup-shaped ears; aplasia of ulna, radius, or humerus; monodactyly; absence of multiple fingers; syndactyly; proximally placed thumbs; ectrodactyly of feet; metatarsus adductus; talipes equinovarus; supernumerary preaxial digit; postaxial polydactyly; absence of entire leg; bifid or hypoplastic femur; contracted knee joint with patellar hypoplasia; hypoplasia of great toe; craniosynostosis; bifid xiphoid.

ETIOLOGY. This disorder has an autosomal dominant inheritance pattern with widely variable expression and frequent examples of nonpenetrance in structurally normal obligate carriers.

COMMENT. Because of the frequency of clinically normal individuals who carry the gene for this disorder, prenatal ultrasonographic studies should be performed in all pregnancies in affected families.

References

Majewski F et al: Aplasia of tibia with split-hand/split-foot deformity: Report of six families with 35 cases and considerations about variability and penetrance. Hum Genet 70:136, 1985.

Hoyme HE et al: Autosomal dominant ectrodactyly and absence of long bones of upper or lower limbs: Further clinical delineation. J Pediatr 111:538, 1987.

Richieri-Costa A et al: Tibial hemimelia: Report on 37 new cases. Clinical and genetic considerations. Am J Med Genet 27:867, 1987.

Majewski F et al: Ectrodactyly and absence (hypoplasia) of the tibia: Are there dominant and recessive types? Am J Med Genet 63:185, 1996.

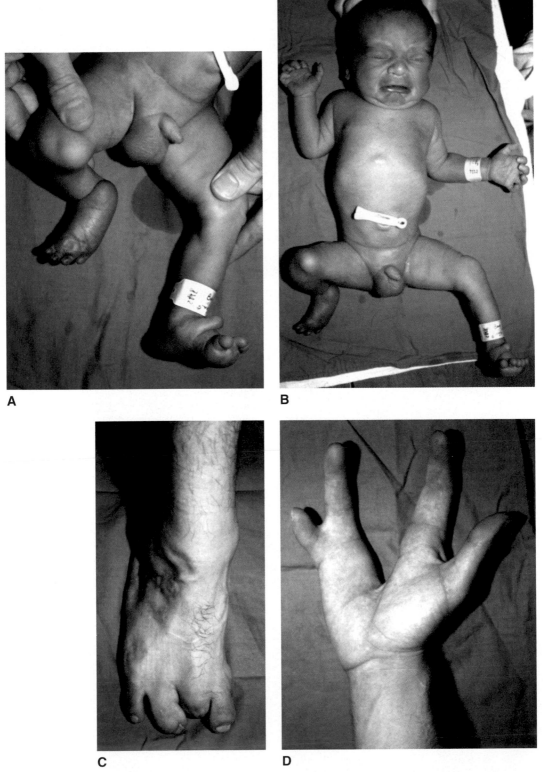

FIGURE 1. Tibial aplasia-ectrodactyly syndrome. **A** and **B**, Newborn infant with absent right tibia and great toe and supernumerary preaxial digit arising from dorsum of right foot. **C** and **D**, Father of newborn infant pictured above. Note the typical split hand. Ectrodactyly of the foot has been surgically repaired. (**A–D**, From Hoyme HE et al: Pediatrics 111:538, 1987, with permission.)

ADAMS-OLIVER SYNDROME

Aplasia Cutis Congenita, Terminal Transverse Defects of Limbs

Adams and Oliver described eight members of a family with this disorder in 1945. More than 85 affected individuals have been reported.

ABNORMALITIES

Growth. Mild growth deficiency (third to tenth percentile).

Scalp. Aplasia cutis congenita over posterior parietal region, with or without an underlying defect of bone; in older individuals, solitary or multiple, round-oval hairless scars are found in the parietal region; tortuous veins over posterior scalp.

Limbs. Variable degrees of terminal transverse defects, including those of lower legs, feet, hands, fingers, toes, or distal phalanges; short fingers; small toenails.

Skin. Cutis marmorata.

OCCASIONAL ABNORMALITIES.
Encephalocele; acrania; microcephaly; arrhinencephaly; defects of neuronal migration with combined focal pachygyria and polymicrogyria; dysplastic cerebral cortex; esotropia; microphthalmia; mental retardation; spastic hemiplegia; epilepsy; cleft lip; cleft palate; cardiovascular defects, obstructive lesions of left heart (29%); syndactyly; talipes equinovarus; accessory nipples; duplicated collecting system; imperforate vaginal hymen; aplasia cutis congenita on trunk and limbs; thin, hyperpigmented skin; Poland sequence; chylothorax; pulmonary and portal hypertension.

NATURAL HISTORY.
Although prognosis is excellent in the vast majority of cases, larger scalp defects are more likely to be associated with underlying defects of bone and, where the superior sagittal sinus or dura are exposed, an increased risk of hemorrhage or meningitis. For those cases, early surgical intervention with grafting is indicated. For the usual case in which the sagittal sinus or dura are not exposed, healing without need for grafting virtually always occurs.

ETIOLOGY.
This disorder has an autosomal dominant inheritance pattern with marked variability in expression and lack of penetrance in some cases. A careful physical examination and radiographs of hands and feet are indicated in first-degree relatives of affected individuals. At least three families have been reported in which more than one affected child has been born to presumably unaffected parents, suggesting autosomal recessive inheritance in some cases.

References

Adams FH, Oliver CP: Hereditary deformities in man due to arrested development. J Hered 36:3, 1945.

Scribanu N, Tamtamy SA: The syndrome of aplasia cutis congenita with terminal transverse defects of limbs. J Pediatr 87:79, 1975.

Bonafede RP, Beighton P: Autosomal dominant inheritance of scalp defects with ectrodactyly. Am J Med Genet 3:35, 1979.

Kuster W et al: Congenital scalp defects with distal limb anomalies (Adams-Oliver syndrome): Report of ten cases and review of the literature. Am J Med Genet 31:99, 1988.

Toriello HW et al: Scalp and limb defects with cutis marmorata telangiectatica congenita: Adams-Oliver syndrome? Am J Med Genet 29:269, 1988.

Der Kaloustian VM et al: Possible common pathogenetic mechanisms for Poland sequence and Adams-Oliver syndrome. Am J Med Genet 38:69, 1991.

Whitely CB, Gorlin RJ: Adams-Oliver syndrome revisited. Am J Med Genet 40:319, 1991.

Bamforth JS et al: Adams-Oliver syndrome: A family with extreme variability in clinical expression. Am J Med Genet 49:393, 1994.

Lin AE et al: Adams-Oliver syndrome associated with cardiovascular malformations. Am J Med Genet 7:235, 1999.

Verdyck P et al: Clinical and molecular analysis of nine families with Adams-Oliver syndrome. Eur J Hum Genet 11:457, 2003.

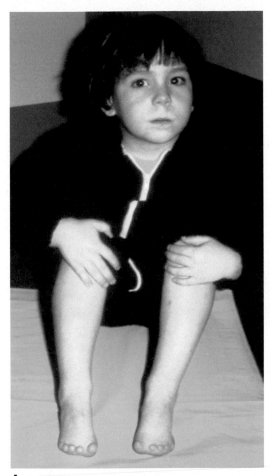

A

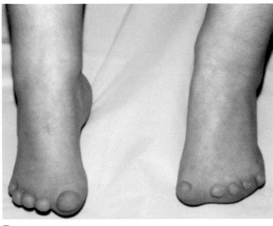

B

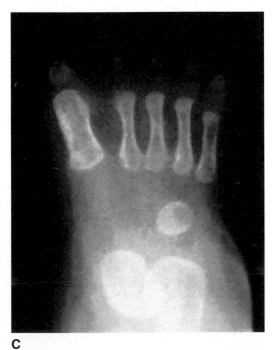

C

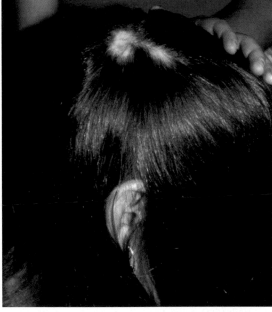

D

FIGURE 1. Adams-Oliver syndrome. **A–D,** Boy, 3½ years old, and his mother's sister. Note the terminal transverse defects involving the toes (**A–C**) and the area of aplasia cutis congenita over his maternal aunt's posterior scalp (**D**). The maternal aunt was otherwise normal.

HOLT-ORAM SYNDROME
(CARDIAC-LIMB SYNDROME)

Upper Limb Defect, Cardiac Anomaly, Narrow Shoulders

This syndrome of skeletal and cardiovascular abnormalities was first described by Holt and Oram in 1960. Over 200 cases have been reported. Its prevalence is approximately 1 in 100,000 live births.

ABNORMALITIES

Skeletal. All gradations of defect in the upper limb and shoulder girdle. The thumbs may be absent, hypoplastic, triphalangeal, or bifid; syndactyly often occurs between thumb and index finger; phocomelia (10%); asymmetric involvement with left side more severely affected is frequently seen; clinodactyly; brachydactyly; hypoplasia to absence of first metacarpal and radius; defects of ulna, humerus, clavicle, scapula, sternum; decreased range of motion at elbows and shoulders, which are often narrow and sloping; carpal anomalies particularly involving the scaphoid, which is often hypoplastic or has a bipartite ossification; proximal as well as distal epiphyses of metacarpals, particularly the first.

Cardiovascular. Ostium secundum atrial septal defect, and ventricular septal defect have been the most common defects, and about one third of patients have had other types of congenital heart defects; conduction defects; hypoplasia of distal blood vessels.

OCCASIONAL ABNORMALITIES.

Hypertelorism, absent pectoralis major muscle, pectus excavatum, thoracic scoliosis, vertebral anomalies, absence of one or more ossification centers in the wrist, Sprengel deformity, postaxial and central polydactyly, lung hypoplasia, refractive errors.

NATURAL HISTORY.
Conduction defects can get worse with time. Pacemakers are sometimes required. Sudden death from heart block has been reported.

ETIOLOGY.
This disorder has an autosomal dominant inheritance pattern with marked intra- and interfamilial variation. A correlation has been observed between the severity of the limb and heart defects in a given patient. Mutations of the TBX5 gene, a member of the T-box transcription factor family, which is linked to chromosome 12q24.1 and is detected in embryonic heart and limb tissues, are detected in approximately 25% of familial cases and in up to 50% of sporadic cases. Consistent with the concept of anticipation, increasing severity has occurred in succeeding generations.

COMMENT.
Because of the marked variability in expression, at-risk individuals with a normal physical exam should have radiographs of wrists, arms, and hands looking for subtle changes of the thumb and carpal bones and an echocardiogram. Skeletal defects involve the upper limbs exclusively. Although bilateral, the limb defects are more prominent on the left.

References

Holt M, Oram S: Familial heart disease with skeletal malformations. Br Heart J 22:236, 1960.

Poznauski A et al: Objective evaluation of the hand in the Holt-Oram syndrome. Birth Defects 8:125, 1972.

Kaufman RL et al: Variable expression of the Holt-Oram syndrome. Am J Dis Child 127:21, 1974.

Hurst JA et al: The Holt-Oram syndrome. J Med Genet 28:406, 1991.

Moens P et al: Holt-Oram syndrome: Postaxial and central polydactyly as variable manifestations in a four generation family. Genet Couns 4:277, 1993.

Basson CT et al: The clinical and genetic spectrum of the Holt-Oram syndrome (heart-hand syndrome). N Engl J Med 330:885, 1994.

Terrett JA et al: Holt-Oram syndrome is a genetically heterogeneous disease with one locus mapping to human chromosome 12q. Nat Genet 6:401, 1994.

Newbury-Ecob RA et al: Holt-Oram syndrome: A clinical genetic study. J Med Genet 33:300, 1996.

Yi Li Q et al: Holt-Oram syndrome is caused by mutations in TBX5, a member of the Brachyury (T) gene family. Nat Genet 15:21, 1997.

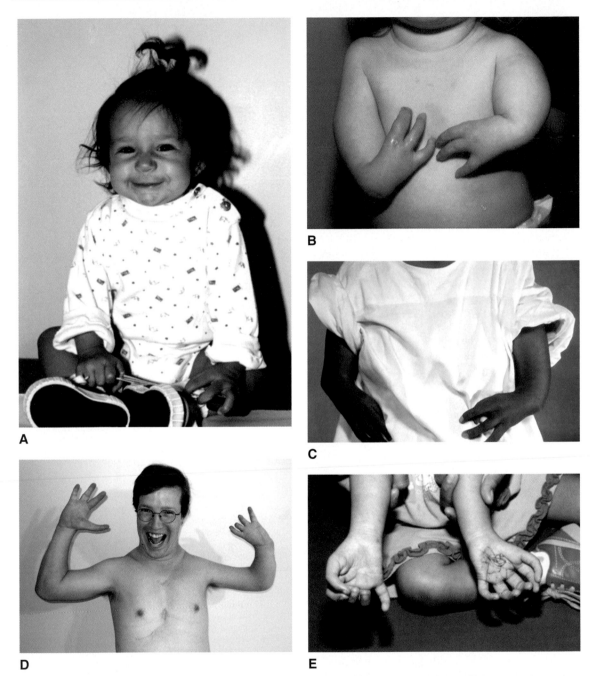

FIGURE 1. Holt-Oram syndrome. **A–E,** Note radial defects that vary from severe forearm hypoplasia to thumb anomalies including absent, hypoplastic, and triphalangeal thumbs, and the altered shoulder girdle. (**A** and **E,** Courtesy of Dr. Marilyn C. Jones, Children's Hospital, San Diego; **C,** courtesy of Dr. Mark Stephan, Madigan General Hospital, Tacoma, Washington; **D,** courtesy of Dr. Michael Bamshad, University of Utah, Salt Lake City.)

LEVY-HOLLISTER SYNDROME
(LACRIMO-AURICULO-DENTO-DIGITAL
SYNDROME, LADD SYNDROME)

Although Levy described the first affected patient in 1967, this disorder was first delineated by Hollister and colleagues in 1973. Well over 20 cases have been reported.

ABNORMALITIES

Lacrimal Anomalies. Nasolacrimal duct obstruction; aplasia or hypoplasia of lacrimal puncta (45%); alacrima due to hypoplasia or aplasia of lacrimal glands (40%).

Ears. Simple, cup-shaped ears with short helix and underdeveloped antihelix (70%).

Hearing. Mild to severe mixed conductive and sensorineural hearing loss (55%).

Dental. Abnormalities in 90%, including hypodontia, peg-shaped incisors, enamel hypoplasia of both deciduous and permanent teeth; delayed eruption of primary teeth.

Limb. Digital abnormalities in 95% including digitalization of thumb; deficiency of bone and soft tissue of thumb and index finger; preaxial polydactyly; triphalangeal thumb; duplication of distal phalanx of thumb; thenar muscle hypoplasia; syndactyly between index and middle fingers; clinodactyly of third and fifth fingers; absent radius and thumb, and broad first toe. Shortening of radius and ulna.

OCCASIONAL ABNORMALITIES.

Absence of parotid glands and Stensen ducts, nasolacrimal fistulae, hypoplastic epiglottis, hypertelorism or telecanthus, downslanting palpebral fissures, coronal hypospadias, renal agenesis or nephrosclerosis, congenital hip dislocation, hiatal hernia, diaphragmatic hernia, 2 to 3 and 3 to 4 syndactyly of toes, cystic ovarian disease.

NATURAL HISTORY. A persistent dry mouth with eating difficulties and a propensity to develop inflammation of the oral mucosa and candidiasis frequently occur early in life. Because of decreased salivation and enamel hypoplasia, severe dental caries occur. A lack of tears and chronic dacryocystitis results from hypoplasia of the nasolacrimal duct system. A decreased tear production also can occur. Although the hearing loss is usually mild to moderate, it has been severe in a few cases. Neonatal death secondary to bilateral renal agenesis has occurred rarely.

ETIOLOGY. This disorder has an autosomal dominant inheritance pattern with marked variability of expression.

References
Levy WJ: Mesoectodermal dysplasia. Am J Ophthalmol 63:978, 1967.
Hollister DW et al: The lacrimo-auriculo-dento-digital syndrome. J Pediatr 83:438, 1973.
Shiang EL, Holmes LB: The lacrimo-auriculo-dento-digital syndrome. Pediatrics 59:927, 1977.
Thompson E, Pembrey M, Graham JM: Phenotypic variation in LADD syndrome. J Med Genet 22:382, 1985.
Wiedemann HR, Drescher J: LADD syndrome: Report of new cases and review of the clincal spectrum. Eur J Pediatr 144:579, 1986.
Heinz GW et al: Ocular manifestations of the lacrimo-auriculo-dento-digital syndrome. Am J Ophthalmol 115:243, 1993.
Horn D, Witkowski R: Phenotype and counseling in lacrimo-auriculo-dento-digital (LADD) syndrome. Genet Couns 4:305, 1993.
Azar T et al: Epiglottic hypoplasia associated with lacrimo-auriclo-dental-digital syndrome. Ann Otol Rhinol Laryngol 109:779, 2000.

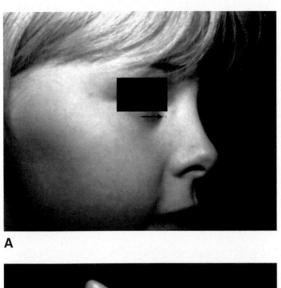

A

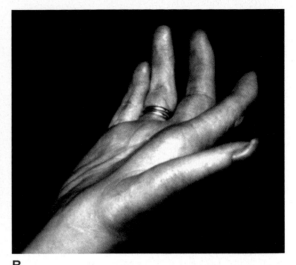

B

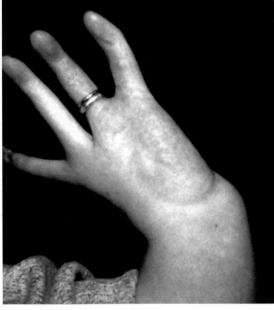

C

FIGURE 1. Levy-Hollister syndrome. A 9-year-old girl showing a nasolacrimal fistula caused by nasolacrimal duct obstruction (**A**; see *arrow*), digitalized thumb plus fifth finger clinodactyly (**B**), and a long tapering thumb with absent creases and surgically removed index finger (**C**). (Courtesy of Dr. H. E. Hoyme, Stanford University, Palo Alto.)

FANCONI PANCYTOPENIA SYNDROME

Radial Hypoplasia, Hyperpigmentation, Pancytopenia

Since Fanconi's original description of three affected siblings in 1927, numerous cases have been reported. Glanz and Fraser as well as Giampietro and colleagues have documented the marked variability of the clinical phenotype. Because 25% of affected individuals are structurally normal, the importance of considering this diagnosis in any anemic child with chromosome breaks, even in the absence of dysmorphic features on the physical examination, has been emphasized. Conversely, since the median age of onset of the hematologic abnormalities is 7 years (range, birth to 31 years), this diagnosis should be considered in all children with the characteristic dysmorphic features even in the absence of hematologic abnormalities.

ABNORMALITIES

Growth. Short stature, frequently of prenatal onset.

Performance. Microcephaly (25 to 37%), mental deficiency in 25%.

Eye. Anomalies in 41%, including ptosis of eyelid, strabismus, nystagmus, and microphthalmos.

Skeletal. Radial ray defect in 49%, including hypoplasia to aplasia of thumb, with supernumerary thumbs in some cases or hypoplastic or aplastic radii.

Urogenital. Renal and urinary tract anomalies in 34%, including hypoplastic or malformed kidneys and double ureters; abnormalities in males, including hypospadias, small penis, small testes, or cryptorchidism in 20%.

Hematologic. Pancytopenia manifested by poikilocytosis, anisocytosis, reticulocytopenia, thrombocytopenia, and leukopenia; decreased bone marrow cellularity; leukemia; myelodysplastic syndrome.

Skin. Brownish pigmentation (64%).

OCCASIONAL ABNORMALITIES

Central Nervous System. Abnormalities in 8% including hydrocephalus, absent septum pellucidum, absent corpus callosum, neural tube closure defect, migration defect, Arnold-Chiari malformation, or single ventricle.

Gastrointestinal. Abnormalities in 14%, including anorectal, duodenal atresia, tracheoesophageal fistula with or without esophageal atresia, annular pancreas, intestinal malrotation, intestinal obstruction, and duodenal web.

Other Skeletal. Defects occurring in 22%, including congenital hip dislocation, scoliosis, rib anomalies, talipes equinovarus, broad base of proximal phalanges, sacral agenesis or hypoplasia, Perthes disease, Sprengel deformity, genu valgum, leg length discrepancy, and kyphosis.

Other. Cardiac defect (13%), auricular anomaly (15%), deafness (11%), syndactyly.

NATURAL HISTORY. The majority of patients are relatively small at birth. Respiratory tract infections may be a frequent problem. The uneven brownish pigmentation of the skin tends to increase with age, being most evident in the anogenital area, groin, axillae, and trunk.

Life expectancy averages 20 years (range, 0 to 50 years). The usual presentation is progressive bone marrow failure and the development of malignancy, especially acute myeloid leukemia and to a lesser extent solid tumors, particularly squamous cell carcinomas. Progressive bone marrow failure, which usually leads to transfusion-dependent anemia, often occurs in the first two decades. Survivors frequently develop solid cancers later in life.

ETIOLOGY. This disorder has an autosomal recessive inheritance pattern. At least eight different complementation groups have been identified, and six of the corresponding genes have been cloned. There is very little correlation between the complementation group and differences in phenotype.

COMMENT. Successful prenatal and postnatal diagnoses of this disorder can be accomplished by demonstrating a high frequency of spontaneous diepoxy-butane–induced chromosomal breakage in peripheral blood lymphocytes as well as in cultured amniotic fluid cells.

References

Fanconi G: Familiäre infantile pernizosaaritige anämie. Z Kinderheilkd 117:257, 1927.

Garriga S, Crosby WH: The incidence of leukemia in families of patients with hypoplasia of the marrow. Blood 14:1008, 1959.

Nilsson LR: Chronic pancytopenia with multiple congenital abnormalities (Fanconi's anaemia). Acta Paediatr 49:518, 1960.

Schmid WK et al: Chromosomenbrueihigkeit bei der familiären Panmyelopathie (Typus Fanconi). Schweiz Med Wochenschr 95:1461, 1965.

Glanz A, Fraser FC: Spectrum of anomalies in Fanconi anemia. J Med Genet 19:412, 1982.

Mann WR et al: Fanconi anemia: Evidence for linkage heterogeneity on chromosome 20q. Genomics 9:329, 1991.

Strathdee CA et al: Cloning of CDNAs for Fanconi anaemia by functional complimentation. Nature 356:763, 1992.

Strathdee CA et al: Evidence for at least four Fanconi anaemia genes including FACC on chromosome 9. Nat Genet 1:196, 1992.

Giampietro PF et al: The need for more accurate and timely diagnosis in Fanconi anemia: A report from the International Fanconi Anemia Registry. Pediatrics 91:1116, 1993.

Joenje H, Patel KJ. The emerging genetic and molecular basis of fanconi anaemia. Nature Rev Genet 2:446, 2001.

Kutler DI et al: A 20-year perspective on the International Fanconi anemia registry (IFAR). Blood 101:1249, 2003.

Rosenberg PS et al: Cancer incidence in persons with Fanconi anemia. Blood 101:822, 2003.

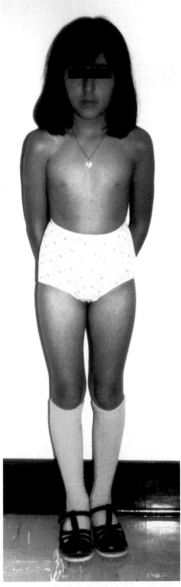

A

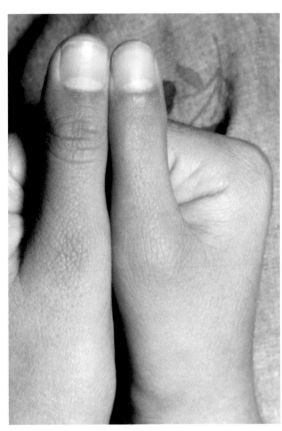

B

FIGURE 1. Fanconi pancytopenia syndrome. **A** and **B,** A 7-year-old child with brownish pigmentation of the skin and hypoplasia of the right thumb with absent creases.

RADIAL APLASIA–THROMBOCYTOPENIA SYNDROME
(TAR Syndrome)

Gross, Groh, and Weippl described this entity in siblings in 1956; subsequently, well over 100 cases have been reported.

ABNORMALITIES

Hematologic. Most severe in early infancy; thrombocytopenia with absence or hypoplasia of megakaryocytes (absent in 66%, decreased in 12%, inactive in 12%); "leukemoid" granulocytosis in 62% of patients, especially during bleeding episodes; eosinophilia in 53%; anemia, often out of proportion to apparent blood loss.

Limbs. Arms: Bilateral absence of radius (100%); abnormalities of ulna including hypoplasia (100%), bilateral absence (20%) or unilateral absence (10%); abnormal humerus (50%) with bilateral absence in 5% to 10%; shoulder joint may be abnormal; the thumbs are always present.

Legs: Abnormalities in 50%, including hip dislocation, subluxation of knees, coxa valga, dislocation of patella, femoral and tibial torsion, abnormal tibiofibular joint, ankylosis of knee, small feet, abnormal toe placement; absence of fibula.

OCCASIONAL ABNORMALITIES.

Cleft palate, congenital heart defect (22% to 33%), primarily tetralogy of fallot and atrial septal defect, small stature, central facial capillary hemangioma, strabismus, ptosis, dysseborrheic dermatitis, excessive perspiration, pedal and dorsal edema, pes valgus, talpes equinovarus, fourth and fifth metatarsal synostosis, fourth and fifth toe syndactyly, agenesis of cruciate ligament and hypoplasia of menisci with knee dysplasia, renal anomaly (23%), absent uterus, ovarian agenesis, spina bifida, scoliosis, brachycephaly, micrognathia, lateral clavicular hook, pancreatic cyst, Meckel diverticulum, hypogammaglobulinemia, sensorineural hearing loss, mental deficiency (7%) that is usually related to intracranial bleeding, delayed myelination, hypoplasia of cerebellum, particularly the vermis and a cavum septum pellucidum on magnetic resonance imaging of brain (one patient).

NATURAL HISTORY. Approximately 40% of the patients have died, usually as a result of hemorrhage during early infancy. Thrombocytopenia during that time, most likely associated with a dysmegakaryocytopoiesis characterized by cells blocked at an early stage of differentiation, is precipitated by viral illness, particularly gastrointestinal. With advancing age, the severity of the hematologic disorder usually becomes less profound, and therefore, vigorous early management is indicated. With the exception of menorrhagia, affected adults usually have no problem. Intracranial bleeding, when present, almost always occurs before 1 year of age. Delayed motor development is due to the skeletal abnormalities. Bracing, splinting, or stabilization of the wrist centrally should be considered. Arthritis of wrist and knees is a late complication. Cow's milk allergy or intolerance (47%) can be a significant problem with introduction of cow's milk precipitating thrombocytopenia, eosinophilia, or leukemoid reactions.

ETIOLOGY. This disorder has an autosomal recessive inheritance pattern. Prenatal diagnosis can be made by demonstrating the defect of the upper limb on sonography.

References

Gross H, Groh C, Weippl G: Congenitale hypoplastische Thrombopenie mit Radialaplasie. Neue Osterr Z Kinderheilkd 1:574, 1956.

Shaw S, Oliver RAM: Congenital hypoplastic thrombocytopenia with skeletal deformities in siblings. Blood 14:374, 1956.

Hall JG et al: Thrombocytopenia with absent radius (TAR). Medicine 48:441, 1969.

Anyane-Yeboa K et al: Brief clinical report: Tetraphocomelia in the syndrome of thrombocytopenia with absent radii (TAR syndrome). Am J Med Genet 20:571, 1985.

Hall JG: Thrombocytopenia and absent radius (TAR) syndrome. J Med Genet 24:79, 1987.

MacDonald MR et al: Hypoplasia of the cerebellar vermis and corpus callosum in thrombocytopenia with absent radius syndrome on MRI studies. Am J Med Genet 50:46, 1994.

Letestu R et al: Existence of a differentiation blockage at the stage of a megakaryocyte precursor in the thrombocytopenia and absent radii (TAR) syndrome. Blood 95:1633, 2000.

Greenhalgh KL et al: Thrombocytopenia-absent radius: a clinical genetic study. J Med Genet 39:876, 2002.

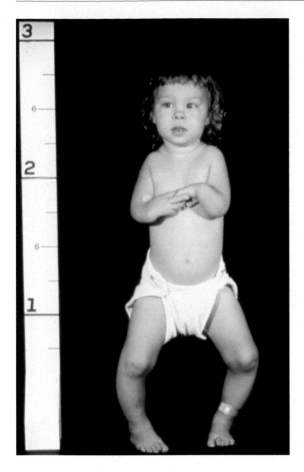

FIGURE 1. Radial aplasia–thrombocytopenia syndrome. Child with serious bleeding and thrombocytopenia as an infant. Note the presence of thumbs despite the bilateral absence of radii, abnormal shoulders, and subluxation of the knees.

AASE SYNDROME

Triphalangeal Thumb, Congenital Anemia

Aase and Smith described two male siblings with triphalangeal thumbs and a congenital anemia in 1969. Diamond-Blackfan anemia, initially described in 1938, is a pure red cell aplasia that is sometimes associated with features seen in the Aase syndrome. It is now clear that the Aase syndrome should not be separated from the Diamond-Blackfan anemia.

ABNORMALITIES

Growth. Mild growth deficiency, about third percentile.
Hematologic. Hypoplastic anemia that tends to improve with age.
Skeletal. Triphalangeal thumbs, mild radial hypoplasia, narrow shoulders, late closure of fontanels.

OCCASIONAL ABNORMALITIES.

Mental retardation; downslanting palpebral fissures; cleft lip; cleft palate; retinopathy; cataracts; glaucoma; webbed neck; 11 pairs of ribs; bifid thoracic vertebra; agenesis of clavicle; underdeveloped ilia, distal sacrum and coccygeal vertebrae; dysplastic middle phalanx of fifth finger; cardiac defects; urogenital anomalies.

NATURAL HISTORY. The anemia, which

has been responsive to prednisone therapy, tends to improve with age.

ETIOLOGY. Although most cases are sporadic, both autosomal dominant and autosomal recessive inheritance patterns have been described. One locus for Diamond-Blackfan anemia has been mapped to chromosome 19q13.2 for both dominant and recessive inherited cases, and the responsible gene, which encodes the ribosomal protein (RP) S19, has been cloned. At least three patients, each of whom were also mentally retarded, had microdeletions in 19q13.2 suggesting the likelihood of a contiguous gene syndrome with a gene for mental retardation and skeletal malformations included in the deletion.

References

Aase JM, Smith DW: Congenital anemia and triphalangeal thumbs: A new syndrome. J Pediatr 74:417, 1969.

Murphy S, Lubin B: Triphalangeal thumbs and congenital erythroid hypoplasia: Report of a case with unusual features. J Pediatr 81:987, 1972.

Higginbottom MC et al: Case report: The Aase syndrome in a female patient. J Med Genet 15:484, 1978.

Muis N et al: The Aase syndrome: Case report and review of the literature. Eur J Pediatr 145:153, 1986.

Hurst JA et al: Autosomal dominant transmission of congenital erythroid hypoplastic anemia with radial abnormalities. Am J Med Genet 40:482, 1991.

Hing AV, Dowton SB: Aase syndrome: Novel radiographic features. Am J Med Genet 45:413, 1993.

Draptchinskaia N et al: The gene encoding ribosomal protein S19 is mutated in Diamond-Blackfan anaemia. Nat Genet 21:169, 1999.

Tentler D et al: A microdeletion in 19q13.2 associated with mental retardation, skeletal malformations, and Diamond-Blackfan anaemia suggests a novel contiguous gene syndrome. J Med Genet 37:128, 2000.

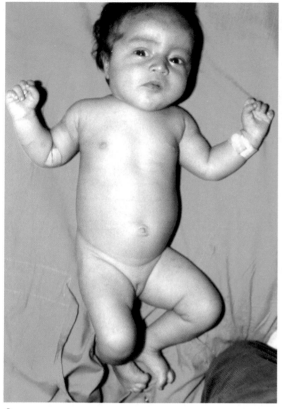

A

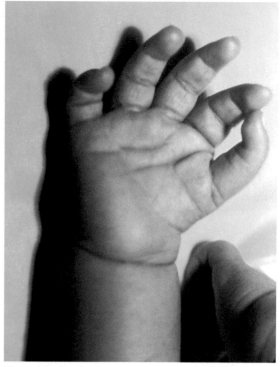

B

FIGURE 1. Aase syndrome. **A** and **B**, Newborn female infant with triphalangeal thumbs and thenar hypoplasia.

J Osteochondrodysplasias

ACHONDROGENESIS, TYPES IA AND IB

Low Nasal Bridge, Very Short Limbs, Incomplete Ossification of Lower Spine

This early lethal disorder was described in 1925 by Donath and Vogl and termed achondrogenesis by Fraccaro in 1952. More than 20 cases have been reported. Studies by Borochowitz and colleagues indicate that achondrogenesis type I (previously referred to as Parenti-Fraccaro type) represents two radiographically and histopathologically distinct disorders, referred to as types IA and IB. In the classification set forth by Whitley and Gorlin, type I is synonymous with type IA and type II with type IB.

ABNORMALITIES

Growth. Extremely small stature (22 to 30 cm).
Craniofacies. Cranium large for gestational age, low nasal bridge, micrognathia.
Limbs. Severe micromelia.
Radiographs. In both types, the skull, vertebral bodies, fibula, talus, and calcaneus are poorly ossified; the ilia are crenated; the long bones are stellate; and the ribs are extremely short. In type IA, multiple rib fractures are present, and the proximal femurs have metaphyseal spikes. Conversely, in type IB, rib fractures do not occur, and the distal femurs have metaphyseal irregularities.

NATURAL HISTORY AND COMMENT.

The defect in the development of cartilage and bone is severe. In type IA, normal-appearing but hypervascular cartilage matrix is present with increased cellular density. Large lacuna surround the chondrocytes, which contain round cytoplasmic inclusion bodies. In type IB, sparse interterritorial cartilaginous matrix is present, with a marked deficiency of collagen fibers. The chondrocytes are large, have a central round nucleus, and are surrounded by a dense collagenous ring. Developmental pathology beyond the skeletal system is implied by the frequent findings of polyhydramnios, hydrops, and early lethality. Most infants are stillborn or die shortly after birth. Occipital encephalocele has been reported in one child with type IA disease.

ETIOLOGY. This disorder has an autosomal recessive inheritance pattern. The molecular basis for type IA is unknown and it may contain as yet unknown subtypes. Achondrogenesis, type IB is due to mutations in the gene for diastrophic dysplasia, which has been shown to encode a sulfate transporter (DTDST) and is located on 5q. Mutations in this gene are responsible for four recessively inherited chondrodysplasias, including achondrogenesis type IB, diastrophic dysplasia, multiple epiphyseal dysplasia, and atelosteogenesis type 2.

References

Donath J, Vogl A: Untersuchungen über den chondrodystrophischen Zwergwuchs. Wien Arch Intern Med 10:1, 1925.

Fraccaro M: Contributo allo studies delle malattie del mesenchima osteopoietico: L'achondrogenesi. Folia Hered Pathol (Milano) 1:190, 1952.

Maroteaux P, Lamy M: Le diagnostic des nanismes chondrodystrophiques chez les nouveaunés. Arch Fr Pediatr 25:241, 1968.

Whitley CB, Gorlin RJ: Achondrogenesis: New nosology with evidence of genetic heterogeneity. Radiology 148:693, 1983.

Borochowitz Z et al: Achondrogenesis type I—further heterogeneity. J Pediatr 112:23, 1988.

Freisinger P et al: Achondrogenesis type IB (Fraccaro): Study of collagen in the tissue and in chondrocytes cultured in agarose. Am J Med Genet 49:439, 1994.

Superti-Furga A: Achondrogenesis type 1B. J Med Genet 33:957, 1996.

Superti-Furga A et al: Achondrogenesis type IB is caused by mutations in the diastrophic dysplasia sulfate transporter gene. Nature Genet 2:100, 1996.

Karniski IP: Mutations in the diastrophic dysplasia sulfate transporter (DTDST) gene: Correlation between sulfate transport activity and chondrodysplasia phenotype. Hum Molec Genet 10:1485, 2001.

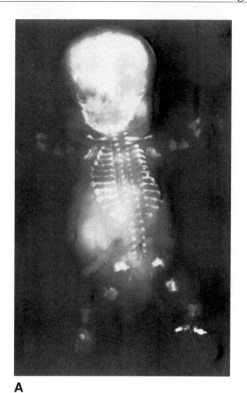

A

Type	Achondrogenesis IA	Achondrogenesis IB
Skull	Poorly ossified	Poorly ossified
Ribs	Short and fractured	Short, no fractures, cupped ends
Spine	Completely unossified	Posterior pedicles only
Illium	Arched	Crenated
Ischium	*Ossified-hypoplastic	Unossified
Femur	Wedged with metaph. spike	Trapezoid
Tibia Fibula	Short with metaph. flare	Crenated Unossified
	*Unossified 30 weeks' gestation	

B

FIGURE 1. **A,** Stillborn infant at 30 weeks' gestation with achondrogenesis, type IA. **B,** Radiographic features that differentiate type IA from type IB are delineated on the drawings. (**A** and **B,** Courtesy of Dr. R. Lachman, Harbor-UCLA Medical Center, and Dr. D. L. Rimoin, Cedars-Sinai Medical Center, Los Angeles.)

TYPE II ACHONDROGENESIS-HYPOCHONDROGENESIS

(Langer-Saldino Achondrogenesis, Hypochondrogenesis)

Initially described by Langer and colleagues and Saldino, this early lethal disorder has been more completely delineated by Chen and colleagues and Borochowitz and colleagues.

ABNORMALITIES

Growth. Extremely short stature (27 to 36 cm).

Craniofacies. Large calvarium with large anterior and posterior fontanels, flat nasal bridge, small anteverted nostrils, micrognathia.

Limbs. Short.

Radiographs. Normal cranial ossification; short ribs without fractures; short, broad long bones with disproportionately long fibula and metaphyseal irregularity of distal ulna; variable degrees of failure of ossification of lumbar spine, cervical spine, sacrum, ischial and pubic bones, and calcaneus and talus.

Other. Polyhydramnios.

OCCASIONAL ABNORMALITIES.

Cleft soft palate, microtia, postaxial polydactyly of feet, cystic hygroma, hydrops, atrial septal defect, AV canal defect.

NATURAL HISTORY.
Although one child survived to 3 months, the majority are stillborn or die in the first few hours of life from pulmonary hypoplasia.

ETIOLOGY.
The vast majority of cases are sporadic. Molecular studies have documented mutations of COL2A1, the gene encoding type II collagen. In all cases where mutations have been identified, they have been heterozygous, indicating an autosomal dominant mode of inheritance; however, autosomal recessive inheritance cannot be ruled out in all cases, particularly those with the most severe radiographic and pathologic features. Mutations in the gene for type II collagen result in disorders with a clinical spectra ranging from mild to perinatal lethal, including Stickler syndrome, spondyloepimetaphyseal dysplasia, Strudwick type, Kniest dysplasia, spondyloepiphyseal dysplasia congenita, and type II achondrogenesis hypochondrogenesis.

COMMENT.
Hypochondrogenesis, previously thought to be a distinct disorder, and achondrogenesis type II represent a spectrum of the same disorder referred to as type II achondrogenesis-hypochondrogenesis. Patients with the most severe radiographic and pathologic features have been labeled achondrogenesis type II, while those with less severe, although similar features, hypochondrogenesis.

References

Langer LO et al: Thanatophoric dwarfism: A condition confused with achondroplasia in the neonate, with brief comments on achondrogenesis and homozygous achondroplasia. Radiology 92:285, 1969.

Saldino RM: Lethal short-limbed dwarfism: Achondrogenesis and thanatophoric dwarfism. AJR 112:185, 1971.

Chen H, Lin CT, Yang SS: Achondrogenesis: A review with special consideration of achondrogenesis type II (Langer-Saldino). Am J Med Genet 10:379, 1981.

Borochowitz Z et al: Achondrogenesis II-hypochondrogenesis: variability versus heterogeneity. Am J Med Genet 24:273, 1986.

Godfrey M, Hollister DW: Type II achondrogenesis-hypochondrogenesis: Identification of abnormal type II collagen. Am J Hum Genet 43:904, 1988.

Horton WA: Characterization of a type II collagen gene (COL2A1) mutation identified in cultured chondrocytes from human hypochondrogenesis. Proc Natl Acad Sci USA 89:4583, 1992.

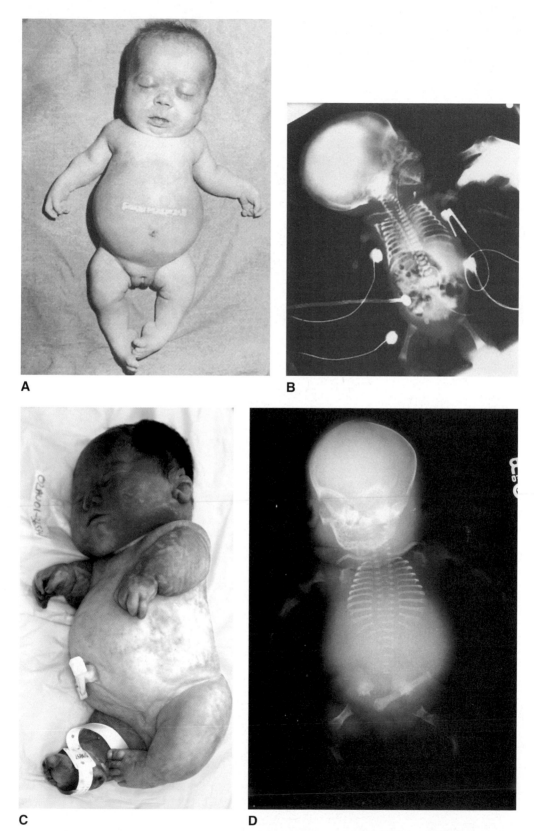

A

B

C

D

FIGURE 1. **A–D,** Two stillborn infants with type II achondrogenesis-hypochondrogenesis, showing the variation in severity of the disorder. Note the relatively normal cranial ossification, short ribs, and variable degrees of failure of ossification of lumbar and cervical spines, sacrum, and ischial and pubic bones. (**A** and **B,** Courtesy of Dr. R. Lachman, Harbor-UCLA Medical Center, and Dr. D. L. Rimoin, Cedars-Sinai Medical Center, Los Angeles; **C** and **D,** courtesy of Dr. Lynne M. Bird, Children's Hospital, San Diego.)

FIBROCHONDROGENESIS

Lazzaroni-Fossati described a patient with this early lethal disorder in 1978. Subsequently, approximately 13 additional patients have been reported. A distinctive fibrosis of the growth-plate cartilage led to the designation fibrochondrogenesis.

ABNORMALITIES

Growth. Short stature.

Craniofacies. Widely patent anterior fontanel, coronal and sagittal sutures; protuberant eyes with large corneae; hypoplastic nose with flat nasal bridge and anteverted nares; long philtrum; small mouth; cleft palate; short neck; low-set, malformed ears.

Trunk. Flattened vertebrae with posterior vertebral hypoplasia and a sagittal midline cleft; short, thin ribs with anterior and posterior cupping; long, thin clavicles; small chest; small/elevated scapula.

Limbs. Rhizomelic shortening; small hands and feet; camptodactyly; fifth finger clinodactyly; hypoplastic finger and toenails; short, dumbbell-shaped long bones with broad, irregular metaphyses; prominent metaphyseal spurs adjacent to growth plates; short fibulae.

Pelvis. Hypoplastic with ovoid ilia, irregular flattened acetabula with medial spikes and narrow sacrosciatic notches; broad, hypoplastic ischii.

Other. Omphalocele, hydrops.

NATURAL HISTORY. All affected individuals have been stillborn or have died in the neonatal period.

ETIOLOGY. This disorder has an autosomal recessive inheritance pattern.

COMMENT. Microscopic examination of long bones demonstrates gross disorganization of growth plate cartilage, fibrous appearance of the matrix, and normal metaphyseal and diaphyseal bone formation.

References

Lazzaroni-Fossati F et al: La fibrochondrogenese. Arch Fr Pediatr 35:1096, 1978.

Eteson DJ et al: Fibrochondrogenesis: Radiologic and histologic studies. Am J Med Genet 19:277, 1984.

Whitely CB et al: Fibrochondrogenesis: Lethal, autosomal recessive chondrodysplasia with distinctive cartilage histopathology. Am J Med Genet 19:265, 1984.

Bankier A et al: Fibrochondrogenesis in male twins at 24 weeks gestation. Am J Med Genet 38:95, 1991.

Al-Gazali LI et al: Fibrochondrogenesis: Clinical and radiological features. Clin Dysmorphol 6:157, 1997.

Al-Gazali LI et al: Recurrence of fibrochondrogenesis in a consanguineous family. Clin Dysmorphol 8:59, 1999.

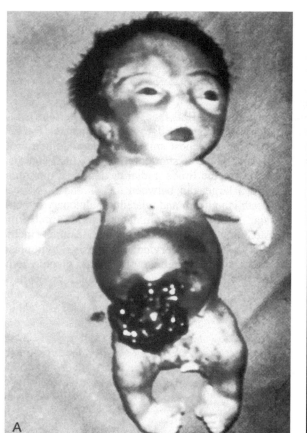 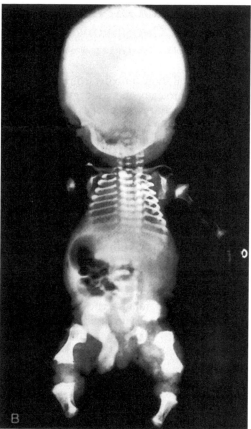

FIGURE 1. **A,** Stillborn infant with fibrochondrogenesis. Note the flat, wide nasal bridge, anteverted nares, short limbs, and equinovarus position of the feet. **B,** The radiograph reveals long, thin clavicles; short, thin ribs; flattened acetabula; narrow sacrosciatic notches; metaphyseal widening of the tibia and fibula; and dumbbell-shaped femora. (**A** and **B,** From Eteson DJ et al: Am J Med Genet 19:277, 1984. Copyright © 1984. Reprinted with permission of Wiley-Liss, Inc., a subsidiary of John Wiley & Sons, Inc.)

SHORT RIB–POLYDACTYLY SYNDROME, TYPE I (SALDINO-NOONAN TYPE)

This disorder was originally described by Saldino and Noonan in 1972. Naumoff and colleagues and Yang and colleagues published cases suggesting that short rib–polydactyly syndrome (SRP) type I represents two separate disorders, referred to as SRP type I and SRP type III. However, clinical, radiographic, and morphologic studies suggest that only one disorder exists, with wide variability in expression. This issue remains to be completely resolved.

ABNORMALITIES

Growth. Short stature.

Limbs. Short; postaxial polydactyly of hands or feet; syndactyly; metaphyseal irregularities of long bones, with spurs extending longitudinally from medial and lateral segments; underossified phalanges.

Trunk. Short, horizontal ribs; notch-like ossification defects around periphery of vertebral bodies.

Pelvis. Small iliac bones with horizontal acetabular roof, triangular ossification defect above lateral aspect of acetabulum.

Other. Cardiac defects, including transposition of great vessels, double-outlet left ventricle, double-outlet right ventricle, endocardial cushion defect, and hypoplastic right heart; polycystic kidneys; hypoplasia of penis; defects of cloacal development; imperforate anus.

OCCASIONAL ABNORMALITIES. Natal teeth, preaxial polydactyly, sex-reversal (phenotypic females with a 46XY karyotype).

NATURAL HISTORY. Death from respiratory insufficiency secondary to pulmonary hypoplasia has occurred in all infants within the first few hours after birth.

ETIOLOGY. This disorder has an autosomal recessive inheritance pattern.

References

Saldino RM, Noonan CD: Severe thoracic dystrophy with striking micromelia, abnormal osseous development, including the spine, and multiple visceral anomalies. AJR 114:257, 1972.

Spranger J et al: Short rib-polydactyly (SRP) syndromes, types Majewski and Saldino-Noonan. Z Kinderheilkd 116:73, 1974.

Naumoff P et al: Short rib-polydactyly syndrome type 3. Radiology 122:443, 1977.

Sillence DO: Invited editorial comment: Non-Majewski short rib–polydactyly syndrome. Am J Med Genet 7:223, 1980.

Yang SS et al: Short rib–polydactyly syndrome, type 3 with chondrocytic inclusions: Report of a case and review of the literature. Am J Med Genet 7:205, 1980.

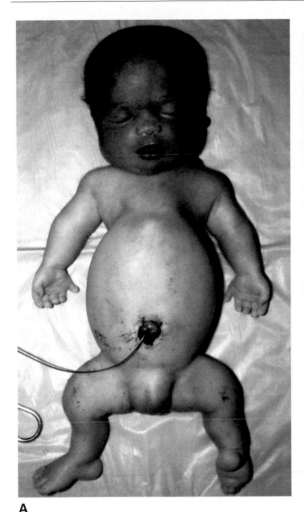

A

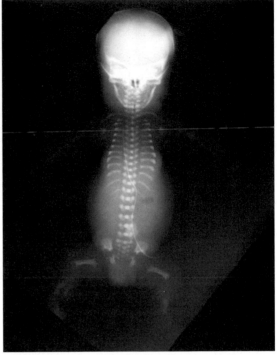

B

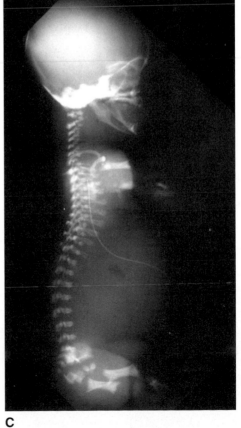

C

FIGURE 1. Short rib–polydactyly syndrome, Saldino-Noonan type. **A,** Stillborn male infant. Note the narrow thorax, short limbs, postaxial polydactyly, and hypoplastic penis. **B** and **C,** Radiographs show short, horizontal ribs; metaphyseal irregularities of long bones, with spurs extending from medial and lateral segments; and triangular ossification defects above lateral aspect of acetabulum.

SHORT RIB–POLYDACTYLY SYNDROME, TYPE II (MAJEWSKI TYPE)

In 1971, Majewski and colleagues described four infants with this early lethal form of short-limb dwarfism. Spranger and colleagues differentiated it from other forms of short rib–polydactyly in 1974, and subsequently a number of additional cases have been described.

ABNORMALITIES

Growth. Short stature with disproportionately short limbs.

Craniofacial. Midline cleft lip; cleft palate; short, flat nose; low-set, small, malformed ears.

Limbs. Both preaxial and postaxial polysyndactyly of hands or feet; brachydactyly; disproportionately short, oval-shaped tibiae; short, rounded metacarpals and metatarsals; premature ossification of proximal epiphyses of humeri, femora, and lateral cuboids; underossified phalanges.

Trunk. Narrow thorax; short, horizontal ribs; high clavicles.

Other. Ambiguous genitalia; hypoplasia of epiglottis and larynx; multiple glomerular cysts and focal dilatation of distal tubules of kidney.

OCCASIONAL ABNORMALITIES.

Microglossia; lobulated tongue; absent gallbladder; brain anomalies, including pachygyria, a small vermis, and absence of olfactory bulbs; persisting left superior vena cava; hydrops; polyhydramnios.

NATURAL HISTORY. Respiratory insufficiency secondary to pulmonary hypoplasia has led to death soon after birth in all cases.

ETIOLOGY. This disorder has an autosomal recessive inheritance pattern.

COMMENT. It has been suggested that this disorder and oro-facial-digital syndrome type II may represent severe and mild ends of the spectrum of the same disorder.

References

Majewski F et al: Polysyndaktylie, verkürzte Gliedmassen und Genitalfehlbildungen: Kennzeichen eines selbaständigen Syndroms? Z Kinderheilkd 111:118, 1971.

Spranger J et al: Short rib-polydactyly (SRP) syndromes, types Majewski and Saldino-Noonan. Z Kinderheilkd 116:73, 1974.

Motegi T et al: Short rib-polydactyly syndrome, Majewski type, in two males. Hum Genet 49:269, 1979.

Chen H et al: Short rib-polydactyly syndrome, Majewski type. Am J Med Genet 7:215, 1980.

Silengo MC et al: Oro-facial-digital syndrome II: Transition types between the Mohr and Majewski syndromes. Report of 2 new cases. Clin Genet 31:331, 1987.

Prudlo J et al: Central nervous system alterations in a case of short–rib polydactyly syndrome, Majewski type. Devel Med Child Neurol 35:158, 1993.

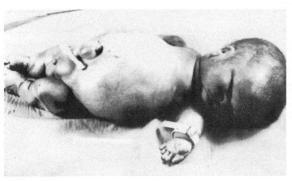

A

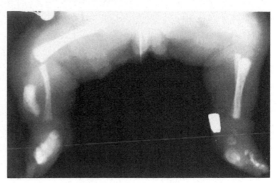

B

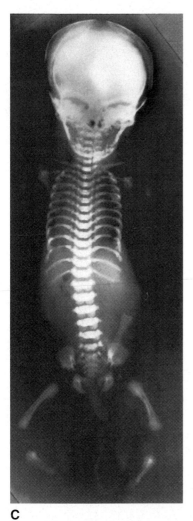

C

FIGURE 1. **A–C,** Neonate with short rib–polydactyly syndrome, Majewski type. Note the disproportionately short limbs, postaxial polydactyly, and, on the radiographs, the narrow thorax with short ribs and disproportionately short, abnormally shaped tibia. (Courtesy of Dr. R. Lachman, Harbor-UCLA Medical Center, and Dr. D. L. Rimoin, Cedars-Sinai Medical Center, Los Angeles.)

THANATOPHORIC DYSPLASIA

Short Limbs, Flat Vertebrae, Large Cranium with Low Nasal Bridge

Maroteaux and colleagues set forth this disorder in 1967 and used the Greek term *thanatophoric* (death-bringing) to emphasize that such patients usually die shortly after birth. Langer and colleagues separated this condition into two types. Type 1 (TD I) is most common and is characterized by curved long bones (most obviously the femora), and very flat vertebral bodies (35% or less of the adjacent disk space in the lumbar region). Type 2 (TD II) is characterized by straight femora and taller vertebral bodies. Almost all cases of thanatophoric dysplasia with a severe cloverleaf skull (the kleeblattschädel anomaly) are TD II.

ABNORMALITIES

Central Nervous System. Severe abnormalities, the most common of which is temporal lobe dysplasia; other defects include megalencephaly, hydrocephalus, brainstem hypoplasia, maldevelopment of inferior olivary and cerebellar dentate nuclei; hypotonia; severe developmental delay in the few survivors.

Growth. Severe growth deficiency; 36 to 46 cm tall, with an average of 40 cm.

Craniofacial. Large cranium and fontanel; 36 to 47 cm, average of 37 cm; small foramen magnum and short base of skull, with full forehead, low nasal bridge, bulging eyes, and small facies; cloverleaf skull.

Limbs. Short, with small sausage-like fingers, bowed long bones with cupped spur-like irregular flaring of metaphyses, and lack of ossification in secondary centers at knee; fibulae are shorter than tibiae; disorganized chondrocytes and bony trabeculae, especially in central epiphyseal-metaphyseal region.

Thorax. Narrow with short ribs.

Spine. Short, flattened vertebrae with relatively wide intervertebral disk space; lack of caudal widening of spinal canal.

Scapulae. Small and square.

Pelvis. Square and short, with small sciatic notch and medial spurs; accessory ossification centers in the ischia and ilia at gestational age younger than 24 weeks.

OCCASIONAL ABNORMALITIES.
Patent ductus arteriosus, atrial septal defect, horseshoe kidney, hydronephrosis, imperforate anus, radioulnar synostosis, soft tissue syndactyly of fingers and toes, acanthosis nigricans in long-term survivors.

NATURAL HISTORY.
Feeble fetal activity and polyhydramnios are frequent in this disorder. These patients usually die shortly after birth, at least partially owing to the small thoracic cage and respiratory insufficiency. Although survival beyond the neonatal period is rare, three affected children, two 9 year olds and one 10 year old, have been reported. All had profound developmental delay, severe growth deficiency, and were ventilatory-dependent.

ETIOLOGY.
This disorder has an autosomal dominant inheritance pattern. All cases represent fresh gene mutations, and most, if not all, are due to mutations in the fibroblast growth factor receptor 3 (FGFR3) gene. All cases with a Lys650Glu substitution had straight femora with craniosynostosis and frequently a cloverleaf skull (TD2). All other mutations were associated with curved femora and cloverleaf skull was only infrequently present (TD1).

References

Maroteaux P, Lamy M, Robert JM: Le nanisme thanatophore. Presse Med 75:2519, 1967.

Giedion A: Thanatophoric dwarfism. Helv Paediatr Acta 23:175, 1968.

Goutières F, Aicardi J, Farkas-Bargeton E: Une Malformation cérébrale particulière associée au nanisme thanatophore. Presse Med 79:960, 1971.

Thompson BH, Parmley TH: Obstetric features of thanatophoric dwarfism. Am J Obstet Gynecol 109:396, 1971.

Horton WA, Harris DJ, Collins DL: Discordance for the kleeblattschädel anomaly in monozygotic twins with thanatophoric dysplasia. Am J Med Genet 15:97, 1983.

Langer LO et al: Thanatophoric dysplasia and cloverleaf skull. Am J Med Genet Suppl 3:167, 1987.

Knisely AS, Amber MW: Temporal lobe abnormalities in thanatophoric dysplasia. Pediatr Neurosci 14:169, 1988.

Martinez-Frias ML et al: Thanatophoric dysplasia: An autosomal dominant condition? Am J Med Genet 31:815, 1988.

MacDonald IM et al: Growth and development in thanatophoric dysplasia. Am J Med Genet 33:508, 1989.

Tavorima PL et al: Thanatophoric dysplasia (types I and II) caused by distinct mutations in fibroblast growth factor receptor 3. Nat Genet 9:321, 1995.

Baker KM et al: Long-term survival in typical thanatophoric dysplasia type I. Am J Med Genet 70:427, 1997.

Wilcox WR et al: Molecular, radiologic, and histologic correlations in thanatophoric dysplasia. Am J Med Genet 78:274, 1998.

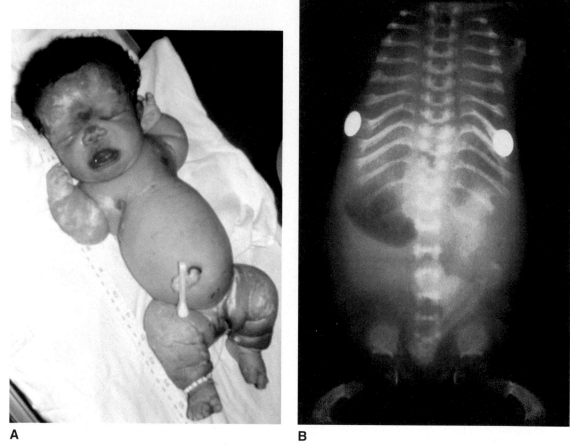

A   **B**

FIGURE 1. Thanatophoric dysplasia, type I. **A,** Note the large cranium with full forehead, low nasal bridge, short limbs, narrow thorax. **B,** Note the curved femurs and very flat vertebrae.

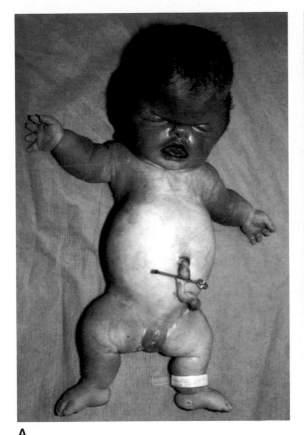

A

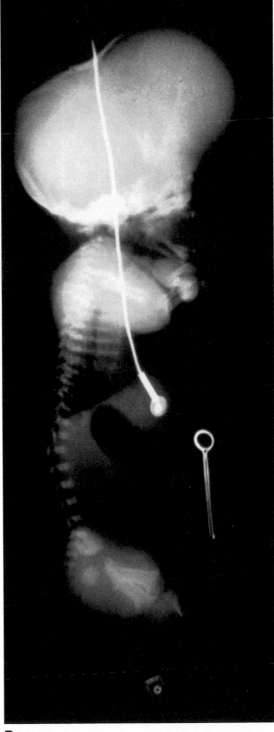

B

FIGURE 2. Thanatophoric dysplasia, type II. **A,** Note the cloverleaf skull in addition to the other features of type I. **B,** Note the straight femurs and taller vertebral bodies.

JEUNE THORACIC DYSTROPHY
(Asphyxiating Thoracic Dystrophy)

Small Thorax, Short Limbs, Hypoplastic Iliac Wings

First described by Jeune and colleagues in 1955, over 100 cases have now been reported.

ABNORMALITIES

Growth. Short stature.

Skeletal. Infancy: Short horizontal ribs with irregular costochondral junctions and small thoracic cage, hypoplastic iliac wings, horizontal acetabular roofs with spur-like projections at lower margins of sciatic notches, early ossification of capital femoral epiphysis. Childhood: Irregular epiphyses and metaphyses with relatively short limbs, especially the hands; ulnae and fibulae relatively short; cone-shaped epiphyses and early fusion between epiphyses and metaphyses of distal and middle phalanges.

Respiratory. Lung hypoplasia, presumably secondary to the small thoracic cage, is the major cause of death in early infancy.

Renal. Cystic tubular dysplasia or glomerular sclerosis.

Hepatic. Biliary dysgenesis with portal fibrosis and bile duct proliferation.

OCCASIONAL ABNORMALITIES.
Polydactyly, usually of hands and feet, notching of distal end of metacarpal and metatarsal bones; lacunar skull; direct hyperbilirubinemia with prolonged jaundice, pancreatic defects including fibrosis and cysts; Hirschsprung disease; retinal degeneration with predominantly cone-type cells remaining; lobation of the tongue and gingiva; cardiac failure; abdominal muscle dysplasia; situs inversus; mental retardation; Dandy-Walker complex.

NATURAL HISTORY.
Early death, usually the consequence of asphyxia with or without pneumonia, occurs frequently. For those who survive, progressive improvement in the relative growth of the thoracic cage occurs and there may be only slight to moderate shortness of stature. Chronic nephritis leading to renal failure is a serious potential feature of this disorder. Renal insufficiency may be evident by 2 years of age. Although infrequent, progressive hepatic dysfunction also occurs and may contribute to the relatively poor long-term prognosis for individuals with this disorder. Survival to the fourth decade has occurred.

ETIOLOGY.
This disorder has an autosomal recessive inheritance pattern. A locus has been mapped to 15q13. Prenatal diagnosis utilizing ultrasonography has been accomplished successfully at 18 weeks' gestation.

References

Jeune M, Beraud C, Carron R: Dystrophie thoracique asphyxiante de caractère familial. Arch Fr Pediatr 12:886, 1955.

Pirnar T, Neuhauser EBD: Asphyxiating thoracic dystrophy of the newborn. Am J Roentgenol Radium Ther Nucl Med 98:358, 1966.

Herdman RC, Langer LO: The thoracic asphyxiant dystrophy and renal disease. Am J Dis Child 116:192, 1968.

Langer LO: Thoracic-pelvic-phalangeal dystrophy. Radiology 91:447, 1968.

Friedman JM, Kaplan HG, Hall JG: The Jeune syndrome in an adult. Am J Med 59:857, 1975.

Okerklaid F et al: Asphyxiating thoracic dystrophy. Arch Dis Child 52:758, 1977.

Allen AW et al: Ocular findings in thoracic-pelvic-phalangeal dystrophy. Arch Ophthalmol 97:489, 1979.

Shah KJ: Renal lesions in Jeune's syndrome. Br J Radiol 53:432, 1980.

Elejalde BR, Mercedes de Elejalde M, Pansch D: Prenatal diagnosis of Jeune syndrome. Am J Med Genet 21:433, 1985.

Hudgins L et al: Early cirrhosis in survivors with Jeune thoracic dystrophy. J Pediatr 120:754, 1992.

Morgan NV et al: A locus for asphyxiating thoracic dystrophy, ATD, maps to chromosome 15q13. J Med Genet 40:431, 2003.

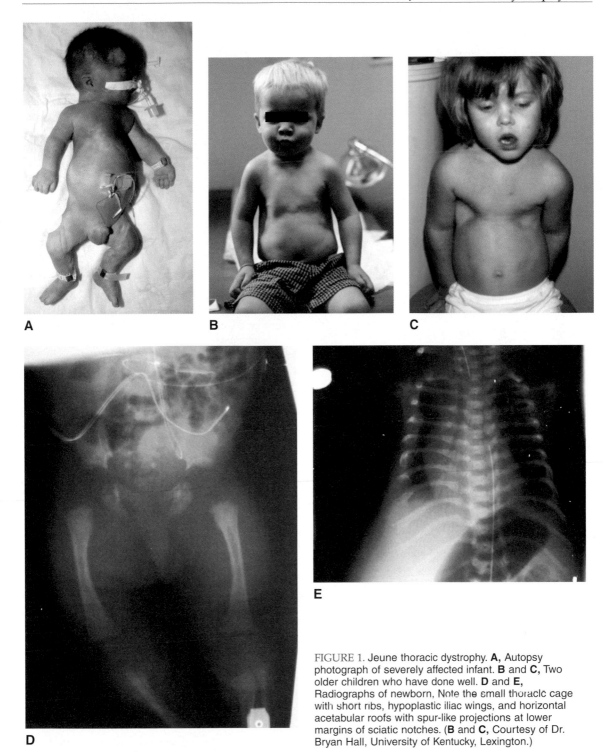

FIGURE 1. Jeune thoracic dystrophy. **A,** Autopsy photograph of severely affected infant. **B** and **C,** Two older children who have done well. **D** and **E,** Radiographs of newborn. Note the small thoracic cage with short ribs, hypoplastic iliac wings, and horizontal acetabular roofs with spur-like projections at lower margins of sciatic notches. (**B** and **C,** Courtesy of Dr. Bryan Hall, University of Kentucky, Lexington.)

CAMPOMELIC DYSPLASIA

Bowed Tibiae, Hypoplastic Scapulae, Flat Facies

Although reports of this condition appeared in the 1950s by Bound and colleagues and Bain and Barrett, it was not until the 1970s that the syndrome became more broadly recognized by Spranger and colleagues and Maroteaux and colleagues, who used the term *camptomelique*, meaning bent limb, to epitomize the disorder.

ABNORMALITIES

Growth. Prenatal onset of growth deficiency with retarded osseous maturation and large head; birth length, 35 to 49 cm; average occipitofrontal circumference is 37 cm.

Central Nervous System. Tendency toward having large brain with gross cellular disorganization, most evident in cerebral cortex, thalamus, and caudate nucleus; absence or hypoplasia of olfactory tract or bulbs; hydrocephalus.

Facies. Flat-appearing small face with high forehead, anterior frontal hair upsweep, large anterior fontanel, low nasal bridge, micrognathia, cleft palate, short palpebral fissures, and malformed or low-set ears.

Limbs. Anterior bowing of tibiae with skin dimpling over convex area, short fibulae, mild bowing of femora and tibiae, congenital hip dislocation, and talipes equinovarus.

Radiographic. Short and somewhat flat vertebrae, particularly cervical; hypoplastic scapulae, small thoracic cage with slender or decreased number of ribs, kyphoscoliosis, small iliac wings with relatively wide pelvic outlet; absent mineralization of sternum; lack of ossification of proximal tibial and distal femoral epiphysis and talus; short first metacarpal.

Tracheobronchial. Incomplete cartilaginous development with tracheobronchiomalacia.

Genitalia. Sex reversal or ambiguous genitalia in 75% of chromosomal males.

OCCASIONAL ABNORMALITIES.
Cardiac defects, renal anomalies, polyhydramnios, hypoplastic cochlea and semicircular canals, anomalies of incus and stapes, hearing loss.

NATURAL HISTORY.
The great majority of patients die in the neonatal period from respiratory insufficiency. Although there have been some survivors with normal intelligence, the vast majority have mild to moderate developmental delay. At birth the limbs are short with a trunk of normal length, but with development of the kyphoscoliosis, which is progressive, the trunk becomes short relative to the arms. Conductive hearing loss, myopia, dental caries, and recurrent apnea and respiratory problems are complications with advancing age.

ETIOLOGY.
This disorder has an autosomal dominant inheritance pattern, with most cases representing fresh gene mutations. The small number of recurrences are due to gonadal mosaicism. Mutations in the SOX9 gene located on 17q are responsible. Chromosomal rearrangements in this region also result in cases of campomelic dysplasia, which have in most cases been phenotypically milder. SOX9 is involved in both bone formation and control of testes development. It regulates the expression of COL2A1 and is a transcription factor essential for chondrocyte differentiation and formation of cartilage.

References

Bound JP, Finlay HVL, Rose FC: Congenital anterior angulation of the tibia. Arch Dis Child 27:179, 1952.

Bain AD, Barrett HS: Congenital bowing of the long bones: Report of a case. Arch Dis Child 34:516, 1959.

Spranger J, Langer LO, Maroteaux P: Increasing frequency of a syndrome of multiple osseous defects? Lancet 2:716, 1970.

Maroteaux P et al: Le syndrome camptomélique. Presse Med 79:1157, 1971.

Hoefnagel D et al: Campomelic dwarfism. Lancet 1:1068, 1972.

Schmickel RD, Heidelberger KP, Poznanski AK: The camptomelique syndrome. J Pediatr 82:299, 1973.

Hall BD, Spranger JW: Campomelic dysplasia. Am J Dis Child 134:285, 1980.

Houston CS et al: The camptomelic syndrome: Review, report of 17 cases, and follow-up on the currently 17 year old boy first reported by Maroteaux et al in 1971. Am J Med Genet 15:3, 1983.

Normann EK et al: Campomelic dysplasia—an underdiagnosed condition? Eur J Pediatr 152:331, 1993.

Foster JW et al: Campomelic dysplasia and autosomal sex reversal caused by mutations in an SRY-related gene. Nature 372:525, 1994.

Mansour S et al: A clinical and genetic study of campomelic dysplasia. J Med Genet 32:415, 1995.

Mansour S et al: The phenotype of survivors of campomelic dysplasia. J Med Genet 39:597, 2002.

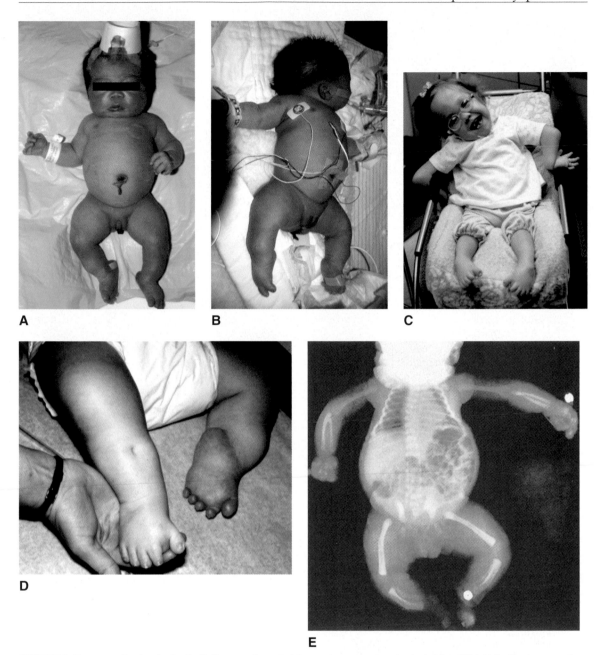

FIGURE 1. Campomelic dysplasia. **A–E,** Two newborn babies and a severely retarded older child. Note the low nasal bridge, micrognathia, small thorax, aberrant hand positioning, and bowed tibiae with dimples at the maximal point of bowing. Roentgenogram shows the slim, poorly developed bones and osseous immaturity (knee and foot). (**C** and **D,** Courtesy of Dr. Bryan Hall, University of Kentucky, Lexington; **E,** from Hoefnagel D et al: Lancet 1:1068, 1972, with permission. Copyrighted by The Lancet Ltd., 1972.)

ACHONDROPLASIA

Short Limbs, Low Nasal Bridge, Caudal Narrowing of Spinal Canal

The most common chondrodysplasia, true achondroplasia, occurs with a frequency of approximately 1 in 15,000.

ABNORMALITIES

Growth. Small stature, mean adult height in males is 131 ± 5.6 cm and in females is 124 ± 5.9 cm.

Craniofacial. Megalocephaly, small foramen magnum, short cranial base with early spheno-occipital closure, low nasal bridge with prominent forehead, mild midfacial hypoplasia with narrow nasal passages.

Skeletal. Small cuboid-shaped vertebral bodies with short pedicles and progressive narrowing of lumbar interpedicular distance; lumbar lordosis, mild thoracolumbar kyphosis with anterior beaking of first or second lumbar vertebra; small iliac wings with narrow greater sciatic notch; short tubular bones, especially humeri; metaphyseal flare with ball-and-socket arrangement of epiphysis to metaphysis; short trident hand, fingers being similar in length, with short proximal and midphalanges; short femoral neck; incomplete extension of elbow.

Other. Mild hypotonia; early motor progress is often slow, although eventual intelligence is usually normal; relative glucose intolerance evident with an oral glucose tolerance test.

OCCASIONAL ABNORMALITIES.

Hydrocephalus, spinal cord or root compression; pulmonary hypertension.

NATURAL HISTORY.

Macrocephaly may represent mild hydrocephaly relating to a small foramen magnum. Therefore, ultrasound studies of the brain should be seriously considered if the fontanel size is particularly large, the occipito-frontal circumference increases too rapidly, or any symptoms of hydrocephalus develop. Respiratory problems secondary to a small chest, upper airway obstruction, and sleep-disordered breathing are common. Although a relatively small foramen magnum is seen in all children with achondroplasia, symptoms related to cord compression at the cervicomedullary junction occur only rarely. For example, sudden death probably caused by brainstem or upper cervical cord compression, a threat particularly during the first year of life, occurs in less than 3%. Significant controversy exists as to when and if decompressive neurosurgery should be performed. It is important to recognize that evaluation of affected children with symptoms relating to cervical cord compression should be performed by individuals experienced with and aware of the natural history of achondroplasia. Computed tomography dimensions for the foramen magnum of children with achondroplasia have been established by Hecht and colleagues. The physician should be alert to detect any neurologic complications caused by bone or disk compression. Osteoarthritis is not a usual feature in the adult. Osteotomies for severe bowlegs are usually deferred until full growth has occurred. By discouraging the sitting position or other positions that cause the trunk to curve anteriorly until an age when good trunk strength has developed, a permanent gibbus or kyphosis which is due to anterior wedging of the first two lumbar vertebrae can be prevented as well as obviating many of the problems with spinal stenosis and spinal cord compression that are so debilitating to adults with this condition. Exercises may also be used in an attempt to flatten the lumbosacral curve. Relative overgrowth of the fibula may accentuate bowing and require early stapling. Short eustachian tubes may lead to middle ear infection and conductive hearing loss. Tympanic membrane tubes may be indicated. Verbal comprehension is frequently impaired. Sleep-related respiratory disturbances, primarily hypoxemia, is common. The mandibular teeth may become crowded, possibly requiring removal of one or more. Todorov and colleagues developed a screening test that establishes normal milestones for children with achondroplasia up to 2 years of age. A history of polyhydramnios seems to be a predictor of more severe growth impairment. There is a tendency toward late childhood obesity, and females are more prone to have menorrhagia, fibroids, and large breasts.

ETIOLOGY. This disorder has an autosomal dominant inheritance pattern; approximately 90% of the cases represent a fresh gene mutation. Older paternal age has been a contributing factor in these cases. Because of gonadal mosaicism, there is a 0.2% recurrence risk for siblings of achondroplastic children with unaffected parents. Mutations in the gene encoding fibroblast growth factor receptor 3 (FGFR3) located at 4p16.3 have been documented in all cases reported to date. Interestingly, virtually all cases demonstrate the same single base pair substitution, possibly accounting for the consistency of the phenotype seen in this disorder.

References

Maroteaux P, Lamy M: Achondroplasia in man and animals. Clin Orthop 33:91, 1964.

Caffey J: Pediatric X-Ray Diagnosis, 5th ed. Chicago: Year Book Medical Publishers, 1967.

Cohen ME, Rosenthal AD, Matson DD: Neurological abnormalities in achondroplastic children. J Pediatr 71:367, 1967.

Nelson MA: Spinal stenosis in achondroplasia. Proc R Soc Med 65:1028, 1972.

Horton WA et al: Standard growth curves for achondroplasia. J Pediatr 93:435, 1978.

Oberklaid F et al: Achondroplasia and hypochondroplasia. J Med Genet 16:140, 1979.

Todorov AB et al: Developmental screening tests in achondroplastic children. Am J Med Genet 9:19, 1981.

Hall JG et al: Letter to the editor. Head growth in achondroplasia: Use of ultrasound studies. Am J Med Genet 13:105, 1982.

Stokes DC et al: Respiratory complications of achondroplasia. J Pediatr 102:534, 1983.

Hecht JT et al: Computerized tomography of the foramen magnum: Achondroplastic values compared to normal standards. Am J Med Genet 20:355, 1985.

Reid CS et al: Cervicomedullary compression in young patients with achondroplasia: Value of comprehensive neurologic and respiratory evaluation. J Pediatr 110:522, 1987.

Hall JG: Kyphosis in achondroplasia: Probably preventable. J Pediatr 112:166, 1988.

Brinkman G et al: Cognitive skills in achondroplasia. Am J Med Genet 47:800, 1993.

Shiang R et al: Mutations in the transmembrane domain of FGFR3 causes the most common genetic form of dwarfism, achondroplasia. Cell 78:335, 1994.

Committee on Genetics: Health supervision for children with achondroplasia. Pediatrics 95:443, 1995.

Pauli RM et al: Prospective assessment of risk for cervicomedullary junction compression in infants with achondroplasia. Am J Hum Genet 56:732, 1995.

Rimoin DL: Invited editorial. Cervicomedullary junction compression in infants with achondroplasia: When to perform neurosurgical decompression. Am J Hum Genet 56:824, 1995.

Hunter AGW et al: Medical complications of achondroplasia: A multicentre patient review. J Med Genet 35:705, 1998.

Mettler G, Fraser FC: Recurrence risk for sibs of children with "sporadic" achondroplasia. Am J Med Genet 90:250, 2000.

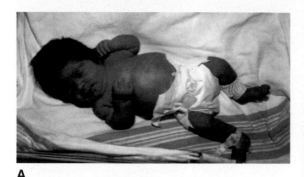

A

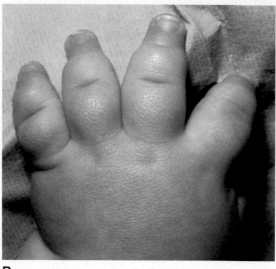

B

FIGURE 1. Achondroplasia. **A,** Newborn infant with achondroplasia, showing macrocephaly, low nasal bridge, relatively small thoracic cage, shortness of humeri and femurs (rhizomelia). (Courtesy of Dr. Lynne M. Bird, Children's Hospital, San Diego.) **B,** "Trident" position of the open, small hand.

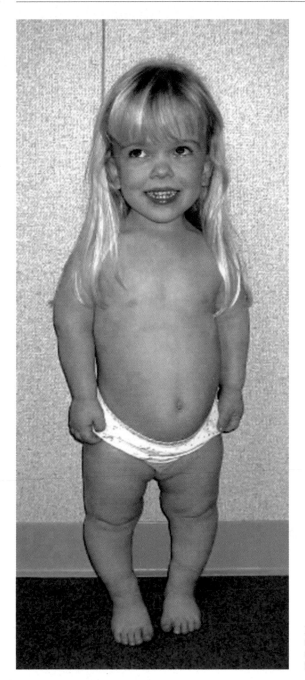

FIGURE 2. Photograph of a 1-year-old girl showing relative macrocephaly, small thoracic cage, and rhizomelic shortening. (Courtesy of Dr. Stephen Braddock, University of Missouri, Columbia.)

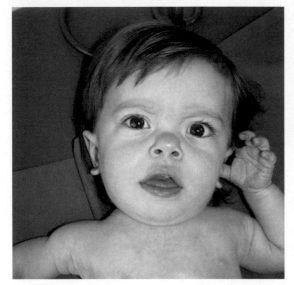

A

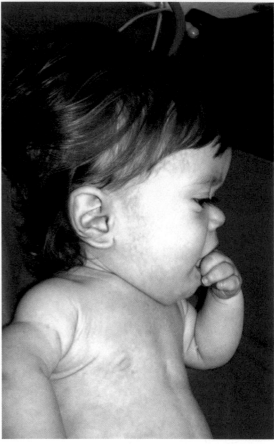

B

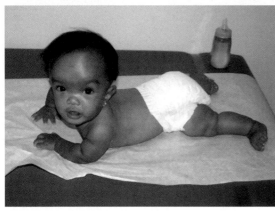

C

FIGURE 3. **A–C,** Two affected 6-month-old children. Note low nasal bridge, relative macrocephaly with prominent forehead and midface hypoplasia. (Courtesy of Dr. Lynne M. Bird, Children's Hospital, San Diego.)

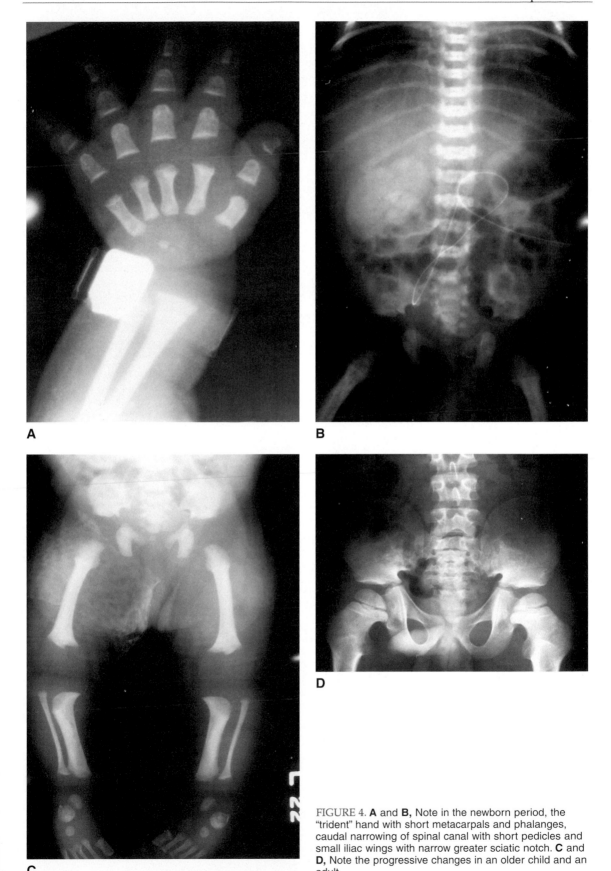

FIGURE 4. **A** and **B,** Note in the newborn period, the "trident" hand with short metacarpals and phalanges, caudal narrowing of spinal canal with short pedicles and small iliac wings with narrow greater sciatic notch. **C** and **D,** Note the progressive changes in an older child and an adult.

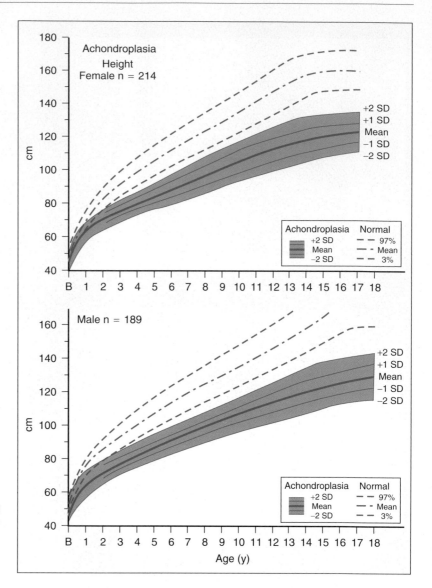

FIGURE 5. Note that approximately one half of the newborn babies with achondroplasia are within normal limits for length at birth, but there is a progressive deceleration of growth rate beginning in infancy. (From Horton WA et al: J Pediatr 93:435, 1978, with permission.)

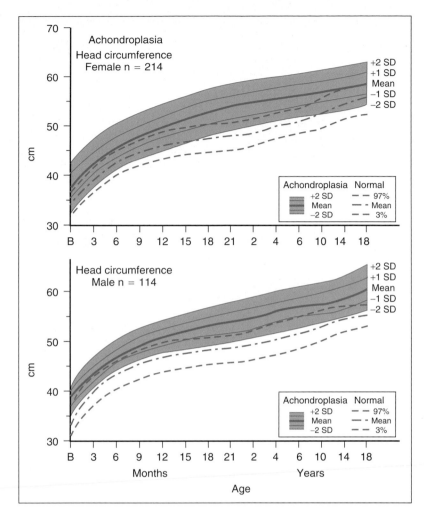

FIGURE 6. Macrocephaly, predominantly caused by a large brain, is a usual feature of individuals with achondroplasia. (From Horton WA et al: J Pediatr 93:435, 1978, with permission.)

HYPOCHONDROPLASIA

Short Limbs, Caudal Narrowing of Spine, Near-Normal Craniofacies

Although the features of this disorder were described by Ravenna in 1913, and its designation as hypochondroplasia and mode of inheritance were set forth in 1924, the majority of cases have been misdiagnosed as achondroplasia until recently.

Hypochondroplasia has an incidence of approxiamtely one twelfth that of achondroplasia and can be distinguished from it by the relative lack of craniofacial involvement and milder features in the hands and spine.

ABNORMALITIES

Growth. Small stature, usually of postnatal onset; mean birth length, 47.7 cm; mean birth weight, 2.9 kg; macrocephaly.

Limbs. Relatively short without rhizomelic, mesomelic, or acromelic predominance; short tubular bones with mild metaphyseal flare; short, broad femoral necks; long distal fibulae, short distal ulnae, and long ulnar styloids; brachydactyly; bowing of legs; stubby hands and feet; mild limitation in elbow extension and supination.

Spine. Anteroposterior shortening of lumbar pedicles on lateral view; spinal canal narrowing or unchanged caudally, with or without lumbar lordosis.

Pelvis. Squared and short ilia.

OCCASIONAL ABNORMALITIES.

Mental deficiency, bilateral dysgenesis of the medial temporal lobe structures, brachycephaly with short base of skull, mild frontal bossing, esotropia, cataract, ptosis, postaxial polydactyly of feet, high vertebrae, flat vertebrae.

NATURAL HISTORY. Slow growth, if not evident by birth, is usually obvious by 3 years of age. Final height attainment in adults ranged from 46.5 to 60 inches. Outward bowing of the lower limbs and genu varum may become pronounced with weight-bearing. Although this may improve in childhood, the condition may merit surgical straightening. The relatively long fibulae can result in inversion of the feet. Exercise may provoke mild aching in the knees, ankles, or elbows during childhood, and such discomfort is usually worse and may include the low back in the adult. Cesarean section is often required for delivery in pregnant women with this disorder. Mental deficiency, a rare feature in achondroplasia, was noted in four of the 13 cases reported by Walker and colleagues, with IQs ranging from 50 to 80, and in 9% of the patients reported by Hall and Spranger.

ETIOLOGY. This disorder has an autosomal dominant inheritance pattern. Older paternal age has been documented in presumed fresh mutation cases. Approximately 50% of affected patients carry an N540K mutation in the fibroblast growth factor receptor 3 (FGFR3) gene located at 4p16.3.

COMMENT. In contrast to achondroplasia, hypochondroplasia is clinically and genetically heterogeneous. Patients with the N540K mutation have a more severe phenotype associated with disproportionate short stature, macrocephaly, and with radiologic evidence of unchanged/narrow interpedicular distance and fibula longer than tibia. In contrast, patients with hypochondroplasia unlinked to chromosome 4p16.3, have milder radiologic anomalies with normal hand and long bones, and no metaphyseal flaring.

References

Ravenna F: Achondroplasie et chondrohypoplasie: Contribution clinique. N Iconog Salpêtrière 26:157, 1913.

Léri A, Linossier (Mlle): Hypochondroplasia héréditaire. Bull Mem Soc Med Hop (Paris) 48:1780, 1924.

Beals RK: Hypochondroplasia: A report of five kindred. J Bone Joint Surg [Am] 51:728, 1969.

Walker BA et al: Hypochondroplasia. Am J Dis Child 122:95, 1971.

Hall BD, Spranger J: Hypochondroplasia: Clinical and radiological aspects in 39 cases. Radiology 133:95, 1979.

Le Merrer M et al: A gene for achondroplasia-hypochondroplasia maps to chromosome 4p. Nat Genet 6:318, 1994.

Bellus GA et al: A recurrent mutation in the tyrosine kinase domain of fibroblast growth factor receptor 3 causes hypochondroplasia. Nat Genet 10:357, 1995.

Prinster C et al: Diagnosis of hypochondroplasia: The role of radiological interpretation. Pediatr Radiol 31:203, 2001.

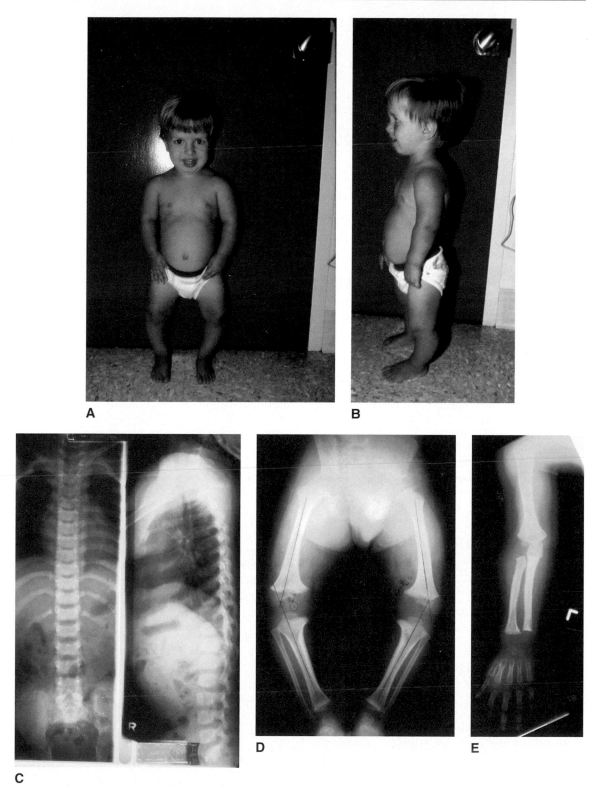

FIGURE 1. Hypochondroplasia. **A** and **B,** A 2½-year-old boy showing short stature, short arms with mild limitation in elbow extension, bowed legs, relative macrocephaly. **C–E,** Radiographs of the same child at 2½ years of age. Note the anterior-posterior shortening of lumbar pedicles on lateral view and mild degree of caudal narrowing of the spinal canal (**C**) and the relatively short tubular bones with mild metaphyseal flare, short, broad femoral necks, long distal fibula, and short distal ulna (**D** and **E**). (**A–E,** Courtesy of Dr. Marilyn C. Jones, Children's Hospital, San Diego.)

PSEUDOACHONDROPLASIA
(Pseudoachondroplastic
Spondyloepiphyseal Dysplasia)

Small Irregular Epiphyses, Irregular Mushroomed Metaphyses, Flattening or Anterior Beaking of Vertebrae, Normal Craniofacial Appearance

Maroteaux and Lamy described three individuals with this pattern of altered bone morphogenesis in 1959. Numerous cases have been published.

ABNORMALITIES

Growth. Postnatal onset of short-limbed growth deficiency that becomes obvious between 18 months and 2 years; adult stature, 82 to 130 cm.

Craniofacies. Normal head size and face.

Limbs. Disproportionately short; hypermobility of major joints except elbows leading to genu varum, valgum, and recurvatum; ulnar deviation of hands; short fingers that are hypermobile.

Radiographs. Short long bones with wide metaphyses; epiphyses are small, irregular, or "fragmented," especially the capital femoral epiphyses; vertebral abnormalities consist of variable degrees of flattening with biconvex end plates and a central anterior bony protrusion from the anterior surface of the body; there is normal widening of the interpedicular distance from upper to lower lumbar spine; odontoid aplasia or hypoplasia; short sacral notches; ribs tend to be spatulate; terminal phalanges small.

Other. Lumbar lordosis, kyphosis, scoliosis.

NATURAL HISTORY. The patients have been described as "normal" at birth, with small size, short arms, and waddling gait becoming evident between 6 months and 4 years of age. Bowed lower extremities with waddling gait and scoliosis are the principal orthopedic problems, and there may be some limitation in joint motility. Intelligence is normal. Odontoid hypoplasia in association with hypermobility can result in increased motion of C1 on C2, leading to cord damage. Although the vertebral changes resolve with age, the epiphyseal changes of the long bones become more severe leading to progressive degeneration and severe osteoarthritis. About one-third to one-half require total hip replacement in their midthirties. Neurologic complications, most commonly numbness or tingling of the limbs, occur in 28%. A mild and severe form have been described.

ETIOLOGY. This disorder has an autosomal dominant inheritance pattern. Mutations in the cartilage oligomeric matrix protein gene (COMP), which has been localized to chromosome 19p13.1, lead to both the mild and severe forms of this disorder. Most of the cases have been sporadic and presumably represent fresh mutations. Based on what may well be an increased risk of gonadal mosaicism in this disorder, it has been estimated that unaffected parents who have had one affected child have a recurrence risk in the range of 4%.

COMMENT. A mutation in the COMP gene also has been identified in multiple epiphyseal dysplasia. It has been suggested that these two disorders comprise a clinical spectrum with mild multiple epiphyseal dysplasia at one end and pseudoachondroplasia at the other.

References

Maroteaux P, Lamy M: Les formes pseudoachondroplastiques des dysplasies spondyloépiphysaires. Presse Med 67:383, 1959.

Ford N, Silverman FN, Kozlowski K: Spondyloepiphyseal dysplasia (pseudoachondroplastic type). Am J Roentgenol Radium Ther Nucl Med 86:462, 1961.

Hall JG et al: Gonadal mosaicism in pseudoachondroplasia. Am J Med Genet 28:143, 1987.

Briggs MD et al: Genetic linkage of mild pseudoachondroplasia (PSACH) to markers in the pericentromeric region of chromosome 19. Genomics 18:656, 1993.

Hecht JT et al: Linkage of typical pseudoachondroplasia to chromosome 19. Genomics 18:661, 1993.

Langer LO et al: Patients with double heterozygosity for achondroplasia and pseudoachondroplasia, with comments on these conditions and the relationship between pseudoachondroplasia and multiple epiphyseal dysplasia, Fairbank type. Am J Med Genet 47:772, 1993.

Hecht JL et al: Mutations in exon 17B of cartilage oligomeric matrix protein (COMP) cause pseudoachondroplasia. Nat Genet 10:325, 1995.

McKeand J et al: Natural history study of pseudoachondroplasia. Am J Med Genet 63:406, 1996.

Mabuchi A et al: Novel types of COMP mutations and genotype-phenotype association in pseudoachondroplasia and multiple epiphyseal dysplasia. Hum Genet 112:84, 2003.

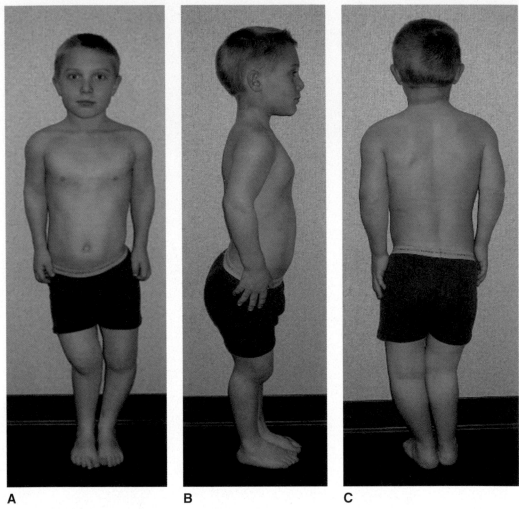

A   B   C

FIGURE 1. Pseudoachondroplasia. **A–C,** A boy with disproportionately short limbs, genu varus and valgus, and scoliosis. (Courtesy of Dr. Stephen Braddock, University of Missouri, Columbia.) *Continued*

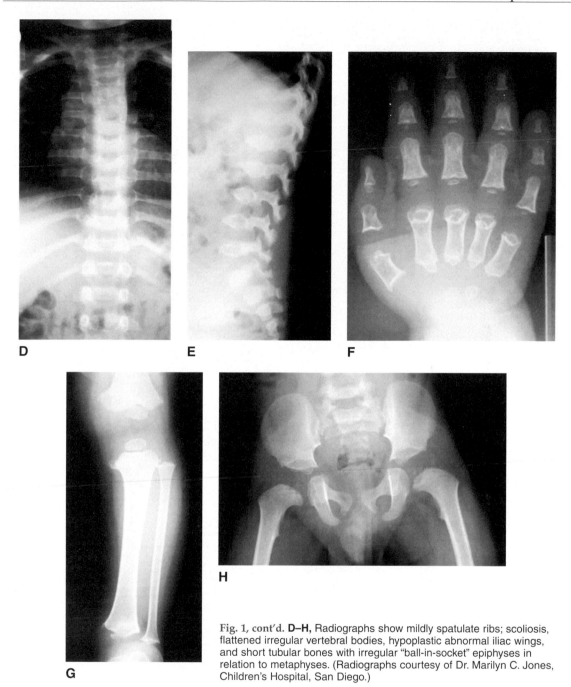

Fig. 1, cont'd. D–H, Radiographs show mildly spatulate ribs; scoliosis, flattened irregular vertebral bodies, hypoplastic abnormal iliac wings, and short tubular bones with irregular "ball-in-socket" epiphyses in relation to metaphyses. (Radiographs courtesy of Dr. Marilyn C. Jones, Children's Hospital, San Diego.)

ACROMESOMELIC DYSPLASIA
(ACROMESOMELIC DWARFISM)

Short Distal Limbs, Frontal Prominence, Low Thoracic Kyphosis

Maroteaux and colleagues recognized this disorder in 1971, and Langer and colleagues summarized the manifestations in 19 patients in 1977. More than 40 cases have been reported.

ABNORMALITIES

Craniofacial. Disproportionately large head with relative frontal prominence, with or without relatively short nose.

Limbs. Short limbs with short hands and feet, bowed forearms that are relatively shorter than upper arms, limited elbow extension, short fingers and toes with short but not dysplastic nails, redundant skin develops over fingers in childhood.

Spine. Development of lower thoracic kyphosis.

Radiographs. Metacarpals and phalanges become increasingly shorter during the first year; middle and proximal phalanges are broad; cone-shaped epiphyses develop; shortening of humerus, radius, and ulna progresses during first year; bowed radius; vertebral bodies are oval shaped in infancy, but with advancing age the lumbar vertebrae become wedge-shaped with the posterior aspect of the bodies shorter than the anterior; by 24 months, a central protrusion of bone develops anteriorly; superiorly curved clavicles that appear located high; flared metaphyses of long tubular bones; hypoplasia of basilar portion of ilia and irregular ossification of lateral superior acetabular region in childhood.

OCCASIONAL ABNORMALITIES.
Relatively large great toe, corneal clouding, hydrocephalus, mild mental retardation.

NATURAL HISTORY.
Birth weight may be normal, and the linear growth deficiency becomes more evident during the first year. Lower thoracic kyphosis, increased lumbar lordosis, and prominent buttocks are common. Most joints tend to be relatively lax. There may be some lag in gross motor performance because of the relatively large head and short limbs but intelligence is normal. Final height in nine adults ranged from 38 to 49 inches.

ETIOLOGY.
This disorder has an autosomal recessive inheritance pattern. The gene for this disorder has been mapped to chromosome 9p13-q12.

References
Maroteaux P, Martinelli B, Campailla E: Le nanisme acromesomelique. Presse Med 79:1838, 1971.
Langer LO et al: Acromesomelic dwarfism: Manifestations in childhood. Am J Med Genet 1:87, 1977.
Langer LO, Garrett RT: Acromesomelic dysplasia. Radiology 137:349, 1980.
Fernandez del Moral R et al: Report of a case: Acromesomelic dysplasia. Radiologic, clinical and pathological study. Am J Med Genet 33:415, 1989.
Kant SG et al: Acromesomelic dysplasia, Maroteaux type, maps to human chromosome 9. J Med Genet 63:155, 1998.

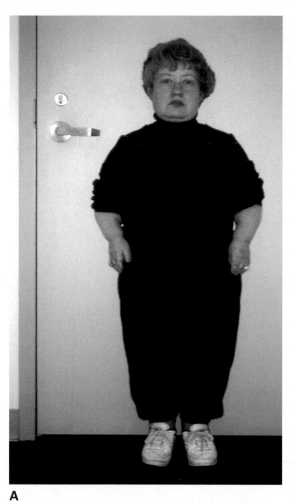

A

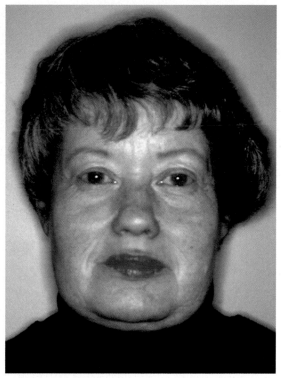

B

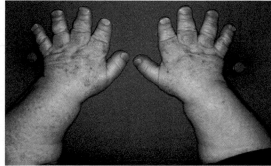

D

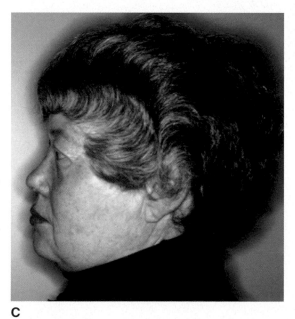

C

FIGURE 1. **A–D,** A 57-year-old woman with acromesomelic dysplasia. Note the relative macrocephaly with frontal prominence without short nose and the short limbs with short hands, particularly the fingers.

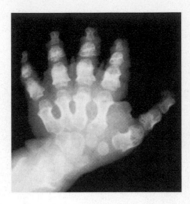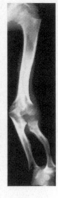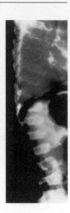

FIGURE 2. Characteristic radiologic findings. (From Langer LO et al: Am J Med Genet 1:87, 1977. Copyright © 1977. Reprinted with permission of Wiley-Liss, Inc., a subsidiary of John Wiley & Sons, Inc.)

SPONDYLOEPIPHYSEAL DYSPLASIA CONGENITA

Short Trunk, Lag in Epiphyseal Mineralization, Myopia

Spranger and Wiedemann established this disorder in 1966 when they reported six new cases and summarized 14 from the literature. Numerous additional cases have been reported subsequently.

ABNORMALITIES

Onset at birth.

Growth. Prenatal onset of growth deficiency; final height, 37 to 52 inches.

Facies. Variable flat facies, malar hypoplasia, cleft palate.

Eyes. Myopia, retinal detachment (50%).

Spine. Short, including neck with ovoid flattened vertebrae with narrow intervertebral disk spaces, odontoid hypoplasia, kyphoscoliosis, lumbar lordosis.

Chest. Barrel chest with pectus carinatum.

Limbs. Lag in mineralization of epiphyses, which tend to be flat, with no os pubis, talus, calcaneus, or knee centers mineralized at birth; coxa vara; diminished joint mobility at elbows, knees, and hips; conductive hearing loss.

Muscles. Weakness, easy fatigability, hypoplasia of abdominal muscles.

OCCASIONAL ABNORMALITIES.

Talipes equinovarus, dislocation of hip.

NATURAL HISTORY. The hypotonic weakness and orthopedic situation contribute to a late onset of walking, usually with a waddling gait. Myopia should be suspected, and frequent ophthalmologic evaluation is merited to guard against retinal detachment. Morning stiffness may be a feature; however, there is usually no undue joint pain.

ETIOLOGY. This disorder has an autosomal dominant inheritance pattern. A variety of alterations in the COL2A1 gene, which codes for type II collagen lead to spondyloepiphyseal dysplasia congenita. Instances of affected siblings born to unaffected parents is most likely due to gonadal mosaicism.

References

Spranger J, Wiedemann HR: Dysplasia spondyloepiphysaria congenita. Helv Paediatr Acta 21:598, 1966.

Spranger J, Langer LO: Spondyloepiphyseal dysplasia congenita. Radiology 94:313, 1970.

Harrod MJE et al: Genetic heterogeneity in spondyloepiphyseal dysplasia congenita. Am J Med Genet 18:311, 1984.

Spranger J et al: The type II collagenopathies: A spectrum of chondrodysplasias. Eur J Pediatr 153:56, 1994.

Dahiya R et al: Spondyloepiphyseal dysplasia congenita associated with conductive hearing loss. Ear Nose Throat J 79:178, 2000.

KNIEST DYSPLASIA

Flat Facies, Thick Joints, Platyspondyly

Though Kniest described this disorder in 1952, it has been more generally recognized only in recent years.

ABNORMALITIES

Growth. Disproportionate short stature with short, barrel-shaped chest.

Craniofacies. Flat facies with prominent eyes, low nasal bridge, myopia that may progress to retinal detachment, vitreoretinal degeneration, cleft palate with frequent ear infections; the head, which is of normal size, is relatively large with respect to height.

Limbs. Enlarged joints with limited joint mobility and variable pain and stiffness; short limbs, often with bowing; some irregularity of epiphyses with late ossification of femoral heads; flexion contractures in hips; inability to form fist secondary to bony enlargements and soft tissue swelling at interphalangeal joints.

Other. Lumbar kyphoscoliosis; inguinal and umbilical hernias, small pelvis, short clavicles; hearing loss; tracheomalacia; cataracts; lens dislocation.

Radiographs. Dumbbell-shaped femurs, hypoplastic pelvic bones, platyspondyly, and vertical clefts of vertebrae in newborn period; by age 3, pelvis becomes "dessert-cup shaped," ends of bones reveal irregular epiphyses, diffuse osteoporosis, and cloud-like radiodensities on both sides of epiphyseal plates; thereafter, platyspondyly remains, intervertebral disk space is narrow, odontoid is large and wide; flared metaphyses; large epiphyses.

Other. Lumbar kyphoscoliosis, inguinal and umbilical hernias, small pelvis, short clavicles, hearing loss, tracheomalacia, cataracts, lens dislocation, glaucoma.

NATURAL HISTORY. Short extremities with stiff joints in neonatal period; respiratory distress associated with tracheomalacia sometimes occurs in infancy; marked lumbar lordosis and kyphoscoliosis lead to disproportionate shortening of trunk in childhood; late walking because of orthopedic disability with contracted hips; limitation of joint motion with pain, stiffness, and flexion contractures of major joints develops; chronic otitis media related to cleft palate; normal intelligence despite delayed motor milestones and speech; final height, 106 to 145 cm; frequent ophthalmologic evaluations are indicated in order to prevent retinal detachment.

ETIOLOGY. This disorder has an autosomal dominant inheritance pattern. Most cases represent a fresh gene mutation. This disorder represents one of a spectrum of chondrodysplasias due to defects in the gene for type II collagen, COL2A1. Others include type II achondrogenesis-hypochondrogenesis, spondyloepiphyseal dysplasia congenita, and Stickler syndrome.

COMMENT. The original patient described by Wilhelm Kniest is now 50 years of age, has short stature, restricted joint mobility, and blindness, but she is mentally alert and leads an active life.

References

Kniest W: Zur Abgrenzung der Dysostosis enchondralis von der Chondrodystrophie. Z Kinderheilkd 70:633, 1952.

Kim HJ et al: Kniest syndrome with dominant inheritance and mucopolysacchariduria. Am J Hum Genet 77:755, 1975.

Rimoin DL et al: Metatropic dwarfism, the Kniest syndrome and the pseudoachondroplastic dysplasias. Clin Orthop 114:70, 1976.

Maumenee IH, Traboulsi EI: The ocular findings in Kniest dysplasia. Am J Ophthalmol 100:155, 1985.

Spranger J et al: The type II collagenopathies: A spectrum of chondrodysplasias. Eur J Pediatr 153:56, 1994.

Cole WG: Abnormal skeletal growth in Kniest dysplasia caused by type II collagen mutations. Clin Orthop 341:162, 1997.

Spranger J et al: Kniest dysplasia: Dr. W. Kniest, his patient, the molecular defect. Am J Med Genet 69:79, 1997.

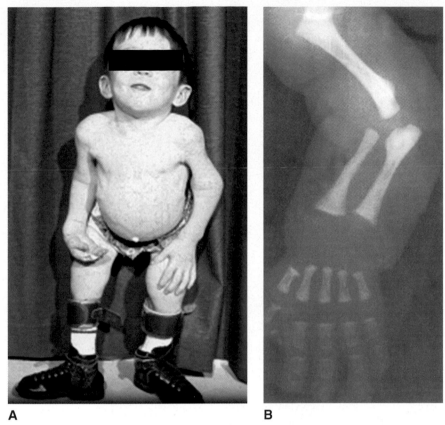

A   **B**

FIGURE 1. **A** and **B,** A 3-year-old boy with Kniest dysplasia. (Courtesy of Dr. D. L. Rimoin, Cedars-Sinai Medical Center, Los Angeles.)

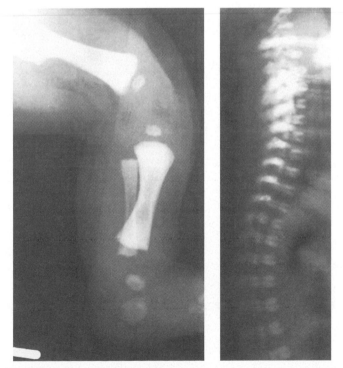

FIGURE 2. Radiographs show altered limb morphogenesis and platyspondyly with coronal clefting. (Courtesy of Dr. J. H. Graham, Cedars-Sinai Medical Center, Los Angeles.)

411

DYGGVE-MELCHIOR-CLAUSEN SYNDROME

Initially described in 1962 by Dyggve and colleagues, the clinical and radiographic features were set forth more completely in 1975 by Spranger and colleagues.

ABNORMALITIES

Growth. Deficiency of postnatal onset, with short trunk dwarfism becoming evident before 18 months.

Performance. Mental deficiency.

Craniofacies. Microcephaly, coarse facies, prognathism, facial bones large for cranium.

Spine. Platyspondyly, vertebral bodies show double-humped appearance with central constriction, short neck, odontoid hypoplasia, scoliosis, kyphosis, lordosis.

Thorax. Sternal protrusion, barrel chest.

Pelvis. Small ilia with irregularly calcified (lace-like) iliac crests in childhood developing into a marginal irregularity in adulthood, lateral displacement of capital femoral epiphyses, sloping, dysplastic acetabulae, pubic ramus is wide.

Limbs. Restricted joint mobility; waddling gait; dislocated hips; genu valga and vera; rhizomelic limb shortening with irregular metaphyses and epiphyses; malformed olecranons and radial heads; broad hands and feet; short metacarpals, particularly the first, and short notched phalanges; cone-shaped epiphyses; small carpals.

NATURAL HISTORY. Manifestations

become evident between 1 and 18 months and are progressive. Feeding problems frequently occur during infancy. Restriction of joint mobility primarily affects the elbows, hips, and knees. Spinal cord compression due to atlantoaxial instability is a preventable complication. The degree of mental retardation has varied from moderate to severe.

Three known adults measured 128 cm, 127 cm, and 119 cm, respectively.

ETIOLOGY. This disorder has an autosomal recessive inheritance pattern. Mutations in a gene referred to as Dymeclin located at chromosome 18q21.1 are responsible. This gene is expressed in brain, cartilage, and bone, the three tissues most affected by Dyggve-Melchior-Clausen syndrome (DMC).

COMMENT. Smith-McCort dysplasia (SMC) has identical radiographic findings, but is associated with normal intelligence. Mutations in Dymeclin are also responsible for SMC indicating that DMC and SMC are allelic. Of particular interest, lower levels of the Dymeclin protein product are found in DMC. This suggests that decreased levels initially lead to abnormalities of cartilage and bone, but once the levels of functional protein drop below a certain threshold, the brain becomes affected.

References

Dyggve HV, Melchior JC, Clausen J: Morquio-Ullrich's disease: An inborn error of metabolism? Arch Dis Child 37:525, 1962.

Spranger J, Maroteaux P, Der Kaloustian VM: The Dyggve-Melchior-Clausen syndrome. Radiology 114:415, 1975.

Naffah J: The Dyggve-Melchior-Clausen syndrome. Am J Hum Genet 28:607, 1976.

Spranger J, Bierbaum B, Herrmann J: Heterogeneity of Dyggve-Melchior-Clausen dwarfism. Hum Genet 33:279, 1976.

Bonafede RP, Beighton P: The Dyggve-Melchior-Clausen syndrome in adult siblings. Clin Genet 14:24, 1978.

Beighton P: Dyggve-Melchior-Clausen syndrome. J Med Genet 27:512, 1990.

Cohn DH et al: Mental retardation and abnormal skeletal development (Dyggve-Melchoir-Clausen) due to mutations in a novel evolutionary conserved gene. Am J Hum Genet 72:419, 2003.

Ghouzzi VE et al: Mutations in a novel gene Dymeclin (FLJ20071) are responsible for Dyggve-Melchior-Clausen syndrome. Mol Genet 12:357, 2003.

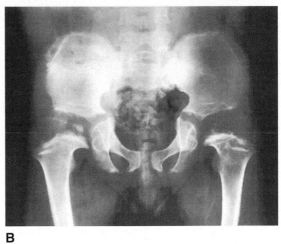

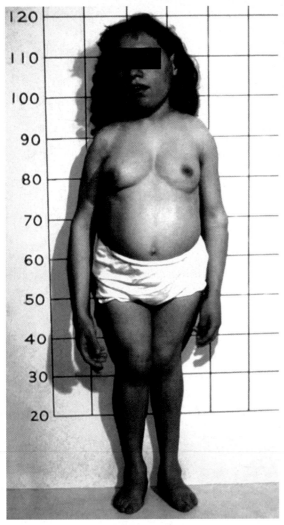

FIGURE 1. **A** and **B,** Adolescent with Dyggve-Melchior-Clausen syndrome. Note the irregularly calcified iliac crests. (Courtesy of Dr. R. Lachman, Harbor-UCLA Medical Center, and Dr. D. L. Rimoin, Cedars-Sinai Medical Center, Los Angeles.)

SPONDYLOMETAPHYSEAL DYSPLASIA, KOZLOWSKI TYPE
(KOZLOWSKI SPONDYLOMETAPHYSEAL CHONDRODYSPLASIA)

Early-Childhood-Onset Short Spine, Irregular Metaphyses, Pectus Carinatum

Kozlowski and colleagues established this disorder in 1967. Spondylometaphyseal dysplasia comprises a group of disorders in which the spine and metaphyses of the tubular bones are affected. At least seven types have been classified based on minor radiographic differences and mode of transmission. The Kozlowski type is the most well known and the most common.

ABNORMALITIES

Growth. Growth deficiency, especially of trunk, with onset from 1 to 4 years of age; adult height, 4 feet 3 inches to 5 feet.

Spine. Short neck and trunk with dorsal kyphosis; generalized platyspondyly with anterior narrowing in thoracolumbar region on lateral roentgenograms; on anteroposterior view, vertebral bodies extend more laterally to pedicles producing an "open-staircase" appearance; odontoid hypoplasia.

Thorax. Pectus carinatum.

Pelvis. Square, short iliac wings; flat, irregular acetabula.

Limbs. Irregular rachitic-like metaphyses, especially the proximal femur with very short femoral necks; short, stocky hands; hypo-plastic carpal bones with late ossification (delayed bone age).

NATURAL HISTORY. Affected patients are usually normal at birth. A noticeably waddling gait with limitation of joint mobility becomes apparent at 15 to 20 months and is often the first sign of the disorder. Degenerative joint changes leading to discomfort occur at a relatively early age. The elbows are often more affected than the knees. Final adult height is 130 to 150 cm.

ETIOLOGY. This disorder has an autosomal dominant inheritance pattern, with most cases representing fresh mutation.

References

Kozlowski K, Maroteaux P, Spranger J: La dysostose spondylo-métaphysaire. Presse Med 75:2769, 1967.

Riggs W Jr, Summitt RL: Spondylometaphyseal dysplasia (Kozlowski): Report of affected mother and son. Radiology 101:375, 1971.

Le Quesne GW, Kozlowski K: Spondylometaphyseal dysplasia. Br J Radiol 46:685, 1973.

Kozlowski K et al: Spondylo-metaphyseal dysplasia. (Report of 7 cases and essay of classification.) In Papadatos CJ, Bartsocas CS (eds): Skeletal Dysplasias. New York: Alan R. Liss, 1982, pp 89–101.

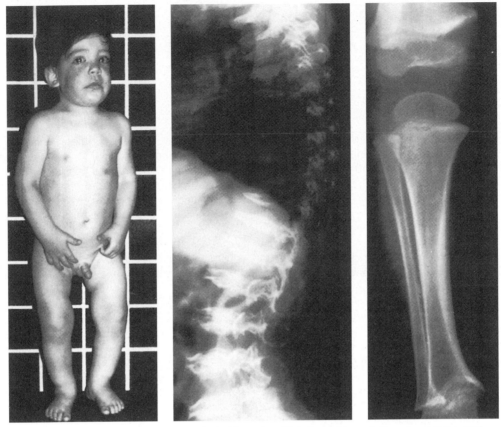

FIGURE 1. Kozlowski spondylometaphyseal dysplasia. Young boy. Note bowed legs, flattened vertebrae, and metaphyseal flare. (From Riggs W Jr, Summitt RL: Radiology 101:375, 1971, with permission.)

METATROPIC DYSPLASIA
(METATROPIC DWARFISM SYNDROME)

Small Thorax, Thoracic Kyphoscoliosis, Metaphyseal Flaring

Maroteaux and colleagues set forth this entity with 5 cases of their own and 12 unrecognized cases from the literature. More than 50 cases have been reported.

ABNORMALITIES

Growth. Birth weight normal; birth length greater than 97th percentile; trunk, initially long relative to the limbs, becomes progressively short with the development of kyphoscoliosis, leading to short-trunk dwarfism.

Skeletal. Early platyspondyly with progressive kyphosis and scoliosis in infancy to early childhood; odontoid hypoplasia; C1–C2 subluxation; narrow thorax with short ribs; short limbs with metaphyseal flaring and epiphyseal irregularity with hyperplastic trochanters; prominent joints with restricted mobility at knee and hip but increased extensibility of finger joints; hypoplasia of basilar pelvis with horizontal acetabula, short deep sacroiliac notch, and squared iliac wings.

OCCASIONAL ABNORMALITIES.
Macrocephaly, enlarged ventricles, small foramen magnum, clinical evidence of cord compression, ocular hypertelorism, thyroid agenesis, excess vertebrae.

NATURAL HISTORY.
Often evident at birth, the vertebral changes become severe during infancy. The trunk, originally long, becomes extremely short secondary to rapidly progressing kyphoscoliosis. Odontoid hypoplasia with C1–C2 subluxation can lead to cord compression, quadriplegia, and sometimes death. Cervical (C1–C2) fusion should be considered in all such cases. Measurements of the foramen magnum are indicated. Pelvic outlet constriction has led to colonic obstruction in at least one case.

ETIOLOGY.
Genetic heterogeneity is suggested by three different presentations: A nonlethal autosomal recessive form, a nonlethal autosomal dominant form with less severe spinal and pelvic changes, and a lethal autosomal recessive form with severe mushrooming and shortening of tubular bones and severe underossification of vertebral bodies.

References

Fleury J et al: Un cas singulier de dystrophie osteochondrale congenitale (nanisme metatrophique de Maroteaux). Ann Pediatr (Paris) 13:453, 1966.

Maroteaux P, Spranger I, Wiedemann HR: Der metatropische Zwergwucks. Arch Kinderheilkd 173:211, 1966.

Larose JH, Gay BG: Metatropic dwarfism. Am J Roentgenol Radium Ther Nucl Med 106:156, 1969.

Beck M et al: Heterogeneity of metatropic dysplasia. Eur J Pediatr 140:231, 1983.

Shohat M et al: Odontoid hypoplasia with vertebral cervical subluxation and ventriculomegaly in metatropic dysplasia. J Pediatr 114:239, 1989.

O'Sullivan MJ et al: Morphologic observations in a case of lethal variant (type I) metatropic dysplasia with atypical features: Morphology of lethal metatropic dysplasia. Pediatr Dev Pathol 1:405, 1998.

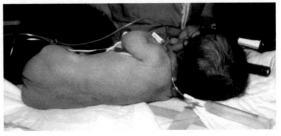

B

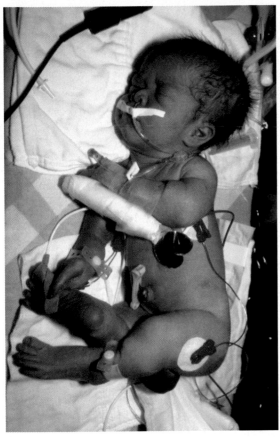

A

FIGURE 1. Metatropic dysplasia. **A** and **B,** Term male infant. Note the midface hypoplasia, large joints, short limbs, relatively large feet and hands, and congenital scoliosis. (Courtesy of Dr. Marilyn C. Jones, Children's Hospital, San Diego.)

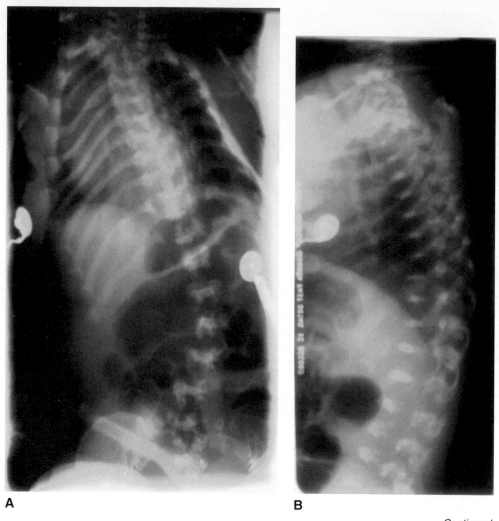

A

B

Continued

FIGURE 2. **A–D,** Radiographs of same child in Figure 1. Note scoliosis, striking platyspondyly, and metaphyseal flaring. (Courtesy of Dr. Marilyn C. Jones, Children's Hospital, San Diego.)

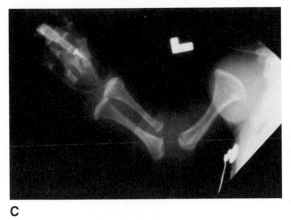

C

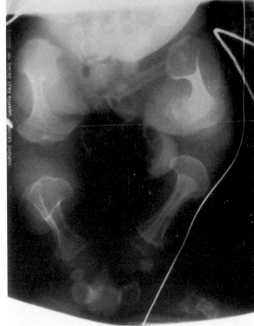

D

Fig. 2, cont'd.

GELEOPHYSIC DYSPLASIA

Initially described by Spranger and colleagues in 1971, approximately 25 cases have now been reported. The term "geleophysic" (*geleos*, meaning "happy" and *physis*, meaning "nature") refers to the happy-natured facial appearance typical of this disorder.

ABNORMALITIES

Growth. Short stature predominantly of postnatal onset with normal upper/lower segment ratio, span is decreased, decreased birth length has been noted in one third of cases in which it was reported.

Craniofacial. Round, full face; short nose with anteverted nares; upslanting palpebral fissures; long, smooth philtrum with thin, inverted vermilion and wide mouth; thickened helix of normally formed ear; "pleasant, happy-natured" appearance; gradual coarsening occurs postnatally.

Limbs. Short limbs and brachydactyly with markedly short tubular bones and relatively normal epiphyses; wide shafts of first and fifth metacarpals and proximal and middle phalanges; progressive contractures of multiple joints, particularly fingers and wrists; small, irregular capital femoral epiphyses (after 4 years), but other epiphyses, metaphyses, and diaphyses are normal; J-shaped sella turcica.

Cardiac. Progressive thickening of heart valves, with incompetence.

Other. Hepatomegaly; thickened, tight skin.

OCCASIONAL ABNORMALITIES.

Narrowing of trachea and mainstem bronchi, pectus excavatum, paralysis of upward gaze caused by abnormality of superior oblique muscle, myopia, ocular hypertelorism, developmental delay, seizures, trigger fingers, Perthes-like changes associated with dysplastic proximal capital femoral epiphysis.

NATURAL HISTORY. Recognizable at birth because of typical face and small hands and feet, growth deficiency and the characteristic facies become more obvious with time. With respect to prognosis, two children have died secondary to tracheal stenosis at 3 and 4 years of age, respectively, and three died of heart failure secondary to progressive valvular disease at 5 months, 1 year, and 5 years of age, respectively. All the survivors have had cardiac involvement, although mild and asymptomatic in some. Two are now young adults. Tracheal narrowing seems to significantly affect outcome as does the extent of the cardiac involvement.

ETIOLOGY. This disorder has an autosomal recessive inheritance pattern. Although the basic biochemical defect is unknown, lysosome-like inclusions have been found in skin epithelial cells, tracheal mucosa, liver, cartilage, and heart valves suggesting that this is a generalized lysosomal storage defect.

References

Spranger JW et al: Geleophysic dwarfism—a "focal" mucopolysaccharidosis? Lancet 2:97, 1971.

Koiffmann CP et al: Brief clinical report: Familial recurrence of geleophysic dysplasia. Am J Med Genet 19:483, 1984.

Spranger J et al: Geleophysic dysplasia. Am J Med Genet 19:487, 1984.

Shohat M et al: Geleophysic dysplasia: A storage disorder affecting the skin, bone, liver, heart and trachea. J Pediatr 117:227, 1990.

Wraith JE et al: Geleophysic dysplasia. Am J Med Genet 35:153, 1990.

Pontz BF et al: Clinical and ultrastructural findings in three patients with geleophysic dysplasia. Am J Med Genet 63:50, 1996.

Titomanlio L et al: Geleophysic dysplasia: 7-year follow-up study of a patient with an intermediate form. Am J Med Genet 86:82, 1999.

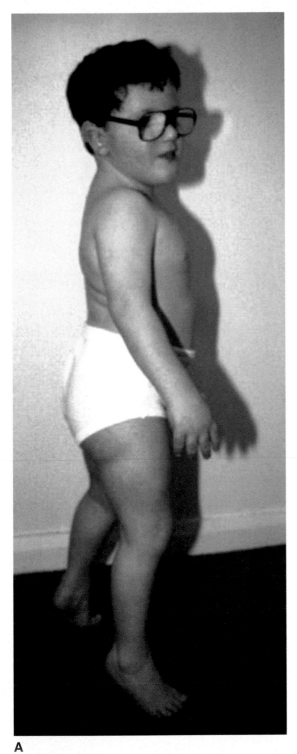

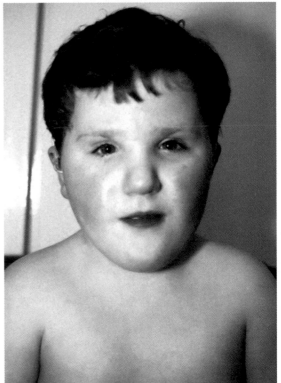

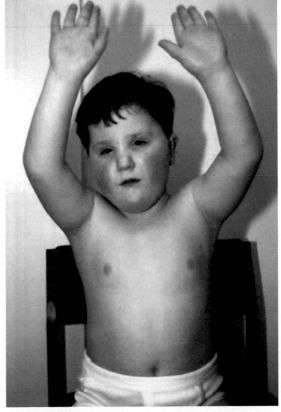

FIGURE 1. Geleophysic dysplasia. **A–C,** Note short palpebral fissures, broad nasal bridge, long upper lip, flat philtrum, and thin vermilion border. He has small hands and feet, limitation of joint movement, and a "tiptoe" gait. (From Rosser EM et al: Am J Med Genet 58:217, 1995, with permission.)

CHONDROECTODERMAL DYSPLASIA
(Ellis–van Creveld Syndrome)

Short Distal Extremities, Polydactyly, Nail Hypoplasia

Ellis and van Creveld set forth this entity in 1940. Approximately 40 cases were reported by 1964 when McKusick and colleagues added 52 cases from an inbred Amish population. More than 200 cases have now been reported.

ABNORMALITIES

Growth. Small stature of prenatal onset.

Skeletal. Disproportionate, irregularly short extremities; polydactyly of fingers, occasionally of toes; short, broad middle phalanges and hypoplastic distal phalanges; malformed carpals, fusion of capitate and hamate, and extra carpal bones; narrow thorax with short, poorly developed ribs; hypoplasia of upper lateral tibia, with knock-knee; pelvic dysplasia with low iliac wings and spur-like, downward projections at the medial and lateral aspects of the acetabula.

Nails. Hypoplastic.

Teeth. Neonatal teeth, partial anodontia, small teeth, or delayed eruption.

Mouth. Short upper lip bound by frenula to alveolar ridge; defects in alveolar ridge with accessory frenula.

Cardiac. Approximately 60% of patients have a cardiac defect, most commonly an atrial septal defect; often with a single atrium.

OCCASIONAL ABNORMALITIES.

Mental retardation, Dandy-Walker malformation, heterotopic masses of gray matter, scant or fine hair, cryptorchidism, epispadias, talipes equinovarus, duplication of primary ulnar ossification center, renal agenesis.

NATURAL HISTORY. Approximately one half of the patients die in early infancy as a consequence of cardiorespiratory problems. The majority of survivors are of normal intelligence. Eventual stature is in the range of 43 to 60 inches. There is usually some limitation in hand function, such as inability to form a clenched fist. Dental problems are frequent.

ETIOLOGY. This disorder has an autosomal recessive inheritance pattern. Mutations in two nonhomologous genes, both located at chromosome location 4p16, are responsible.

References

Ellis RWB, van Creveld S: A syndrome characterized by ectodermal dysplasia, polydactyly, chondro-dysplasia and congenital morbus cordis: Report of three cases. Arch Dis Child 15:65, 1940.

McKusick VA et al: Dwarfism in the Amish. The Ellis–van Creveld syndrome. Bull Johns Hopkins Hosp 115:306, 1964.

Feingold M et al: Ellis–van Creveld syndrome. Clin Pediatr (Phila) 5:431, 1966.

Rosemberg S et al: Brief clinical report: Chondroectodermal dysplasia (Ellis–van Creveld) with anomalies of CNS and urinary tract. Am J Med Genet 15:291, 1983.

Taylor GA et al: Polycarpaly and other abnormalities of the wrist in chondroectodermal dysplasia: The Ellis–van Creveld syndrome. Radiology 151:393, 1984.

Quereshi F et al: Skeletal histopathology in fetus with chondroectodermal dysplasia (Ellis–van Creveld syndrome). Am J Med Genet 45:471, 1993.

Ruiz-Perez VL et al: Mutations in a new gene in Ellis–van Creveld syndrome and Weyers acrodental dysostosis. Nat Genet 24:283, 2000.

Ruiz-Perez VL et al: Mutations in two nonhomologous genes in a head-to-head configuration cause Ellis–van Creveld syndrome. Am J Hum Genet 72:728, 2003.

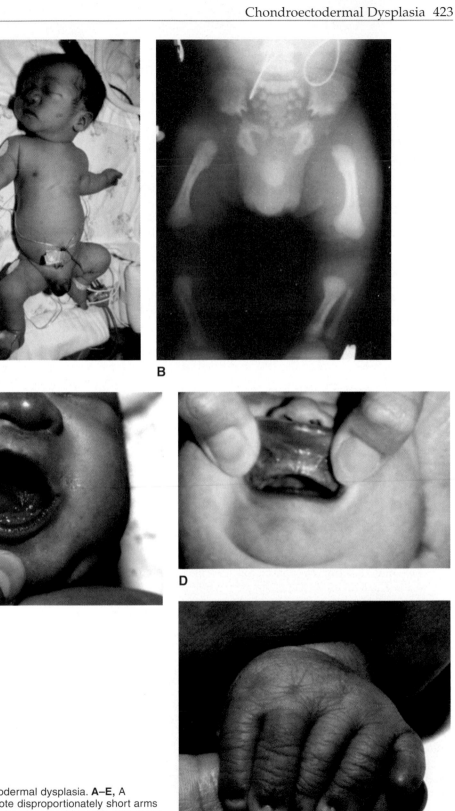

FIGURE 1. Chondroectodermal dysplasia. **A–E,** A newborn male infant. Note disproportionately short arms and legs, hypoplasia of the alveolar ridge with accessory frenula, polydactyly, hypoplastic fingernails, and on radiograph, the hypoplastic tibia and the low iliac wings with spur-like, downward projections of the medial and lateral aspects of the acetabula. (Courtesy of Dr. Marilyn C. Jones, Children's Hospital, San Diego.)

DIASTROPHIC* DYSPLASIA
(DIASTROPHIC NANISM SYNDROME)

*Short Tubular Bones (Especially First Metacarpal),
Joint Limitation with Talipes Equinovarus
Hypertrophied Auricular Cartilage*

The 1960 report of Lamy and Maroteaux concerning three cases of their own and 11 similar cases from the literature established this pattern of malformation as a distinct entity. It is now recognized with frequency.

ABNORMALITIES

Growth. Disproportionate short stature of prenatal onset; mean birth length, 42 cm.

Limbs. Talipes equinovarus plus limitation of flexion at proximal phalangeal joints and of extension at elbow, with or without dislocation of hip or knee with weight-bearing; short and thick tubular bones with development of broad metaphyses and flattened irregular epiphyses that are late in mineralizing; carpal bones may be accelerated in ossification in contrast with the remainder of the hand; first metacarpal unduly small; abduction of thumbs (hitchhiker thumbs) and great toes; variable symphalangism of proximal interphalangeal joints; variable webbing at joints.

Spine. Scoliosis; cervical spine abnormalities including anterior hypoplasia of vertebrae C3 to C5, kyphosis, subluxation, spina bifida occulta, and hyperplastic and dysmorphic odontoid process; interpedicular narrowing from L1 to L5; accessory ossification centers of manubrium sterni.

Pinnae. Soft cystic masses in auricle develop into hypertrophic cartilage in early infancy in 84% of patients.

OCCASIONAL ABNORMALITIES.

Thick pectinate strands at root of iris, cleft palate (25%), micrognathia, lateral displacement of patellae, elbow dislocation, hyperelasticity of skin, cryptorchidism; early mineralization of ribs, intra-cranial calcification; deafness secondary to fusion or lack of ossicles, stenosis of the external auditory canal; laryngotracheal stenosis; midfacial capillary hemangiomata.

NATURAL HISTORY. Two affected infants with cleft palate and micrognathia, similar in this respect to those with the Robin sequence, died of respiratory obstruction. The mortality rate related to respiratory obstruction, including laryngeal stenosis, can be as high as 25% in early infancy. For the survivors, general health is usually good, and the patients have normal intelligence, although there is a risk for development of neurologic complications from cervical spine anomalies. Motor milestones are delayed with onset of walking at 24.4 ± 9.2 months. The possibility of atlantoaxial instability must always be considered. Unfortunately, the talipes equinovarus and the scoliosis that develop have been rather resistant to corrective orthopedic measures, and the functional problem is aggravated by the limitation in joint motility. Spinal cord compression may occur as a consequence of severe kyphoscoliosis. When present, the unusual defect of hypertrophied auricular cartilage may eventually give way to ossification. Growth failure is progressive. The pubertal growth spurt is often weak or absent. Final height varies from 100 to 140 cm, with a mean of 125 cm. Adults tend to be overweight.

ETIOLOGY. This disorder has an autosomal recessive inheritance pattern. Mutations in the diastrophic dysplasia sulfate transporter (DTDST) gene, located at chromosome 5q32-q33.1, are responsible. It is likely that impaired function of its product leads to the production of undersulfated proteoglycans in cartilage matrix, the presumed basis for the clinical phenotype in this disorder.

---

*Diastrophic = crooked.

References
Lamy M, Maroteaux P: Le nanisme diastrophique. Presse Med 68:1977, 1960.

Langer LO: Diastrophic dwarfism in early infancy. Am J Roentgenol Radium Ther Nucl Med 93:399, 1965.

Walker BA et al: Diastrophic dwarfism. Medicine 51:41, 1972.

Horton WA et al: The phenotypic variability of diastrophic dysplasia. J Pediatr 93:608, 1978.

Hastbacka J et al: Diastrophic dysplasia gene maps to the distal long arm of chromosome 5. Proc Natl Acad Sci USA 87:8056, 1990.

Hastbacka J et al: The diastrophic dysplasia gene encodes a novel sulfate transporter: Positional cloning by fine-structure linkage disequilibrium mapping. Cell 78:1073, 1994.

Makitie O, Kaitila I: Growth in diastrophic dysplasia. J Pediatr 130:641, 1997.

Crockett MM et al: Motor milestones in children with diastrophic dysplasia. J Pediatr Orthop 20:437, 2000.

Remes V et al: Scoliosis in patients with diastrophic dysplasia: A new classification. Spine 26:1689, 2001.

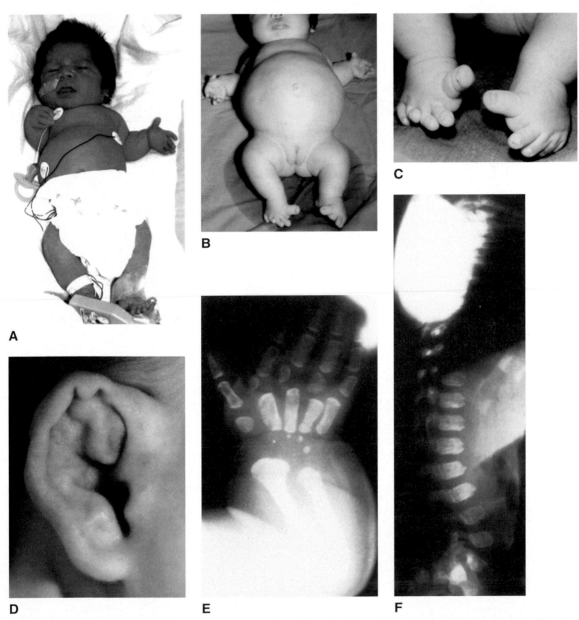

FIGURE 1. Diastrophic dysplasia. **A–C,** Two newborn infants. Note the disproportionate short stature and abduction of thumbs and great toes. (**A,** Courtesy of Dr. Marilyn C. Jones, Children's Hospital, San Diego.) **D,** Note the cystic swelling of the ear. **E** and **F,** Radiographs showing small first metacarpal.

X-LINKED RECESSIVE SPONDYLOEPIPHYSEAL DYSPLASIA TARDA

Flattened Vertebrae of Midchildhood, Small Iliac Wings, Short Femoral Neck

This disorder was recognized in 1939 by Jacobsen.

ABNORMALITIES. Onset between 5 and 10 years of age; affected males are clinically and radiographically normal at birth.

Growth. Short stature; final height, 52 to 62 inches with an average of 55 inches; trunk is disproportionately short and there is a barrel chest.

Spine. Flattened vertebrae with hump-shaped mound of bone in central and posterior portions of vertebral end plates; narrowing of disk spaces usually posteriorly; lumbar spine is primarily affected; kyphosis, mild scoliosis, short neck.

Pelvis. Small iliac wings.

Limbs. Short femoral neck, mild epiphyseal irregularity with flattening of femoral head.

Joints. Eventual pain and stiffness in hips, shoulders, cervical and lumbar spine.

OCCASIONAL ABNORMALITIES.
Corneal opacities.

NATURAL HISTORY. Symptoms usually occur between 5 and 10 years of age; vague back pain in adolescence is frequently the initial symptom and the radiologic defects of the spine are most pronounced during periods of maximum growth; back, knee, and especially hip pain caused by osteoarthritis by 40 years of age, often disabling by 60 years; total hip arthroplasty is commonly needed before 40 years of age.

ETIOLOGY. This disorder has an X-linked recessive inheritance pattern. A defect in a gene located at Xp22.2-22.1 is responsible. In some cases, obligate carrier females have been suspected based on minor radiographic changes, including mild alterations in the shape of the pelvis and knees as well as premature degenerative changes in the spine, and the development of arthralgia in middle age. In addition, both autosomal dominant and autosomal recessive late-onset spondyloepiphyseal dysplasia have been reported. A more severe degree of truncal shortening is evident in the X-linked recessive form.

References

Jacobsen AW: Hereditary osteochondrodystrophia deformans: A family with twenty members affected in five generations. JAMA 113:121, 1939.

Maroteaux P, Lamy M, Bernard J: La dysplasie spondylo-epiphysaire tardive: Description clinique et radiologique. Presse Med 65:1205, 1957.

Langer LO: Spondyloepiphyseal dysplasia tarda: Hereditary chondrodysplasia with characteristic vertebral configuration in the adult. Radiology 82:833, 1964.

Bannerman RM, Ingall GB, Mohn JF: X-linked spondyloepiphyseal dysplasia tarda. J Med Genet 8:291, 1971.

Wells JA et al: Corneal opacities in spondyloepiphyseal dysplasia tarda. Cornea 13:280, 1994.

Heuertz S et al: Genetic mapping of Xp22.12-p22.31, with refined localization for spondyloepiphyseal dysplasia (SEDL). Hum Genet 96:407, 1995.

Whyte MP et al: X-linked recessive spondyloepiphyseal dysplasia tarda: Clinical and radiographic evolution in a 6-generation kindred and review of the literature. Medicine 78:9, 1999.

Gedeon AK et al: The molecular basis of X-linked spondyloepiphyseal dysplasia tarda. Am J Hum Genet 68:1386, 2001.

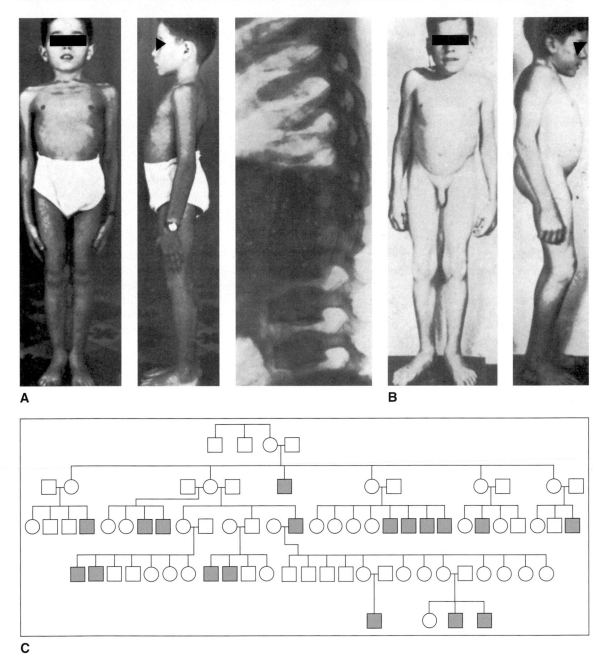

C

FIGURE 1. Spondyloepiphyseal dysplasia tarda. **A,** A 12-year-old child. Note shortening of trunk caused by flattened vertebrae, each of which has a central "hump" in the area of its epiphyses. (Courtesy of P. Maroteaux, Hospital for Sick Infants, Paris.) **B,** A 15-year-old child. (From Jacobsen AW. JAMA 113:121, 1939, with permission.) **C,** Pedigree, of which patient shown in **B** is a member, showing evidence of X-linked recessive inheritance. (Courtesy of R. Bannaman, Buffalo General Hospital, Buffalo, New York.)

MULTIPLE EPIPHYSEAL DYSPLASIA

*Small Irregular Epiphyses, Pain
and Stiffness in Hips, Short Stature*

This condition was described by Ribbing in 1937 and by Fairbank in 1947. It is frequently misdiagnosed as bilateral Legg-Perthes disease.

ABNORMALITIES

Growth. Normal to slight shortness of stature; adult stature, 145 to 170 cm.

Limbs. Late ossifying, small, irregular, mottled epiphyses with eventual osteoarthritis caused by loss of articular cartilage in many large joints, especially in hips and knees; short femoral neck; mild metaphyseal flare; shortness of metacarpals and phalanges leading to short stubby fingers; approximately one third have symmetrical shoulder problems; double-layered patellae that often dislocate laterally; genu varum or genu valgus.

Spine. Although vertebral bodies are usually spared, they can be blunted, slightly ovoid, sometimes flattened.

NATURAL HISTORY.
Evident from 2 to 10 years because of waddling gait, easy fatigue, joint pain after exercise and slow growth; back pain is common; slowly progressive pain and stiffness in joints, particularly in the hips, may be a complaint as early as 5 years, but usually not until 30 to 35 years; joint replacement is often required.

ETIOLOGY.
This disorder has an autosomal dominant inheritance pattern with wide variability in expression. Mutations in the cartilage oligomeric matrix protein (COMP) gene, which has been localized to chromosome 19p13.1, have been identified in some cases. Point mutations in the three type IX collagen genes (COL9A1, COL9A2, and COL9A3) located on 6q13, 1p33-p32.2, and 20q13.3, respectively cause a milder phenotype. In addition, mutations in a gene encoding matrilin-3 located on chromosome 2p24-23 can cause a distinctive mild type. Finally, mutations in the diastrophic dysplasia sulfate transporter (DTDST) gene located on chromosome 5q32-q33.1 and mutations in solute carrier family 26, member 2 gene (SLC26A2) located at 5q32-33.1 are responsible for autosomal recessive forms of multiple epiphyseal dysplasia.

COMMENT.
Radiographic abnormalities are correlated with genotype. Type IX collagen defects are associated with more severe joint involvement at the knees and relative hip sparing. Significant involvement at the capital femoral epiphysis and irregular acetabuli are associated with COMP mutations. Radiographic evidence of a "double layered" patella is characteristic of mutations in the DTDST gene.

References

Ribbings S: Studien über hereditäre multiple ëpiphysenstörungen. Acta Radiol [Suppl] 34, 1937.

Fairbank T: Dysplasia epiphysealis multiplex. Br J Surg 34:225, 1947.

Maudsley RH: Dysplasia epiphysialis multiplex: A report of fourteen cases in three families. J Bone Joint Surg 37B:228, 1955.

Hoefnagel D et al: Hereditary multiple epiphyseal dysplasia. Ann Hum Genet 30:201, 1967.

Spranger J: The epiphyseal dysplasias. Clin Orthop Rel Res 114:46, 1976.

Ingram RR: The shoulder in multiple epiphyseal dysplasia. J Bone Joint Surg 73B:277, 1991.

Unger SL et al: Multiple epiphyseal dysplasia: radiographic abnormalities correlated with genotype. Pediatr Radiol 31:10, 2001.

Briggs MD, Chapman KL: Pseudoachondroplasia and multiple epiphyseal dysplasia: Mutation review, molecular interactions, and genotype to phenotype correlations. Hum Mutat 19:465, 2002.

Chapman KL et al: Review: Clinical variability and genetic heterogeneity in multiple epiphyseal dysplasia. Pediatr Pathol Molec Med 22:53, 2003.

Makitie O et al: Autosomal recessive multiple epiphyseal dysplasia with homozygosity for C653S in the DTDST gene: Double-layer patella as a reliable sign. Am J Med Genet 122A:187, 2003.

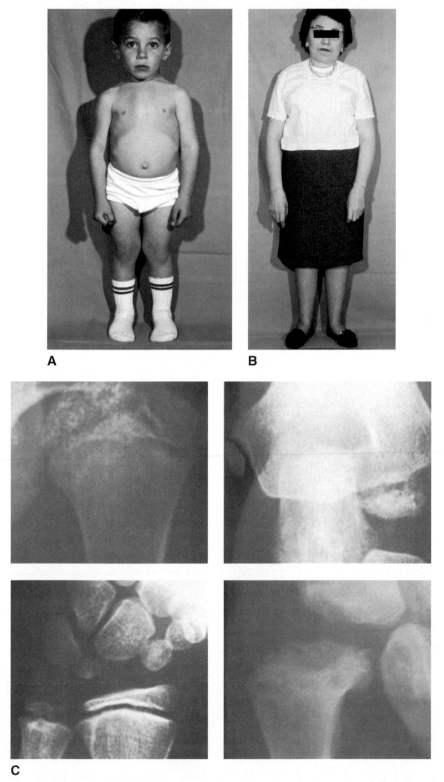

FIGURE 1. Multiple epiphyseal dysplasia. **A,** A 5-year-old child with height age of 2½ years. Patient had occasional aching in legs. **B,** Affected mother of patient shown in **A**. She is short of stature and has hip discomfort. **C,** Late and irregular mineralization of epiphyses, which may be small or aberrant in shape or both.

METAPHYSEAL DYSPLASIA, SCHMID TYPE

Since the initial description by Schmid in 1949, several large pedigrees of affected individuals have been reported.

ABNORMALITIES

Growth. Mild to moderate shortness of stature; adult height, 130 to 160 cm.

Skeletal. Relatively short tubular bones; tibial bowing, especially at ankle; waddling gait with coxa vara and genu varum; flare to lower rib cage.

Radiographic. Enlarged capital femoral epiphyses before 10 years of age; coxa vara beginning at 3 years; femoral bowing; metaphyseal abnormalities of distal and proximal femurs, proximal tibias, proximal fibulas, distal radius and ulna; anterior cupping, splaying, and sclerosis of ribs; metacarpals and phalanges as well as spine are normal in the majority of cases; there is mild irregularity of acetabular roof.

OCCASIONAL ABNORMALITIES.

Mild platyspondyly, vertebral body abnormalities, and end-plate irregularities.

NATURAL HISTORY.

Bowed legs with waddling gait, the usual presenting sign, is usually evident in second year; height, usually less than the fifth percentile, is rarely less than 7 SD below the mean; pain in legs during childhood; symptomatic and radiographic improvement beginning as early as 3 years of age, with orthopedic measures indicated only for unusual degrees of deformity and usually not until growth is complete; because the epiphyses are not affected, there are usually no osteoarthritic symptoms; intelligence and life expectancy are not affected.

ETIOLOGY.

This disorder has an autosomal dominant inheritance pattern with variable expression. Mutations of the type X collagen (COL10A1) gene, which has been mapped to 6q22.3, are responsible for this pattern of malformation. Type X collagen expression is restricted to hypertrophic chondrocytes in areas undergoing endochondral ossification, such as growth plates. It has been suggested that reduction in the amount of normal type X collagen results in the phenotype.

References

Schmid F: Beitrag zur Dysostosis Enchondralis Metaphysaria. Monatsschr Kinderheilkd 97:393, 1949.

Stickler GB et al: Familial bone disease resembling rickets (hereditary metaphyseal dysostosis). Pediatrics 29:996, 1962.

Rosenbloom AL, Smith DW: The natural history of metaphyseal dysostosis. J Pediatr 66:857, 1965.

Lachman RS et al: Metaphyseal chondrodysplasia: Schmid type. Clinical and radiographic delineation with review of the literature. Pediatr Radiol 18:93, 1988.

Warman ML et al: A type X collagen mutation causes Schmid metaphyseal chondrodysplasia. Nat Genet 5:79, 1993.

Savarirayan R et al: Schmid type metaphyseal chondrodysplasia: A spondylometaphyseal dysplasia identical to the "Japanese" type. Pediatr Radiol 30:460, 2000.

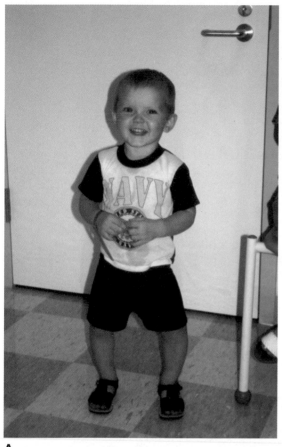

A

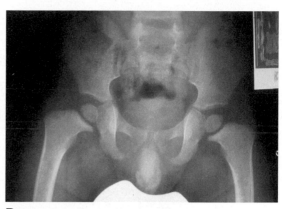

B

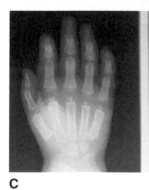
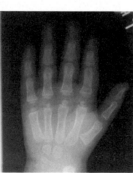

C

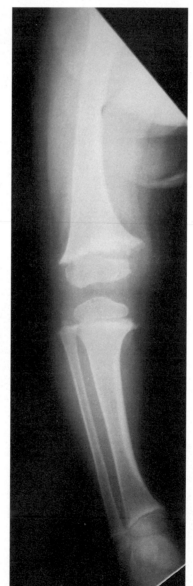

D

FIGURE 1. Metaphyseal dysplasia, Schmid type. **A–D,** Image of a 27-month-old boy. Note the bowing of legs, enlarged capital femoral epiphyses, and metaphyseal abnormalities. (Courtesy of Dr. Marilyn C. Jones, Children's Hospital, San Diego.)

METAPHYSEAL DYSPLASIA, McKUSICK TYPE
(CARTILAGE-HAIR HYPOPLASIA SYNDROME)

Mild Bowing of Legs, Wide Irregular Metaphyses, Fine Sparse Hair

Discovered by McKusick and colleagues among an inbred Amish population, this condition has subsequently been detected in non-Amish individuals, particularly in the Finnish population.

ABNORMALITIES

Growth. Prenatal onset of short limb, long trunk, short stature evident neonatally in 76% of cases and in 98% by 1 year; adult height, 104 to 149 cm; decreased or absent pubertal growth spurt; obesity in adults.

Hair. Fine, sparse, light, relatively fragile; eyebrows, eyelashes, and body hair are also affected.

Skeletal. Relatively short limbs, mild bowing of legs; prominent heel; flat feet; short hands, fingernails, toenails; loose-jointed "limp" hands and feet; incomplete extension of elbow; mild flaring of lower rib cage with prominent sternum; lumbar lordosis, scoliosis, small pelvic inlet.

Radiographic. Flared, scalloped, irregularly sclerotic metaphyses noted before closing of epiphyses primarily in knees and ankles, less frequently in hips; epiphyses only minimally affected; short tibia in relation to fibula.

Other. Diminished cellular immune response manifest by lymphopenia, decreased delayed hypersensitivity, and impaired in vitro responsiveness of lymphocytes to PHA; mild macrocytic anemia; neutropenia.

OCCASIONAL ABNORMALITIES.
Brachycephaly; malignancies (6% to 10%), particularly non-Hodgkin lymphoma; esophageal atresia; Hirschsprung disease, particularly in severe cases; intestinal malabsorption in infancy; impaired humoral immunity; congenital hypoplastic anemia; impaired spermatogenesis.

NATURAL HISTORY. The early history is often indicative of an intestinal malabsorption problem, which tends to improve with time. Postoperative mortality following surgery for Hirschsprung disease is as high as 38%, primarily related to severe enterocolitis-related septicemia. The diminished cellular immunity often leads to severe or fatal response to varicella as well as other infections. Even those patients for whom in vitro immunologic competence has been documented should be followed carefully. The rare congenital hypoplastic anemia can occasionally be fatal. However, in most cases spontaneous recovery occurs before adulthood. The presence of anemia correlates with severity of the immunodeficiency and growth failure and to the neutropenia.

ETIOLOGY. This disorder has an autosomal recessive inheritance pattern. Mutations in the RMRP gene, which encodes the untranslated RNA that is a component of mitochondrial RNA-processing endoribonuclease and is mapped to the proximal part of 9p, are responsible.

COMMENT. The diagnosis is difficult in infancy. Widened metaphyses, short long bones, elongated fibulae, and anterior angulation of the sternum should raise concern regarding this disorder in the neonatal period.

References
McKusick VA et al: Dwarfism in the Amish. II. Cartilage-hair hypoplasia. Bull Johns Hopkins Hosp 116:285, 1965.
Lux SE et al: Chronic neutropenia and abnormal cellular immunity in cartilage-hair hypoplasia. N Engl J Med 282:231, 1970.
Van der Burgt I et al: Cartilage hair hypoplasia, metaphyseal chondrodysplasia type McKusick: Description of seven patients and review of the literature. Am J Med Genet 41:371, 1991.

Makitie O, Kaitila I: Cartilage-hair hypoplasia—clinical manifestations in 108 Finnish patients. Eur J Pediatr 152:211, 1993.

Sulisalo T et al: Cartilage-hair hypoplasia gene assigned to chromosome 9 by linkage analysis. Nat Genet 3:338, 1993.

Makitie O et al: Cartilage-hair hypoplasia. J Med Genet 32:39, 1995.

Glass RBJ et al: Radiologic changes in infancy in McKusick cartilage hair hypoplasia. Am J Med Genet 86:312, 1999.

Ridanpaa M et al: Mutations in the RNA component of RNase MRP cause a pleiotropic human disease, cartilage hair hypoplasia. Cell 104:195, 2001.

Makitie O et al: Hirschsprung's disease in cartilage-hair hypoplasia has poor prognosis. J Pediatr Surg 37:1585, 2002.

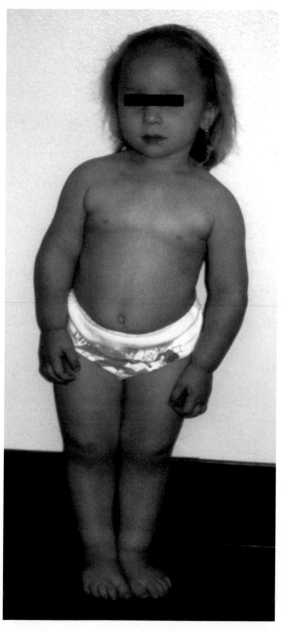

FIGURE 1. Metaphyseal dysplasia, McKusick type. Note the fine, sparse hair and short limbs.

METAPHYSEAL DYSPLASIA, JANSEN TYPE
(METAPHYSEAL DYSOSTOSIS, JANSEN TYPE)

Wide Irregular Metaphyses, Flexion Joint Deformity, Small Thorax

Since Jansen described this severe type of metaphyseal dysostosis, at least 14 cases have been reported.

ABNORMALITIES

Growth. Severe short stature of postnatal onset; adult stature approximately 125 cm.

Facies. Small, immature in appearance, with prominent eyes; mild supraorbital and frontonasal hyperplasia in the adult; micrognathia.

Skeletal and Joint. Small thoracic cage; flexion deformities of joints, especially at knee and hip, yielding a squatting stance with symmetric para-articular widening.

Radiographic. Severe metaphyseal dysplasia, large epiphyses, wide distance between the epiphyses and metaphyses in the long bones and a sclerotic skull base.

Other. Waddling gait; clinodactyly; short clubbed fingers; hyperostosis of calvarium with thick dense base of skull; hypercalcemia and hypophosphatemia despite lack of parathyroid gland abnormalities; variable deafness.

NATURAL HISTORY. Skeletal changes have been noted at birth or in early infancy; the defective growth and joint dysfunction are severe.

ETIOLOGY. This disorder has an autosomal dominant inheritance pattern, with most cases being fresh mutations. The responsible gene, which is the parathyroid hormone–related peptide receptor, has been localized to chromosome 3p22-p21.

COMMENT. Radiographic features change with age. At birth, diffuse radiolucency and irregularity of metaphyses of long bones. Wide growth plates of tubular bones. In childhood, cupping of metaphyses with a wide zone of irregular calcification. In adult, the large calcified masses in the metaphyses turn into bone, resulting in bulbous deformities at the ends of short, bowed long bones.

References

Jansen M: Über atypische Chondrodystrophie (Achondroplasia) und über eine noch nicht beschriebene angeborene Wachstummsstörung des Knochensystems: Metaphysäre Dysostosis. 2. Orthop Chir 61:253, 1934.

Charrow J, Poznanski AK: The Jansen type of metaphyseal chondrodysplasia: Confirmation of dominant inheritance and review of radiographic manifestations in the newborn and adult. Am J Med Genet 18:321, 1984.

Frezal J et al: Osteochondrodysplasias, dysostosis, disorders of calcium metabolism, congenital malformations with skeletal involvement mapped on human chromosomes. Pediatr Radiol 27:366, 1997.

Kozlowski K et al: Metaphyseal chondrodysplasia, type Jansen. Aust Radiol 43:544, 1999.

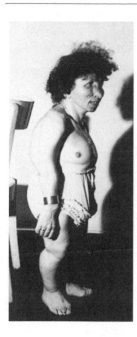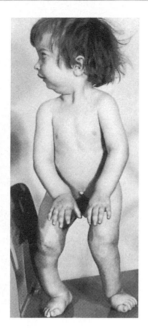

FIGURE 1. Metaphyseal dysplasia, Jansen type. Affected mother and daughter. (Courtesy of W. Lenz, Münster, Germany.)

SHWACHMAN-DIAMOND SYNDROME
(METAPHYSEAL DYSPLASIA WITH PANCREATIC INSUFFICIENCY AND NEUTROPENIA)

Metaphyseal Chondrodysplasia, Neutropenia, Exocrine Pancreatic Insufficiency

In 1963, Shwachman and colleagues described five children with evidence of pancreatic insufficiency and leukopenia, none of whom had cystic fibrosis of the pancreas. Burke and colleagues subsequently documented the association of metaphyseal chondrodysplasia with this syndrome. More than 300 cases have been reported.

ABNORMALITIES

Growth. Short stature of prenatal onset, failure to thrive.

Performance. IQ significantly lower than that in siblings, mild mental retardation in one third.

Pancreas. Lack of exocrine pancreas, which is replaced by adipose tissue; pancreatic trypsin, lipase, and amylase are absent.

Radiographic. Skeletal changes, including short ribs with widely flared costochondral junctions, ovoid vertebral bodies, widening and irregularity of metaphyses of long bones, which are short, and focal lack of mineralization in epiphyses; narrow sacroiliac notch.

Hematologic. Neutropenia, impaired neutrophil chemotaxis, anemia, thrombocytopenia, pancytopenia, bone marrow dysfunction.

OCCASIONAL ABNORMALITIES.
Delayed dentition of permanent teeth, dental dysplasia, dental caries, periodontal disease, hepatomegaly, elevated liver enzymes, myocardial fibrosis, nephrocalcinosis, intermittent and variable glycosuria, generalized aminoaciduria, type I renal tubular acidosis.

NATURAL HISTORY. Failure to thrive with diarrhea and malabsorption is the most common presenting sign, usually between 2 and 10 months of age. Of interest is the observation that there is no steatorrhea; presumably the intestinal lipases are adequate in the absence of pancreatic lipase. The viscosity of duodenal secretions is also normal in contrast with cystic fibrosis of the pancreas, which can be excluded readily by sweat electrolyte studies. The diarrhea tends to improve with age even without pancreatic enzyme replacement therapy. The therapy is followed by dramatic response in some patients but not in others. The leukopenia can occur intermittently and may be accompanied by a high frequency of bacterial infections. There is a high risk of development of myelodysplastic syndrome.

ETIOLOGY. This disorder has an autosomal recessive inheritance pattern. Mutations in an uncharacterized gene (SBDS), located at chromosome 7q11, are responsible.

References
Shwachman H et al: Pancreatic insufficiency and bone marrow dysfunction: A new clinical entity. J Pediatr 63:835, 1963.

Burke V et al: Association of pancreatic insufficiency and chronic neutropenia in childhood. Arch Dis Child 42:147, 1967.

McLennan TW, Steinbach HL: Shwachman's syndrome: The broad spectrum of bone abnormalities. Radiology 112:167, 1974.

Danks DM et al: Metaphyseal chondrodysplasia, neutropenia, and pancreatic insufficiency presenting with respiratory distress in the neonatal period. Arch Dis Child 51:697, 1976.

Woods WG et al: The occurrence of leukemia in patients with the Shwachman syndrome. J Pediatr 99:425, 1981.

Kent A et al: Psychological characteristics of children with Shwachman syndrome. Arch Dis Child 65:1349, 1990.

Rothbaum R et al: Shwachman-Diamond syndrome: Report from an international conference. J Pediatr 141:266, 2002.

Boocock GRB et al: Mutations in SBDS are associated with Shwachman-Diamond syndrome. Nat Genet 33:97, 2003.

CHONDRODYSPLASIA PUNCTATA, X-LINKED DOMINANT TYPE

(CONRADI-HÜNERMANN SYNDROME)

Asymmetric Limb Shortness, Early Punctate Mineralization, Large Skin Pores

Initially described by Conradi and later by Hünermann, this disorder was clearly distinguished from the autosomal recessive type of chondrodysplasia punctata by Spranger and colleagues.

ABNORMALITIES

Growth. Mild to moderate growth deficiency.

Facies. Variable low nasal bridge with flat facies; hypoplasia of malar eminences with downslanting palpebral fissures; cataracts.

Limbs. Asymmetric shortening related to areas of punctate mineralization in epiphyses, variable joint contractures.

Spine. Frequent scoliosis, even in infancy, related to areas of punctate mineralization.

Skin. Erythema and thick adherent scales in newborn period; in older children, variable follicular atrophoderma with large pores resembling "orange peel" and ichthyosis predominate; sparse hair that tends to be coarse, and patchy areas of alopecia.

OCCASIONAL ABNORMALITIES.

Dysplastic auricles; minor nail anomalies; nystagmus; hazy cornea; microphthalmos; glaucoma; atrophy of retina and optic nerve; short neck; hydramnios; hydrops; mild to moderate mental deficiency; tracheal calcifications with associated tracheal stenosis; cardiac defects; dislocated patella; hexadactyly; vertebral anomalies including clefting, wedging, or absence.

NATURAL HISTORY.

Failure to thrive and infection may occur in early infancy. If the patient survives the first few months, the prognosis for survival is good. Stippling of the epiphyses of the long bones frequently resolves by 9 months. Orthopedic problems including scoliosis are frequent, and there is an enhanced risk of cataract formation.

ETIOLOGY. This disorder has an X-linked dominant inheritance pattern. Mutations of an X-linked gene encoding Δ^8,Δ^7 sterol isomerase emopamil-binding protein (EBP), leading to a deficiency of sterol-Δ^1-isomerase, are responsible. Recognition that abnormal cholesterol biosynthesis is a feature of this disorder permits a definitive biochemical diagnosis.

COMMENT. In addition to this disorder and the autosomal recessive chondrodysplasia punctata, an X-linked recessive type exists. That condition is characterized by skeletal manifestation of chondrodysplasia punctata, ichthyosis caused by steroid sulfatase deficiency, short stature, microcephaly, developmental delay, cataracts, and hearing loss. In addition, some affected males have anosmia and hypogonadism (Kallmann syndrome). The majority of patients have documented deletions and translocations of Xp22.3. Point mutations in the gene encoding arylsulfatase E (ARSE), which maps to Xp22.3, have been identified in a number of patients with this disorder, suggesting that the skeletal abnormalities are the result of altered ARSE activity.

References

Conradi E: Vorzeitiges Auftreten von Knochen und eigenartigen Verkalkungskernen bei Chondrodystrophia foetalis hypoplastica. Jahrb Kinderheilkd 80:86, 1914.

Hünermann C: Chondrodystrophia calcificans congenita als abortive Form der Chondrodystrophie. Z Kinderheilkd 51:1, 1931.

Spranger J, Opitz JM, Bidder U: Heterogeneity of chondrodysplasia punctate. Humangenetik 11:190, 1971.

Happle R: X-linked dominant chondrodysplasia punctata: Review of literature and report of a case. Hum Genet 53:65, 1979.

Curry CJR et al: Inherited chondrodysplasia punctata due to a deletion of the terminal short arm of an X chromosome. N Engl J Med 311:1010, 1984.

Ballabio A, Andria G: Deletions and translocations involving the distal short arm of the human X chromosome: Review and hypothesis. Hum Mol Genet 1:221, 1992.

Wulfsberg EA et al: Chondrodysplasia punctata: A boy with

X-linked recessive chondrodysplasia punctata due to an inherited X-Y translocation with a current classification of these disorders. Am J Med Genet 43:823, 1992.

Franco B et al: A cluster of sulfatase genes on Xp22.3: Mutations in chondrodysplasia punctata (CDPX) and implications for warfarin embryopathy. Cell 81:15, 1995.

Derry JM et al: Mutations in a delta 8-delta 7 sterol isomerase in the tattered mouse and X-linked dominant chondrodysplasia punctata. Nat Genet 22:286, 1999.

Kelley RI et al: Abnormal sterol metabolism in patients with Conradi-Hünermann-Happle syndrome and sporadic lethal chondrodysplasia punctata. Am J Med Genet 83:213, 1999.

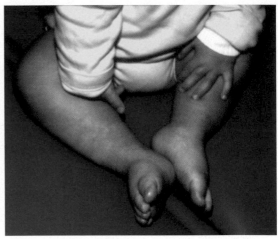

B

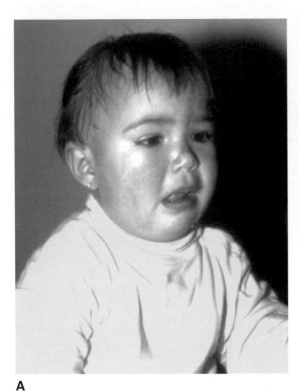

A

FIGURE 1. Chondrodysplasia punctata, X-linked dominant type. **A** and **B,** Image of a 19-month-old girl. Note the flat face, low nasal bridge, sparse hair with patchy alopecia and leg asymmetry. (Courtesy of Marilyn C. Jones, Children's Hospital, San Diego.)

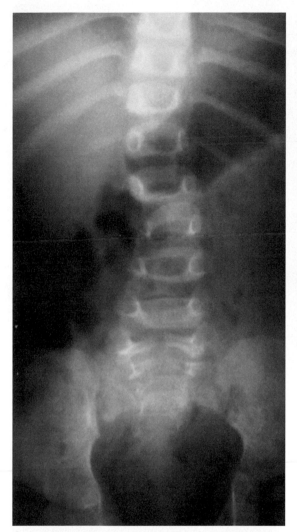

A

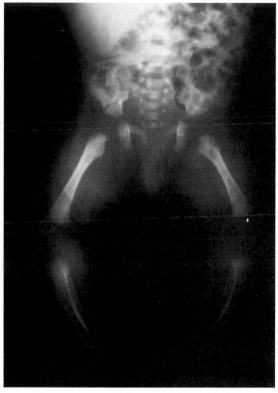

B

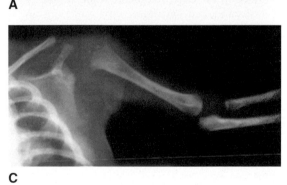

C

FIGURE 2. **A–C,** Radiographs of child in Figure 1. Note the scoliosis and ectopic calcifications, most evident in the shoulder. (Courtesy of Marilyn C. Jones, Children's Hospital, San Diego.)

AUTOSOMAL RECESSIVE CHONDRODYSPLASIA PUNCTATA

(Chondrodysplasia Punctata, Rhizomelic Type)

Short Humeri and Femora, Coronal Cleft in Vertebrae, Punctate Epiphyseal Mineralization

Spranger and colleagues clearly distinguished the rhizomelic (short proximal limb) type of chondrodysplasia punctata as a separate entity from the Conradi-Hünermann or X-linked dominant type of chondrodysplasia punctata. Besides nine personal cases, Spranger and colleagues were able to find 33 additional cases from the literature.

ABNORMALITIES

Growth. Mean birth weight 2.9 kg; birth length 46.6 cm and OFC 32.4 cm; postnatal growth slow, averaging 1 kg in the first 6 months, 0.5 kg in the second 6 months, and 0.5 kg per year thereafter to at least 3 years of age.

Central Nervous System. Mental deficiency, with or without spasticity, microcephaly; although delayed, skills such as smiling, laughing and recognition of familiar voices do develop; more advanced milestones such as walking, sitting without support, speaking in phrases, and toilet training never occur; seizures.

Craniofacies. Low nasal bridge and flat facies with or without upward slanting palpebral fissures; cataracts.

Limbs. Symmetric proximal shortening of humeri and femora; metaphyseal splaying and cupping, especially at the knee, with sparse and irregular trabeculae; epiphyseal and extra-epiphyseal foci of calcification in early infancy with later epiphyseal irregularity; multiple joint contractures.

Spine. Coronal cleft noted on lateral roentgenogram with dysplasia and irregularity of vertebrae.

Pelvis. Trapeziform dysplasia of upper ilium.

OCCASIONAL ABNORMALITIES.

Ichthyosiform skin dysplasia (28%), lipomas, craniocervical junction anomalies, cardiac defects, hip dislocation, delayed myelination, cerebellar atrophy, hemifacial paralysis, diaphragmatic hernia, cleft palate, hypospadias, cryptorchidism.

NATURAL HISTORY. Survival beyond infancy occurs in 90% and to age 6 to 6½ years in 50% of children. Respiratory problems are the major cause of death. Severe feeding problems are common. In children who live beyond 2 months of age, seizures occur in over 80%. Temperature instability is common. Cataract extraction is recommended for visual stimulation and to improve environmental interaction. Otitis media with hearing loss is common. Delayed eruption of teeth as well as dental caries occur frequently. Joint contractures improve with time, and benefit from physical therapy. Curvature of the spine occurs in the majority of children who live beyond 2 months of age.

ETIOLOGY. This disorder has an autosomal recessive inheritance pattern. Three types, all of which are associated with alterations of peroxisomal metabolism and are clinically indistinguishable, have been identified: (1) Those with mutations in the PEX7 gene that encodes peroxin 7, the cytosolic PTS2-receptor protein required for targeting a subset of enzymes to peroxisomes; (2) those with mutations in the gene that encodes peroxisomal dihydroxyacetonephosphate acyltransferase; and (3) those with mutations in the gene that encodes peroxisomal alkyl-dihydroxy-acetonephosphatate synthase.

References

Spranger JW, Opitz JM, Bidder U: Heterogeneity of chondrodysplasia punctata. Humangenetik 11:190, 1970.

Spranger JW, Bidder U, Voelz C: Chondrodysplasia punctata (Chondrodystrophia calcifans). II. Der rhizomele Type. Fortschr Geb Roentgenstr Nuklearmed 114:327, 1971.

Gilbert EF et al: Chondrodysplasia punctata: Rhizomelic form. Eur J Pediatr 123:89, 1976.

Heselson NG, Cremin BJ, Beighton P: Lethal chondrodysplasia punctata. Clin Radiol 29:679, 1978.

Schutgens RBH et al: Peroxisomal disorders: A newly recognized group of genetic diseases. Eur J Pediatr 144:430, 1986.

Schutgens RBH et al: Prenatal and perinatal diagnosis of peroxisomal disorders. J Inherit Metab Dis 12(Suppl 1):118, 1989.

Braverman N et al: Human PEX7 encodes the peroxisomal PTS2 receptor and is responsible for rhizomelic chondrodysplasia punctata. Nat Genet 15:369, 1997.

White AL et al: Natural history of rhizomelic chondrodysplasia punctata. Am J Med Genet 118:332, 2003.

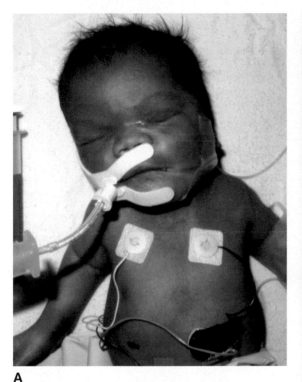

A

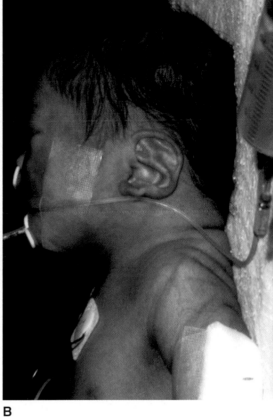

B

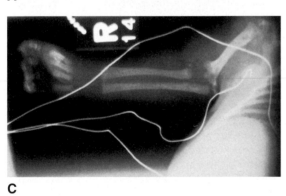

C

FIGURE 1. Autosomal recessive chondrodysplasia punctata syndrome. **A** and **B,** Newborn showing flat face and low nasal bridge. **C,** Radiographs of his arm, showing proximal shortening with aberrant form and punctate mineralization.

HYPOPHOSPHATASIA
(Perinatal Lethal Hypophosphatasia)

Poorly Mineralized Cranium, Short Ribs, Hypoplastic Fragile Bones

Rathbun recognized this disease in 1948, and numerous cases of this autosomal recessive, invariably lethal condition have been documented subsequently.

ABNORMALITIES

Growth. Short limb dwarfism.

Radiographic. Generalized lack of ossification; poorly mineralized globular cranium; poorly formed teeth; hypoplastic fragile bones of varying density with irregular lack of metaphyseal mineralization, bowed lower extremities, characteristic "spurs" in midshaft of ulna and fibula sometimes protruding through skin, and short ribs with rachitic rosary and fractures; small thoracic cage; vertebral bodies, frequently unossified, but sometimes dense, rectangular/round, flattened, sagitally clefted, or butterfly shaped; posterior elements are poorly ossified; clavicles are least affected bones.

OCCASIONAL ABNORMALITIES.
Polyhydramnios, blue sclera.

NATURAL HISTORY.
Death secondary to respiratory insufficiency during early infancy is usual; of those who survive, early failure to thrive, hypotonia, irritability and occasionally seizures, anemia or hypercalcemia, and nephrocalcinosis are common.

ETIOLOGY.
This disorder has an autosomal recessive inheritance pattern with marked radiographic variability. Affected infants have a severe deficiency of tissue and serum alkaline phosphatase and an excessive urinary excretion of phosphoethanolamine. Carriers may have a low value for serum alkaline phosphatase and mildly elevated phosphoethanolamine excretion. This disorder is due to various mutations in the tissue-nonspecific alkaline phosphatase (TNSALP) gene located at chromosome 1p36.1-1p34. Prenatal diagnosis has been accomplished successfully with midtrimester ultrasonography and measurement of the liver/bone/kidney isoenzyme of alkaline phosphatase in chorionic villus sample taken between 10 and 12 weeks of gestation.

COMMENT.
Based on age of onset and major clinical findings, six forms of hypophosphatasia have been characterized: A perinatal lethal form described above; an infantile form that presents within the first 6 months with growth deficiency, rachitic-like skeletal defects resulting in recurrent respiratory infection, increased intracranial pressure, and death in approximately 50% of cases; a milder childhood type that presents after 6 months and is associated with premature loss of deciduous teeth, rachitic-appearing skeletal findings, and craniosynostosis; an adult type that presents later in life with premature loss of adult teeth, recurrent fractures, and pseudofractures; odonto-hypophosphatasia; and a "benign prenatal" form in which angulation or bowing of long bones improves spontaneously prenatally. Autosomal recessive inheritance has been implicated for both the lethal and infantile forms while the mild forms may be dominantly or recessively inherited.

References

Rathbun JC: "Hypophosphatasia": A new developmental anomaly. Am J Dis Child 75:822, 1948.

Rathbun JC et al: Hypophosphatasia: A genetic study. Arch Dis Child 36:540, 1961.

Kellsey DC: Hypophosphatasia and congenital bowing of the long bones. JAMA 179:187, 1962.

MacPherson RI, Kroeker M, Houston CS: Hypophosphatasia. J Can Assoc Radiol 23:16, 1972.

Greenberg CR et al: Infantile hypophosphatasia: Localization within chromosome region 1p36.1-34 and prenatal diagnosis using linked DNA markers. Am J Hum Genet 46:286, 1990.

Brock DJH, Barron L: First-trimester diagnosis of hypophosphatasia: Experience with 16 cases. Prenat Diagn 11:387, 1991.

Shohat M et al: Perinatal lethal hypophosphatasia: Clinical, radiologic and morphologic findings. Pediatr Radiol 21:421, 1991.

Henthorn PS et al: Different missense mutations at the tissue-nonspecific alkaline phosphatase gene locus in autosomal recessively inherited forms of mild and severe hypophosphatasia. Proc Natl Acad Sci USA 89:9924, 1992.

Pauli RM et al: Mild hypophosphatasia mimicking severe osteogenesis imperfecta in utero: Bent but not broken. Am J Med Genet 86:434, 1999.

Zurutuza L et al: Correlations of genotype and phenotype in hypophosphatasia. Hum Mol Genet 8:1039, 1999.

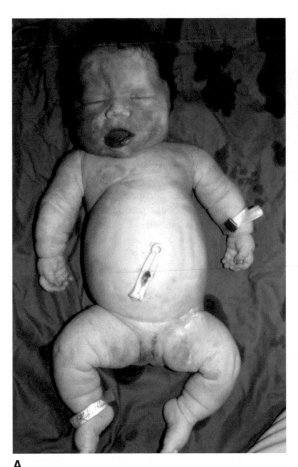

A

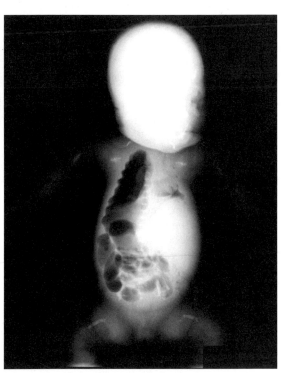

B

FIGURE 1. Hypophosphatasia. **A** and **B,** Stillborn infant with almost complete lack of mineralization of bony skeleton. Serum alkaline phosphatase was low, and there was an increased urinary phosphoethanolamine.

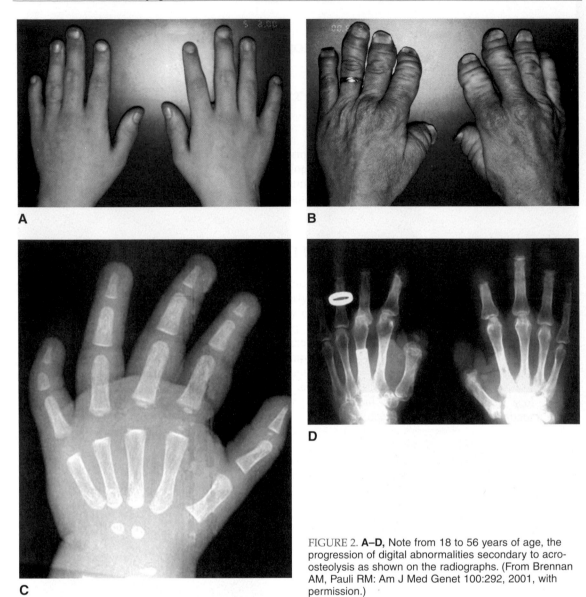

FIGURE 2. **A–D,** Note from 18 to 56 years of age, the progression of digital abnormalities secondary to acro-osteolysis as shown on the radiographs. (From Brennan AM, Pauli RM: Am J Med Genet 100:292, 2001, with permission.)

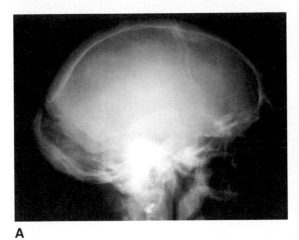

A

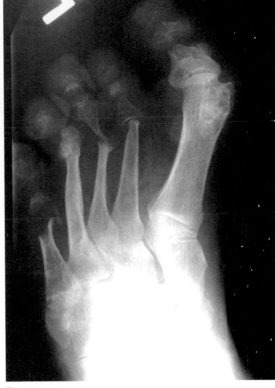

B

FIGURE 3. **A** and **B,** Lateral skull and foot in 56-year-old man showing thickening of the calvarium, prominent occiput and platybasia, and severe acro-osteolysis of virtually all phalanges and metatarsals. (From Brennan AM, Pauli RM: Am J Med Genet 100:292, 2001, with permission.)

CRANIOMETAPHYSEAL DYSPLASIA

Bony Wedge over Bridge of Nose, Mild Splaying of Metaphyses

Often confused with the Pyle metaphyseal dysplasia syndrome, this disorder has more profound craniofacial hyperostosis and less metaphyseal broadening than in Pyle disease. An autosomal dominant and a much rarer and more severe autosomal recessive form have been reported.

ABNORMALITIES

Craniofacial. Thick calvarium with dense base of cranial vault, facial bones, and mandible; macrocephaly; variable absence of pneumatization; unusual thick bony wedge over bridge of nose and supraorbital area with hypertelorism and relatively small nose; variable proptosis of eyes; compression of foramina with cranial nerve deficits, headache, and narrow nasal passages with rhinitis.

Limbs. Mild to moderate metaphyseal broadening with diaphyseal sclerosis, most evident in the distal femora; genu valgum.

OCCASIONAL ABNORMALITIES.

Chiari I malformation, syringomyelia, mental retardation.

NATURAL HISTORY.

Evident from infancy in both forms, in adults with autosomal dominant craniometaphyseal dysplasia, the typical craniofacial appearance becomes less obvious. Clinical features, if present, are mild and consist of compression of cranial nerves, particularly the seventh and eighth. Sclerosis along the suture lines may be the only findings. In the autosomal recessive form, the craniofacial features progress. The skull base becomes more sclerotic with overgrowth and the calvarium becomes progressively hyperostotic with bony encroachment around the orbits and nasal bones. In those cases, severe visual handicaps, bilateral hearing loss, malocclusion, and facial paralysis occur. Prognathism becomes more pronounced with age. Truncal ataxia, responsive to posterior cranial fossa decompression, occurs.

ETIOLOGY.

Both autosomal dominant and autosomal recessive types of disease have been delineated, the latter being more severe in degree. The autosomal dominant type is caused by mutations in the human homologue (ANKH) of the mouse progressive ankylosis gene located on human chromosome 5p15.2-p14.1. The ANK protein spans the outer cell membrane and shuttles inorganic pyrophosphate, a major inhibitor of physiologic and pathologic calcification, bone mineralization, and bone resorption.

References

Spranger J, Paulsen K, Lehmann W: Die Kraniometaphysare Dysplasia. Z Kinderheilkd 93:64, 1965.

Millard DR Jr et al: Craniofacial surgery in craniometaphyseal dysplasia. Am J Surg 113:615, 1967.

Gorlin RJ, Spranger J, Koszalka M: Genetic craniotubular bone dysplasias and hyperostoses: A critical analysis. Birth Defects 5:79, 1969.

Gorlin RJ et al: Pyle's disease (familial metaphyseal dysplasia). J Bone Joint Surg (Am) 52:347, 1970.

Penchaszadeh VB, Gutierrez ER, Figuero P: Autosomal recessive craniometaphyseal dysplasia. Am J Med Genet 5:43, 1980.

Beighton P: Pyle disease (metaphyseal dysplasia). J Med Genet 24:321, 1987.

Hudgins RJ, Edwards MSB: Craniometaphyseal dysplasia associated with hydrocephalus: Case report. Neurosurgery 20:617, 1987.

Cole DEC, Cohen MM: A new look at craniometaphyseal dysplasia. J Pediatr 112:577, 1988.

Elcioglu N, Hall CM: Temporal aspects in craniometaphyseal dysplasia: Autosomal recessive type. Am J Med Genet 76:245, 1998.

Nurnberg P et al: Heterozygous mutations in ANKH, the human ortholog of the mouse progressive ankylosis gene, result in craniometaphyseal dysplasia. Nat Genet 28:37, 2001.

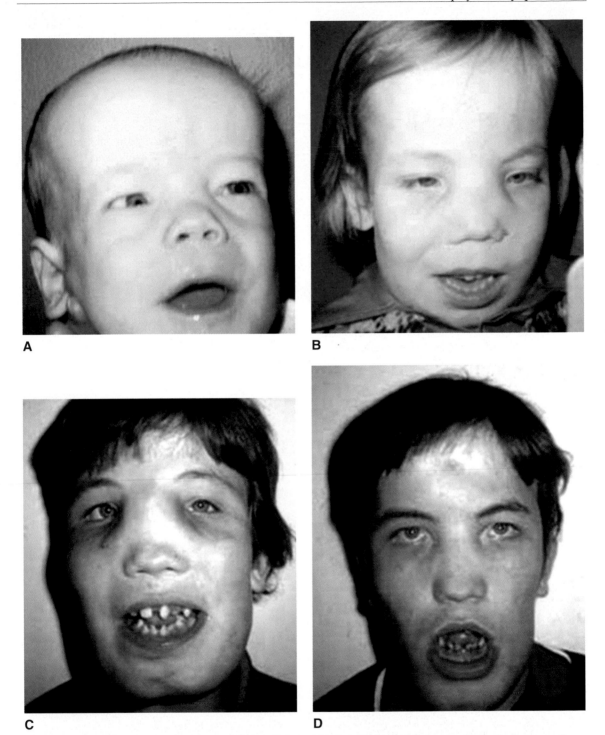

FIGURE 1. Craniometaphyseal dysplasia. **A–D,** An affected child showing the facial changes that took place over time. Note the craniofacial findings at 7 months, 3 years, 12 years, and 16 years of age, respectively. (From Feingold M: Am J Med Genet 86:501, 1999, with permission.)

FRONTOMETAPHYSEAL DYSPLASIA

Prominent Supraorbital Ridges, Joint Limitations, Splayed Metaphyses

More than 30 cases of this disorder have been reported since Gorlin and Cohen's initial description in 1969.

ABNORMALITIES

Craniofacial. Coarse facies with wide nasal bridge and prominent supraorbital ridges; incomplete sinus development; partial anodontia, delayed eruption, and retained deciduous teeth; high palate; small mandible with decreased angle and prominent antigonial notch.

Limbs. Flexion contracture of fingers, wrists, elbows, knees, and ankles; arachnodactyly with disproportionately wide and elongated phalanges; increased density in diaphyseal region with lack of modeling in metaphyseal region, giving Erlenmeyer-flask appearance to femur and tibia; partial fusion of carpal and of tarsal bones.

Other Skeletal. Wide foramen magnum with various cervical vertebral anomalies and wide interpedicular distance of vertebrae; flared pelvis with constriction of supra acetabular area; chest cage deformities; winged scapulae; scoliosis.

Other. Mixed conductive and sensorineural hearing loss, which progresses; wasting of muscles of arms and legs, especially hypothenar and interosseous muscles of hands.

OCCASIONAL ABNORMALITIES.

Mental retardation; ocular hypertelorism with downslanting palpebral fissures; myopia; obstructive uropathy; cardiac murmur, cause unknown; subglottic tracheal narrowing.

NATURAL HISTORY. Affected individuals are usually asymptomatic at birth. The restriction of joint mobility and development of contractures are progressive. Respiratory difficulties including subglottic stenosis can lead to significant morbidity and even death. Severe progressive scoliosis has occurred. Anesthesia can be a significant problem. All patients should be evaluated to rule out urologic abnormalities.

ETIOLOGY. This disorder has an X-linked inheritance pattern with severe manifestations in males and variable but more mildly affected females. Mutations in the gene (FLNA) located at Xq28 are responsible. FLNA codes for filamin A, a widely expressed protein that regulates reorganization of the actin cytoskeleton.

COMMENT. Mutations in FLNA are responsible for three additional X-linked disorders, otopalatodigital syndrome, types 1 and 2, and Melnick-Needles syndrome. All four of these disorders have a number of clinically overlapping features.

References

Gorlin RJ, Cohen MM: Frontometaphyseal dysplasia: A new syndrome. Am J Dis Child 118:487, 1969.

Danks DM et al: Fronto-metaphyseal dysplasia: A progressive disease of bone and connective tissue. Am J Dis Child 123:254, 1972.

Gorlin RJ, Winder RB: Frontometaphyseal dysplasia—evidence for X-linked inheritance. Am J Med Genet 5:81, 1980.

Fitzsimmons JS et al: Frontometaphyseal dysplasia: Further delineation of the clinical syndrome. Clin Genet 22:195, 1982.

Verloes A et al: Fronto-otopalatodigital dysplasia: Clinical evidence for a single entity encompassing Melnick-Needles syndrome, otopalatodigital syndromes, type 1 and 2, and frontometaphyseal dysplasia. Am J Med Genet 90:407, 2000.

Morava E et al: Clinical and genetic heterogeneity in frontometaphyseal dysplasia: Severe progressive scoliosis in two families. Am J Med Genet 116:272, 2003.

Robertson SP et al: Localized mutations in the gene encoding the cytoskeletal protein filamin A cause diverse malformations in humans. Nat Genet 33:487, 2003.

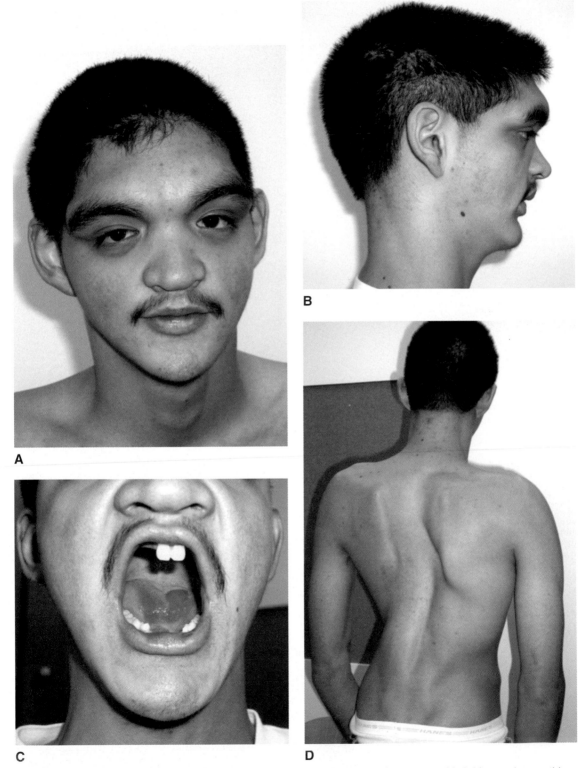

FIGURE 1. Frontometaphyseal dysplasia. **A–D,** Note wide nasal bridge, prominent supraorbital ridges, micrognathia, partial anodontia, and scoliosis. (Courtesy of Dr. H. Eugene Hoyme, Stanford University, Palo Alto.)

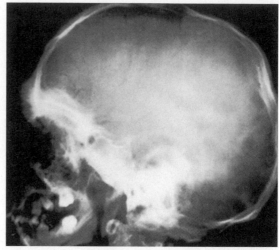

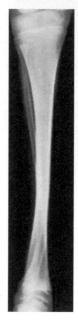

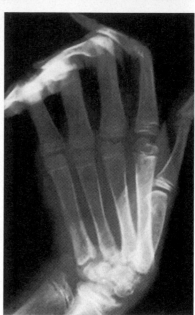

FIGURE 2. The skull shows supraorbital bossing with small paranasal sinuses. Note metaphyseal flaring of tibia; long, poorly modeled tubular bones of hands; and partial lysis of carpal bones. (From Danks DM et al: Am J Dis Child 123:254, 1972, with permission.)

K Osteochondrodysplasia with Osteopetrosis

OSTEOPETROSIS: AUTOSOMAL RECESSIVE—LETHAL
(SEVERE OSTEOPETROSIS)

Dense, Thick, Fragile Bone; Secondary Pancytopenia; Cranial Nerve Compression

More than 100 cases of this lethal disorder have been reported since its initial description. Two different cellular anomalies occur—prevention of the formation of osteoclasts through a defect in differentiation of osteoclast progenitors or a failure to activate differentiated mature osteoclasts. In both cases there is absence of proper bone resorption and an increased bone mass. It is estimated to occur in 1 of 200,000 births.

ABNORMALITIES

Skeletal. Thick, dense, fragile bone with modeling alterations such as obtuse mandibular angle, partial aplasia of distal phalanges, straight femora, block-like "bone within a bone" metacarpals, and macrocephaly with frontal bossing; marrow compression leads to pancytopenia, and compression of cranial foramina may lead to deafness, blindness, vestibular nerve dysfunction, extraocular muscle paralysis, other cranial nerve palsies, blindness, and/or hydrocephalus; primary molars and permanent dentition tend to be distorted and teeth fail to erupt; periodontal attachment is poor, allowing for exfoliation; early decay; fractures are common.

Metabolic. Serum calcium level may be low and serum phosphorus level elevated, increased alkaline phosphatase.

Other. Hepatosplenomegaly, mental retardation, growth deficiency.

NATURAL HISTORY. Often evident at birth, with subsequent severe complications and death from anemia, bleeding, or overwhelming infection in infancy or childhood. Ocular involvement, occurring at a median age of 2 months, is the most common presenting sign followed by

seizures from hypocalcemia. The natural course of the disease results in survival of 30% of patients at 6 years of age. Without treatment, life expectancy rarely exceeds adolescence. Problems of dentition and dental infection may become serious. Neurologic deterioration occurs infrequently. Tests of cognition, adaptation, and language development revealed widely scattered abilities from profound delay to average. Gross motor skills were mildly to moderately delayed in the first 2 years; however, for those who survive beyond 4 years, the majority were ambulatory.

ETIOLOGY. This disorder has an autosomal recessive inheritance pattern. Mutations in two genes involved in ion transport, ATP6i (TCIRG1), located at 11q13, responsible for about 50% of cases and CLCN7 chloride channel gene, located at 16p13.3 have been identified. In addition, a mutation in GL, homologous to mouse gray-lethal, leads to a subset of affected infants. Gray-lethal function in the mouse is critical for osteoclast and melanocyte function and maturation. Two less severe forms of osteopetrosis exist: a rare autosomal recessive disorder that usually presents in the second year of life with fractures and is associated with renal tubular acidosis, cerebral calcifications, and low levels of carbonic anhydrase II and a relatively common mild form of osteopetrosis with delayed manifestations and autosomal dominant inheritance referred to as Albers-Schonberg disease. In addition to the autosomal recessive lethal form, mutations in the CLCN7 chloride channel gene on 16p13.3 are responsible for Albers-Schonberg disease. In this latter form, diagnosis is often made by chance when radiographs are taken for other reasons. Bone pain occurs in 25% of cases. Facial palsy and deafness, as well as involvement of the optic and trigeminal nerves, occur infrequently. Osteomyelitis, particularly of the mandible, occurs frequently. Mild skeletal changes become apparent in childhood. Life span is normal.

COMMENT. Hematopoietic stem cell transplantation (HSCT) is the only potentially curative approach for this disorder. After successful HSCT, no further deterioration in vision was noted in the majority of children involved in a long-term outcome study, particularly in those in whom the procedure was performed before 3 months of age.

References

Albers-Schönberg H: Eine bisher nicht beschriebene Allgemeinekrankung des Skelettes im Röntgenbilde. Fortschr Geb Roentgenstrahlen Nuklearmed 11:261, 1907.

Beighton P, Horan F, Hamersma H: A review of the osteopetroses. Postgrad Med J 53:507, 1977.

Shapiro F: Osteopetrosis: Current clinical considerations. Clin Orthop 294:34, 1993.

Gerritsen EJA et al: Autosomal recessive osteopetrosis: Variability of findings at diagnosis and during the natural course. Pediatrics 93:247, 1994.

Charles JM, Key LL: Developmental spectrum of children with osteopetrosis. J Pediatr 132:371, 1998.

Cleiren E et al: Albers-Schonberg disease (autosomal dominant osteopetrosis, type II) results from mutations in the (CLCN7) chloride channel gene. Hum Mol Genet 10:2861, 2001.

Sobacchi C et al: The mutational spectrum of human malignant autosomal recessive osteopetrosis. Hum Mol Genet 10:1767, 2001.

Driessen GJA et al: Long-term outcome of haematopoietic stem cell transplantation in autosomal recessive osteopetrosis: An EBMT report. Bone Marrow Transplant 32:637, 2003.

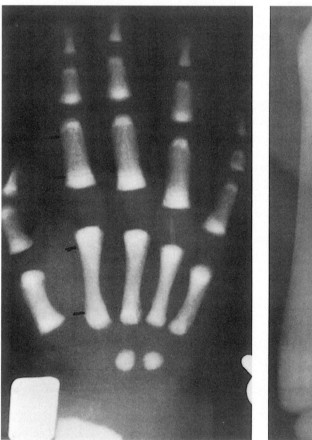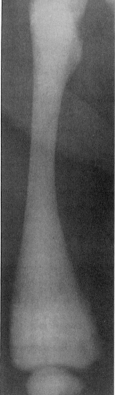

FIGURE 1. Osteopetrosis: autosomal recessive—lethal. An 8-month-old child. The sclerotic skeleton shows the "bone within a bone" (endobone) appearance, vertical striations at the metaphyseal-diaphyseal juncture, and broad metaphyses.

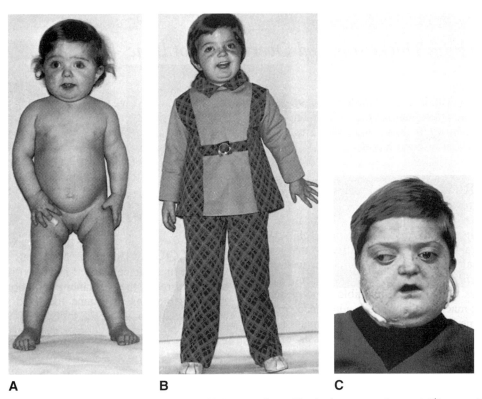

A   **B**   **C**

FIGURE 2. Same child at 2 years (**A**), with length at third percentile and beginning genu valgum; at 3½ years (**B**), with vision lost, despite attempted decompression of optic nerve; and at 10½ years (**C**), with proptosis and mandibular osteitis. Her death at 11 years resulted from carotid artery compression. (Courtesy of Dr. Dag Aarskog, Bergen, Norway.)

LENZ-MAJEWSKI HYPEROSTOSIS SYNDROME

Dense, Thick Bone; Symphalangism; Hypotrophic Skin

Since 1974, when Lenz and Majewski first proposed this condition as a distinct syndrome, only seven patient reports have appeared in the literature. However, at least three other isolated cases have been published as "unknown" multiple malformation syndromes. The features in infancy differ greatly from those in older childhood, producing difficulties in early diagnosis.

ABNORMALITIES

Growth. Intrauterine growth retardation, postnatal short stature, eventual severe emaciation.
Performance. Moderate to severe mental retardation.
Craniofacial. Disproportionately large cranium with broad and prominent forehead late closure of large fontanels; hypertelorism with protuberant eyes; frequent choanal stenosis or atresia, nasolacrimal duct stenosis.
Skin. Cutis laxa in infancy; later, skin becomes hypotrophic and thin with prominent, subcutaneous veins, especially over the scalp; cutaneous syndactyly of the digits; absence of elastic fibers on skin biopsy.
Hair. Sparse in infancy.
Teeth. Dysplastic enamel.
Limbs. Syndactyly, brachydactyly.
Skeletal. Proximal symphalangism, delayed ossification of ulnar rays, short or absent middle phalanges, and dorsiflexion of fingers; broad, thick ribs and clavicles; widespread cortical sclerosis and thickening of bone in diaphyses, calvarium, vertebrae, and skull base; shallow and distorted orbits; long, flared, and radiolucent metaphyses, osteopenic epiphyses, long bone hyperostosis; delayed bone age.
Genitalia. Cryptorchidism and inguinal hernia in boys.

OCCASIONAL ABNORMALITIES.

Large, floppy ears, small tongue, micrognathia, cerebral atrophy, dysgenesis of corpus callosum, flexion contractures at elbows and knees, hypospadias/chordee, inguinal hernia, dislocated hips (one case), early death.

NATURAL HISTORY. At birth, cutis laxa, large fontanels, and syndactyly are the most prominent features. Progressive hyperostosis becomes evident only after the first 6 months of life, often leading to erroneous diagnosis in infancy. Choanal stenosis may cause respiratory insufficiency and repeated episodes of pneumonia. Later, this problem may be aggravated by relative thoracic immobility caused by rib widening. Poor weight gain and slow statural growth persist even after resolution of infantile feeding difficulties. The original patient described by Lenz and Majewski is now 30 years of age. She is 120 cm tall, speaks only a few words, and is ambulatory.

ETIOLOGY. The cause of this disorder is unknown. All cases have been sporadic. New mutation for a dominant gene has been suggested because of a tendency toward increased parental age.

References

Kaye CI, Fischer DE, Esterly BE: Cutis laxa, skeletal anomalies and ambiguous genitalia. Am J Dis Child 127:115, 1974.

Lenz WD, Majewski FA: A generalized disorder of the connective tissues with progeria, choanal atresia, symphalangism, hypoplasia of dentine and craniodiaphyseal hyperostosis. Birth Defects 10(12):133, 1974.

Robinow M, Johanson AJ, Smith TH: The Lenz-Majewski hyperostotic dwarfism: A syndrome of multiple congenital anomalies, mental retardation and progressive skeletal sclerosis. J Pediatr 91:417, 1977.

Gorlin RJ, Whitley CB: Lenz-Majewski syndrome. Radiology 149:129, 1983.

Majewski F: Lenz-Majewski hyperostotic dwarfism: Reexamination of the original patient. Am J Med Genet 93:335, 2000.

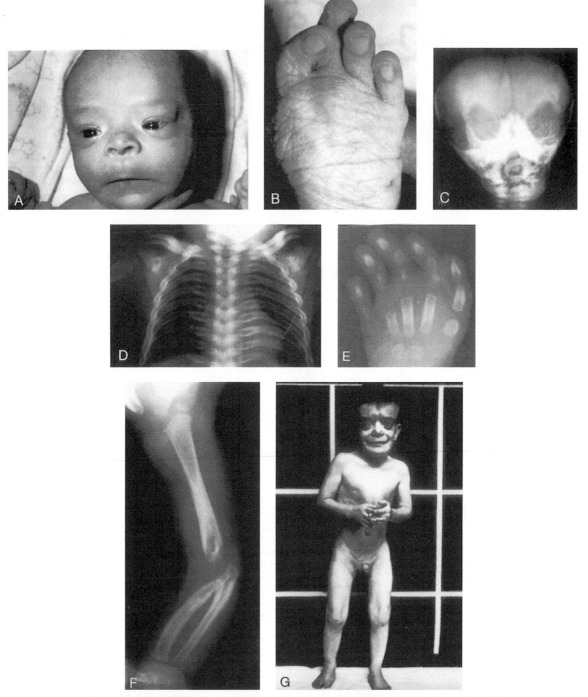

FIGURE 1. Lenz-Majewski hyperostosis syndrome. **A** and **B,** A 2-month-old boy with broad, prominent forehead; ocular hypertelorism; cutaneous syndactyly with dorsiflexed fingers; and cutis laxa. Radiographs of the same patient at 1 year reveal sclerosis of skull base (**C**), broad ribs and clavicles (**D**), symphalangism and hypoplasia of middle phalanges (**E**), and diaphyseal undermodeling and cortical thickening with radiolucent metaphyses and epiphyses (**F**). (**A–F**, Courtesy of Dr. Jon Aase, University of New Mexico, Albuquerque.) **G,** The changing phenotype is demonstrated by a boy, 4½ years old, who has a square forehead with bifrontal bossing, ocular hypertelorism, and flexion contractures at elbows and knees. (**G**, Courtesy of Dr. Meinhard Robinow, Children's Medical Center, Dayton, Ohio.)

PYKNODYSOSTOSIS

Osteosclerosis, Short Distal Phalanges, Delayed Closure of Fontanels

Though cleidocranial dysostosis associated with osteosclerosis and bone fragility had been recognized before 1962, this condition was not well clarified until Maroteaux and Lamy described it as pyknodysostosis (*pyknos* meaning dense).

ABNORMALITIES

Growth. Small stature with adult height of less than 150 cm.

Skeletal. Osteosclerosis with tendency toward transverse fracture.

Craniofacial. Frontal and occipital prominence, delayed closure of sutures, persistence of anterior fontanel, wormian bones, lack of frontal sinus; facial hypoplasia with prominent nose and narrow grooved palate; obtuse angle to mandible, which may be small.

Dentition. Irregular permanent teeth with or without partial anodontia, delayed eruption, caries.

Clavicle. Dysplasia to loss of acromion end.

Digits. Acro-osteolytic dysplasia of distal phalanges, especially of index finger; wrinkled skin over dorsa of distal fingers; flattened and grooved nails.

OCCASIONAL ABNORMALITIES.
Mental retardation, scoliosis, vertebral arch defects in the interarticular parts or pedicles, most frequently at L5.

NATURAL HISTORY. Approximately two thirds of the patients have had fractures, most commonly the mandible, clavicle, and lower extremities, including the metatarsals. There may be a progressive degeneration of the distal phalanges and outer clavicle and persistent open fontanels, especially posteriorly. Special dental care is often indicated. Osteomyelitis of the jaw occurs frequently.

ETIOLOGY. This disorder has an autosomal recessive inheritance pattern. Mutations in the cathepsin K gene located at chromosome 1q21 are responsible. Cathepsin K is involved in the process of bone resorption.

COMMENT. The artist Toulouse-Lautrec may have had pyknodysostosis.

References

Thomsen G, Guttadauro M: Cleidocranial dysostosis associated with osteosclerosis and bone fragility. Acta Radiol 37:559, 1952.

Maroteaux P, Lamy M: La pycnodysostose. Presse Med 70:999, 1962.

Shuler SE: Pycnodysostosis. Arch Dis Child 38:620, 1963.

Elmore SM: Pycnodysostosis: A review. J Bone Joint Surg [Am] 49A:153, 1967.

Mills KLG, Johnson AW: Pyknodysostosis. J Med Genet 25:550, 1988.

Gelb BD et al: Pycnodysostosis, a lysosomal disease caused by cathepsin K deficiency. Science 273:1236, 1996.

Bathi RJ, Masur VN: Pyknodysostosis—a report of two cases with a brief review of the literature. Int J Oral Maxillofac Surg 29:439, 2000.

Haagerup A et al: Cathepsin K gene mutations and 1q21 haplotypes in patients with pyknodysostosis in an outbred population. Eur J Hum Genet 8:431, 2000.

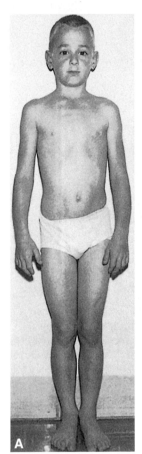

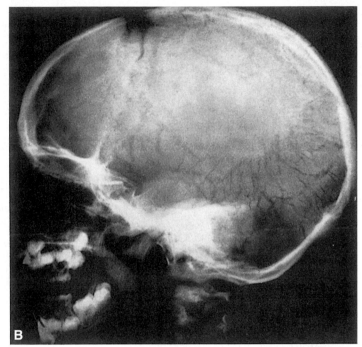

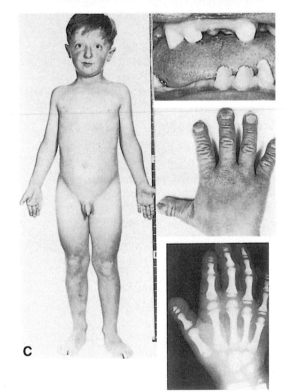

FIGURE 1. Pyknodysostosis. **A,** A 10-year-old child with height age of 8½ years. **B,** Same patient shown in **A**. Note the open fontanel and lamboid suture, absence of frontal sinus or mastoid air cells, obtuse angle of mandible, and delay in eruption of permanent dentition. **C,** A 7½-year-old with height age of 4½ years. Note the generally dense bone and partial loss of several distal phalanges. (**C,** From Shuler SE: Arch Dis Child 38:620, 1963, with permission.)

CLEIDOCRANIAL DYSOSTOSIS

Defect of Clavicle, Late Ossification of Cranial Sutures, Delayed Eruption of Teeth

A possible example of this rather generalized dysplasia of osseous and dental tissues was detected in the skull of a Neanderthal man. The more obvious features of the defect in the clavicle and cranium prompted Marie and Sainton to use the term cleidocranial dysostosis for this condition. However, the more generalized dysplasia of bone and teeth has been emphasized, and the term cleidocranial dysostosis depicts only a portion of the abnormal development. Well over 500 cases have been reported.

ABNORMALITIES

Growth. Slight to moderate shortness of stature.

Craniofacial. Brachycephaly with bossing of frontal, parietal, and occipital bones; late closure of fontanels and mineralization of sutures; late or incomplete development of accessory sinuses and mastoid air cells; wormian bones; small sphenoid bones; calvarial thickening; midfacial hypoplasia with low nasal bridge, narrow high-arched palate; hypertelorism.

Dentition. Late eruption, especially the permanent teeth, which are often abnormal with aplasia, malformed roots, retention cysts, enamel hypoplasia, enhanced caries, supernumerary teeth.

Clavicle and Chest. Partial to complete aplasia of clavicle with associated muscle defects, small thorax with short oblique ribs.

Hands. Hand anomalies including asymmetric length of fingers with long second metacarpal, short middle phalanges of second and fifth fingers, short and tapering distal phalanges with or without down-curving nails, cone-shaped phalangeal epiphyses in childhood, accessory proximal metacarpal epiphyses that fuse in childhood, and slow rate of carpal ossification.

Other Skeletal. Delayed mineralization of pubic bone with wide symphysis pubis, narrow pelvis, broad femoral head with short femoral neck, with or without coxa vara, lateral notching of proximal femoral ossification centers, spondylolysis, spondylolisthesis.

OCCASIONAL ABNORMALITIES.
Cervical rib, small scapulae, syringomyelia, scoliosis, kyphosis, flat acetabula, genu valga, scoliosis, pes planus, osteosclerosis, increased bone fragility, deafness, cleft palate, micrognathia.

NATURAL HISTORY.
Although stature is often reduced, mentality is usually normal. Hearing should be assessed, and dental problems should be anticipated. Removal of deciduous teeth does not seem to hasten the eruption of permanent teeth, and the permanent teeth may be difficult to extract because of malformed roots. A narrow pelvis may necessitate cesarean section in the pregnant woman with this condition. A narrow thorax may lead to respiratory distress in early infancy. Upper respiratory complications and sinus infections are common.

ETIOLOGY.
Autosomal dominant inheritance with wide variability in expression. Mutations in RUNX2, formerly known as the core-binding factor α-1 (CBFA1) gene, located at 6p21, are responsible. RUNX2 plays an important role in osteogenesis, and differentiation of precursor cells of the clavicular anlage as well as having an important role in regulating many osteogenesis genes and chondrocyte differentiation.

References

Marie P, Sainton P: Observation d'hydrocéphalie héréditaire (père et fils) par vice de développement du crane et du cerveau. Bull Mem Soc Med Hop (Paris) 14:706, 1897.

Grieg DM: Neanderthal skull presenting features of cleidocranial dysostosis and other peculiarities. Edinburgh Med J 40:407, 1933.

Lasker GW: The inheritance of cleidocranial dysostosis. Hum Biol 18:103, 1946.

Jackson WPU: Osteo-dental dysplasia (cleidocranial dysostosis). The "Arnold head." Acta Med Scand 139:292, 1951.

Forland M: Cleidocranial dysostosis: A review of the syndrome and report of a sporadic case, with hereditary transmission. Am J Med 33:792, 1962.

Fauré C, Maroteaux P: Cleidocranial dysplasia. In Kaufman HJ (ed): Progress in Pediatric Radiology, vol. 4. Basel: Karger, 1973, pp 211–238.

Jarvis JL, Keats TE: Cleidocranial dysostosis: A review of 40 new cases. AJR 121:5, 1974.

Mundlos S et al: Genetic mapping of cleidocranial dysplasia and evidence of a microdeletion in one family. Hum Mol Genet 4:71, 1995.

Mundlos S: Cleidocranial dysplasia: Clinical and molecular genetics. J Med Genet 36:177, 1999.

Cohen MM: RUNX genes, neoplasia, and cleidocranial dysplasia. Am J Med Genet 104:185, 2001.

Cooper SC et al: A natural history of cleidocranial dysplasia. Am J Med Genet 104:1, 2001.

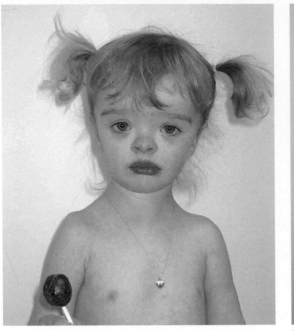

A

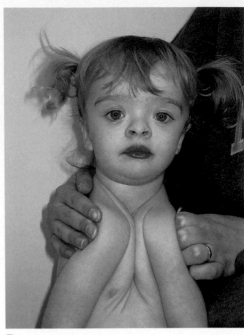

B

FIGURE 1. **A–E,** Cleidocranial dysostosis in a 4-year-old girl and 11-year-old boy. Note the absent clavicles and hypoplasia of the ilia with widespread pubic rami. (**A** and **B,** Courtesy of Dr. Stephen Braddock, University of Missouri, Columbia.) *Continued*

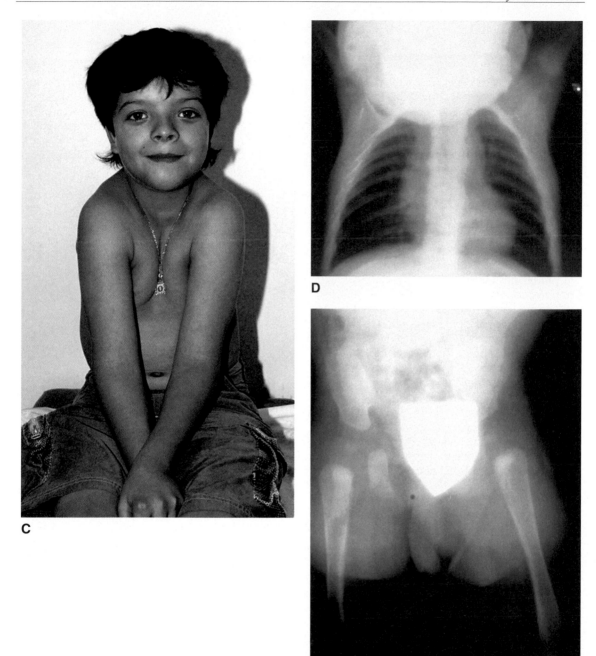

Fig. 1, cont'd. (**C,** Courtesy of Dr. Marilyn C. Jones, Children's Hospital, San Diego.)

YUNIS-VARON SYNDROME

Yunis and Varon reported five patients from three families with this disorder in 1980. An additional nine affected children have been described subsequently.

ABNORMALITIES

Performance. Severe developmental delay in two out of three children who survived the neonatal period.

Growth. Prenatal growth deficiency (approximately 50% of patients); severe failure to thrive postnatally.

Craniofacial. Microcephaly; sparse scalp hair, eyebrows, and eyelashes; wide calvarial sutures and enlarged fontanels; short upslanting palpebral fissures; anteverted nares; labiogingival retraction; short philtrum; thin lips; low-set/dysplastic ears with hypoplastic lobes; loose nuchal skin; broad secondary alveolar ridge; micrognathia.

Limbs. Agenesis/hypoplasia of thumbs and great toes; short tapering fingers and toes with nail hypoplasia; agenesis/hypoplasia of distal phalanges of fingers and toes, middle phalanges of fingers and first metatarsals; simian crease.

Other Skeletal. Absence or hypoplasia of one or both clavicles; absent sternal ossification; pelvic dysplasia; hip dislocation; abnormal scapula.

OCCASIONAL ABNORMALITIES.

Absent nipples; external genital anomalies; sclerocornea; cataracts; mild ocular hypertelorism; premature loss of deciduous teeth; cystic dental follicles; glossoptosis; central nervous system malformations including arrhinencephaly, agenesis of the corpus callosum, abnormality of cerebellar vermis, hydrocephalus, delayed brain maturation; tetralogy of Fallot; cardiomyopathy; hypertension; atrophy of left lobe of liver and anomalous hepatic vessel; syndactyly of fingers and toes.

NATURAL HISTORY. Death in the neonatal period has occurred in 8 of 11 live-born infants. Although intellectual performance was normal in one mildly affected 3-year-old boy, the other two children who survived the neonatal period had severe developmental delay at 1 and 4 years of age, respectively.

ETIOLOGY. This disorder has an autosomal recessive inheritance pattern. Prominent intraneuronal inclusions with vacuolar degeneration, noted in the thalamic, dentate nuclei, cerebellar cortex, and inferior olivary nuclei, were noted in one patient on autopsy, and are suggestive of a lysosomal storage disease.

References

Yunis E, Varon H: Cleidocranial dysostosis, severe micrognathism, bilateral absence of thumbs and first metatarsal bones, and distal aphlangia: A new genetic syndrome. Am J Dis Child 134:649, 1980.

Hughes HE, Partington MW: Brief clinical report: The syndrome of Yunis and Varon—report of a further case. Am J Med Genet 14:539, 1983.

Garrett G et al: Yunis-Varon syndrome with osteodysplasia. J Med Genet 27:114, 1990.

Ades LD et al: Congenital heart malformation in Yunis-Varon syndrome. J Med Genet 30:788, 1993.

Walch E et al: Yunis-Veron syndrome: Evidence for a lysosomal storage disease. Am J Med Genet 95:157, 2000.

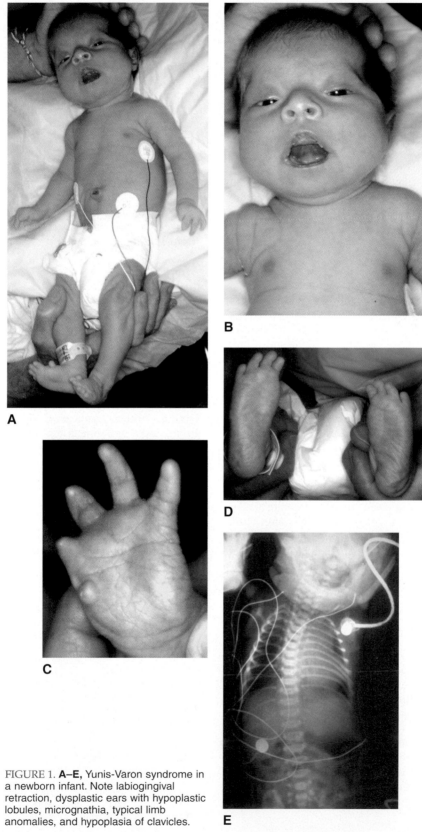

FIGURE 1. **A–E,** Yunis-Varon syndrome in a newborn infant. Note labiogingival retraction, dysplastic ears with hypoplastic lobules, micrognathia, typical limb anomalies, and hypoplasia of clavicles.

L Craniosynostosis Syndromes

SAETHRE-CHOTZEN SYNDROME

Brachycephaly with Maxillary Hypoplasia, Prominent Ear Crus, Syndactyly

Originally described by Saethre and by Chotzen in the early 1930s, this disorder was more recently appreciated as a distinct entity.

ABNORMALITIES

Craniofacial. Disturbance of cranial development including craniosynostosis of coronal, lambdoid, or metopic sutures; late closing fontanels, parietal foramina; and both ossification defects and hyperostosis of the calvarium; brachycephaly with high flat forehead; low frontal hairline; maxillary hypoplasia with narrow palate; facial asymmetry with deviation of nasal septum; shallow orbits; hypertelorism; ptosis of eyelids; lacrimal duct abnormalities; prominent ear crus extending from the root of the helix across the concha; small, posteriorly rotated ears.

Limbs. Cutaneous syndactyly, usually partial, most commonly of second and third fingers or third and fourth toes; mild to moderate brachydactyly with small distal phalanges and clinodactyly of fifth finger; single upper palmar crease; short angulated or flattened thumbs; broad great toes with valgus deformity; finger-like thumbs; limited elbow extension; delayed bone age.

Other. Short clavicles with distal hypoplasia.

OCCASIONAL ABNORMALITIES.
Increased intracranial pressure; mental deficiency; small stature; cleft palate; teeth with broad, bulbous crowns, thin, narrow tapering roots, and diffuse pulp stones in the pulp chambers of all posterior teeth; deafness; strabismus; radioulnar synostosis, vertebral anomalies, particularly of the cervical spine; short fourth metacarpals; hallucal reduplication; triangular shape of the epiphysis and duplicated terminal phalanges of great toe; presumed cardiac anomaly (murmur); cryptorchidism; renal anomaly.

NATURAL HISTORY. Although most patients are apparently of normal intelligence, mental deficiency of mild to moderate degree has been a feature. Facial appearance tends to improve during childhood.

ETIOLOGY. This disorder has an autosomal dominant inheritance pattern. Mutations of the TWIST gene located at 7p21-p22 are responsible. An extremely wide variance in expression exists, and craniosynostosis is a variable feature. A significant number of affected individuals have deletions in 7p21.1 that encompass the TWIST gene. Those with large deletions in this region have, in addition to the characteristic features of Saethre-Chotzen syndrome, significant learning difficulties, thus delineating a new microdeletion or contiguous gene syndrome.

References

Saethre H: Ein Beitrag zum Turmschaedelproblem (Pathogenese, Erblichkeit und Symptomatologie). Z Nervenheilkd 117:533, 1931.

Chotzen F: Eine eigenartige familiare Entwicklungs-störung (Akrocephalosyndaktylie, Dysostosis craniofacialis und Hypertelorismus). Monatsschr Kinderheilkd 55:97, 1932.

Aase JM, Smith DW: Facial asymmetry and abnormalities of palms and ears: A dominantly inherited developmental syndrome. J Pediatr 76:928, 1970.

Pantke OA et al: The Saethre-Chotzen syndrome. Birth Defects 11(2):190, 1975.

Friedman JM et al: Saethre-Chotzen syndrome: A broad and variable pattern of skeletal malformations. J Pediatr 91:929, 1977.

Reardon W, Winter RM: Saethre-Chotzen syndrome. J Med Genet 31:393, 1994.

El Ghouzzi V et al: Mutations of the TWIST gene in the Saethre-Chotzen syndrome. Nat Genet 15:42, 1997.

Howard TD et al: Mutations in TWIST, a basic helix-loop-helix transcription factor, in Saethre-Chotzen syndrome. Nat Genet 15:36, 1997.

Johnson D et al: A comprehensive screen for TWIST mutations in patients with craniosynostosis identified a new microdeletion syndrome of chromosome band 7p21.1. Am J Hum Genet 63:1282, 1998.

Trusen A et al: The pattern of skeletal anomalies in the cervical spine, hands, and feet in patients with Saethre-Chotzen syndrome. Pediatr Radiol 33:168, 2003.

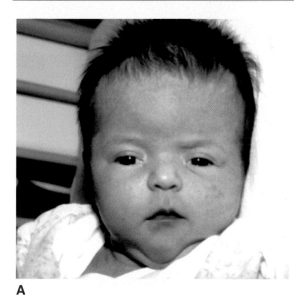

A

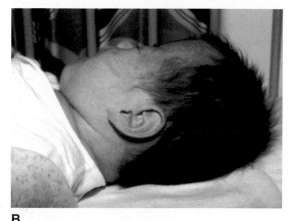

B

C

FIGURE 1. Saethre-Chotzen syndrome. **A–C,** A 1-month-old child showing brachycephaly with high flat forehead, shallow orbits, prominent ear crus, and brachydactyly. (Courtesy of Dr. Marilyn C. Jones, Children's Hospital, San Diego.)

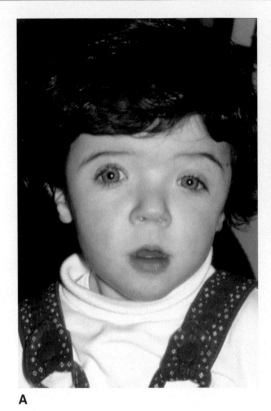

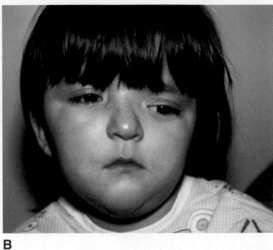

B

Continued

A

FIGURE 2. **A–E,** Two children and an adult. Note ocular hypertelorism, high flat forehead, maxillary hypoplasia, ptosis, prominent ear crus extending from the root of the helix across the concha, cutaneous syndactyly, and fifth finger clinodactyly. (Courtesy of Dr. Michael Cohen, Dalhousie University, Halifax, Nova Scotia.)

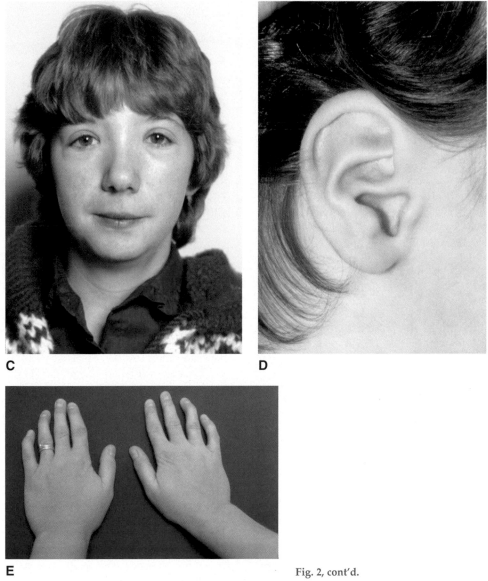

C

D

E

Fig. 2, cont'd.

PFEIFFER SYNDROME
(Pfeiffer-Type Acrocephalosyndactyly)

Brachycephaly, Mild Syndactyly, Broad Thumbs and Toes

Since this disorder was reported by Pfeiffer in 1964, many cases have been published.

ABNORMALITIES

Craniofacial. Brachycephaly with craniosynostosis of coronal, with or without sagittal sutures with full high forehead, ocular hypertelorism, shallow orbits, proptosis, strabismus, small nose with low nasal bridge, narrow maxilla.

Hands and Feet. Broad, medially deviated distal phalanges of thumb and big toe, proximal phalanx of thumb and great toe is frequently a delta phalanx, small middle phalanges of fingers, partial syndactyly of second and third fingers and second, third, and fourth toes.

Other. Hearing loss secondary to anatomic abnormalities of external auditory canal and middle ear.

OCCASIONAL ABNORMALITIES.

Choanal atresia; ocular anterior chamber dysgenesis; cartilaginous trachea; laryngo-, tracheo-, and bronchomalacia; kleeblattschädel anomaly (cloverleaf skull); radiohumeral synostosis of elbow; symphalangism of index finger; fused vertebrae; mental retardation; hydrocephalus; Arnold-Chiari malformation; seizures; fifth finger clinodactyly; intestinal malrotation; imperforate anus; cryptorchidism.

NATURAL HISTORY AND COMMENT.

Three clinical subtypes have been delineated by Cohen that are significant with respect to prognosis. Patients with type 1 have the "classic" phenotype with craniosynostosis, broad thumbs and great toes, variable degrees of syndactyly, and normal to near normal intelligence. This type is compatible with life. Type 2 is associated with cloverleaf skull, severe ocular proptosis, severe central nervous system involvement, elbow ankylosis/synostosis, broad thumbs and great toes, and a variety of low-frequency visceral anomalies. Affected children generally do poorly, with early death. Type 3 Pfeiffer syndrome is similar to type 2 but lacks cloverleaf skull. Although the vast majority of children with types 2 and 3 do very poorly, a favorable outcome is possible, especially with aggressive medical and surgical treatment particularly as it relates to the upper airway.

ETIOLOGY. Autosomal dominant inheritance as well as sporadic cases presumably caused by fresh gene mutation have been seen in type 1. All cases of types 2 and 3 Pfeiffer syndrome reported to date have been sporadic. Pfeiffer syndrome is genetically heterogeneous. Mutations of the fibroblast growth factor receptor 1 (FGFR1) gene, which maps to chromosome 8p11.22-p12 and to the fibroblast growth factor receptor 2 (FGFR2) gene, which maps to chromosome 10q25-q26, have been documented. Changes of the hands and feet tend to be less severe in children with FGFR1 than in those with FGFR2 mutations. It is presently unclear what relationship if any exists between the clinical subclassification of Pfeiffer syndrome set forth by Cohen and the molecular genetics. The value of the subclassification relates primarily to providing the family with a realistic prognosis.

References

Pfeiffer RA: Dominant erbliche Akrocephalosyndactylie. Z Kinderheilkd 90:301, 1964.

Martsolf JT et al: Pfeiffer syndrome: An unusual type of acrocephalosyndactyly with broad thumbs and great toes. Am J Dis Child 121:257, 1971.

Cohen MC: Pfeiffer syndrome update, clinical subtypes, and guidelines for differential diagnosis. Am J Med Genet 45:300, 1993.

Muenke M et al: A common mutation in the fibroblast growth factor receptor 1 gene in Pfeiffer syndrome. Nat Genet 8:268, 1994.

Rutland P et al: Identical mutations in the FGFR2 gene cause both Pfeiffer and Crouzon syndrome phenotypes. Nat Genet 9:173, 1995.

Gripp KW et al: Phenotype of the fibroblast growth factor receptor 2 ser351cys mutation: Pfeiffer syndrome type III. Am J Med Genet 78:356, 1998.

Robin NH et al: Favorable prognosis for children with Pfeiffer syndrome types 2 and 3: Implications for classification. Am J Med Genet 75:240, 1998.

Cornejo-Roldan LR et al: Analysis of the mutational spectrum of the FGFR2 gene in Pfeiffer syndrome. Hum Genet 104:425, 1999.

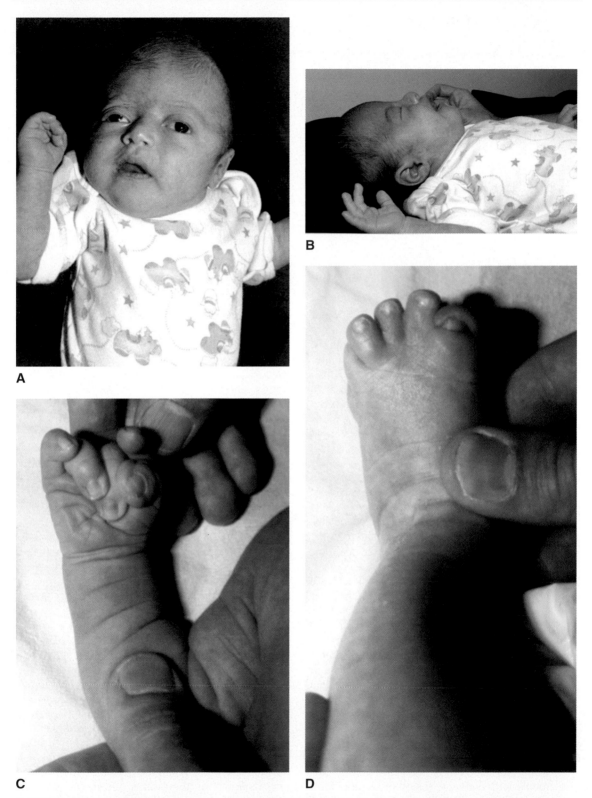

FIGURE 1. Pfeiffer syndrome. **A–D,** A 1-month-old child. Note the brachycephaly, high forehead, ocular hypertelorism, broad thumbs and great toes with syndactyly of feet. (**A** and **B,** Courtesy of Dr. Marilyn C. Jones, Children's Hospital, San Diego.)

APERT SYNDROME
(ACROCEPHALOSYNDACTYLY)

Irregular Craniosynostosis, Midfacial Hypoplasia, Syndactyly, Broad Distal Phalanx of Thumb and Big Toe

The condition was reported by Wheaton in 1894. In 1906, Apert summarized nine cases, and in 1920, Park and Powers published an exceptional essay on this entity. Numerous cases have been reported. The birth prevalence is 1 in every 65,000 live births.

ABNORMALITIES

Growth. Mean birth length and weight above the 50th percentile; in childhood, deceleration of linear growth occurs such that most values are between the 5th and 50th percentiles; deceleration becomes more pronounced after adolescence.

Performance. Mental deficiency is present in a significant number of patients. In two separate studies mean IQ was 74 with a range from 52 to 89, and 61 with a range from 44 to 90, respectively; in a third study, 52% had an IQ less than 70.

Central Nervous System. Although their incidence is unknown, the following defects occur: Agenesis of corpus callosum, nonprogressive ventriculomegaly, progressive hydrocephalus, absent or defective septum pellucidum, gyral abnormalities, hippocampal abnormalities, and megalencephaly.

Craniofacial. Short anteroposterior diameter with high, full forehead and flat occiput; irregular craniosynostosis, especially of coronal suture; fontanels may be large and late in closure; flat facies, supraorbital horizontal groove, shallow orbits, hypertelorism, strabismus, downslanting of palpebral fissures, small nose, maxillary hypoplasia; narrow palate with median groove, with or without cleft palate or bifid uvula; dental anomalies include delayed or ectopic eruption and shovel-shaped incisors; malocclusion.

Limbs. Osseous or cutaneous syndactyly, varying from total fusion to partial fusion, most commonly with complete fusion of second, third, and fourth fingers; distal phalanges of the thumbs are often broad and in valgus position; fingers may be short; cutaneous syndactyly of all toes with or without osseous syndactyly; distal hallux may be broad and malformed.

Skin. Moderate to severe acne, including the forearms, at adolescence.

Other. Fusion of cervical vertebrae usually at C5 to C6.

OCCASIONAL ABNORMALITIES.
Short humerus, synostosis of radius and humerus, limitation of joint mobility, genu valga; gastrointestinal anomalies in 1.5% including pyloric stenosis, esophageal atresia, and ectopic anus; respiratory anomalies in 1.5% including pulmonary aplasia and anomalous tracheal cartilage; cardiac defects in 10% including pulmonic stenosis, overriding aorta, ventricular septal defect, and endocardial fibroelastosis; genitourinary anomalies in 10% including polycystic kidney, hydronephrosis, bicornuate uterus, vaginal atresia, and cryptorchidism; diaphragmatic hernia.

NATURAL HISTORY.
Early surgery for craniosynostosis is indicated when there is evidence of increased intracranial pressure. However, early neurosurgical treatment does not prevent mental retardation, which is most likely related to malformations of the central nervous system. Moderate to severe language problems, as well as expressive language difficulties, occur frequently. Clinically significant social problems, attentional problems, and social withdrawal are common. Upper airway compromise caused by a combination of reduction in size of the nasopharynx and reduction in patency of the choanae as well as lower airway compromise caused by anomalies of the tracheal cartilage may be responsible for early death. There should be vigorous early management of the syndrome. When the thumb is immobilized, early surgery to allow for a pincer grasp is indicated, with later attempts at further improvement of hand function. Hearing loss secondary to chronic

otitis media or congenital fixation of the stapedial footplate is not uncommon. An increased risk exists for development of corneal ulcers because of exophthalmos. Newer techniques allow for vastly improved facial cosmetic reconstruction.

ETIOLOGY.

ETIOLOGY. This disorder has an autosomal dominant inheritance pattern. The vast majority of cases are sporadic and have been associated with older paternal age. Mutations in the fibroblast growth factor receptor 2 gene (FGFR2), which maps to chromosome 10q25-10q26, cause Apert syndrome. Individuals with the P253R mutation respond better to craniofacial surgery but have more pronounced severity of syndactyly than those with the S252W mutation. Different mutations in the same gene cause Crouzon syndrome as well as Pfeiffer syndrome. The recurrence risk for the unaffected parents of a child with Apert syndrome is negligible, whereas the recurrence risk for the affected individual is 50%.

References

Wheaton SW: Two specimens of congenital cranial deformity in infants associated with fusion of the fingers and toes. Trans Pathol Soc Lond 45:238, 1894.

Apart E: De l'Acrocephalosyndactylie. Bull Soc Med 23:1310, 1906.

Park EA, Powers GF: Acrocephaly and scaphocephaly with symmetrically distributed malformations of the extremities: A study of the so-called "acrocephalosyndactylism." Am J Dis Child 20:235, 1920.

Blank CE: Apert's syndrome (a type of acrocephalosyndactyly). Observations on British series of thirty-nine cases. Ann Hum Genet 24:151, 1960.

Cohen MM, Kreiborg S: The central nervous system in the Apert syndrome. Am J Med Genet 35:36, 1990.

Cohen MM et al: An updated pediatric perspective on the Apert syndrome. Am J Dis Child 147:989, 1993.

Wilkie AOM et al: Apert syndrome results from localized mutations of FGFR2 and is allelic with Crouzon syndrome. Nat Genet 9:165, 1995.

Sarimski K: Social adjustment of children with a severe craniofacial anomaly (Apert syndrome). Child Care Health Dev 27:538, 2001.

Shipster C et al: Speech and language skills and cognitive functioning in children with Apert syndrome: A pilot study. Int J Lang Commun Disord 37:325, 2002.

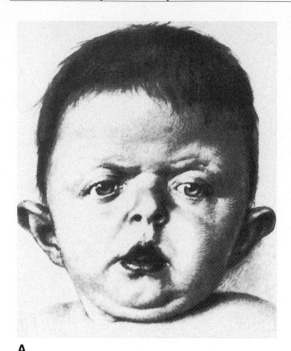

A

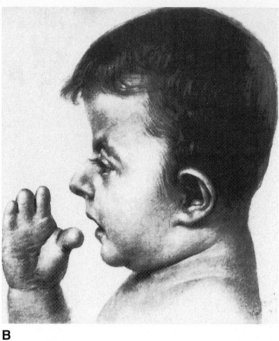

B

FIGURE 1. Apert syndrome. **A** and **B,** A girl, drawn by the late M. Brödel. (**A** and **B,** From Park EA, Powers GF: Am J Dis Child 20:235, 1920.)   *Continued*

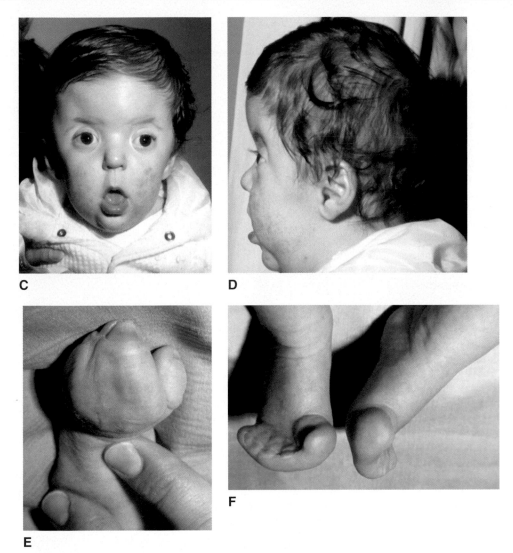

Fig. 1, cont'd. **C–F,** A 6-month-old child. Note the short anterior-posterior diameter of the head with high full forehead and flat occiput, shallow orbits with proptosis, maxillary hypoplasia, and syndactyly of hands and feet.

CROUZON SYNDROME
(CRANIOFACIAL DYSOSTOSIS)

Shallow Orbits, Premature Craniosynostosis, Maxillary Hypoplasia

Originally described in 1912 by Crouzon in a mother and her daughter, this condition usually has an adverse effect on craniofacial development alone. With complete examination, including the hands and feet, many of the patients who have been diagnosed as having Crouzon syndrome in the past have been recognized as having Saethre-Chotzen syndrome or Muenke syndrome. Furthermore, others are due to fetal head constraint, a nongenetic cause of craniosynostosis.

ABNORMALITIES

Craniofacial. Ocular proptosis caused by shallow orbits with or without divergent strabismus, hypertelorism; frontal bossing; exposure conjunctivitis or keratitis; unexplained poor visual acuity; optic atrophy; nystagmus; hypoplasia of maxilla with or without curved parrot-like nose, inverted V shape to palate; conductive hearing loss; craniosynostosis, especially of coronal, lambdoid, and sagittal sutures with palpable ridging; short antero-posterior and wide lateral dimensions of the cranium may occur.

OCCASIONAL ABNORMALITIES.

Mental retardation; hydrocephalus; seizures; agenesis of corpus callosum; Chiari I malformation; syringomyelia; keratoconus; iris coloboma; jugular foraminal stenosis; atresia of auditory meatus; cleft lip with or without cleft palate; bifid uvula; pulmonary valve stenosis; tracheobroncho-malacia; subluxation of radial heads; acanthosis nigricans involving eyelids, perioral, perialar, and neck skin predominantly.

NATURAL HISTORY.

The degree of cranio-synostosis, as well as the age of onset, is variable. One infant is described who showed no radiologic evidence of craniosynostosis at 4 months but complete sutural closure by 11 months of age. Surgical morcellation procedures to allow for more normal brain development are indicated when there is increased intracranial pressure. Otherwise, the indications are usually cosmetic, and the decision toward surgery is usually mitigated by the severity of the aberrant shape plus the competency of the surgeon who will perform the procedure. Newer techniques allow for cosmetic reconstruction of the facial bones. Obstruction of the upper airway frequently results in obligatory mouth breathing but rarely leads to acute respiratory distress.

ETIOLOGY.

This disorder has an autosomal dominant inheritance pattern with variable expression. Approximately one fourth of the reported cases have had a negative family history and presumably represent fresh mutations. Mutations in the fibroblast growth factor receptor 2 gene (FGFR2), which maps to chromosome 10q25-q26, are responsible for greater than 90% of cases. Crouzon syndrome with acanthosis nigricans (CAN) is due to a specific substitution (Ala391Glu) in the FGFR3 gene. CAN is associated with cranio-synostosis, ocular proptosis, midface hypoplasia, choanal atresia, hydrocephalus, and acanthosis nigricans, the latter initially develops during childhood.

COMMENT.

Mutations of FGFR2 are responsible for Crouzon syndrome, Pfeiffer syndrome, Apert syndrome, and Beare-Stevenson cutis gyrate syndrome.

References

Crouzon O: Dysostose cranio-faciale héréditaire. Bull Mem Soc Med Hop (Paris) 33:545, 1912.

Bertelsen TI: The premature synostosis of the cranial sutures. Acta Ophthalmol [Suppl 51] (Kbh) 1:176, 1958.

Dodge HW Jr, Wood MW, Kennedy RLJ: Craniofacial dysostosis: Crouzon's disease. Pediatrics 23:98, 1959.

Kreiborg S: Crouzon syndrome: A clinical and roentgen-cephalometric study. Scand J Plast Reconstr Surg [Suppl 18] 1981.

Jabs EW et al: Jackson-Weiss and Crouzon syndromes are allelic with mutations in fibroblast growth factor receptor 2. Nat Genet 8:275, 1994.

Perlman JM, Zaidman GW: Bilateral keratoconus in Crouzon's syndrome. Cornea 13:80, 1994.

Reardon W et al: Mutations in the fibroblast growth factor

receptor 2 gene cause Crouzon syndrome. Nat Genet 8:98, 1994.

Rutland P et al: Identical mutations in the FGFR2 gene cause both Pfeiffer and Crouzon syndrome phenotypes. Nat Genet 9:173, 1995.

Przylepa KA et al: Fibroblast growth factor receptor 2 mutations in Beare-Stevenson cutis gyrata syndrome. Nat Genet 13:492, 1996.

Schweitzer DN et al: Subtle radiographic findings of achondroplasia in patients with Crouzon syndrome with acanthosis nigricans due to an Ala391glu substitution in FGFR3. Am J Med Genet 98:75, 2001.

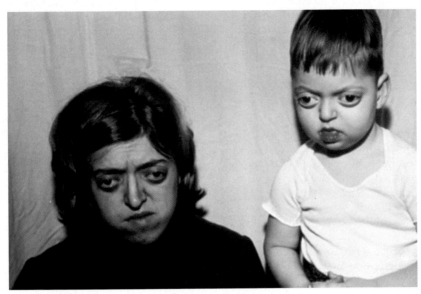

FIGURE 1. Mother and son with Crouzon syndrome. (Courtesy of Dr. Michael Cohen, Dalhousie University, Halifax, Nova Scotia.)

FGFR3-ASSOCIATED CORONAL SYNOSTOSIS SYNDROME
(Muenke Craniosynostosis)

Initially defined by a mutation in the fibroblast growth factor receptor (FGFR) gene located on chromosome 4p, the clinical phenotype of this disorder is variable. Therefore, all patients with coronal synostosis, who lack a confirmed diagnosis of another condition, should be tested for this mutation.

ABNORMALITIES

Craniofacial. Coronal craniosynostosis, either unilateral or bilateral; mild maxillary hypoplasia; downslanting palpebral fissures; ocular hypertelorism.

Hands and Feet. Brachydactyly, fifth finger clinodactyly, thimble-like middle phalanges, cone-shaped epiphyses, carpal/tarsal fusion, broad halluces.

Other. Ptosis, hearing loss, developmental delay/mental retardation.

OCCASIONAL ABNORMALITIES.

Macrocephaly, cloverleaf skull, broad great toe, absent/fused middle phalanx of fifth finger, growth deficiency.

ETIOLOGY. This disorder has an autosomal dominant inheritance pattern. A single point mutation in the FGFR3 gene on chromosome 4p is causative. Marked variability of expression is the rule and nonpenetrance has been documented. All parents of mutation positive patients should be tested for the mutation whether they have clinical features or not. The phenotype seems to be more severe in females.

COMMENT. Mutations in the FGFR3 gene also result in achondroplasia, hypochondroplasia, thanatophoric dysplasia, Crouzon syndrome with acanthosis nigricans and SADDAN (severe achondroplasia with developmental delay and acanthosis nigricans) dysplasia.

References

Bellus GA et al: Identical mutations in three different fibroblast growth factor receptor genes in autosomal dominant craniosynostosis syndromes. Nat Genet 14:174–176, 1996.

Muenke M et al: A unique point mutation in the Fibroblast Growth Factor Receptor 3 gene (FGFR3) defines a new craniosynostosis syndrome. Am J Hum Genet 60:555–564, 1997.

Graham JM et al: Syndrome of coronal craniosynostosis with brachydactyly and carpal/tarsal coalition due to Pro250 Arg mutation in FGFR3 gene. Am J Med Genet 77:322–329, 1998.

Lajeunie E et al: Sex related expressivity of the phenotype in coronal craniosynostosis caused by the recurrent P250R FGFR3 mutation. J Med Genet 36:9–13, 1999.

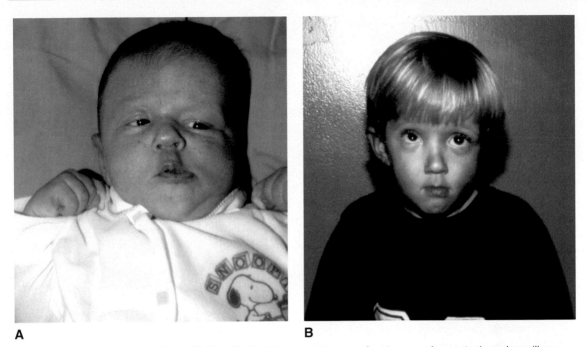

A   **B**

FIGURE 1. Muenke syndrome. **A** and **B,** Note the facial asymmetry secondary to coronal synostosis and maxillary hypoplasia. (Courtesy of Dr. Marilyn C. Jones, Children's Hospital, San Diego.)

CRANIOFRONTONASAL DYSPLASIA

The name craniofrontonasal dysplasia was introduced by Cohen in 1979 to designate this condition. Through analysis of 58 families and 8 males from 18 families, Grutzner and Gorlin have set forth the differences in the clinical phenotype between males and females with this disorder. This is one of the few conditions in which females are more severely affected than males.

ABNORMALITIES

Cranial. Females—craniosynostosis, brachycephaly, and frontal bossing; males—increased bony interorbital distance; craniosynostosis is only rarely seen.

Facial. Females and males—hypertelorism, facial asymmetry, broad nasal root, bifid nasal tip.

Limbs. Females and males—longitudinal splitting of nails, syndactyly of toes, broad first toe, clinodactyly; females—syndactyly of fingers.

OCCASIONAL ABNORMALITIES.

Females—telecanthus, exotropia, nystagmus, strabismus, hearing loss, axillary pterygium, Sprengel deformity, restriction of joint motion, Poland sequence, and dry, curly hair. Females and males—cleft lip/palate, webbed neck, and mental retardation. Males—short stature, pectus excavatum, pseudoarthrosis of clavicles, brachydactyly, pre- and postaxial polydactyly, deviated distal phalanges of fingers and toes, wide space between first and second toes, hypospadias, shawl scrotum, and diaphragmatic hernia.

ETIOLOGY. This disorder has a probable X-linked dominant inheritance pattern. All daughters of affected males have been affected and no male-to-male transmission has been documented. The responsible gene has been mapped to Xp22. The far milder manifestations of the disorder in males is unusual and not adequately explained.

COMMENT. This condition is primarily diagnosed in females. All reported males have been identified based on a confirmed diagnosis in a female relative.

References

Cohen MM: Craniofrontonasal dysplasia. Birth Defects 15(5B):85, 1979.

Slover R, Sujanski E: Frontonasal dysplasia with coronal craniosynostosis in three sibs. Birth Defects 15(5B):75, 1979.

Young ID: Craniofrontonasal dysplasia. J Med Genet 24:193, 1987.

Grutzner E, Gorlin RJ: Craniofrontonasal dysplasia: Phenotypic expression in females and males and genetic considerations. Oral Surg Oral Med Oral Pathol 65:436, 1988.

Feldman GJ et al: A nove phenotypic pattern in x-linked inheritance: Craniofrontalnasal syndrome maps to Xp22. Hum Mol Genet 6:1937, 1997.

Pulleyn LJ et al: Further evidence from two families that craniofrontonasal dysplasia maps to Xp22. Clin Genet 55:473, 1999.

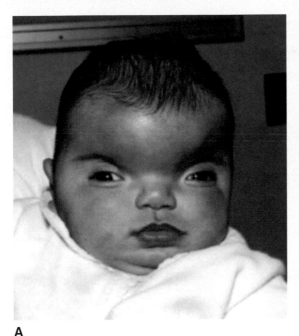

A

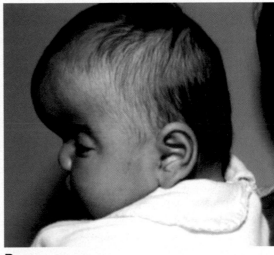

B

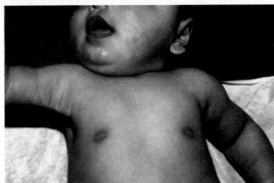

C

FIGURE 1. Craniofrontonasal dysplasia. **A–C,** A 3-month-old female infant with ocular hypertelorism, facial asymmetry, and right coronal craniosynostosis. Note axillary pterygium. (Courtesy of Dr. Marilyn C. Jones, Children's Hospital, San Diego.)

CARPENTER SYNDROME

Acrocephaly, Polydactyly and Syndactyly of Feet, Lateral Displacement of Inner Canthi

Although Carpenter described this condition in 1901, it was not firmly established as an entity until Temtamy's report in 1966. More than 45 cases have been reported.

ABNORMALITIES

Growth. Postnatal growth less than 25th percentile, obesity.

Performance. Variable delay in intellectual performance, IQs have ranged from 52 to 104.

Craniofacial. Brachycephaly with variable synostosis of coronal, sagittal, and lambdoid sutures; shallow supraorbital ridges; flat nasal bridge; lateral displacement of the inner canthi with or without inner canthal folds; corneal opacity, maldeveloped or microcornea, optic atrophy and/or blurring of disk margins; low-set and malformed ears; hypoplastic mandible or maxilla; narrow, highly arched palate.

Limbs. Brachydactyly of hands with clinodactyly, partial syndactyly, and camptodactyly; single flexion crease; subluxation at distal interphalangeal joints; angulation deformities at knees; preaxial polydactyly of the feet with partial syndactyly; short or missing middle phalanges of fingers and toes.

Cardiovascular. Defects in 50% including ventricular septal defect, atrial septal defect, patent ductus arteriosus, pulmonic stenosis, tetralogy of Fallot, and transposition of great vessels.

Other. Hypogenitalism, cryptorchidism, umbilical hernia, omphalocele.

OCCASIONAL ABNORMALITIES.

Brain abnormalities including atrophy, partial absence of corpus callosum, abnormal gyral patterns, enlarged foramen magnum; polydactyly, preauricular pits, short muscular neck, delayed loss of deciduous teeth, partial anodontia, duplication of second phalanx of thumb, metatarsus varus, flat acetabulum, flare to pelvis, coxa valga, genu valgum, lateral displacement of patellae, pilonidal dimple, accessory spleen; hydronephrosis with or without hydroureter; obesity; precocious puberty; conductive and neurosensory hearing loss.

NATURAL HISTORY. Recent reports indicate that mental retardation is not an obligate feature of this condition and probably does not relate to the timing of craniofacial surgery. Fine motor dysfunction secondary to the digital anomalies is a continuing problem. Articulation errors attributed to inability to perform rapidly alternating movements of the lips and tongue can lead to speech problems. Eustachian tube dysfunction is secondary to the short cranial base.

ETIOLOGY. This disorder has an autosomal recessive inheritance pattern.

References

Carpenter G: Two sisters showing malformations of the skull and other congenital abnormalities. Rep Soc Study Dis Child Lond 1:110, 1901.

Temtamy SA: Carpenter's syndrome: Acrocephalo-polysyndactyly, an autosomal recessive syndrome. J Pediatr 69:111, 1966.

Frias JL et al: Normal intelligence in two children with Carpenter syndrome. Am J Med Genet 2:191, 1978.

Robinson LK et al: Carpenter syndrome: Natural history and clinical spectrum. Am J Med Genet 20:461, 1985.

Cohen DM et al: Acrocephalopolysyndactyly type II—Carpenter syndrome: Clinical spectrum and an attempt at unification with Goodman and Summit syndromes. Am J Med Genet 28:311, 1987.

Richieri-Costa A et al: Carpenter syndrome with normal intelligence: Brazilian girl born to consanguineous parents. Am J Med Genet 47:281, 1993.

Islek I et al: Carpenter syndrome: Report of two siblings. Clin Dysmorphol 7:185, 1998.

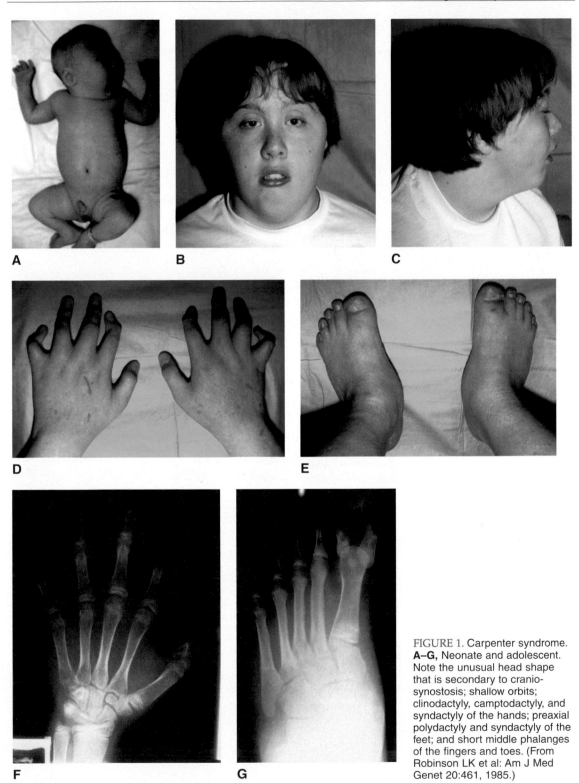

FIGURE 1. Carpenter syndrome. **A–G,** Neonate and adolescent. Note the unusual head shape that is secondary to craniosynostosis; shallow orbits; clinodactyly, camptodactyly, and syndactyly of the hands; preaxial polydactyly and syndactyly of the feet; and short middle phalanges of the fingers and toes. (From Robinson LK et al: Am J Med Genet 20:461, 1985.)

GREIG CEPHALOPOLYSYNDACTYLY SYNDROME

Preaxial and Postaxial Polydactyly, Syndactyly, Frontal Bossing

Initially described by Greig in 1926, additional cases were reported by Temtamy and McKusick, Marshall and Smith, and Hootnick and Holmes. Subsequently, more than 50 cases have been published.

ABNORMALITIES

Craniofacies. High forehead (70%); frontal bossing (58%); macrocephaly (52%); apparent hypertelorism; broad nasal root (79%).

Hands. Postaxial polydactyly (78%); broad thumbs (90%); syndactyly, primarily fingers 3 and 4 (82%).

Feet. Preaxial polydactyly (81%); broad halluces (89%); syndactyly, primarily toes 1 to 3 (90%).

OCCASIONAL ABNORMALITIES.

Broad, late-closing cranial sutures, advanced bone age, downslanting palpebral fissures, mild mental deficiency, seizures, muscle fiber anomalies, agenesis of corpus callosum, mild degrees of hydrocephaly, craniosynostosis, camptodactyly, cardiac defect, hyperglycemia, hirsutism, radiographic evidence of preaxial polydactyly of hands and postaxial polydactyly of feet, osseous syndactyly, inguinal and umbilical hernia, cryptorchidism, hypospadias.

ETIOLOGY.

This disorder has an autosomal dominant inheritance pattern. Mutations in the GLI3 gene located on chromosome 7p13 are responsible. In addition to mutations, translocations that interrupt the gene, microdeletions, and large cytogenetically detectable deletions have been described. The latter are associated with a more complex phenotype, involving some of the occasional abnormalities noted previously, as a result of deletion of additional genes.

COMMENT. Pallister-Hall syndrome is also due to mutations of GLI3.

References

Greig DM: Oxycephaly. Edinburgh Med J 33:189, 1926.

Temtamy S, McKusick VA: Synopsis of hand malformation with particular emphasis on genetic factors. Birth Defects 5(3):125, 1969.

Marshal RE, Smith DW: Frontodigital syndrome: A dominant inherited disorder with normal intelligence. J Pediatr 77:129, 1970.

Hootnick D, Holmes LB: Family polysyndactyly and craniofacial anomalies. Clin Genet 3:128, 1972.

Tommerup N, Nielsen F: A familial translocation t(3;7)(p21.1;p13) associated with the Greig polysyndactyly-craniofacial anomalies syndrome. Am J Med Genet 16:313, 1983.

Gollop TR, Fontes LR: The Greig cephalopolysyndactyly syndrome: Report of a family and review of the literature. Am J Med Genet 22:59, 1985.

Pettigrew AL et al: Greig syndrome associated with an interstitial deletion of 7p: Confirmation of the localization of Greig syndrome to 7p13. Hum Genet 87:452, 1991.

Ausems MGEM et al: Greig cephalopolysyndactyly syndrome in a large family: A comparison of the clinical signs with those described in the literature. Clin Dysmorphol 3:21, 1994.

Kroisel PM et al: Phenotype of five patients with Greig syndrome and microdeletion of 7p13. Am J Med Genet 102:243, 2001.

Debeer P et al: Variable phenotype in Grieg cephalopolysyndactyly syndrome: Clinical and radiological findings in four independent families and three sporadic cases with identified GLI3 mutations. Am J Med Genet 120:49, 2003.

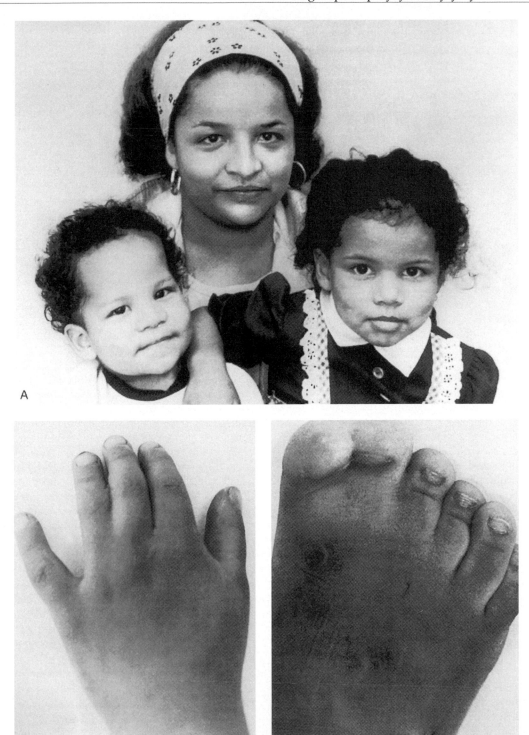

FIGURE 1. **A–C,** Mother and her children with Greig cephalopolysyndactyly syndrome. Note the high forehead, syndactyly of fingers 3 and 4, and preaxial polydactyly of foot. (From Duncan PA et al: Am J Dis Child 133:818, 1979, with permission.)

ANTLEY-BIXLER SYNDROME
(Multisynostotic Osteodysgenesis,
Trapezoidcephaly/Multiple Synostosis)

Craniosynostosis, Choanal Atresia, Radiohumeral Synostosis

First described by Antley and Bixler in 1975, subsequent cases have been reported by DeLozier and colleagues and Robinson and colleagues. Schinzel and colleagues documented the first instance of affected siblings. Approximately 50 cases have been reported.

ABNORMALITIES

Craniofacial. Brachycephaly, frontal bossing, large anterior fontanel, craniosynostosis, midfacial hypoplasia, depressed nasal bridge, proptosis, choanal stenosis or atresia, dysplastic ears, stenotic external auditory canals.

Limbs. Radiohumeral synostosis; joint contractures, including inability to extend fingers and decreased range of motion at wrists, hips, knees, and ankles; arachnodactyly associated with enlarged interphalangeal joints, increased numbers of flexion creases, and distal tapering with narrow nails; femoral bowing; femoral fractures; rocker-bottom feet.

OCCASIONAL ABNORMALITIES.

Hydrocephalus, Arnold-Chiari malformation, preauricular tags, ambiguous genitalia, vaginal atresia, hypoplastic labia majora, fused labia minora, clitoromegaly, atrial septal defects, renal defect, multiple hemangiomata, partial cutaneous syndactyly, narrow chest and pelvis.

NATURAL HISTORY.

Respiratory compromise secondary to upper airway obstruction has varied from severe nasal congestion to multiple apneic episodes leading to death in the first few months of life. Survivors frequently require tracheostomy, and the placement of a gastrostomy tube is often necessary. Although gross and fine motor function have been difficult to assess because of joint contractures, prognosis may be reasonably good once the difficult perinatal period

has passed. Joint contractures have improved with age and passive range-of-motion exercises. There has been no propensity to fracture postnatally. Resection of the radiohumeral synostosis was attempted in one child at 6 months of age. However, recurrence of the bone fusion recurred within 3 months. That same child, now 10 years of age, functions intellectually and socially as a normal fifth grader.

ETIOLOGY.

The cause of the Antley-Bixler syndrome (ABS) is heterogeneous. There are at least four different causes of the ABS phenotype: (1) Autosomal dominant mutations in the fibroblast growth factor receptor 2 (FGFR2) gene associated with a phenotype that includes the skeletal abnormalities and lacks manifestations of altered steroidogenesis or genital ambiguity. (2) Mutations in the cytochrome P450 oxidoreductase gene (POR) located on chromosome 7q11.23 resulting in autosomal recessive inheritance and an ABS phenotype that includes genital ambiguity and a characteristic urinary steroid profile. (Elevated excretion of metabolites of pregnenolone and progesterone; elevated metabolite levels associated with 17-α-hydroxylase deficiency; and elevated metabolites characteristic of 21-hydroxylase deficiency.) POR mutations may also lead to the skeletal defects as a result of decreased lanosterol 14-α-demethylase activity. (3) In utero exposure to fluconazole, an antifungal medication that inhibits lanosterol 14-α-demethylase, an enzyme critical in sterol biosynthesis. (4) Digenic inheritance where FGFR2 mutations account for the skeletal abnormalities and different mutations causing altered steroidogenesis contribute to the genital anomalies.

COMMENT.

Undetectable unconjugated estriol implying abnormal fetal steroid or sterol metabolism has been demonstrated at midgestation maternal serum screening and may provide a prenatal marker for this disorder in some cases.

References

Antley RM, Bixler D: Trapezoidcephaly, midface hypoplasia, and cartilage abnormalities with multiple synostoses and skeletal fractures. Birth Defects 11(2):397, 1975.

DeLozier CD et al: The syndrome of multisynostotic osteodysgenesis with long-bone fractures. Am J Med Genet 7:391, 1980.

Robinson LK et al: The Antley-Bixler syndrome. J Pediatr 101:201, 1982.

Schinzel A et al: Antley-Bixler syndrome in sisters: A term newborn and a prenatally diagnosed fetus. Am J Med Genet 14:139, 1983.

Escobar LF et al: Antley-Bixler syndrome from a prognostic perspective: Report of a case and review of the literature. Am J Med Genet 29:829, 1988.

DeLozier CD: Antley-Bixler syndrome from a prognostic perspective. Am J Med Genet 32:262, 1989.

Reardon W: Evidence for digenic inheritance in some cases of Antley-Bixler syndrome? J Med Genet 37:26, 2000.

Kelley RJ et al: Abnormal sterol metabolism in a patient with Antley-Bixler syndrome and ambiguous genitalia. Am J Med Genet 110:95, 2002.

Adachi M et al: Compound heterozygous mutations of cytochrome P450 oxidoreductase gene (POR) in two patients with Antley-Bixler syndrome. Am J Med Genet 128:333, 2004.

Cragun DL et al: Undetectable maternal serum uE3 and postnatal abnormal sterol and steroid metabolism in Antley-Bixler syndrome. Am J Med Genet 129:1, 2004.

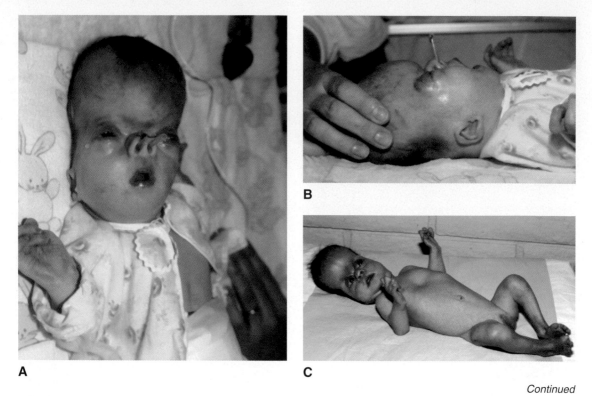

A

B

C

Continued

FIGURE 1. Antley-Bixler syndrome. **A–E,** Newborn female infant with severe maxillary hypoplasia, depressed nasal bridge, proptosis, and dysplastic ears. Note the multiple joint contractures, radiohumeral synostosis, and femoral bowing. (From Robinson LK et al: J Pediatr 101:201, 1982, with permission.)

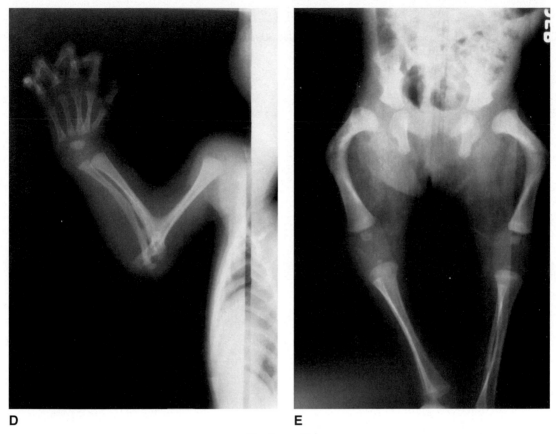

D E

Fig. 1, cont'd.

BALLER-GEROLD SYNDROME
(Craniosynostosis–Radial Aplasia Syndrome)

Baller described a 26-year-old woman in 1950, and Gerold subsequently reported affected siblings. More than 30 cases have been reported.

ABNORMALITIES

Performance. Fifty percent of those followed beyond infancy have been mentally deficient.

Growth. Prenatal and postnatal growth deficiency.

Craniofacial. Craniosynostosis involving any or all sutures (100%), low-set and posteriorly rotated ears (64%), micrognathia (50%), prominent nasal bridge (32%), downslanting palpebral fissures (32%), microstomia (32%), epicanthal folds (27%), flattened forehead (27%).

Limbs. Radial aplasia/hypoplasia (77%); short, curved ulna (68%); missing carpals, metacarpals, and phalanges; fused carpals; absent or hypoplastic thumbs (100%).

Anal. Anomalies in 40%, including imperforate anus or anteriorly placed anus.

Urogenital. Anomalies in 35%, including ectopic, hypoplastic, dysplastic, or absent kidney, and persistence of the cloaca.

OCCASIONAL ABNORMALITIES.

Epicanthal folds; bifid uvula; cleft palate; choanal stenosis; strabismus; optic atrophy; myopia; seizures; polymicrogyria; hydrocephalus; absent corpus callosum; conductive hearing loss; capillary hemangiomata over nose and philtrum; hypoplastic ala nasi; vertebral defects; rib fusions; scoliosis; hypoplastic humerus; decreased range of motion at shoulders, elbows, and knees; hypoplastic patellae; coxa valga; spina bifida occulta; cardiac defects (25%) include subaortic valvular hypertrophy, ventricular septal defect, and tetralogy of Fallot; congenital portal venous malformation.

NATURAL HISTORY. Twenty percent of the live-born infants died unexpectedly during the first year of life. For the remainder, postnatal growth deficiency is common. Of the 13 affected individuals for whom developmental performance was mentioned, six were mentally retarded; two, both of whom were less than 2 years of age, had moderate motor delay; and five were normal.

ETIOLOGY. This disorder has an autosomal recessive inheritance pattern.

COMMENT. Before diagnosis of this disorder, other conditions with overlapping clinical features, including Fanconi pancytopenia syndrome and Roberts syndrome, should be excluded.

References

Baller F: Radiusaplasie und Inzucht. Z Menschl Vererb-Konstit-Lehre 29:782, 1950.

Gerold M: Frakturheilung bei einem seltenen Fall kongenitaler Anomalie der oberen Gliedmassen. Zentralbl Chir 84:831, 1959.

Greitzer LJ et al: Craniosynostosis–radial aplasia syndrome. J Pediatr 84:723, 1974.

Lin AE et al: Further delineation of the Baller-Gerold syndrome. Am J Med Genet 45:519, 1993.

Ramos Fuentes FJ et al: Phenotypic variability in the Baller-Gerold syndrome: Report of a mildly affected patient and review of the literature. Eur J Pediatr 153:483, 1994.

Quarrell OWJ et al: Baller-Gerold syndrome and Fanconi anaemia. Am J Med Genet 75:228, 1998.

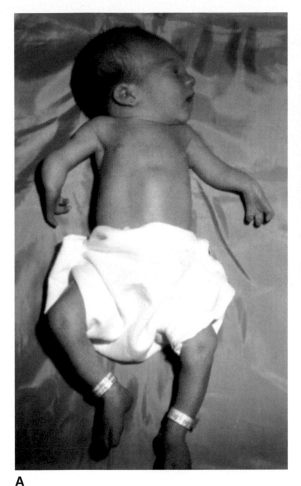

A

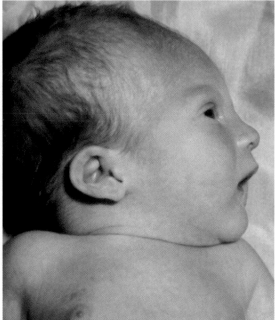

B

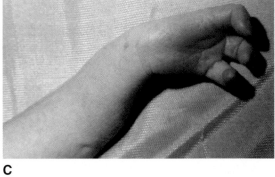

C

FIGURE 1. Baller-Gerold syndrome. **A–C,** Newborn infant with metopic craniosynostosis, mildly dysplastic ears, and radial dysplasia with absent thumbs. (From Greitzer LJ: J Pediatr 84:723, 1974, with permission.)

M Other Skeletal Dysplasias

MULTIPLE SYNOSTOSIS SYNDROME
(Symphalangism Syndrome)

Symphalangism, Hypoplasia of Alae Nasi

In the past, this disorder was generally termed symphalangism (synostosis of finger joints), a nonspecific anomaly. The multiple synostosis character of the disorder herein set forth was emphasized by Maroteaux and colleagues.

ABNORMALITIES

Facies. Narrow, with hypoplasia of alae nasi, hypoplastic nasal septum, fusion of the nasal bone and the frontal process of the maxilla, short philtrum, thin vermilion of upper lip, occasional strabismus.

Limbs. Multiple fusion of proximal and middle phalangeal joints, elbows, and carpal and tarsal bones (especially navicular to talus); variable clinodactyly, brachydactyly, and distal bone hypoplasia or aplasia in phalanges; aplasia/hypoplasia of fingernails/toenails; cutaneous syndactyly; limited forearm pronation/supination, rotation of hips, and abduction of shoulders; short feet and hallux.

Spine. Vertebral anomalies.

Middle Ear. Variable fusion of middle ear ossicles, with conductive deafness, most commonly fusion of stapes to the round window.

Other. Pectus excavatum, prominent costochondral junction.

OCCASIONAL ABNORMALITIES.
Moderate mental deficiency, Klippel-Feil anomaly, short sternum, humeroradial synostosis, good muscle development, short arms and legs.

NATURAL HISTORY. Potential for significant partial or complete restoration of hearing by otologic surgery is excellent. Symphalangism is not always present in childhood. Bony fusions are progressive, lead to increasing stiffness, and limitation of movement of the spine and/or limbs. Neurologic complications secondary to spinal canal stenosis occurred in one patient.

ETIOLOGY. This disorder has an autosomal dominant inheritance pattern with appreciable variance in expression. Mutations in the human homologue of the gene encoding noggin, located on chromosome 17q21-q22, are responsible. Noggin is an antagonist of bone morphogenetic protein (BMP). Mice lacking noggin fail to initiate joint development suggesting that excess BMP leads to enhanced recruitment of cells into cartilage, resulting in oversized growth plates and failure of normal joint development.

References

Vesell ES: Symphalangism, strabismus and hearing loss in mother and daughter. N Engl J Med 263:839, 1960.

Fuhrmann W et al: Dominant erbliche Brachydaktylie mit Gelenksaplasien. Humangenetik 1:337, 1965.

Strasburger AK et al: Symphalangism: Genetic and clinical aspects. Bull Johns Hopkins Hosp 117:108, 1965.

Elkington SG, Huntsman RG: The Talbot fingers: A study in symphalangism. BMJ 1:407, 1967.

Maroteaux P, Bouvet JP, Briard ML: La maladie des synostoses multiples. Nouv Presse Med 1:3041, 1972.

Herrmann J: Symphalangism and brachydactyly syndrome. Birth Defects 10(5):23, 1974.

de-Silva EO, Filho SM, de Albuquerque SC: Multiple synostosis syndrome: Study of a large Brazilian kindred. Am J Med Genet 18:237, 1984.

Hurvitz SA et al: The facio-audio-symphalangism syndrome: Report of a case and review of the literature. Clin Genet 28:61, 1985.

Gong Y et al: Heterozygous mutations in the gene encoding noggin affect human joint morphogenesis. Nat Genet 21:302, 1999.

Edwards MW et al: Herrman multiple synostosis syndrome with neurological complications caused by spinal canal stenosis. Am J Med Genet 95:118, 2000.

Takahashi T et al: Mutations of the NOG gene in individuals with proximal symphalangism and multiple synostosis syndrome. Clin Genet 60:447, 2001.

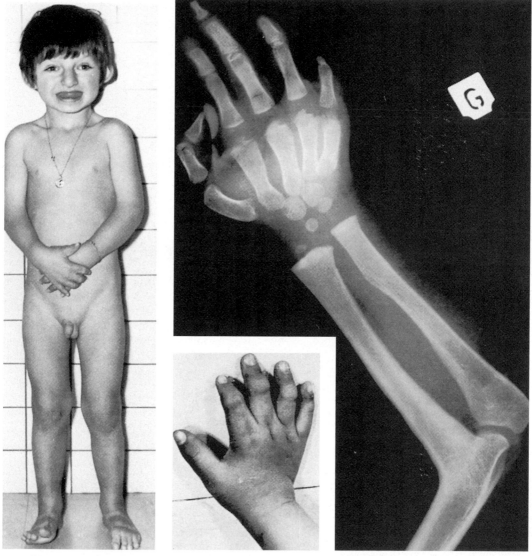

FIGURE 1. Multiple synostosis syndrome. Note the narrow nose; prominent external ear; and variable brachydactyly, aplasia of distal phalanges, and synostoses. (From Maroteaux P et al: Nouv Presse Med 1:3041, 1972, with permission.)

SPONDYLOCARPOTARSAL SYNOSTOSIS SYNDROME

Disproportionate Short Stature, Block Vertebrae, Carpal Synostosis

This disorder was delineated in 1994 by Langer and colleagues, who described six affected individuals and reviewed an additional six from the literature.

ABNORMALITIES

Growth. Disproportionate short stature with short trunk.

Thorax. Failure of normal spinal segmentation, which when symmetric leads to block vertebrae, and when asymmetric leads to mild scoliosis and lordosis; the presence of a unilateral unsegmented bar results in severe scoliosis and lordosis; the thoracic spine is most commonly involved.

Hands and Feet. Carpal synostosis, most commonly capitate-hamate and lunate-triquetrum; tarsal synostosis; pes planus.

OCCASIONAL ABNORMALITIES.

Cleft palate; sensorineural or mixed hearing loss; preauricular skin tag; round broad face with ocular hypertelorism, and short nose with anteverted nares and broad, square nasal tip; enamel hypoplasia; decreased range of motion at elbows; postaxial polydactyly; renal cyst; odontoid hypoplasia; delayed ossification of many epiphyses as well as in carpal ossification.

NATURAL HISTORY. Progressive scoliosis and lordosis are the major complications and are sometimes associated with restrictive impairment of total lung capacity. Cervical vertebral instability has been described. The unsegmented bar is difficult to identify on radiographs in early life because it is cartilaginous. Serial follow-up radiographs are indicated. Tomography is often helpful.

ETIOLOGY. This disorder has an autosomal recessive inheritance pattern. Mutations in the gene encoding Filamin B (FLNB) localized to chromosome 3p14 are responsible. FLNB seems to have an important role in vertebral segmentation, joint formation, and endochondral ossification.

References

Langer LO, Moe JM: A recessive form of congenital scoliosis different from spondylothoracic dysplasia. Birth Defects 11(6):83, 1975.

Wiles CR et al: Congenital synspondylism. Am J Med Genet 42:288, 1992.

Langer LO et al: Spondylocarpotarsal synostosis syndrome (with or without unilateral unsegmented bar). Am J Med Genet 51:1, 1994.

Seaver LH, Boyd E: Spondylocarpotarsal synostosis syndrome and cervical instability. Am J Med Genet 91:340, 2000.

Honeywell C et al: Spondylocarpotarsal synostosis syndrome with epiphyseal dysplasia. Am J Med Genet 109:318, 2002.

Krakow D et al: Mutations in the gene encoding filamin B disrupt vertebral segmentation, joint formation, and skeletogenesis. Nat Genet 36:405, 2004.

Steiner C et al: A locus for spondylocarpotarsal synostosis syndrome at chromosome 3p14. J Med Genet 41:266, 2004.

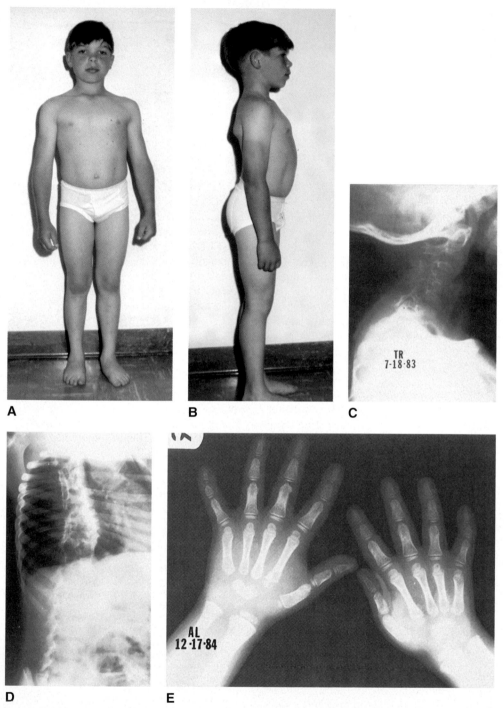

A

B

C

D

E

FIGURE 1. Spondylocarpotarsal synostosis syndrome. **A–E,** Note the disproportionate short stature and short neck, synostosis of the cervical vertebrae, the unilateral unsegmented bar and the carpal synostosis. (**A** and **B,** From Jones KL, Smith DW: Syndrome Identification 1:10, 1973; **C–E,** radiographs from Langer LL et al: Am J Med Genet 51:1, 1994. Copyright © 1994. Reprinted with permission of Wiley-Liss, Inc., a subsidiary of John Wiley & Sons, Inc.)

LARSEN SYNDROME

Multiple Joint Dislocation, Flat Facies, Short Fingernails

Larsen and colleagues described six sporadic cases of this condition in 1950.

ABNORMALITIES

Facies. Flat, with depressed nasal bridge and prominent forehead, hypertelorism; cleft palate.

Joints. Dislocations of elbows, hips, knees, and wrists, with dysplastic epiphyseal centers developing in childhood.

Hands. Long, nontapering fingers with spatulate thumbs, short nails, short metacarpals, and multiple carpal ossification centers.

Feet. Talipes equinovalgus or varus. Delayed coalescence of the two calcaneal ossification centers.

Spine. Cervical kyphosis; spina bifida and hypoplastic bodies of cervical vertebrae; scoliosis, wedged vertebrae, lordosis, and anomalies of posterior elements of thoracic spine; dysraphism, spondylolysis, and scoliosis of lumbar spine; spina bifida occulta of sacral spine.

OCCASIONAL ABNORMALITIES.

Mental retardation; cleft lip; hypodontia; conductive and sensorineural hearing loss; hypoplastic humerus; entropion of lower eyelids; anterior cortical lens opacities; simian crease; cardiovascular defect; mobile, infolding arytenoid cartilage; tracheomalacia; bronchomalacia; tracheal stenosis; cryptorchidism.

NATURAL HISTORY. Evaluations of

adults in four generations of one family indicate that prognosis is relatively good following aggressive orthopedic management. Many patients begin walking late. Osteoarthritis involving large joints and progressive kyphoscoliosis are potential complications. Airway obstruction caused by tracheomalacia and bronchomalacia may be life-threatening. All affected individuals should be evaluated for cervical spine instability. Particular care should be exercised during anesthesia because

of the mobile arytenoid cartilage as well as the potentially dangerous spinal anomalies.

ETIOLOGY. Although autosomal dominant is the most commonly reported mode of inheritance, autosomal recessive inheritance also has been suggested. Mutations in the gene encoding Filamin B (FLNB) localized to chromosome 3p14 are responsible for autosomal dominant Larsen syndrome. FLNB seems to have an important role in vertebral segmentation, joint formation, and endochondral ossification.

COMMENT. A rare lethal form of this disorder has been described. The principal features include a flat facies, cleft soft palate, redundant neck skin, multiple joint dislocations, rhizomelic shortening of the upper limbs, hypoplasia of the fibula, and hypoplastic vertebral bodies. Death is secondary to pulmonary hypoplasia.

References

Larsen LJ, Schottstaedt ER, Bost FC: Multiple congenital dislocations associated with characteristic facial abnormality. J Pediatr 37:574, 1950.

Latta RJ et al: Larsen's syndrome: A skeletal dysplasia with multiple joint dislocations and unusual facies. J Pediatr 78:291, 1971.

Striscinglio P et al: Severe cardiac anomalies in sibs with Larsen syndrome. J Med Genet 20:422, 1983.

Bowen JR et al: Spinal deformities in Larsen's syndrome. Clin Orthop 197:159, 1985.

Stanley D, Seymoor N: The Larsen syndrome occurring in four generations of one family. Int Orthop 8:267, 1985.

Clayton-Smith J, Donnai D: A further patient with the lethal type of Larsen syndrome. J Med Genet 25:499, 1988.

Patrella R et al: Long-term follow-up of two sibs with Larsen syndrome possibly due to parental germ-line mosaicism. Am J Med Genet 47:187, 1993.

Vujic M et al: Localization of a gene for autosomal dominant Larsen syndrome to chromosome region 3p21.1-14.1 in the proximity of, but distinct from, the COL7A1 locus. Am J Hum Genet 57:1104, 1995.

Johnston CE et al: Cervical kyphosis in patients who have Larsen syndrome. J Bone Joint Surg [Am] 78A:538, 1996.

Malik P, Choudhry DK: Larsen syndrome and its anaesthetic considerations. Paediatr Anaesth 12:632, 2002.

Krakow D et al: Mutations in the gene encoding filamin B disrupt vertebral segmentation, joint formation, and skeletogenesis. Nat Genet 36:405, 2004.

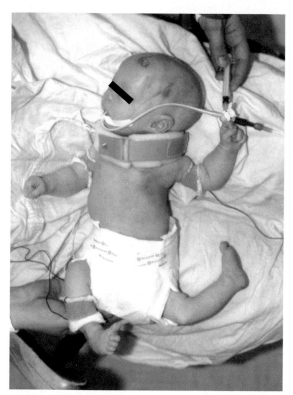

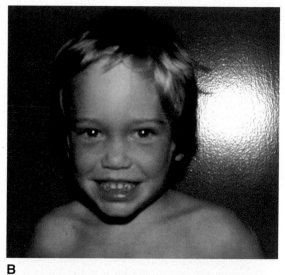

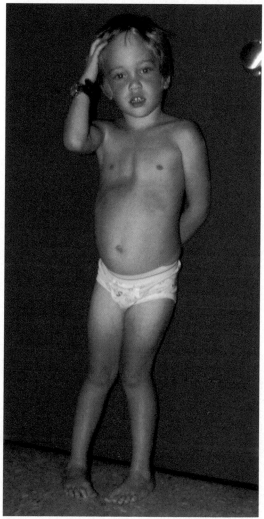

FIGURE 1. Larsen syndrome. **A,** A newborn with dislocation of knees and hypoplastic bodies of cervical vertebrae for which he is wearing a neck collar. (Courtesy of Dr. David Weaver, Indiana University, Indianapolis.) **B–D,** A 5-year-old boy. Note the flat face with depressed nasal bridge, and prominent forehead. (**B–D,** Courtesy of Dr. Marilyn C. Jones, Children's Hospital, San Diego.)

MULTIPLE EXOSTOSES SYNDROME
(DIAPHYSEAL ACLASIS, EXTERNAL
CHONDROMATOSIS SYNDROME)

Diaphyseal Outgrowths Leading to Limb Deformity, with or without Short Metacarpals

More than 1000 cases have been reported. Prevalence is estimated to be 1/50,000.

ABNORMALITIES

Skeletal. Multiple benign cartilage-capped tumors (osteochondromas or exostosis) located most commonly around the knee, followed in frequency by the wrist, the proximal humerus, the proximal fibula, and the ribs; variable involvement of the scapula and pelvis occurs; neither the mandible nor the calvarium are involved; lesions are usually not present at birth, but become obvious between 2 and 10 years of age; there is a slowing in their growth at adolescence, and no further growth occurs in the adult; remodeling defects caused by disruption of normal epiphyseal growth plate of the long bones leads to limb discrepancy and angular deformities; involved bone may be relatively short, especially the ulna, with consequent bowing of the forearm; shortness of stature with a mean male adult height of 170 cm with a range of 155 to 190.5 cm and a mean female adult height of 155 cm with a range of 127 to 173 cm; 37% of male and 44% of female heights less than the fifth percentile.

NATURAL HISTORY.
New outgrowths and enlargement of old exostoses may occur through adolescence. Thereafter, growth or pain in the lesion should raise concern with respect to malignant transformation, which occurs in 3% to 5% with an age ranging from 11 to 64 years. In a retrospective review of 43 affected individuals and 137 of their affected relatives, Luckert-Wicklund and colleagues documented the following: Approximately two thirds of patients have surgery for removal of at least one exostosis; for those patients 21 years or older the mean number of exostosis removed was 3.5; compression of peripheral nerves occurred in 22.6%, of blood vessels in 11.3%, and of the spinal cord in one patient; arthritis with mean age of onset of 36 years occurred in 14%; and during pregnancy changes in the exostosis occurred in 10.5%. Other complications include bursa formation, usually presenting as a painful enlarging mass simulating malignant transformation, osteomyelitis, muscle impingement, and hemarthrosis.

ETIOLOGY.
This disorder has an autosomal dominant inheritance pattern. Three loci for hereditary multiple exostosis (HME) have been identified; EXT1 at 8q23-24, EXT2 at 11p11-p12, and EXT3 at 19p. Both EXT1 and EXT2 have been cloned. Studies of some chondrosarcomas have demonstrated loss of heterozygosity of chromosomes 8q and 11p but not of 19p suggesting that the EXT1 and EXT2 genes may behave as tumor-suppressor genes.

COMMENT.
It has been suggested that the development of exostosis in HME is the consequence of a two-hit mutational model in which a single germline mutation results in predisposition for tumor development and a second somatic mutational hit is necessary for the development of the exostosis.

References
Solomon L: Hereditary multiple exostosis. Am J Hum Genet 16:351, 1964.
Shapiro F, Simon S, Glimcher MJ: Hereditary multiple exostosis. J Bone Joint Surg 61A:815, 1979.
Cook A et al: Genetic heterogeneity in families of hereditary multiple exostoses. Am J Hum Genet 53:71, 1993.
Le Merrer M et al: A gene for hereditary multiple exostoses maps to chromosome 19p. Hum Mol Genet 3:717, 1994.
Wu Y-Q et al: Assignment of a second locus for multiple exostoses to the pericentric region of chromosome 11. Hum Mol Genet 3:167, 1994.
Ahn J et al: Cloning of the putative tumour suppressor gene for hereditary multiple exostosis (EXT 1). Nat Genetics 11:137, 1995.

Hecht JT et al: Hereditary multiple exostoses and chondrosarcoma: Linkage to chromosome 11 and loss of heterozygosity for EXT-linked markers on chromosome 11 and 8. Am J Hum Genet 56:1125, 1995.

Luckert-Wicklund C et al: Natural history study of hereditary multiple exostoses. Am J Med Genet 55:43, 1995.

Vanhoenacker FM et al: Hereditary multiple exostosis; from genetics to clinical syndrome and complications. Eur J Radiol 40:208, 2001.

Hall CR et al: Reevaluation of a genetic model for the development of exostosis in hereditary multiple exostosis. Am J Med Genet 112:1, 2002.

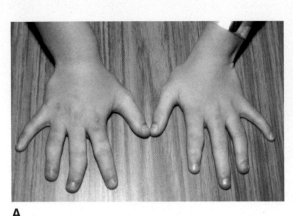

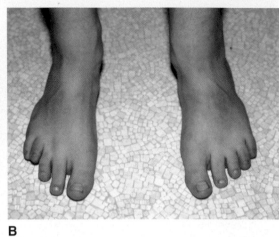

A

B

Continued

FIGURE 1. Multiple exostoses syndrome. **A–F,** Note the grossly evident exostosis in the hand; altered angulation of the finger; short fourth and fifth toes, which are due to short fourth and fifth metatarsals; and, in the radiographs, the presence of exostoses at the ends of long bones as well as in the pelvis.

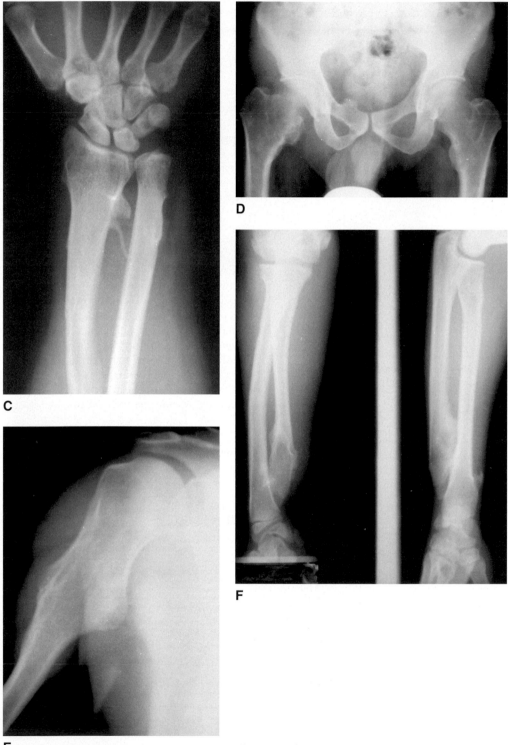

Fig. 1, cont'd.

NAIL-PATELLA SYNDROME
(HEREDITARY OSTEO-ONYCHODYSPLASIA)

Nail Dysplasia, Patella Hypoplasia, Iliac Spurs

Little's report in 1897, limited to a presentation of the patellar defect, is usually credited as the initial description of this syndrome, whereas this pattern includes multiple other dysplasias of osseous as well as nonosseous mesenchymal tissues. More than 400 cases have been reported.

ABNORMALITIES

Nails. Hypoplasia, splitting, most commonly of thumbnail; discoloration, longitudinal ridging, poorly formed lunulae and triangular lunulae.

Knees. Hypoplastic to absent patella, hypoplasia of lateral femoral condyle, small head of fibula, and prominent tibial tuberosity.

Elbows. Incomplete extension, pronation and supination, cubitus valgus, hypoplastic capitellum, small head of radius (90%).

Ilia. Spur in midposterior ilium, 71% palpable (81%).

Scapulae. Hypoplasia, convex thick outer border (44%).

Irides. Dark pigmentation centrally in cloverleaf or flower shape, particularly noticeable in blue eyes.

Renal. Proteinuria with or without hematuria, casts, renal insufficiency.

Other Frequent Features. Absence of distal phalangeal joints, delayed ossification of secondary centers of ossification, valgus deformity of femoral neck, talipes, Madelung deformity, calcaneovalgus, equinovalgus, tight Achilles tendons, scoliosis, lumbar lordosis.

OCCASIONAL ABNORMALITIES

Skeletal. Prominent outer clavicle, hypoplasia of first ribs, malformed sternum, spina bifida, scoliosis, enlarged ulnar styloid process, clinodactyly of fifth finger, dislocation of head of radius, antecubital or axillary pterygia, polyarteritis-like vasculitis, congenital hip dislocation.

Eyes. Glaucoma, keratoconus, microcornea, microphakia, cataract, ptosis.

Muscles. Aplasia of pectoralis minor, biceps, triceps, quadriceps.

Central Nervous System. Occasional mental deficiency, psychosis.

Other. Cleft lip/palate, weak crumbling teeth, sensorineural hearing loss, irritable bowel or constipation, peripheral neurologic symptoms.

NATURAL HISTORY. Patients may have problems resulting from limitation of joint mobility, dislocation, or both, especially at the elbows and knee, where osteoarthritis may eventually limit function. Children should be closely followed for scoliosis. Proteinuria with or without hematuria is the most common early indication of a renal problem. Once proteinuria is present, it can remit spontaneously, remain asymptomatic, progress to nephrotic syndrome or nephritis, and occasionally to renal failure. Renal involvement occurs in approximately 25% of cases, and in one third of those older than 40 years. Mean age at which renal involvement is detected is 22 years. It may be exacerbated during pregnancy.

ETIOLOGY. This disorder has an autosomal dominant inheritance pattern. Mutations in the LIM-homeodomain gene, LMX1B, located at 9q34 are responsible.

References

Little EM: Congenital absence or delayed development of the patella. Lancet 2:781, 1897.

Carbonara P, Alpert M: Hereditary osteoonychodysplasia (Hood). Am J Med Sci 248:139, 1964.

Lucas GL, Optiz JM: The nail-patella syndrome: Clinical and genetic aspects of 5 kindreds with 38 affected family members. J Pediatr 68:273, 1966.

Darlington D, Hawkins CF: Nail-patella syndrome with iliac horns and hereditary nephropathy: Necropsy report and anatomical dissection. J Bone Joint Surg [Br] 49-B:164, 1967.

Beals RK, Eckardt AL: Hereditary onychoosteodysplasia: A report of nine kindreds. J Bone Joint Surg [Am] 51:505, 1969.

Daniel CR, Osment LS, Noojin RO: Triangular lunulae. Arch Dermatol 116:448, 1980.

Looij BJ et al: Genetic counseling in hereditary osteo-onychodysplasia (HOOD, nail-patella syndrome) with nephropathy. J Med Genet 25:682, 1988.

Rizzo R et al: Familial bilateral pterygia with severe renal involvement in nail-patella syndrome. Clin Genet 44:1, 1993.

Dreyer SD et al: Mutations in LMX1B cause abnormal skeletal patterning and renal dysplasia in nail patella syndrome. Nat Genet 19:47, 1998.

Sweeney E et al: Nail patella syndrome: A review of the phenotype aided by developmental biology. J Med Genet 40:153, 2003.

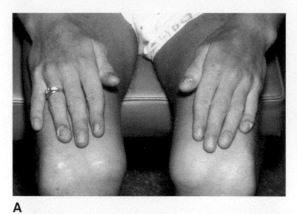

A

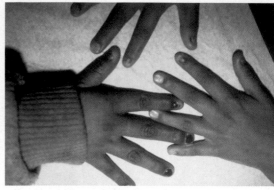

B

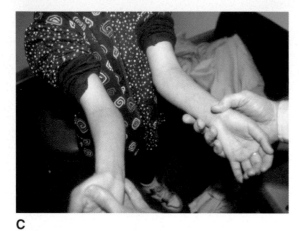

C

FIGURE 1. Nail-patella syndrome. **A,** Adolescent showing nail hypoplasia, especially of thumbs, and displacement of small patellae. **B,** Two affected children showing nail dysplasia. **C,** Incomplete extension of the elbows.

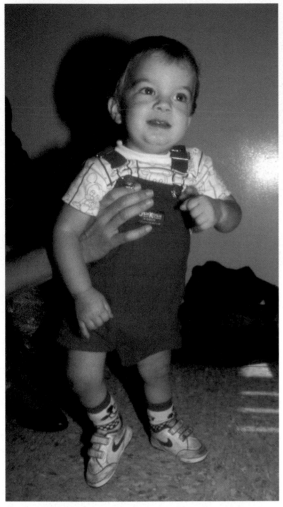

A

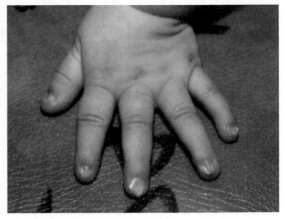

B

FIGURE 2. **A** and **B,** A 15-month-old child. Note the striking nail dysplasia and evidence of joint dislocation at the knees. (Courtesy of Dr. Marilyn C. Jones, Children's Hospital, San Diego.)

MEIER-GORLIN SYNDROME

Absent/Hypoplastic Patella, Microtia, Short Stature

Initially described in two separate case reports in 1959 and by Gorlin and colleagues in 1975, this disorder has now been reported in approximately 30 patients. An excellent review has been published by Bongers and colleagues.

ABNORMALITIES

Growth. Prenatal and postnatal growth deficiency, delayed bone age.

Performance. IQ is usually normal although moderate mental retardation has been described in some cases; expressive language delay, usually associated with normal hearing, occurs occasionally; a cheerful, friendly personality has been described.

Craniofacial. Microcephaly, microtia, low-set abnormally formed ears, atretic/small external auditory canals, small mouth with full lips, micrognathia, high-arched palate.

Skeletal. Absent/hypoplastic patella; slender long bones; abnormal flattened epiphysis; hyperextensible joints; thoracic abnormalities including absent, hypoplastic, slender or short ribs; lack of sternal ossification; pectus carinatum; and chest asymmetry.

Genitalia. Cryptorchidism, hypoplastic labia majora/minora, clitoromegaly.

OCCASIONAL ABNORMALITIES.

Early closure of cranial sutures, maxillary hypoplasia, cleft palate, deafness with congenital labyrinthine anomalies, prominent veins over nose and forehead, thin skin, breast hypoplasia, micropenis, hypospadias, hypoplastic corpora cavernosa and medial segment of urethra, decreased arm span for height, restriction of joint motion, camptodactyly, fifth finger clinodactyly, hyperconvex nails, growth hormone deficiency.

NATURAL HISTORY. Failure to thrive secondary to feeding problems is common throughout the first 2 years. Respiratory difficulties improve after the neonatal period. The typical facial features seen in infancy including micrognathia, a small mouth and full lips change over time such that by adolescence, a high vertical forehead, narrow nose and high nasal bridge are most characteristic.

ETIOLOGY. This disorder has an autosomal recessive inheritance pattern.

References

Meier Z et al: Ein fall von arthrogryposis multilex congenita Kombiniert mit dyostosis mandibulofacialis (Franceschetti syndrome). Helv Pediatr Acta 14:213, 1959.

Gorlin RJ et al: A selected miscellany. Birth Defects 11(2):39, 1975.

Fryns JP: Meier-Gorlin syndrome: The adult phenotype. Clin Dysmorphol 7:231, 1998.

Bongers E et al: Meier-Gorlin syndrome: Report of eight additional cases and review. Am J Med Genet 102:115, 2001.

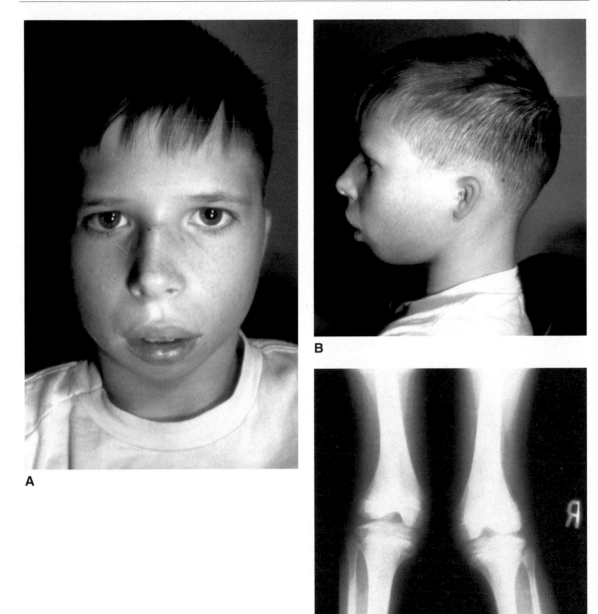

FIGURE 1. Meier-Gorlin syndrome. **A–C,** A 16-year-old boy, Note the small mouth with full lips, micrognathia, microtia, and absent patella. (From Gorlin RJ et al: Birth Defects 11:39, 1975.)

LERI-WEILL DYSCHONDROSTEOSIS

Short Forearms with Madelung Deformity, with or without Short Lower Leg

Leri and Weill described this condition in 1929. Most patients previously categorized as having Madelung deformity have Leri-Weill dyschondrosteosis.

ABNORMALITIES

Growth. Variable small stature, adult height from 135 cm to normal.

Extremities. Short forearm with bowing of radius and distal hypoplasia of the dorsally dislocated ulna leading to a widened gap between radius and ulna, and altered osseous alignment at wrist (Madelung deformity); may have partial dislocation of ulna at wrist, elbow, or both, with limitation of movement; short lower leg.

OCCASIONAL ABNORMALITIES.

Short hands and feet with metaphyseal flaring in metacarpal and metatarsal bones, short fourth metacarpal or metatarsal bones, curvature of tibia, exostoses from proximal tibia and/or fibula, abnormal femoral neck, coxa valga, abnormal tuberosity of humerus.

NATURAL HISTORY. Associated para-
myotonia has been noted in affected individuals in one family; whether this is a frequent feature remains to be determined. Otherwise, the only problems are moderate shortness of stature and limitation of joint mobility at the wrist, elbow, or both.

ETIOLOGY. Autosomal dominant, with an excess of affected females in the recorded cases. Mutations and more commonly deletions of the SHOX (short stature homeobox containing) gene located at Xp22.3 in the pseudoautosomal region of the X and Y chromosomes are responsible. Genes within this region escape X-inactivation and are thus normally expressed on both sex chromosomes in males and females.

References

Leri A, Weill J: Une affection congenitale et symétrique du développement osseus: La dyschondrosteose. Bull Mem Soc Med Hop (Paris) 45:1491, 1929.

Langer LO: Dyschondrosteosis, a hereditary bone dysplasia with characteristic roentgenographic features. Am J Roentgenol Radium Ther Nucl Med 45:178, 1965.

Herdman RC, Langer LO, Good RA: Dyschondrosteosis. The most common cause of Madelung's deformity. J Pediatr 68:432, 1966.

Felman AH, Kirkpatrick JA: Dyschondrosteose. Am J Dis Child 120:329, 1970.

Beals RK: Dyschondrosteosis and Madelung's deformity: Report of three kindreds and review of the literature. Clin Orthop 116:24, 1976.

Belin V et al: SHOX mutations in dyschodrosteosis (Leri-Weill syndrome). Nat Genet 19:67, 1998.

Shears DJ et al: Mutations and deletions of the pseudoautosomal gene SHOX causes Leri-Weill dyschondrosteosis. Nat Genet 19:70, 1998.

Ross JL et al: Phenotypes associated with SHOX deficiency. J Clin Endocrinol Metab 86:5674, 2001.

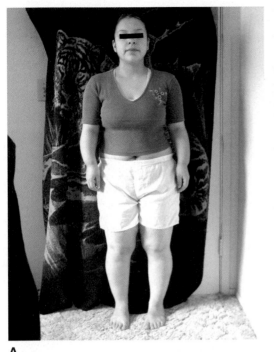

A

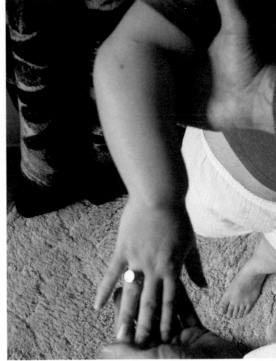

B

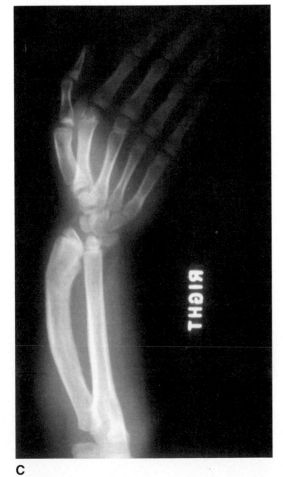

C

FIGURE 1. Leri-Weill dyschondrosteosis. **A–C,** A 20-year-old woman. Note the short forearms with bowing of the radius and distal hypoplasia of the dorsally dislocated ulna.

LANGER MESOMELIC DYSPLASIA
(Homozygous Leri-Weill Dyschondrosteosis Syndrome)

Mesomelic Dwarfism, Rudimentary
Fibula, Micrognathia

Langer delineated this disorder as a distinct entity in 1967, citing numerous cases from past literature. The original report was presented by Brailsford. Espiritu and colleagues first suggested that Langer mesomelic dysplasia represents the homozygous form of Leri-Weill dyschondrosteosis.

ABNORMALITIES

Growth. Disproportionate short stature with decreased arm span and increased upper/lower segment ratio.

Facies. High-arched palate, mandibular hypoplasia.

Limbs. Short, especially forearms and lower legs (mesomelia); the fibula is rudimentary, the tibia is short with proximal hypoplasia, the ulna is reduced distally, and the radius is dorsolaterally bowed and short; increased carrying angle; Madelung deformity in adults.

NATURAL HISTORY. Normal intelligence with surprisingly good function is the rule. One individual, homozygous for a complete SHOX gene deletion, had additional abnormalities including mental retardation. It has been suggested that the associated defects could be attributed to concomitant deletion of an adjacent gene or genes.

ETIOLOGY. The homozygous state of the autosomal dominant gene for Leri-Weill dyschondrosteosis (LWD). Leri-Weill dyschondrosteosis is caused by mutations and deletions of the SHOX (short stature homeobox containing) gene. Whereas Leri-Weill dyschondrosteosis is the result of SHOX haploinsufficiency, individuals with Langer mesomelic dysplasia have complete or nearly complete loss of SHOX function. Although heterozygous SHOX deletions are the most common cause of Leri-Weill dyschondrosteosis, the vast majority of individuals with Langer mesomelis dysplasia are homozygous for SHOX mutations.

References

Brailsford JF: Dystrophies of the skeleton. Br J Radiol 8:533, 1935.

Blockey NJ, Lawrie JH: An unusual symmetrical distal limb deformity in siblings. J Bone Joint Surg [Br] 45:745, 1963.

Langer LO: Mesomelic dwarfism of the hypoplastic ulna, fibula, mandible type. Radiology 89:654, 1967.

Espiritu C, Chen H, Woolley PV Jr: Probable homozygosity for the dyschondrosteosis genes. Am J Dis Child 129:375, 1975.

Kunze J, Klemm T: Mesomelic dysplasia, type Langer—a homozygous state for dyschondrosteosis. Eur J Pediatr 134:269, 1980.

Shears DJ et al: Pseudodominant inheritance of Langer mesomelic dysplasia caused by a SHOX homeobox missense mutation. Am J Med Genet 110:153, 2002.

Zinn AR et al: Complete SHOX deficiency causes Langer mesomelic dysplasia. Am J Med Genet 110:158, 2002.

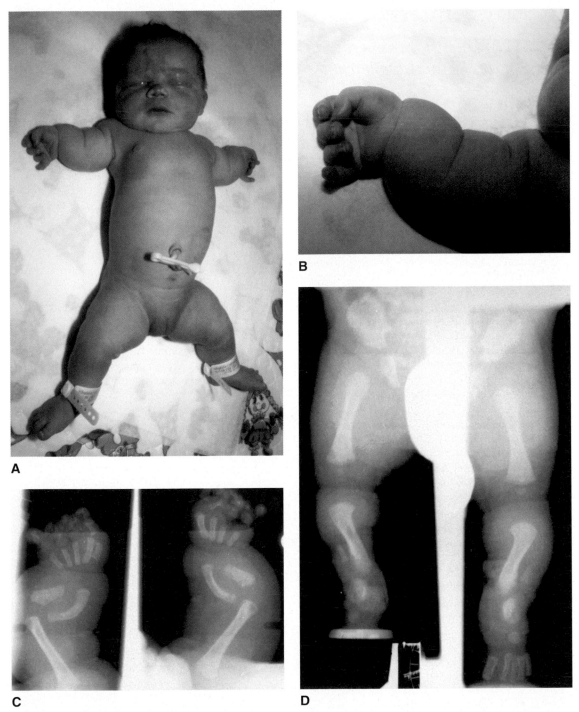

FIGURE 1. Langer mesomelic dysplasia. **A–D,** A newborn with unusual shortness of stature with disproportionate smallness of forearms and lower legs, especially the ulnae and fibulae. (Courtesy of Dr. Marilyn C. Jones, Children's Hospital, San Diego.)

ACRODYSOSTOSIS

Short Hands with Peripheral Dysostosis, Small Nose, Mental Deficiency

Maroteaux and Malamut first described this disorder in three patients in 1968, and there are now over 50 published cases.

ABNORMALITIES

Growth. Mild to moderate prenatal onset of growth deficiency, short stature (55%).

Performance. Mental deficiency in 77%, average IQ of 61 with a range from 24 to 85, hearing deficit (67%).

Craniofacial. Brachycephaly, low nasal bridge, broad and small upturned nose (97%), tendency to hold mouth open, hypoplastic maxilla (100%) with prognathism, increased mandibular angle (68%).

Limbs. Short, especially distally, with progressive deformity in distal humerus, radius, and ulna, and cone-shaped epiphyses that fuse prematurely in hands and feet; hands appear short and broad, with wrinkling of dorsal skin; large great toe.

Other. Vertebral defects including loss of normal caudal widening of the lumbar interpedicular distance (75%), small vertebrae that may collapse, spinal canal stenosis, and scoliosis; advanced bone age; epiphyseal stippling noted in neonatal period principally involving the lumbosacral and cervical vertebral bodies, the carpal and tarsal bones, proximal humeri, terminal phalanges, knees, and hips; stippling regresses by 4 months and is almost always gone by 8 months of age.

OCCASIONAL ABNORMALITIES.

Hydrocephalus, epicanthal folds (39%), hypertelorism (35%), optic atrophy, hearing loss, dimpled nasal tip, malocclusion of teeth, delayed tooth eruption (23%), hypodontia (3%), calvarial hyperostosis, pigmented nevi, hypoplastic genitalia (29%), cryptorchidism (29%), irregular menses (18%), hypogonadism, dislocated radial heads, renal anomalies (3%), hypothyroidism.

NATURAL HISTORY. Most patients with this disorder do relatively well except for the problems of mental deficiency and arthritic complaints. Progressive restriction of movement of the hands, elbows, and spine may occur. Decompressive laminectomy for spinal stenosis is not uncommonly required.

ETIOLOGY. This disorder has an autosomal dominant inheritance pattern.

COMMENT. Radiographic features that distinguish this disorder from Albright hereditary osteodystrophy include decreased interpediculate distance and a characteristic metacarpophalangeal pattern profile for the brachydactyly including metacarpals 2 to 5 that are more severely affected than the corresponding phalanges as well as sparing of the thumbs and halluces. Futhermore, no patient with acrodysostosis has had a mutation in the gene encoding the α subunit of the membrane-bound G_s protein (GNAS1) which is responsible for Albright hereditary osteodystrophy.

References

Maroteaux P, Malamut GL: L'acrodysostose. Presse Med 76:2189, 1968.

Robinow M et al: Acrodysostosis: A syndrome of peripheral dysostosis, nasal hypoplasia, and mental retardation. Am J Dis Child 121:195, 1971.

Butler MG et al: Acrodysostosis: Report of a 13 year old boy with review of literature and metacarpophalangeal pattern profile analysis. Am J Med Genet 30:971, 1988.

Viljoen D, Beighton P: Epiphyseal stippling in acrodysostosis. Am J Med Genet 38:43, 1991.

Davies SJ, Hughes HE: Familial acrodysostosis: Can it be distinguished from Albright's hereditary osteodystrophy? Clin Dysmorphol 1:207, 1992.

Steiner RD, Pagon RA: Autosomal dominant transmission of acrodysostosis. Clin Dysmorphol 1:201, 1992.

Graham JM et al: Radiographic findings and Gs-alpha bioactivity studies and mutation screening in acrodysostosis indicate a different etiology from pseudohypoparathyroidism. Pediatr Radiol 31:2, 2001.

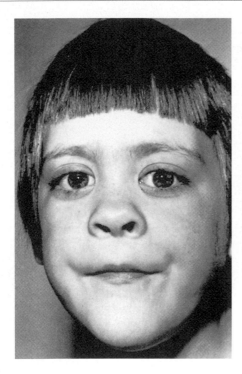

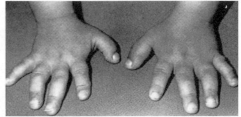

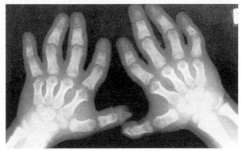

FIGURE 1. Acrodysostosis. A 5-year-old girl. Note the low nasal bridge, epicanthal folds, prominent mandible, short, broad fingers with skin wrinkling, and the broad and short metacarpals and phalanges with cone-shaped epiphyses.

ALBRIGHT HEREDITARY OSTEODYSTROPHY

(Pseudohypoparathyroidism, Pseudopseudohypoparathyroidism)

Short Metacarpals, Rounded Facies, with or without Hypocalcemia or Vicarious Mineralization

Albright described this condition in 1942 and referred to it as pseudohypoparathyroidism (PHP) because of hypocalcemia and hyperphosphatemia that were unresponsive to parathormone. Two variants have been described: PHP type-Ia (PHP-Ia) and pseudopseudohypoparathyroidism (PPHP). Individuals with PHP-Ia have features of Albright hereditary osteodystrophy (AHO) and present with hypocalcemia and hyperphosphatemia, despite elevated serum parathyroid hormone levels. Resistance to thyroid-stimulating hormone and gonadotropins as well as growth hormone–releasing hormone and calcitonin also occur. Individuals with PPHP have the characteristic features of Albright hereditary osteodystrophy but show no evidence of resistance to parathyroid hormone or any other hormone. Both variants result from decreased activity of the alpha subunit of the trimeric G_s regulatory protein, the function of which is to couple membrane receptors to adenyl cyclase, an action that stimulates cyclic adenosine monophosphate.

ABNORMALITIES

Growth. Small stature; final height, 54 to 60 inches; occasionally normal; moderate obesity; span decreased for height.

Performance. Mental deficiency, IQs of 20 to 99, mean IQ of approximately 60; occasionally normal.

Face and Neck. Rounded, low nasal bridge; short neck; cataracts.

Dentition. Delayed dental eruption, aplasia, or enamel hypoplasia.

Limbs. Short metacarpals and metatarsals, especially the fourth and fifth; short distal phalanx of thumb; cone-shaped epiphyses; osteoporosis.

Extraskeletal Calcification. Areas of mineralization in subcutaneous tissues, basal ganglia.

Calcium and Phosphorus. Variable hypocalcemia and hyperphosphatemia.

OCCASIONAL ABNORMALITIES.

Hypothyroidism, hypogonadism with or without gonadal dysgenesis, peripheral lenticular opacities, nystagmus, unequal size of pupils, blurring of disk margins, tortuosity of vessels, diplopia, microphthalmia, optic atrophy, macular degeneration, hypertelorism, thick calvarium, short ulna, short phalanges, genu valgum, fibrous dysplasia, exostosis, osteitis fibrosa cystica, epiphyseal dysplasia, advanced bone age, clavicular abnormalities, cervical vertebral anomalies with associated spinal cord compression, osteochondroma, pancreatic dysfunction.

NATURAL HISTORY.
The shortened metacarpal or phalangeal bones represent early epiphyseal fusion and may not be evident until several years of age. Hypocalcemia, when present, usually becomes evident in childhood, seizures being the most common presenting symptom. Hypocalcemia may become manifest during periods of increased calcium utilization, as in adolescence or in pregnancy. Reproductive dysfunction is common and most likely represents partial resistance to gonadotropins.

ETIOLOGY.
This disorder has an autosomal dominant inheritance pattern. Documentation of more than one affected child born to unaffected parents is an indication of germline mosaicism. A variety of different mutations in the gene encoding the α subunit of the membrane-bound G_s protein (GNAS1) that stimulates adenyl cyclase activity are responsible for both the PHP-Ia and the PPHP variants. The gene is localized to chromosome 20q13.11. PHP-Ia and PPHP have been reported in the same family and are dependent on the parent of origin. Inheritance of the altered gene from a father affected by either PHP-Ia or PPHP leads to PPHP, whereas inheritance of the same mutation from the mother with either variant leads to PHP-Ia.

References

Albright F et al: Pseudohypoparathyroidism—an example of "Seabright-bantam syndrome": Report of three cases. Endocrinology 30:922, 1942.

Christiaen L et al: Le pseudohypoparathyroidisme chronique: A propos de trois cas familiaux. Acta Paediatr Belg 21:5, 1967.

Spranger JW: Skeletal dysplasia and the eye: Albright's hereditary osteodystrophy. Birth Defects 5:122, 1969.

Poznanski AK, Werder EA, Giedion A: The patterning of shortening of the bones of the hand in PHP and PPHP. Pediatr Radiol 123:707, 1977.

Fitch N: Albright's hereditary osteodystrophy: A review. Am J Med Genet 11:11, 1982.

Levine MA et al: Genetic deficiency of the α subunit of the guanine nucleotide-binding protein G_s as the molecular basis for Albright hereditary osteodystrophy. Proc Natl Acad Sci USA 85:615, 1988.

Patten JL et al: Mutation in the gene encoding the stimulatory G protein of adenylate cyclase in Albright's hereditary osteodystrophy. N Engl J Med 322:1412, 1990.

Gejman PV et al: Genetic mapping of the G_s-α subunit gene (GNAS1) to the distal long arm of chromosome 20 using a polymorphism detected by denaturing gradient gel electrophoresis. Genomics 9:782, 1991.

Wilson LC, Trembath RC: Albright's hereditary osteodystrophy. J Med Genet 31:779, 1994.

Levine MA: Clinical spectrum and pathogenesis of pseudohypoparathyroidism. Rev Endocr Metab Disord 1:265, 2000.

Ahrens W et al: Analysis of the GNAS1 gene in Albright's hereditary osteodystrophy. J Clin Endocrinol Metab 86:4630, 2001.

Bastepe M, Juppner H: Editorial: Pseudohypoparathyroidism and mechanisms of resistance toward multiple hormones: Molecular evidence to clinical presentation. J Clin Endocrinol Metab 88:4055, 2003.

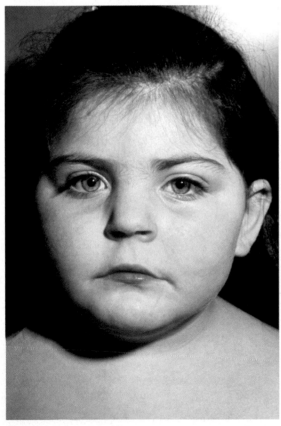

A

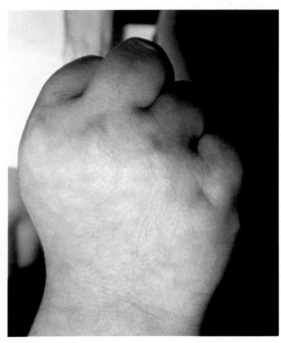

B

FIGURE 1. Albright hereditary osteodystrophy. **A** and **B,** Moderately retarded girl showing rounded face and indications of short fourth and fifth metacarpal bones in fisted hand.

N Storage Disorders

GENERALIZED GANGLIOSIDOSIS SYNDROME, TYPE I (SEVERE INFANTILE TYPE)
(CAFFEY PSEUDO-HURLER SYNDROME, FAMILIAL NEUROVISCERAL LIPIDOSIS)

Coarse Facies, Joint Limitation, Kyphosis in Early Infancy

In 1951, Caffey described two neonates who had many of the features of Hurler syndrome, but of prenatal onset. Landing and colleagues reported pathologic studies in similar cases showing foamy histiocytes in the liver and spleen, swollen neurons, and vacuoles in the glomerular epithelium. They interpreted the storage material as a glycolipid and set forth the name "familial neurovisceral lipidosis," which was changed to "generalized gangliosidosis" by Okada and O'Brien on the basis of finding elevated levels of ganglioside GM_1 in the liver, spleen, and brain tissue from a patient. The molecular defect has been shown to be a deficiency of ganglioside GM_1 β-galactosidase.

ABNORMALITIES

Growth. Deficiency, with relatively low birth weight and severe postnatal growth deficit.

Performance. Severe early defect in developmental performance with hypotonia, poor coordination, and later, spasticity.

Orofacial. Coarse features with low nasal bridge, broad nose, flaring alae nasi, frontal bossing, long philtrum, hypertrophied alveolar ridges with prominent maxilla and mild macroglossia, hirsutism.

Eyes. Cherry-red macular spot in approximately one half of the patients.

Skeletal. Moderate joint limitation with thick wrists, contractures at the elbows and knees, and development of clawhand; early radiographs show poorly mineralized, coarsely trabeculated long bones with medullary midshaft broadening and a "cloak" of subperiosteal new bone formation, especially evident in the humerus; some metaphyseal cupping and epiphyseal irregularity are usually present; with time, the bones appear more like those of the Hurler syndrome, including kyphosis with anterior bullet wedging of vertebrae; ribs are thick, legs may be bowed, and talipes may be present; short broad hands; kyphoscoliosis.

Viscera. Variable hepatosplenomegaly with some foamy histiocytes, vacuolation in glomerular epithelial cells containing swollen lysosomes.

Leukocytes. Vacuolation within cytoplasm of leukocytes and foam cells in marrow.

Urinary Excretion. Mucopolysaccharides occasionally may be increased with the excretion of keratan sulfate–like materials.

Other. Facial and peripheral edema in early infancy; inguinal hernia; angiokeratoma corporis diffusum (telangiectases or warty growths, in groups, together with thickening of the epidermis); dermal melanocytosis.

NATURAL HISTORY. Severe developmental lag with hypotonia, feeding problems with failure to thrive, and frequent infections usually culminate in death during early infancy. Deterioration of cerebral function is rapid if the patient survives the first year, leading to a decerebrate status with seizures and death before 2 years of age. The mean age of survival for 17 patients was 13.5 months, with a range from 3.5 to 25 months. No form of therapy other than life-supportive tube feeding and antibiotic management of infections has been effective.

ETIOLOGY. This disorder has an autosomal recessive inheritance pattern. The human β-galactosidase gene has been assigned to chromosome 3p21.33. Okada and O'Brien detected a deficit (one twentieth of normal) of the lysosomal enzyme β-galactosidase in the liver from these patients. The presumed developmental pathology of the disease is as follows: (1) the inability to cleave the terminal galactose from ganglioside and mucopolysaccharide, (2) the accumulation of these products within lysosomes where they would normally be degraded, and (3) the storage disease.

The diagnosis is confirmed by the assay of β-galactosidase in the peripheral leukocytes or in cultured skin fibroblasts. Prenatal diagnosis has been established based on the appearance of cultured amniotic fluid cells.

COMMENT. In patients with GM$_1$ gangliosidosis, and Morquio syndrome, type B, there is a deficiency of β-galactosidase. Different mutations in the β-GAL gene result in both disorders.

References

Caffey J: Gargoylism (Hunter-Hurler disease, dysostosis multiplex, lipochondrodystrophy): Prenatal and neonatal bone lesions and their early postnatal evolution. Bull Hosp Joint Dis 12:38, 1951.

Landing BH et al: Familial neurovisceral lipidosis: An analysis of eight cases of a syndrome previously reported as "Hurler-variant," "Pseudo-Hurler disease," and "Tay-Sachs disease with visceral involvement." Am J Dis Child 108:503, 1964.

Okada S, O'Brien JS: Generalized gangliosidosis: Beta-galactosidase deficiency. Science 160:1002, 1968.

Kaback MM et al: Gangliosidosis type I: In-utero detection and fetal manifestations. J Pediatr 82:1037, 1973.

Takano T, Yamanouchi Y: Assignment of human β-galactosidase-A gene to 3p21.33 by fluorescence in situ hybridization. Hum Genet 92:403, 1993.

Hanson M et al: Association of dermal melanocytosis with lysosomal storage disease: Clinical features and hypothesis regarding pathogenesis. Arch Dermatol 139:916, 2003.

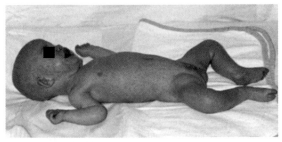

A

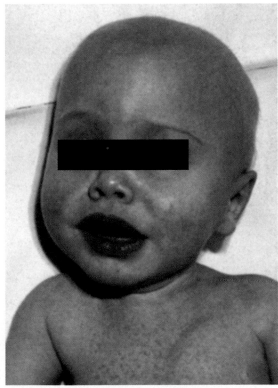

B

FIGURE 1. Generalized gangliosidosis syndrome, type I. **A** and **B,** A 4-week-old infant with coarse facies, hypertrophied alveolar ridges, and broad wrist. (Courtesy of Dr. Jules Leroy, Gent University Hospital, Gent, Belgium.)

LEROY I-CELL SYNDROME
(Mucolipidosis II)

Early Alveolar Ridge Hypertrophy, Joint Limitation, Thick Tight Skin in Early Infancy

This disorder was recognized by Leroy and DeMars when they noted unusual cytoplasmic inclusions in the cultured fibroblasts of a girl who had been considered to have the Hurler syndrome despite the fact that she did not have cloudy corneas or excessive acid mucopolysaccharide in the urine.

ABNORMALITIES

Growth. Birth weight less than $5\frac{1}{2}$ pounds, marked growth deficiency with lack of linear growth after infancy.

Performance. Slow progress from early infancy, reaching a plateau at approximately 18 months with no apparent deterioration subsequently.

Craniofacial. High, narrow forehead; thin eyebrows, puffy eyelids, inner epicanthal folds, clear or faintly hazy corneas; low nasal bridge, anteverted nostrils; long philtrum.

Mouth. Progressive hypertrophy of alveolar ridges.

Skeletal and Joints. Moderate joint limitation in flexion, especially of hips; dorsolumbar kyphosis; broadening of wrists and fingers; roentgenographic findings in the later phases similar to those seen in children with the Hurler syndrome; in early infancy, periosteal new bone formation leading to a "cloaking" of the long tubular bones is best seen in femora and humeri.

Skin. Thick, relatively tight skin during early infancy that becomes less tight as the patients become older; cavernous hemangiomata.

Other. Minimal hepatomegaly, diastasis recti, inguinal hernia (one case), systolic murmurs after 1 year of age, cardiac valve insufficiency, dilated cardiomyopathy, neonatal cholestasis, proximal tubular dysfunction.

Note. No metachromatic granules noted in leukocytes, urinary mucopolysaccharides normal to mildly increased.

NATURAL HISTORY. By 18 months of age, most patients can sit with support, and some stand with support. However, severe progressive retardation of growth and development occur. Recurrent bouts of bronchitis, pneumonia, and otitis media are frequent during early childhood. Death, which usually occurs by 5 years of age, is often associated with congestive heart failure.

ETIOLOGY. This disorder has an autosomal recessive inheritance pattern. The diagnosis is made by detection of deficient lysosomal enzymes in leukocytes and skin fibroblasts and an increase in lysosomal enzyme activity in plasma, cerebrospinal fluid, and urine. This defective processing of lysosomal enzymes is the result of a deficiency of phospho-N-acetylglucosamine transferase seen in this disorder as well as in pseudo-Hurler polydystrophy (mucolipidosis III). A marked increase in serum activity of beta-hexosaminidase, iduronate sulfatase, and aryl-sulfatase A is seen in both disorders.

Heterozygous disease cannot be detected. Prenatal diagnosis can be based on the findings of early amniocentesis and demonstration of elevated lysosomal enzyme activity in cell-free amniotic fluid as well as by demonstrating vacuolation on electron microscopy of chorionic villus cells.

COMMENT. Bone marrow transplant, reported in only a few children with I-cell disease, has prevented progressive cardiac and pulmonary disease and allowed the attainment of neurodevelopmental milestones, although at a much slower than normal rate 5 years following transplantation, in one 7-year-old child.

References

Leroy JG, DeMars RI: Mutant enzymatic and cytological phenotypes in cultured human fibroblasts. Science 157:804, 1967.

Matalon R et al: Lipid abnormalities in a variant of the Hurler syndrome. Proc Natl Acad Sci USA 59:1097, 1968.

Leroy JG, DeMars RI, Opitz JM: "I-cell" disease. In Bergsma DS (ed): The First Conference on the Clinical Delineation of Birth Defects, Part IV. Baltimore: Williams & Wilkins, 1969.

Leroy JG et al: I-cell disease, a clinical picture. J Pediatr 79:360, 1971.

Hickman S, Neufeld EF: A hypothesis for I-cell disease: Defective hydrolases that do not enter lysosomes. Biochem Biophys Res Commun 49:992, 1972.

Kaplan A, Achord DT, Sly WS: Phosphohexosyl components of a lysosomal enzyme are recognized by pinocytosis receptors on human fibroblasts. Proc Natl Acad Sci USA 74:2026, 1977.

Neufeld EF: Lysosomal storage diseases. Ann Rev Biochem 60:257, 1991.

Grewal S et al: Continued neurocognitive development and prevention of cardiopulmonary complications after successful BMT for I-cell disease: A long-term follow-up report. Bone Marrow Transplant 32:957, 2003.

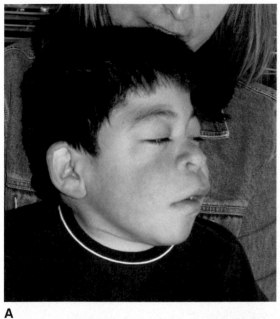

A

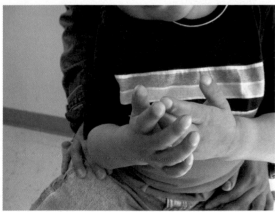

C

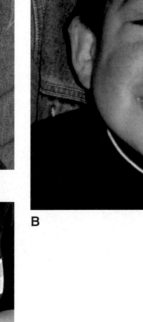

B

FIGURE 1. Leroy I-cell syndrome. **A–C,** A 9-year-old child. Note the high, narrow forehead, puffy eyelids, anteverted nares, long philtrum, hypertrophy of alveolar ridges, and joint contractures. (Courtesy of Dr. Lynne M. Bird, Children's Hospital, San Diego.)

PSEUDO-HURLER POLYDYSTROPHY SYNDROME
(MUCOLIPIDOSIS III)

Coarse Facies, Stiff Joints by 2 to 4 Years, No Mucopolysacchariduria

This disorder was recognized by Maroteaux and Lamy in 1966. Clinically, the disorder is of milder degree than the Hurler syndrome and is similar to the Scheie syndrome, but the patients do not have hepatosplenomegaly, cloudy corneas, or mucopolysacchariduria.

ABNORMALITIES. Onset usually appreciated at 4 to 5 years.
Growth. Decreasing growth rate in early childhood.
Performance. Mild mental retardation; IQs of 64 to 85.
Facies. Development of mildly coarse facies by 6 years.
Eyes. Mild corneal opacities, evident by slit lamp, by 6 to 8 years; mild retinopathy.
Joints. Stiffness and decreased range of motion, especially in hands, elbows, shoulders, and knees; clawhand.
Skeletal. Mild platyspondyly, flaring iliac wings, flattening of femoral epiphyses, changes in hands.
Cardiac. Aortic valve disease, often with regurgitation.
Other. Inguinal hernia, acne.

NATURAL HISTORY. Stiffness of joints usually becomes evident by 4 to 5 years of age, and is the most common early manifestation. Mild facial coarsening, corneal opacities, mild retinopathy, astigmatism, and cardiac valve involvement become evident by 10 years. Approximately 50% have learning disabilities or mild mental retardation. Destruction of hip joints can be a serious problem. Significant variability in clinical expression is common. Carpal tunnel syndrome is common. Mild-to-moderate deterioration of central nervous system function occurs. Some patients have lived into adulthood.

ETIOLOGY. This disorder has an autosomal recessive inheritance pattern. Marrow plasma cells show vacuolations with swollen lysosomes, but without mucopolysacchariduria. Lysosomal enzymes are elevated in the serum and decreased in cultured fibroblasts. The disorder is considered similar to I-cell disease, but is of a milder nature. As with mucolipidosis II, there is a marked increase in serum beta-hexosaminidase, iduronate sulfatase, and arylsulfatase A and a deficiency of phospho-*N*-acetylglucosamine transferase. These two disorders are best differentiated by their clinical courses.

COMMENT. Mucolipidosis III (ML III) is genetically heterogeneous with three complementation groups identified. Group A, the classic mucolipidosis III; group B represented by a single patient; and group C. A mutation in a gene mapped to 16p is responsible for MP IIIC.

References
Maroteaux P, Lamy M: La pseudopolydystrophie de Hurler. Presse Med 74:2889, 1966.
Scott CI Jr, Grossman MS: Pseudo-Hurler polydystrophy. Birth Defects 4(5):349, 1969.
McKusick VA: Heritable Disorders of Connective Tissue, 4th ed. St. Louis: Mosby, 1972.
Melhem R et al: Roentgen findings in mucolipidosis III (pseudo-Hurler polydystrophy). Radiology 106:153, 1973.
Thomas GH et al: Mucolipidosis III (pseudo-Hurler polydystrophy): Multiple lysosomal enzyme abnormalities in serum and cultured fibroblast cells. Pediatr Res 7:751, 1973.
Lang L et al: Lysosomal enzyme phosphorylation in human fibroblasts: Kinetic parameters offer a biochemical rationale for two distinct defects in the uridine diphospho-*N*-acetylglucosamine: Lysosomal enzymic precursor *N*-acetylglucosamine-1-phosphotransferase. J Clin Invest 76:2191, 1985.
Raas-Rothchild A et al: Molecular basis of variant pseudo-Hurler polydystrophy (mucolipidosis IIIC). J Clin Invest 105:673, 2000.
Tylki-Szymanska A et al: Clinical variability in mucolipidosis III (pseudo-Hurler polydystrophy). Am J Med Genet 108:214, 2002.

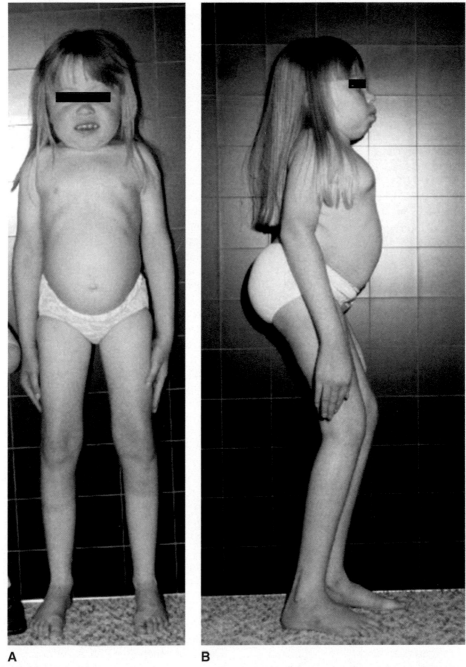

A   **B**

FIGURE 1. Pseudo-Hurler polydystrophy syndrome. **A** and **B,** Early adolescent girl showing facial coarsening, joint contractures, and lumbar lordosis. (Courtesy of Dr. Jules Leroy, Gent University Hospital, Gent, Belgium.)

HURLER SYNDROME
(Mucopolysaccharidosis I H)

Coarse Facies, Stiff Joints, Mental Deficiency, Cloudy Corneas by 1 to 2 Years

Hurler set forth the disorder mucopolysaccharidosis I H (MPS I H) in 1919, 2 years after the Hunter syndrome was described.

ABNORMALITIES

Growth. Deceleration of growth between 6 and 18 months; maximal stature, 110 cm.

Performance. Grossly retarded progress at 6 to 12 months, with failure of advancement by 2 to 5 years.

Craniofacial and Eyes. Scaphocephalic macrocephaly with frontal prominence, coarse facies with full lips, flared nostrils, low nasal bridge, and tendency toward hypertelorism; inner epicanthal folds; hazy corneas; retinal pigmentation.

Mouth. Hypertrophied alveolar ridge and gums with small malaligned teeth, enlarged tongue.

Skeletal and Joints. Diaphyseal broadening of short misshapen bones and joint limitation result in the clawhand and other joint deformities, with more limitation of extension than flexion; flaring of the rib cage; kyphosis and thoracolumbar gibbus secondary to anterior vertebral wedging, short neck; odontoid hypoplasia; J-shaped sella turcica; widening of medial end of clavicle.

Cardiac. Murmurs; cardiac failure may be due to intimal thickening in the coronary vessels or the cardiac valves.

Other. Hirsutism, hepatosplenomegaly, inguinal hernia, umbilical hernia, dislocation of hip, mucoid rhinitis, deafness.

Urinary Excretion. Dermatan sulfate and heparan sulfate.

OCCASIONAL ABNORMALITIES.
Communicating hydrocephalus, presumably a result of thickened meninges; arachnoid cysts; retinal dysfunction; open-angle glaucoma; cardiomyopathy; hydrocele; nephrotic syndrome; carpal tunnel syndrome; hypoplasia of mandibular condyles.

NATURAL HISTORY. Growth during the first year actually may be more rapid than usual, with subsequent deterioration. Subtle changes in the facies, macrocephaly, hernias, limited hip motility, noisy breathing, and frequent respiratory tract infections may be evident during the first 6 months.

Upper airway obstruction secondary to thickening of the epiglottis and tonsillar and adenoidal tissues as well as tracheal narrowing caused by mucopolysaccharide accumulation can lead to sleep apnea and serious airway compromise. Because of the upper airway problems as well as odontoid hypoplasia with or without C1–C2 subluxation, anesthesia is a significant risk. Deceleration of developmental and mental progress is evident during the latter half of the first year. Hearing loss is almost always present. These patients are usually placid, easily manageable, and often lovable. Hypertension frequently occurs and is either centrally mediated or secondary to aortic coarctation. Death usually occurs in childhood secondary to respiratory tract or cardiac complications, and survival past 10 years of age is unusual.

ETIOLOGY. This disorder has an autosomal recessive inheritance pattern. The primary defect is an absence of the lysosomal hydrolase α-L-iduronidase (IDUA), which is responsible for the degradation of the glycosaminoglycans, heparan sulfate and dermatan sulfate. The pathologic consequence is an accumulation of mucopolysaccharides in parenchymal and mesenchymal tissues and the storage of lipids within neuronal tissues. The gene encoding IDUA is located on chromosome 4p16.3. Diagnosis is confirmed by the physical appearance, the excretion of dermatan sulfate and heparan sulfate in the urine, and the absence of α-L-iduronidase in cultured fibroblasts. Heterozygote detection is available. Prenatal diagnosis is possible by measuring α-L-iduronidase in cultured amniotic fluid cells.

COMMENT. Bone marrow transplantation has been effective in the treatment of selected patients.

Engraftment has resulted in resolution of hepato-splenomegaly, an improved airway and improved cardiac function, although valvular abnormalities often progress. Cartilage and bone respond less well and corneal clouding never clears completely. In children with baseline Mental Developmental Index greater than 70, who are engrafted before 24 months, a favorable neurobehavioral outcome has occurred. Enzyme replacement therapy using recombinant human α-L-iduronidase shows some potential. However, its lack of central nervous system penetration is a major drawback to its use in patients with α-L-iduronidase deficiency for whom the central nervous system is severely involved. Potential uses could be while awaiting bone marrow transplantation, in the immediate post-transplantation period, and in successfully transplanted patients who have a heterozygote donor or unfavorable chimerism.

References

Hurler G: Ueber einen Typ multipler Abartungen, vorwiegend am Skelettsystem. Z Kinderheilkd 24:220, 1919.

Leroy JG, Crocker AC: Clinical definition of the Hurler-Hunter phenotypes: A review of 50 patients. Am J Dis Child 112:518, 1966.

Matalon R, Dorfman A: Hurler's syndrome, and α-L-iduronidase deficiency. Biochem Biophys Res Commun 47:959, 1972.

Muenzer J: Mucopolysaccharidoses. Adv Pediatr 33:269, 1989.

Adachi K, Chole RA: Management of tracheal lesions in Hurler syndrome. Arch Otolaryngol Head Neck Surg 116:1205, 1990.

Scott HS et al: Chromosomal localization of the human α-L-iduronidase gene (IDUA) to 4p16.3. Am J Hum Genet 47:802, 1990.

Belani KG et al: Children with mucopolysaccharidosis: Perioperative care, morbidity, mortality and new findings. J Pediatr Surg 28:403, 1993.

Peters C et al: Hurler syndrome: II. Outcome of HLA-genotypically identical siblings and HLA-haploidentical related bone marrow transplantation in fifty-four children. Blood 91:2601, 1998.

Kakkis ED et al: Enzyme replacement therapy in mucopolysaccharidosis I. N Engl J Med 344:182, 2001.

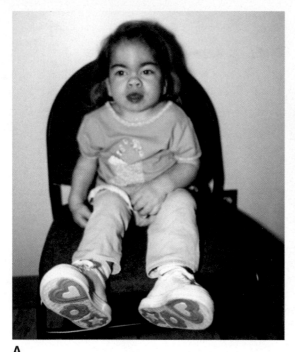

A

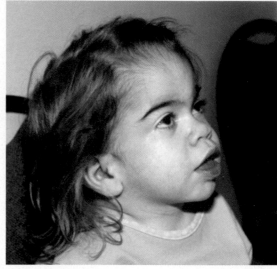

B

FIGURE 1. Hurler syndrome. **A** and **B,** A 4-year-old girl. (**A–E,** Courtesy of Dr. Marilyn C. Jones, Children's Hospital, San Diego.) *Continued*

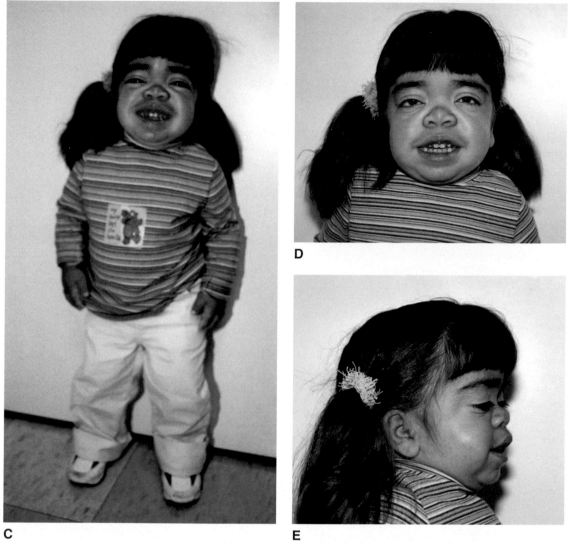

Fig. 1, cont'd. **C–E,** A 6-year-old girl. Note the coarse facies and contractures of the hands.

SCHEIE SYNDROME
(Mucopolysaccharidosis I S, MPS I S)

Broad Mouth with Full Lips, Early Corneal Opacity, Normal Mentality

This disorder was originally described by Scheie and colleagues in 1962.

ABNORMALITIES

Performance. Little, if any, impairment of intelligence.

Facies. Broad mouth with full lips by 5 to 8 years of age, mandibular prognathism.

Corneas. Uniform clouding of cornea in early stage, becoming most dense in periphery.

Limbs. Joint limitation leading to clawhand, small carpal bones, femoral head dysplasia; broad and short hands and feet.

Cardiac. Aortic valvular defect.

Other. Body hirsutism, retinal pigmentation, inguinal and umbilical hernias, short neck.

Urinary Excretion. Proportionately more dermatan sulfate than usual.

OCCASIONAL ABNORMALITIES.

Edema-like swelling of optic disk and macula, carpal tunnel narrowing may cause median nerve compression, trigger thumb, myopathy, psychosis and possible mental deterioration may occur, mild impairment of growth, hearing loss, hepatomegaly, macroglossia, glaucoma, myopia, sleep apnea, progressive juxta-articular cystic lesions in hands and feet, mitral valve stenosis.

NATURAL HISTORY.
Onset of symptoms usually occurs after 5 years of age. Diagnosis made in most cases between 10 and 20 years. Cardiac evaluation is suggested at regular intervals because of the increased incidence of aortic valvular disease. Visual impairment is the most significant handicap, although joint disease is also a problem. Life span is relatively normal.

ETIOLOGY.
This disorder has an autosomal recessive inheritance pattern, with excess urinary excretion of dermatan sulfate and absence of α-L-iduronidase in cultured fibroblasts. The α-L-iduronidase gene, different mutations of which lead to Hurler syndrome, Scheie syndrome, and Hurler-Scheie syndrome, is located at chromosome 4p16.3. Differentiation between these three disorders by biochemical measurements is difficult.

COMMENT.
Enzyme replacement therapy using recombinant human α-L-iduronidase has its greatest potential in children with less severe phenotypes, that is, Scheie syndrome and MPS I H/S (Hurler-Scheie). Improvement in bone and joint disease as well as stabilization of cardiac status and reduction in hepatosplenomegaly can be expected.

References

Scheie HG, Hambrick GW Jr, Barness LA: A newly recognized forme fruste of Hurler's disease (gargoylism). Am J Ophthalmol 53:753, 1962.

Emerit I, Maroteaux P, Vernant P: Deux observations de mucopolysaccharidose avec atteinte cardiovasculaire. Arch Fr Pediatr 23:1075, 1966.

Scott HS et al: Identification of mutations in the α-L-iduronidase gene (IDUA) that cause Hurler and Scheie syndromes. Am J Hum Genet 53:973, 1993.

Summers CG et al: Dense peripheral corneal clouding in Scheie syndrome. Cornea 13:277, 1994.

Kakkis ED et al: Enzyme-replacement therapy in mucopolysaccharidosis I. N Engl J Med 344:182, 2001.

Wraith JE et al: Enzyme replacement therapy in mucopolysaccharidosis I: Progress and emerging difficulties. J Inherit Metab Dis 24:245, 2001.

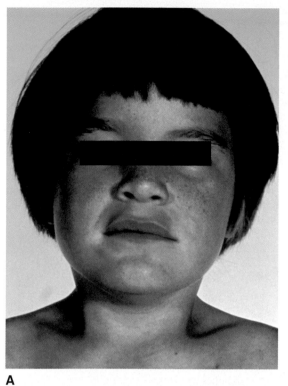

A

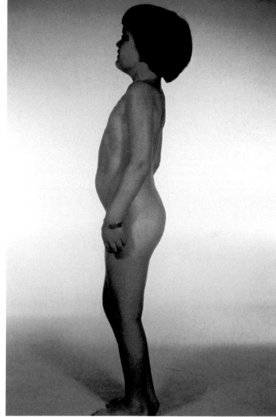

B

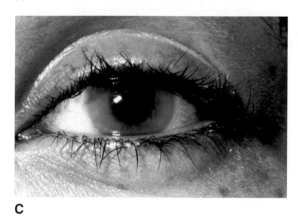

C

FIGURE 1. Scheie syndrome. **A–C,** Child, 9½ years old, with height age of 9 years and IQ of 102. Mild-to-moderate limitation of shoulder, elbow, and hand movement. Mild corneal opacity. (Courtesy of R. Scott, University of Washington, Seattle.)

HURLER-SCHEIE SYNDROME
(MUCOPOLYSACCHARIDOSIS I H/S)

Stevenson and colleagues set forth the disorder Mucopolysaccharidosis I H/S (MPS I H/S) in 1976 and suggested that it represented a genetic compound of the Hurler syndrome and the Scheie syndrome. However, the birth of children with this disorder to consanguineous parents indicates that, like MPS I S and MPS I H, some patients with MPS I H/S represent a different mutation of the α-L-iduronidase (IDUA) gene. The clinical phenotype is intermediate between the severe MPS I H and the mild MPS I S.

ABNORMALITIES

Performance. Mild mental deficiency to normal.

Growth. During the first year, growth may be accelerated; thereafter, it decelerates to growth deficiency; short trunk.

Craniofacial. Development of scaphocephaly with macrocephaly, low nasal bridge, prominent lips, corneal clouding, micrognathia.

Skin. Thickened, with fine hirsutism.

Skeletal. Moderate joint limitation, mild-to-moderate dysostosis multiplex changes with broadening of bones, pectus carinatum, kyphoscoliosis.

Other. Chronic rhinorrhea, middle ear fluid, inguinal hernia with or without umbilical hernia, hepatosplenomegaly, with or without cardiac valvular changes; deafness; arachnoid cyst; tuberous breast deformity; tracheal stenosis.

NATURAL HISTORY. The progression is intermediate between that of Hurler syndrome and that of Scheie syndrome. Onset of symptoms usually between 3 and 8 years with survival into the twenties is common. Onset of corneal clouding, joint limitations, cardiac valvular abnormalities, and hearing impairment frequently develop by the early to midteens. Tonsillar hypertrophy is common. Compression of the cervical spinal cord occurs. Anesthesia can be associated with significant complications.

ETIOLOGY. This disorder has an autosomal recessive inheritance pattern, with excess urinary excretion of dermatan sulfate and heparan sulfate and a deficiency of α-L-iduronidase (IDUA) in cultured fibroblasts. Different mutations in the IDUA gene located at chromosome 4p16.3 lead to MPS I H/S as well as MPS I H and MPS I S.

COMMENT. Enzyme replacement therapy using recombinant human α-L-iduronidase has its greatest potential in children with the less severe phenotype (i.e., Scheie syndrome and MPS I H/S [Hurler-Scheie]). Improvement in bone and joint disease as well as stabilization of cardiac status and reduction of hepatosplenomegaly can be expected.

References

Stevenson RE et al: The iduronidase-deficient mucopolysaccharidoses: Clinical and roentgenographic features. Pediatrics 57:111, 1976.

Roubicek M et al: The clinical spectrum of α-L-iduronidase deficiency. Am J Med Genet 20:471, 1985.

Schmidt H et al: Radiological findings in patients with mucopolysaccharidosis I H/S (Hurler-Scheie syndrome). Pediatr Radiol 17:409, 1987.

Nicholson SC et al: Management of a difficult airway in a patient with Hurler-Scheie syndrome during cardiac surgery. Anesth Analg 75:830, 1992.

Scott HS et al: Identification of mutations in the α-L-iduronidase gene (IDUA) that cause Hurler and Scheie syndromes. Am J Hum Genet 53:973, 1993.

Kakkis ED et al: Enzyme replacement therapy in mucopolysaccharidosis I. N Engl J Med 344:182, 2001.

Wraith JE et al: Enzyme replacement therapy in mucopolysaccharidosis I: Progress and emerging difficulties. J Inherit Metab Dis 24:245, 2001.

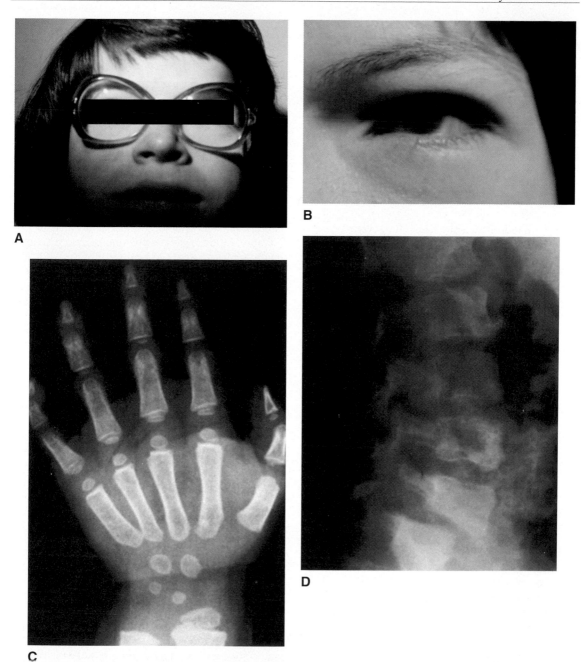

FIGURE 1. Hurler-Scheie syndrome. **A** and **B,** Young girl showing mildly altered facies and corneal clouding. (Courtesy of Dr. Jules Leroy, Gent University Hospital, Gent, Belgium.) **C** and **D,** Subtle dysostosis multiplex type of changes in hand and in lumbar spine. (**C** and **D,** From Stevenson RE et al: Pediatrics 57:111, 1976, with permission.)

HUNTER SYNDROME
(Mucopolysaccharidosis II)

Coarse Facies, Growth Deficiency, Stiff Joints by 2 to 4 Years, Clear Corneas

Hunter described this condition found in two brothers in 1917. A mild and severe type have been delineated, based on the age of onset, degree of central nervous system involvement, and rapidity of deterioration. Both types have the same deficiency of iduronate sulfatase. The severe type is outlined subsequently.

ABNORMALITIES. Onset at approximately 2 to 4 years.

Growth. Deficiency, onset at 1 to 4 years; adult height, 120 to 150 cm.

Performance. Mental and neurologic deterioration at approximately 2 to 5 years of age to the point of severe mental deficiency with aggressive hyperactive behavior and spasticity.

Craniofacial. Coarsening of facial features, full lips, macrocephaly, macroglossia.

Joints and Skeletal. Stiff partial contracture of joints, clawhand; broadening of bones.

Other. Hepatosplenomegaly, hypertrichosis, inguinal hernias, mucoid nasal discharge, progressive deafness, delayed tooth eruption, dentigerous cysts, hoarse voice.

OCCASIONAL ABNORMALITIES.

Diarrhea, nodular skin lesions over scapular area and on arms, dermal melanocytosis/mongolian spots (excessive), kyphosis, pes cavus, osteoarthritis of head of femur, retinal pigmentation, chronic disk edema, ptosis, congestive heart failure, coronary occlusion, hydrocephalus, airway obstruction, seizures, neurogenic bladder secondary to a narrow cervical spinal canal with myelopathy.

IMPORTANT DIFFERENCES IN CONTRAST WITH THE HURLER SYNDROME. (1) Clear corneas, (2) less severe gibbus, (3) no affected females, and (4) more gradual onset of features.

NATURAL HISTORY. Gradual decline in growth rate from 2 to 6 years. Deafness frequently is evident by 2 to 3 years. Severe neurologic complications develop in the late stages. Cardiac complications resulting from valvular, myocardial, and ischemic factors as well as airway obstruction caused by macroglossia, a deformed pharynx, a short thick neck, and gradual deformation and collapse of the trachea not uncommonly lead to death before 15 years of age.

In the mild type, maintenance of intelligence occurs into adult life. Survival into the fifth and sixth decades is not unusual. Adult hearing loss is frequent. Carpal tunnel syndrome and joint contractures are common. Somatic involvement occurs in patients with the mild type but the rate of progression is much less rapid.

ETIOLOGY. The primary defect is a deficiency of iduronate sulfatase, which can be measured in peripheral white blood cells. Excess dermatan sulfate and heparan sulfate are found in urine. The gene for Hunter syndrome has been mapped to Xq27-q28. A number of disease-causing mutations have been identified. The broad variability of expression, which includes the severe and mild types, is due to different mutations in the same gene. Carrier females may be determined by assaying for iduronate sulfatase in peripheral white blood cells. However, results have been ambiguous in approximately 15% of obligate carriers.

COMMENT. Of 10 patients who underwent bone marrow transplantation, three survived more than 7 years. A steady progression of disease occurred in two of the survivors, while maintenance of normal intellectual development occurred in one.

References

Hunter C: A rare disease in two brothers. Proc R Soc Med 10:104, 1917.

Leroy JG, Crocker AC: Clinical definition of the Hurler-Hunter phenotypes: A review of 50 patients. Am J Dis Child 112:518, 1966.

Muenzer J: Mucopolysaccharidoses. Adv Pediatr 33:269, 1986.

Upadhyaya M et al: Localization of the gene for Hunter

syndrome on the long arm of X chromosome. Hum Genet 74:391, 1986.

Sasaki CT: Hunter's syndrome: A study in airway obstruction. Laryngoscope 97:280, 1987.

Wilson PJ: Frequent deletions at Xq28 indicate genetic heterogeneity in Hunter syndrome. Hum Genet 86:505, 1991.

Froissart R et al: Identification of iduronate sulfatase gene alterations in 70 unrelated Hunter patients. Clin Genet 53:362, 1998.

Vellodi A et al: Long-term follow-up following bone marrow transplantation for Hunter disease. J Inherit Metab Dis 22:638, 1999.

Ochiai T et al: Significance of extensive Mongolian spots in Hunter's syndrome. Br J Derm 148:1173, 2003.

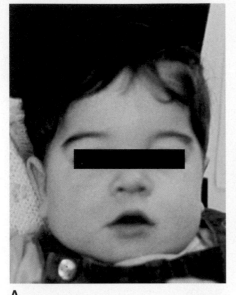

A

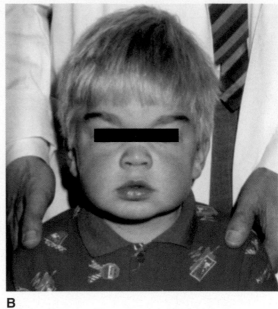

B

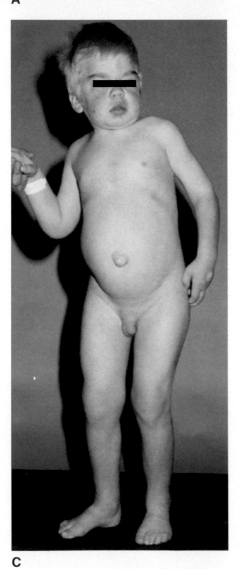

C

FIGURE 1. Hunter syndrome. **A–C,** Three boys with coarsening of the face and evidence of joint contractures who presumably have a mild type of disease. (Courtesy of Dr. Jules Leroy, Gent University Hospital, Gent, Belgium.)

534

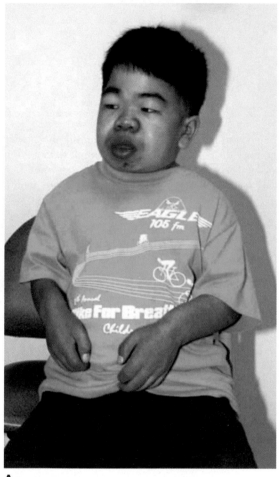

A

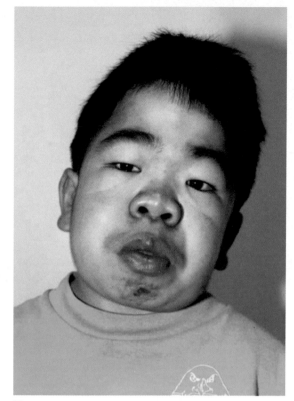

B

FIGURE 2. **A** and **B,** A 14-year-old boy with the severe type of disease. (Courtesy of Dr. Marilyn C. Jones, Children's Hospital, San Diego.)

SANFILIPPO SYNDROME
(MUCOPOLYSACCHARIDOSIS III, TYPES A, B, C, AND D)

Mild Coarse Facies, Mild Stiff Joints, Mental Deficiency

This clinical disorder was recognized by Sanfilippo and colleagues in 1963 and appears to be the most common mucopolysaccharidosis. The excess urinary excretion of mucopolysaccharide is heparan sulfate alone. These individuals usually have clear corneas.

ABNORMALITIES. Onset in early childhood.
Growth. Normal to accelerated growth for 1 to 3 years, followed by slow growth.
Performance. Slowing mental development by 1½ to 3 years, followed by deterioration, including gait, speech, and behavior; hyperactivity.
Craniofacial. Dense calvarium, mildly coarse facies with synophrys.
Other. Variable hepatosplenomegaly, obliteration of pulp chambers of teeth by irregular secondary dentin, ovoid dysplasia of vertebrae, mild cardiac involvement.

NATURAL HISTORY. Sleep disturbances and frequent upper respiratory tract infections may be early evidence of the disorder before the slowing of growth and mental deterioration. Unfortunately, the usual result is severe mental retardation in a strong, often difficult to manage, individual. Serious behavioral problems have improved with use of cerebrospinal shunts. The syndrome may be compatible with long survival, but many die of pneumonia by 10 to 20 years of age.

ETIOLOGY. This disorder has an autosomal recessive inheritance pattern. Sanfilippo A is a deficiency of heparan *N*-sulfatase; Sanfilippo B, a deficiency of *N*-acetyl-α-D-glucosaminidase; Sanfilippo C, a deficiency of acetyl-CoA:α-glucosaminide-*N*-acetyltransferase; and Sanfilippo D, a deficiency of *N*-acetyl-α-D-glucosaminide-6-sulfatase. Excess heparan sulfate is excreted in the urine in all four types, and the clinical phenotype is identical in each. The gene for MPS IIIA has been localized to chromosome 17p25.3, for MPS IIIB to 17q21, and for MPS IIID to 12q14.

COMMENT. In one patient with type IIIA, bone marrow transplantation was not successful in affecting the course of the disease.

References
Sanfilippo SJ et al: Mental retardation associated with acid mucopolysacchariduria (heparitin sulfate type). J Pediatr 63:837, 1963.
Spranger J et al: Die HS-Mucopolysaccharidose von Sanfilippo (Polydystrophe Oligophrenie): Bericht über 10 Patienten. Z Kinderheilkd 101:71, 1967.
Kriel RL et al: Neuroanatomical and EEG correlations in Sanfilippo syndrome, type A. Arch Neurol 35:838, 1978.
Andria G et al: Sanfilippo B syndrome. Clin Genet 15:500, 1979.
Nidiffer FD, Kelly TE: Developmental and degenerative patterns associated with cognitive, behavioral and motor difficulties in Sanfilippo syndrome: An epidemiology study. J Ment Defic Res 27:185, 1983.
Van Schrojenstein-de Valk HMJ et al: Follow-up on seven adult patients with mild Sanfilippo B disease. Am J Med Genet 28:125, 1987.
Robertson SP et al: Cerebrospinal fluid shunts in the management of behavioral problems in Sanfilippo syndrome (MPS III). Eur J Pediatr 157:653, 1998.
Sivakumur P, Wraith JE: Bone marrow transplantation in mucopolysaccharidosis type IIIA: A comparison of an early treated patient with his untreated sibling. J Inherit Metab Dis 22:849, 1999.

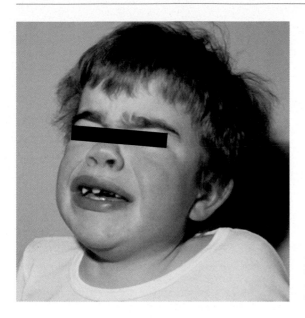

FIGURE 1. Sanfilippo syndrome. An 8-year-old boy whose capabilities have been regressing rapidly. (Courtesy of Dr. Jules Leroy, Gent University Hospital, Gent, Belgium.)

MORQUIO SYNDROME
(Mucopolysaccharidosis IV, Types A and B)

Onset at 1 to 3 Years of Age, Mild Coarse Facies, Severe Kyphosis and Knock-Knees, Cloudy Corneas

Mistakenly interpreted by Osler in 1898, this condition was described by Morquio in 1919; it was recognized as a mucopolysaccharidosis in 1963. Deficiencies of two different enzymes leading to a severe form, mucopolysaccharidosis IV A, and a mild form, mucopolysaccharidosis IV B, are now recognized. Within both forms, marked clinical heterogeneity has been documented that is most likely due to different mutations of the same gene.

ABNORMALITIES. Onset between 1 and 3 years of age.

Growth. Severe limitation with cessation by later childhood, adult stature 82 to 115 cm.

Craniofacial. Mild coarsening of facial features, with broad mouth and short anteverted nose.

Eyes. Glaucoma; cloudy cornea evident by slit lamp examination, usually after 5 to 10 years of age.

Skeletal and Joints. Marked platyspondyly, with vertebrae changing to ovoid, ovoid with anterior projection, to flattened form with short neck and trunk plus kyphoscoliosis; odontoid hypoplasia; early flaring of rib cage progressing to bulging sternum; short, curved long bones with irregular tubulation, widened metaphyses, abnormal femoral neck, flattening of femoral head, knock-knee with medial spur of tibial metaphysis, conical bases of widened metacarpals, irregular epiphyseal form, osteoporosis; short, stubby hands; joint laxity, most evident at wrists and small joints, and joint restriction in some of the larger joints, especially the hips.

Mouth. Widely spaced teeth with thin enamel that tends to become grayish.

Cardiac. Late onset of aortic regurgitation.

Other. Hearing loss, inguinal hernia, hepatomegaly.

Urinary Excretion. Keratan sulfate.

OCCASIONAL ABNORMALITIES.
Macrocephaly, mental deficiency, pigmentary retinal degeneration in older patients, glaucoma, hydrops fetalis.

NATURAL HISTORY. The earliest recognized indications of the disease have been flaring of the lower rib cage, prominent sternum, frequent upper respiratory tract infections (including otitis media), hernias, and growth deficiency, all becoming evident by 18 to 24 months of age. Severe defects of vertebrae may result in cord compression or respiratory insufficiency. These and cardiac complications may result in death before 20 years of age. In the milder form, longer survival is the rule, dental enamel is normal, and C2–C3 subluxation has been documented in addition to C1–C2 subluxation. Mentality is usually normal in both the severe and the mild forms.

ETIOLOGY. Autosomal recessive. In type IV A the basic defect is a deficiency of *N*-acetylgalactosamine-6-sulfatase, whereas in type IV B there is a deficiency of β-galactosidase. The gene for *N*-acetylgalactosamine-6-sulfatase has been isolated and mapped to 16q24.3. The gene for β-galactosidase, different mutations of which cause type IV B Morquio syndrome and generalized gangliosidosis syndrome, type I, has been mapped to 3p21.33. Confirmation of the diagnosis is dependent upon two-dimensional electrophoresis or thin-layer chromatography of isolated urinary glycosaminoglycans, since false-negative screening tests for urinary mucopolysaccharides occur or the deficiency of the enzyme in cultured skin fibroblasts or leukocytes. Heterozygote detection is possible. Prenatal diagnosis has been performed using both amniotic fluid cells and chorionic villi.

References

Osler W: Sporadic cretinism in America. Trans Congr Am Phys 4:169, 1898.

Morquio L: Sur une forme de dystrophie osseuse familiale. Arch Med Enf 32:129, 1929.

Robins MM, Stevens HF, Linker A: Morquio's disease: An abnormality of mucopolysaccharide metabolism. J Pediatr 62:881, 1963.

Langer LO, Carey LS: The roentgenographic features of the KS mucopolysaccharidosis of Morquio (Morquio-Brailsford's disease). Am J Roentgenol Radium Ther Nucl Med 97:1, 1966.

Linker A, Evans LR, Langer LO: Morquio's disease and mucopolysaccharide excretion. J Pediatr 77:1039, 1970.

Matalon R et al: Morquio's syndrome: Deficiency of a chondroitin sulfate N-acetylhexosamine sulfatase. Biochem Biophys Res Commun 61:759, 1974.

Muenzer J: Mucopolysaccharidoses. Adv Pediatr 33:269, 1986.

Applegarth DA et al: Morquio disease presenting as hydrops fetalis and enzyme analysis of chorionic villus tissue in a subsequent pregnancy. Pediatr Pathol 7:593, 1987.

Morris CP et al: Morquio A syndrome: Cloning, sequence and structure of the human N-acetylgalactosamine 6-sulfatase (GALNS) gene. Genomics 22:652, 1994.

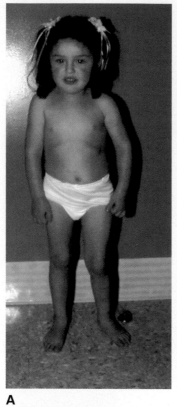

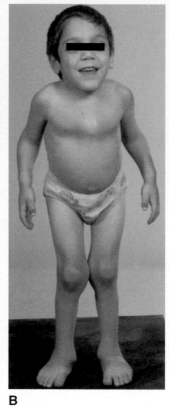

A

B

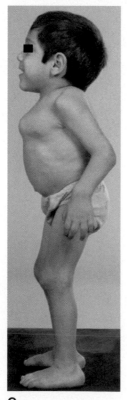

C

FIGURE 1. Morquio syndrome. **A–C,** Two affected children. Note the joint contractures and prominent sternum. (**A,** Courtesy of Dr. Marilyn C. Jones, Children's Hospital, San Diego; **B** and **C,** courtesy of Dr. Jules Leroy, Gent University Hospital, Gent, Belgium.)

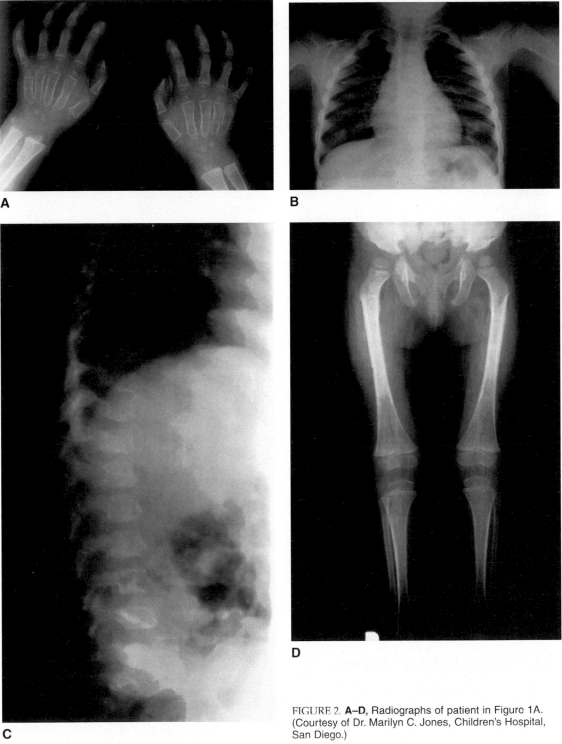

FIGURE 2. **A–D,** Radiographs of patient in Figure 1A. (Courtesy of Dr. Marilyn C. Jones, Children's Hospital, San Diego.)

MAROTEAUX-LAMY MUCOPOLYSACCHARIDOSIS SYNDROME (MILD, MODERATE, AND SEVERE TYPES)
(Mucopolysaccharidosis VI)

Coarse Facies, Stiff Joints, Cloudy Corneas in Infancy, No Mental Deterioration

Maroteaux and colleagues recognized this disorder as being distinct from Hurler syndrome in that mental deterioration did *not* occur during early childhood. Three clinical subtypes have been indicated, based on age of onset, rate of progression, and the extent of involvement of affected organs. Symptoms begin by 1 to 3 years in the severe type, by late childhood in the intermediate type, and after the second decade in the mild type.

ABNORMALITIES

Growth. Deficiency.

Craniofacial. Coarse facies with large nose and thick lips, low nasal bridge.

Eyes. Fine corneal opacity, cornea may be thick or large.

Skeletal and Joints. Mild stiffness of joints; metaphyses, slightly broad and irregular; epiphyseal irregularity, especially femoral epiphysis; hip dysplasia; vertebrae flattened with anterior wedging of T12 and L1; prominent sternum; broad ribs; elongated sella turcica; odontoid hypoplasia; lumbar kyphosis, genu valgum.

Other. Umbilical and inguinal hernias; skin, thick and tight; small, widely spaced teeth with late eruption; hepatosplenomegaly; varying degrees of deafness; cytoplasmic granules in leukocytes.

OCCASIONAL ABNORMALITIES.

Mental retardation, macroglossia, macrocephaly, hydrocephalus secondary to meningeal involvement, involvement of heart valves, glaucoma, hearing impairment, cervical myopathy caused by thickening of the cervical dura mater.

NATURAL HISTORY.

Macrocephaly; frequent upper respiratory tract infections; diarrhea; hernias; and limitation of knee, hip, and elbow movement may be present in infancy. Those with the severe type rapidly deteriorate physically and by 3 to 6 years have serious deformity. The longest survivor of the severe type is into the twenties. Most die from cardiopulmonary complications by the second or third decade. Mental retardation occurs only infrequently. The data on prognosis for the mild and intermediate types are inadequate. Anesthesia, caused by airway management, can pose a significant risk.

ETIOLOGY. This disorder has an autosomal recessive inheritance pattern. The molecular defect is a deficiency of *N*-acetylgalactosamine-4-sulfatase (arylsulfatase B). The enzyme is missing in all tissues, including cultured fibroblasts. The gene for *N*-acetylgalactosamine-4-sulfatase maps to chromosome 5q13-q14. There is an increased urinary excretion of mucopolysaccharides consisting predominantly of dermatan sulfate. Heterozygote detection and prenatal diagnosis may be feasible in selected laboratories.

References

Maroteaux P et al: Une nouvelle dysostose avec élimination urinaire de chondroitine-sulfate B. Presse Med 71:1849, 1963.

Maroteaux P, Lamy M: Hurler's disease, Morquio's disease, and related mucopolysaccharidoses. J Pediatr 67:312, 1965.

Fallis N, Barnes FL II, di Ferrante N: A case of polydystrophic dwarfism with urinary excretion of dermatan sulfate and heparan sulfate. J Clin Endocrinol Metab 28:26, 1968.

O'Brien JF, Cantz M, Spranger J: Maroteaux-Lamy disease, subtype A: Deficiency of an *N*-acetylgalactosamine-4-sulfatase. Biochem Biophys Res Commun 60:1170, 1974.

Litgens T et al: Chromosomal localization of ARSB, the gene for human *N*-acetylygalactosamine-4-sulfatase. Hum Genet 82:67, 1989.

Tan CTT et al: Valvular heart disease in four patients with Maroteaux-Lamy syndrome. Circulation 85:188, 1992.

Isbrandt D et al: Mucopolysaccharidosis VI (Marteaux-Lamy syndrome): Six unique arylsulfatase B gene alleles causing variable disease phenotypes. Am J Hum Genet 54:454, 1994.

Litjens T, Hopwood JJ: Mucopolysaccharidosis type VI: Structural and clinical implications of mutations in *N*-acetylgalactosamine-4-sulfatase. Hum Mutat 18:282, 2001.

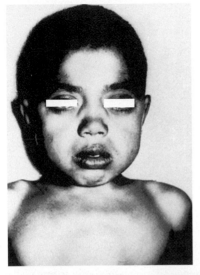
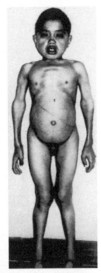
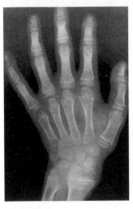
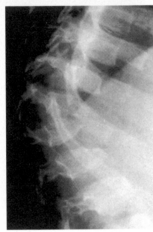

FIGURE 1. Maroteaux-Lamy mucopolysaccharidosis syndrome. Boy who is short of stature, with normal intelligence. (Courtesy of P. Maroteaux, Hôpital des Enfants-Malades, Paris.)

MUCOPOLYSACCHARIDOSIS VII
(Sly Syndrome, β-Glucuronidase Deficiency)

Initially described by Sly and colleagues in an infant with short stature, skeletal deformities, hepatosplenomegaly, and mental deficiency, approximately 32 cases have been reported subsequently. A widely variable clinical phenotype has been noted from severely affected infants to mildly affected adults.

ABNORMALITIES

Growth. Postnatal growth deficiency.
Performance. Moderately severe mental deficiency.
Craniofacial. Macrocephaly, coarsened facies.
Eyes. Corneal clouding in the severe form.
Skeletal. Thoracolumbar gibbus, metatarsus adductus, flaring of lower ribs, prominent sternum, J-shaped sella turcica, acetabular dysplasia, narrow sciatic notches, and hypoplastic basilar portions of ilia, widening of ribs, pointed proximal metacarpals.
Other. Inguinal hernia, hepatosplenomegaly.

OCCASIONAL ABNORMALITIES.
Joint contractures; hydrocephalus; involvement of heart valves; odontoid hypoplasia; shortening and anterior irregularities of vertebral bodies, wedge deformities of lumbar vertebrae; anterior, inferior beaking of lower thoracic and lumbar vertebrae; hip dysplasia; hydrops fetalis.

NATURAL HISTORY.
Unlike the other known mucopolysaccharidoses, MPS VII is sometimes recognizable in the neonatal period, associated with hydrops fetalis and hepatosplenomegaly. For them, death occurs in the first few months. A more mild form, also presenting in the newborn period, is associated with developmental delay, much less rapid deterioration, and survival into adolescence. In addition, there exists at least one further form of β-glucuronidase deficiency that presents during the second decade of life and is characterized by mild skeletal abnormalities and normal intelligence.

ETIOLOGY.
This disorder has an autosomal recessive inheritance pattern. The basic defect is a deficiency of β-glucuronidase, which can be documented in fibroblasts and leukocytes. Mutations in the gene for β-glucuronidase (GUSB) located at chromosome 7q11.21-q11.22 are responsible. The existence of multiple allelic forms of this disorder most likely explains the wide variability in the clinical phenotype.

COMMENT.
Bone marrow transplantation in one patient, a 12-year-old girl, resulted in improved motor function, decreased respiratory and ear infections, but no improvement in cognition.

References

Sly WS et al: Beta glucuronidase deficiency: Report of clinical radiologic, and biochemical features of a new mucopolysaccharidosis. J Pediatr 82:249, 1973.

Daves BS, Degnan M: Different clinical and biochemical phenotype associated with beta glucuronidase deficiency. In Bergsma D (ed): Skeletal Dysplasias. New York: National Foundation March of Dimes, 1974, p 251.

Hoyme HE et al: Presentation of mucopolysaccharidosis VII (β-glucuronidase deficiency) in infancy. J Med Genet 18:237, 1981.

Wallace SP et al: Degeneration of speech, language, and hearing in a patient with mucopolysaccharidosis VII. Int J Pediatr Otorhinolaryngol 19:97, 1990.

Speleman F et al: Localization by fluorescence in situ hybridization of the human functional beta-glucuronidase gene (GUSB) to 7q11.21-q11.22 and two pseudogenes to 5p13 and 5q13. Cytogenet Cell Genet 72:53, 1996.

Yamada Y et al: Treatment of MPS VII (Sly syndrome) by allogeneic BMT in a female with a homozygous A619V mutation. Bone Marrow Transplant 21:629, 1998.

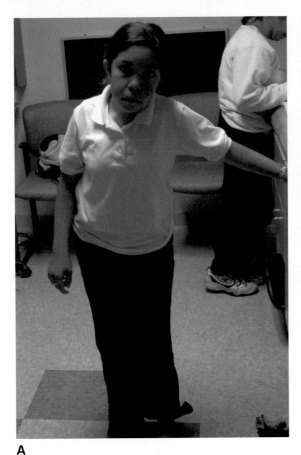

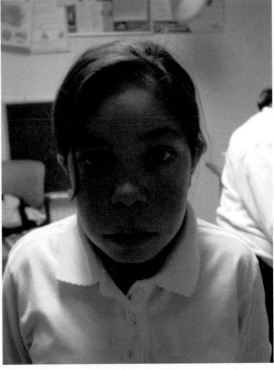

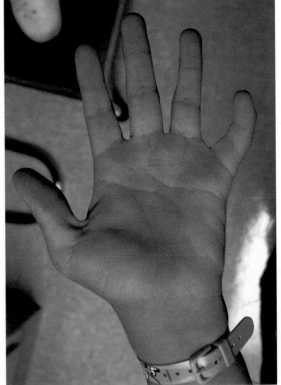

FIGURE 1. Mucopolysaccharidosis VII. **A–C,** A mildly affected adolescent girl. Note the coarse facies and joint contractures. She has a mild degree of mental retardation.

O | Connective Tissue Disorders

MARFAN SYNDROME

Arachnodactyly with Hyperextensibility, Lens Subluxation, Aortic Dilatation

Described as dolichostenomelia in the initial report by Marfan, this disorder has been extensively studied and recognized as a connective tissue disorder by McKusick. Diagnosis is based on criteria established in 1996. It requires, for the index case, major criteria in at least two systems and involvement of a third. For a family member, diagnosis requires presence of a major criterion in the family history and one major criterion in an organ system and involvement of a second system. For the skeletal system, at least four of the eight typical manifestations are required to designate it a major criteria. For all others, only one is required. Abnormalities of growth are not considered as criteria for diagnosis.

ABNORMALITIES

Growth. Tendency toward tall stature with long slim limbs, little subcutaneous fat, and muscle hypotonia; mean birth length and final height 53 cm and 191 cm, respectively, in males and 52.5 cm and 175 cm, respectively, in females; peak growth velocity 2.4 years earlier than normal in boys and 2.7 years earlier in girls; mean age at menarche 11.7 years.

Skeletal. Major criterion: pectus carinatum; pectus excavatum requiring surgery; decreased upper to lower segment ratio or span-height ratio greater than 1:05; wrist and thumb sign; scoliosis > 20 degrees or spondylolisthesis; reduced elbow extension (<170 degrees); pes planus; protrusio acetabuli (protrusion/dislocation of acetabulum). Minor criterion: pectus excavatum of moderate severity; hypermobile joints; high palate with dental crowding; characteristic face including dolichocephaly, malar hypoplasia, enophthalmos, downslanting palpebral fissures.

For the skeletal system to be considered involved, at least two components comprising the major criterion or one comprising the major plus two of the minor criterion must be present.

Ocular. Major criteria: lens subluxation, usually upward, with defect in suspensory ligament. Minor criteria: flat cornea, increased axial globe length, hypoplastic iris or ciliary muscle causing decreased miosis.

For the ocular system to be involved, at least two of the minor criteria must be present.

Cardiovascular. Major criteria: dilatation of ascending aorta with or without aortic regurgitation, dissection of ascending aorta. Minor criteria: mitral valve prolapse, dilated pulmonary artery (below age 40), calcified mitral annulus (below age 40), dilatation or dissection of descending thoracic or abdominal aorta (below age 50).

For the cardiovascular system to be involved, a major criterion or only one minor criteria must be present.

Pulmonary. Major criteria: none. Minor criteria: spontaneous pneumothorax, apical blebs.

For the pulmonary system to be involved, one of the minor criteria must be present.

Skin and Integument. Major criterion: lumbosacral dural ectasia on computed tomography or magnetic resonance imaging. Minor criteria: striae not associated with marked weight changes, recurrent or incisional herniae.

For the skin and integument to be involved, one of the minor criteria must be present.

Family/Genetic History. Major criteria: positive. Minor criteria: none.

For the family history to be contributory, the major criteria must be present.

OCCASIONAL ABNORMALITIES.

Large ears, cataracts, retinal detachment, glaucoma, strabismus, refractive errors, diaphragmatic hernia, hemivertebrae, colobomata of iris, cleft palate, incomplete rotation of colon, ventricular dysrhythmias, cardiomyopathy, intracranial aneurysms, sleep apnea, neuropsychologic impairment including learning disability and attention deficit disorder in 42% of 19 individuals (5 to 18 years of age) despite normal IQ, schizophrenia.

NATURAL HISTORY.

During childhood and adolescence, special care should be directed toward prevention of scoliosis. The serious vascular complications may develop at any time from fetal life through old age and are the chief cause of death. Mitral valve changes may be the earliest feature and mitral regurgitation may require surgery even before the aorta is widely dilated. A significantly reduced rate of aortic dilatation and its associated complications has been documented in affected individuals treated with β-adrenergic blocking agents, leading to the recommendation that patients with Marfan syndrome be seriously considered for treatment with β-adrenergic blockers as soon as the diagnosis is made. Antibiotic prophylaxis should be used before any dental procedure. Children with a slightly dilated aortic root probably need no outright restriction of activity although avoidance of strenuous activity as well as competitive athletics should be avoided. Secondary glaucoma may occur, especially when the lens dislocates into the anterior chamber of the eye. The third trimester of pregnancy, labor and delivery, and the first postpartum month represent a particularly vulnerable time for dissection. For many patients treated prophylactically, life expectancy now approaches normal. Health supervision guidelines for children with Marfan syndrome have been established by the American Academy of Pediatrics.

ETIOLOGY.

This disorder has an autosomal dominant inheritance pattern, with sufficiently wide variability in expression that the diagnosis is often tenuous in sporadic nonfamilial cases. Mutations in the fibrillin (FBN1) gene located on chromosome 15q15-21.3 are responsible. Fibrillin-1 is a glycoprotein that is a major component of extracellular microfibrils. Microfibrils act as a principal component of elastic fibers, as anchoring fibers between dermis and epidermis, and as the ocular zonules. Although a defect in fibrillin metabolism occurs in Marfan syndrome, not all patients with alterations in fibrillin have Marfan syndrome. Because multiple FBN1 mutations have been identified, there is no screening test for a common mutation. Linkage analysis is used only in families in which there are multiple affected members to identify probable carriers of the FBN1 gene.

COMMENT.

Severe Marfan syndrome diagnosed in the first 3 months of life is the result of point mutations or small deletions in the middle third of the fibrillin-1 protein. Serious cardiac defects including mitral valve prolapse, valvular regurgitation, and aortic root dilatation occur in approximately 80% of cases, and congenital contractures are present in 64%. A characteristic facies, dolichocephaly, a high-arched palate, micrognathia, hyperextensible joints, arachnodactyly, pes planus, chest deformity, iridodonesis, megalocornea, and lens dislocation are also frequently present. Fourteen percent of affected children die during the first year.

References

Marfan AB: Un cas de déformation congénitales des quatre membres plus prononcée aux extrémités caractérisée par l'allongement des os avec un certain degré d'amincissement. Bull Mem Soc Med Hop (Paris) 13:220, 1896.

Pyeritz RE, McKusick VA: The Marfan syndrome: Diagnosis and management. N Engl J Med 300:772, 1979.

Hofman KJ, Bernhardt BA, Pyeritz RE: Increased incidence of neuropsychologic impairment in the Marfan syndrome. Am J Hum Genet 37:4A, 1985.

Gott VL et al: Surgical treatment of aneurysms of the ascending aorta in the Marfan syndrome: Results of composite-graft repair in 50 patients. N Engl J Med 314:1070, 1986.

Morse RP et al: Diagnosis and management of infantile Marfan syndrome. Pediatrics 86:888, 1990.

Lee B et al: Linkage of Marfan syndrome and a phenotypically related disorder to two different fibrillin genes. Nature 352:330, 1991.

Kainulainen K et al: Mutations in the fibrillin gene responsible for dominant ectopia lentis and neonatal Marfan syndrome. Nat Genet 6:64, 1994.

American Academy of Pediatrics: Health supervision for children with Marfan syndrome. Pediatrics 98:978, 1996.

DePaepe A et al: Revised diagnostic criteria for the Marfan syndrome. Am J Med Genet 62:417, 1996.

Pyeritz RE: The Marfan syndrome. Annu Rev Med 51:481, 2000.

Dean JCS: Management of Marfan syndrome. Heart 88:97, 2002.

Jones EG et al: Growth and maturation in Marfan syndrome. Am J Med Genet 109:100, 2002.

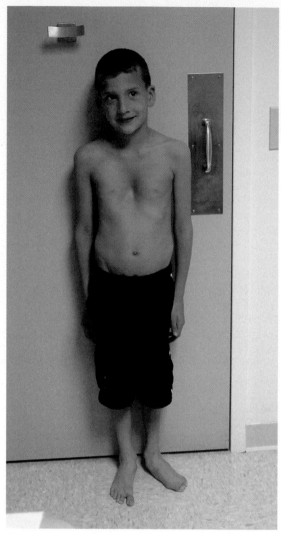

FIGURE 1. Marfan syndrome. **A–C,** Unrelated 9- and 13-year-old boys. Note the long slim limbs, pectus excavatum, narrow face, and reduced elbow extension.

A

Continued

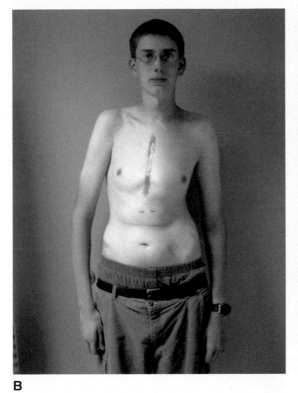

B

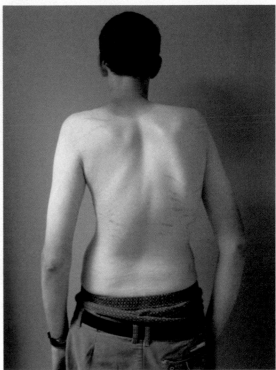

C

Fig. 1, cont'd.

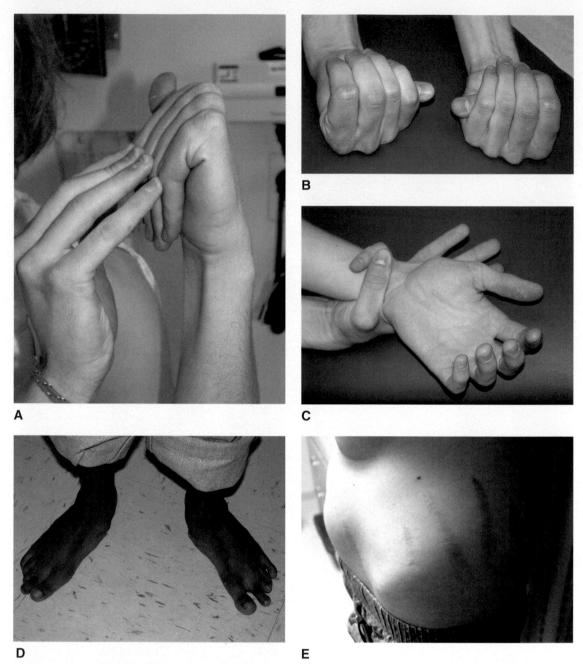

FIGURE 2. Note the joint laxity (**A**), Steinberg thumb sign (**B**), ability to join thumb and fifth finger around the wrist (Walker-Murdock sign) (**C**), pes planus (**D**), and striae over hips and back (**E**). (**A–D,** Courtesy of Dr. Lynne M. Bird, Children's Hospital, San Diego.)

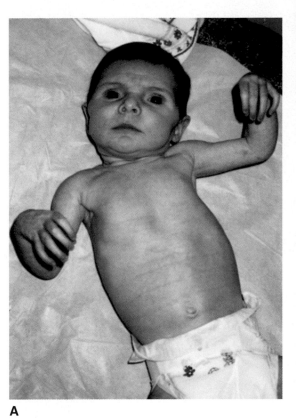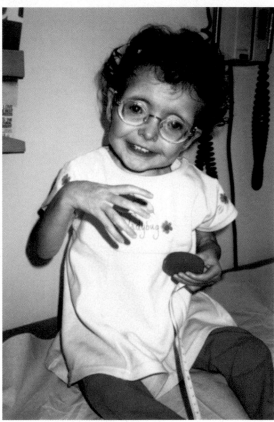

A **B**

FIGURE 3. **A** and **B,** Child with neonatal form of Marfan syndrome. (Courtesy of Dr. Stephen Braddock, University of Missouri, Columbia.)

BEALS SYNDROME
(BEALS CONTRACTURAL ARACHNODACTYLY SYNDROME)

Joint Contractures, Arachnodactyly, "Crumpled" Ear

Beals and Hecht described this syndrome in 1971. They found 11 probable past reports of the same entity, including the original Marfan report.

ABNORMALITIES

Limbs. Long slim limbs (dolichostenomelia) with arachnodactyly (86%); camptodactyly (78%); ulnar deviation of fingers; joint contractures, especially of knees (81%), elbows (86%), and hips (26%).

Other Skeletal. Kyphoscoliosis (46%), relatively short neck, metatarsus varus, mild talipes equinovarus (32%), hypoplasia of calf muscles (65%).

Ears. "Crumpled" appearance with poorly defined conchas and prominent crura from the root of the helix (75%).

Other. Mitral valve prolapse with regurgitation.

OCCASIONAL ABNORMALITIES.
Micrognathia (26%); cranial abnormalities including scaphocephaly, brachycephaly, dolichocephaly, and frontal bossing (29%); iris coloboma; keratoconus; myopia; pectus excavatum and carinatum; subluxation of patella; atrial septal defect; ventricular septal defect; aortic root dilatation; mitral valve prolapse.

NATURAL HISTORY. There tends to be
gradual improvement in the joint limitations, but the scoliosis may be progressive. The long-term prognosis for aortic root dilatation is unknown. Echocardiography to assess the heart and ascending aorta is recommended.

ETIOLOGY. This disorder has an autosomal
dominant inheritance pattern. Linkage of Beals syndrome families to a fibrillin locus on chromosome 5q23-31 (FBN2) has been documented. Mutations in the FBN2 gene have been demonstrated.

COMMENT. A severe form of this disorder,
lethal in the neonatal period, has been described. In addition to the characteristic features of Beals syndrome, severe cardiac defects including interrupted aortic arch, VSD, ASD, and aortic root dilatation, as well as gastrointestinal anomalies including duodenal and esophageal atresia and intestinal malrotation occur.

References

Beals RK, Hecht F: Delineation of another heritable disorder of connective tissue. J Bone Joint Surg [Am] 53:987, 1971.

Hecht F, Beals RK: "New" syndrome of congenital contractural arachnodactyly originally described by Marfan in 1896. Pediatrics 49:574, 1972.

Anderson RA, Koch S, Camerini-Otero RD: Cardiovascular findings in congenital contractural arachnodactyly: Report of an affected kindred. Am J Med Genet 18:265, 1984.

Ramos Arroyo MA, Weaver DD, Beals RK: Congenital contractural arachnodactyly. Report of four additional families and review of literature. Clin Genet 25:570, 1985.

Lee B et al: Linkage of Marfan syndrome and a phenotypically related disorder to two different fibrillin genes. Nature 352:330, 1991.

Viljoen D: Congenital contractural arachnodactyly (Beals syndrome). J Med Genet 31:640, 1994.

Putnam EA et al: Fibrillin-2 (FBN2) mutations result in the Marfan-like disorder, congenital contractural arachnodactyly. Nat Genet 11:456, 1995.

Wang M et al: Familial occurrence of typical and severe lethal contractural arachnodactyly caused by missplicing of exon 34 of fibrillin-2. Am J Hum Genet 59:1027, 1996.

Gupta PA et al: Ten novel FBN-2 mutations in congenital contractural arachnodactyly: Delineation of the molecular pathogenesis and clinical phenotype. Hum Mutat 19:39, 2002.

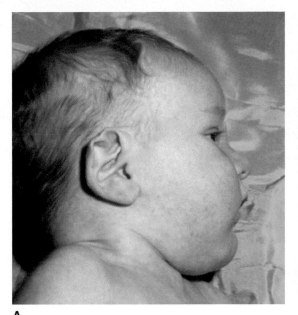

A

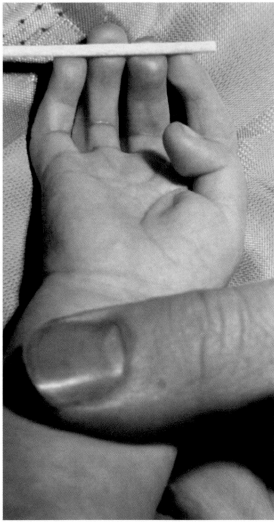

B

FIGURE 1. Beals syndrome. **A** and **B,** Young infant showing folded helices of ears, and relative arachnodactyly with camptodactyly. Severe scoliosis developed by 2 years of age.

SHPRINTZEN-GOLDBERG SYNDROME

Marfanoid Habitus, Dolichocephaly, Ocular Proptosis

In 1982, Shprintzen and Goldberg described two unrelated males with craniosynostosis and marfanoid habitus. A patient with similar findings but lacking craniosynostosis had been reported in 1971 by Sugarman and Vogel. Of the 15 patients who have been reported, 40% have craniosynostosis. The article by Greally and colleagues provides an excellent review.

ABNORMALITIES

Growth. Birth length tends to be increased; with increasing age, weight frequently drops below the third percentile and is associated with decreased subcutaneous fat.

Performance. Hypotonia, delayed developmental milestones, mental retardation.

Craniofacial. Craniosynostosis (40%); dolichocephaly; large anterior fontanel; high prominent forehead; ocular proptosis; strabismus; hypertelorism; downslanting palpebral fissures; maxillary hypoplasia; broad secondary alveolar ridge; micrognathia; low-set, posteriorly rotated ears.

Skeletal. Arachnodactyly, camptodactyly, genu recurvatum, pectus excavatum, pectus carinatum, hyperextensible joints, joint contractures, metatarsus adductus, talipes equinovarus, scoliosis.

Radiologic. Thin ribs; 13 pairs of ribs; square, box-like vertebral bodies; bowing of femora; hypoplastic hooked clavicles; osteopenia.

Other. Hydrocephalus (40%), myopia, umbilical hernia, cryptorchidism.

OCCASIONAL ABNORMALITIES.

Fine sparse hair; ptosis; Chiari-I malformation; C1–C2 abnormality; bifid uvula; choanal atresia/stenosis; vocal cord paralysis; dental malocclusion; prominent/malformed ears; aortic root dilatation; mitral valve prolapse; inguinal hernia; hyperelastic skin; joint dislocation; bowing of ribs, ulna, radii, tibiae, or fibulae; fusion of vertebrae; hypospadias; growth hormone deficiency.

NATURAL HISTORY. Feeding difficulties, often requiring nasogastric tube feeding, stridorous breathing during sleep, cyanosis, and respiratory compromise are frequent in infancy. Obstructive apnea is common and infrequently requires tracheostomy. With advancing age, linear growth rate begins to decrease. Delay in attainment of developmental milestones is usual. Mild-to-moderate degrees of mental retardation have occurred in all but one patient, a boy who at 2 years of age was described as hypotonic with joint contractures but no cognitive dysfunctions.

ETIOLOGY. The cause of this disorder is unknown. Analysis of the Fibrillin-1 (FBN1) gene has been carried out in a few patients, because of the clinical similarity between Shprintzen-Goldberg syndrome and Marfan syndrome. Those studies have been inconclusive.

References

Sugarman G, Vogel MW: Case report 76: Craniofacial and musculoskeletal abnormalities—a questionable connective tissue disease. Synd Ident 7:16–17, 1981.

Shprintzen RJ, Goldberg RB: A recurrent pattern syndrome of craniosynostosis associated with arachnodactyly and abdominal hernias. J Craniofac Genet Dev Biol 2:65–74, 1982.

Adès LC et al: Distinct skeletal abnormalities in four girls with Shprintzen Goldberg syndrome. Am J Med Genet 57:565–572, 1995.

Sood S et al: Mutation in fibrillin-1 and Marfanoid-craniosynostosis (Shprintzen Goldberg) syndrome. Nat Genet 12:209–211, 1996.

Greally MT et al: Shprintzen-Goldberg syndrome: A clinical analysis. Am J Med Genet 76:202–212, 1998.

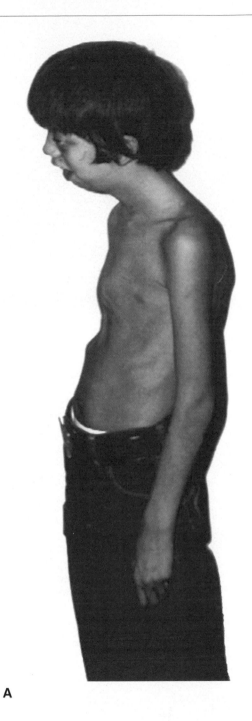

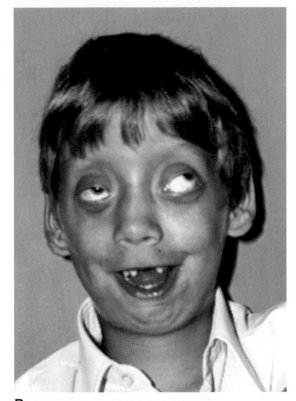

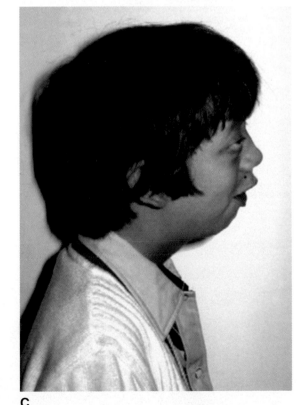

FIGURE 1. Shprintzen-Goldberg syndrome. **A–C,** A 4-year-old boy. Note the marked exophthalmos, micrognathia, and pectus carinatum. (**A–C,** From Shprintzen RJ, Goldberg RB: J Craniofacial Genet Dev Biol 2:65, 1982.) *Continued*

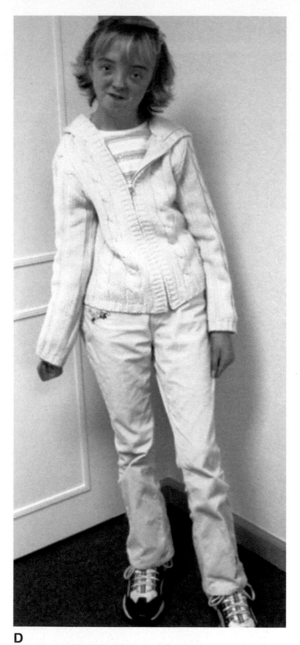

D

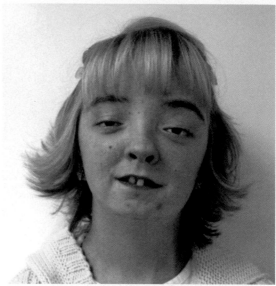

E

F

Fig. 1, cont'd. **D–F,** A 7-year-old girl. Note the low-set, posteriorly rotated ears, micrognathia, and downslanting palpebral fissures. (**D–F,** Courtesy of Dr. Cynthia Curry, University of California, San Francisco.)

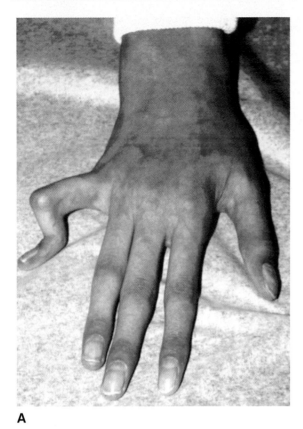

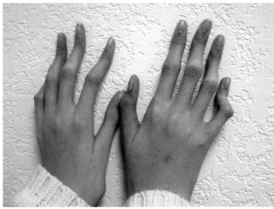

FIGURE 2. **A** and **B,** Note the arachnodactyly and camptodactyly. (**A,** From Shprintzen RJ, Goldberg RB: J Craniofacial Genet Dev Biol 2:65, 1982.)

EHLERS-DANLOS SYNDROME

Hyperextensibility of Joints, Hyperextensibility of Skin, Poor Wound Healing with Thin Scar

Originally described by Van Meekeren in 1682, this condition was further clarified by Ehlers in 1901 and Danlos in 1908. The possibility has been raised that the celebrated violinist Paganini may have had Ehlers-Danlos syndrome, thus accounting for his unusual dexterity and reach.

A simplified classification into six major types has been set forth by Beighton and colleagues. For each type, major and minor criteria have been delineated. The presence of at least one major criterion is necessary for consideration of a diagnosis. One or more minor criteria are contributory to diagnosis of a specific type, but without a major criterion are not sufficient to establish the diagnosis.

Classical Type

ABNORMALITIES

Diagnostic Criteria

Major: Skin hyperextensibility; widened atrophic scars; joint hypermobility leading to sprains, dislocations/subluxation, pes planus.

Minor: Smooth, velvety skin; molluscous pseudotumors (fleshy lesions associated with scars, frequently found over pressure points); subcutaneous spheroids (small subcutaneous spherical hard bodies, often mobile and palpable on forearms and shins; may calcify and become detectable radiographically); muscle hypoplasia; easy bruising; tissue extensibility and fragility manifest by hiatal hernia, anal prolapse, cervical insufficiency; postoperative hernia; mitral valve prolapse; aortic root dilatation; premature rupture of amniotic membranes.

ETIOLOGY. This disorder has an autosomal dominant inheritance pattern. Genetic heterogeneity has been documented. Abnormalities in fibrillar type V collagen encoded by COL5A1 and COL5A2 genes have been documented as well as type I collagen defects resulting from mutations of COL1A1.

COMMENT. The classical type has been separated into type I (gravis) and type II (mitis), which are allelic and best considered the same disorder with variable phenotype.

Hypermobile Type

ABNORMALITIES

Diagnostic Criteria

Major: Hyperextensible or smooth velvety skin; generalized joint hypermobility, most frequently involving the shoulder, patella, and temporomandibular joints.

Minor: Recurring joint dislocations, chronic joint/limb pain, positive family history, mitral valve prolapse, aortic root dilatation.

ETIOLOGY. This disorder has an autosomal dominant inheritance pattern.

Vascular Type

ABNORMALITIES

Diagnostic Criteria

(The presence of two or more major criteria is extremely suggestive.)

Major: Thin translucent skin; arterial/intestinal/uterine fragility or rupture; extensive bruising; characteristic facial appearance including a thin pinched nose, thin lips, tight skin, hallow cheeks, and prominent eyes secondary to a deficiency of adipose tissue.

Minor: Hypermobility of small joints, tendon and muscle rupture, bladder rupture, talipes equinovarus, varicose veins, arteriovenous and carotid-cavernous sinus fistula, pneumothorax/pneumohemothorax, gingival recession, positive family history.

ETIOLOGY. This disorder has an autosomal dominant inheritance pattern. Mutations in COL3A1 leading to defects in the proα1(III) chain of type III collagen are responsible.

Arthrochalasia Type

ABNORMALITIES

Diagnostic Criteria

Major: Severe generalized joint hypermobility with recurrent subluxations, congenital hip dislocation.

Minor: Skin hyperextensibility, tissue fragility, easy bruising, muscle hypotonia, kyphoscoliosis, osteopenia.

ETIOLOGY. This disorder has an autosomal dominant inheritance pattern. Mutations in the COL1A1 and COL1A2 genes that encode the α1 and α2 chains of type I collagen are responsible.

Dermatosparaxis Type

ABNORMALITIES

Diagnostic Criteria

Major: Severe skin fragility, sagging redundant skin.

Minor: Soft, doughy skin; easy bruising; premature rupture of amniotic membranes; umbilical and inguinal hernias.

ETIOLOGY. This disorder has an autosomal recessive inheritance pattern. Homozygous or compound heterozygous mutations in the gene encoding procollagen I N-terminal peptidase are responsible. Electrophoretic demonstration of pNα1 (I) and pNα2 (I) chains from type I collagen extracted from dermis in the presence of protease inhibitors or obtained from fibroblasts is diagnostic.

COMMENT. Although skin fragility and bruising are significant, wound healing is normal.

Kyphoscoliosis Type

ABNORMALITIES

Diagnostic Criteria

(The presence of three major criteria in infancy is diagnostic.)

Major: Generalized joint laxity, severe muscle hypotonia at birth, progressive scoliosis with onset at birth, scleral fragility and rupture of ocular globe.

Minor: Tissue fragility, easy bruising, arterial rupture, marfanoid habitus, microcornea, osteopenia.

ETIOLOGY. This disorder has an autosomal recessive inheritance pattern. Deficiency of lysyl hydroxylase (PLOD), a collagen-modifying enzyme, is responsible.

COMMENT. Loss of ambulation is frequent in the second and third decades.

References

Van Meekeren JA: De dilatabiltate extraordinaria cutis. In Observations Medicochirogicae. Amsterdam, 1682.

Ehlers E: Cutis laxa, Neigung zu Harmorrhagien in der Haut, Lockerung mehrer Artikulationen. Dermat Ztschr 8:173, 1901.

Danlos H: Un cas de cutis laxa avec tumeurs par contusion chronique des coudes et des genoux (santhome juvenile pseudodiabetique de MM. Hallopeau et Mace de Lepinay). Bull Soc Fr Dermat Syph 19:70, 1908.

Barabas AP: Ehlers-Danlos syndrome: Associated with prematurity and premature rupture of foetal membranes; possible increase in incidence. BMJ 2:682, 1966.

Leier CV et al: The spectrum of cardiac defects in Ehlers-Danlos syndrome, types I and III. Ann Intern Med 92:171, 1980.

Yeowell HN, Pinnell SR: The Ehlers-Danlos syndrome. Semin Dermatol 12:229, 1993.

Schievink WI et al: Neurovascular manifestations of heritable disorders of connective tissue. Stroke 25:889, 1994.

Tilstra DJ, Byers PH: Molecular basis of hereditary disorders of connective tissue. Annu Rev Med 45:149, 1994.

Beighton P et al: Ehlers-Danlos syndrome. Revised nosology, Villefranche, 1997. Am J Med Genet 77:31, 1998.

Burrows NP et al: The molecular genetics of the Ehlers-Danlos syndrome. Clin Exp Dermatol 24:99, 1999.

Nuytinck L et al: Classical Ehlers-Danlos syndrome caused by a mutation in type I collagen. Am J Hum Genet 66:1398, 2000.

Pepin M et al: Clinical and genetic features of Ehlers-Danlos syndrome type IV, the vascular type. N Engl J Med 342:673, 2000.

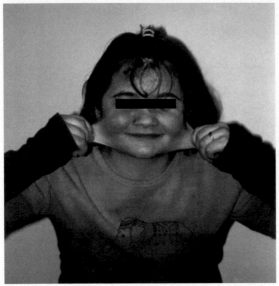

A

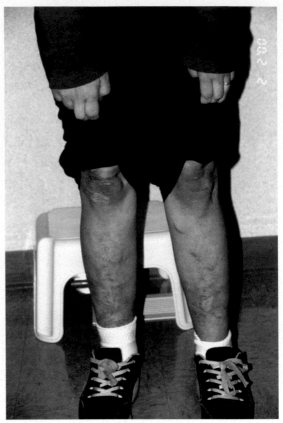

B

FIGURE 1. Ehlers-Danlos syndrome. **A** and **B,** A 12-year-old girl showing hyperelasticity of skin and persistence of scars. (Courtesy of Dr. Stephen Braddock, University of Missouri, Columbia.)

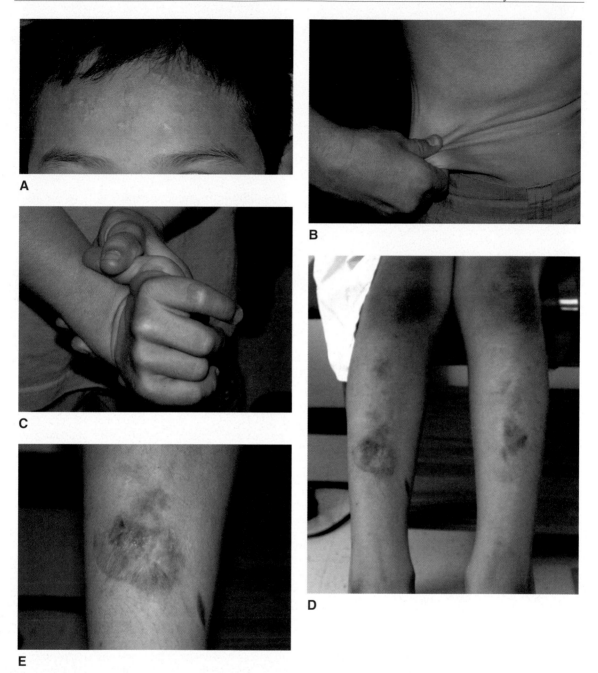

FIGURE 2. Note the persistence of scars over the forehead (**A**), hyperelasticity of the skin of the abdomen (**B**), hyperextensibility of the joints (**C**), and parchment-thin scars (**D** and **E**). (Courtesy of Dr. Lynne M. Bird, Children's Hospital, San Diego.)

OSTEOGENESIS IMPERFECTA SYNDROME, TYPE I
(AUTOSOMAL DOMINANT OSTEOGENESIS IMPERFECTA, LOBSTEIN DISEASE)

Fragile Bone, Blue Sclerae, Hyperextensibility, Presenile Deafness

Six types of osteogenesis imperfecta exist. Only type I and type II are discussed in detail in this text.

ABNORMALITIES

Growth. Normal or near-normal.

Dentition. Hypoplasia of dentin and pulp with translucency of teeth, which have a yellowish or bluish gray color, and susceptibility to caries, irregular placement, and late eruption.

Sclerae and Skin. The skin and sclerae tend to be thin and translucent; partial visualization of the choroid gives the sclerae a blue appearance; easy bruising (75%).

Skeletal. Postnatal onset of mild limb deformity, primarily anterior or lateral bowing of femora and anterior bowing of tibiae (20%), fractures (92%), scoliosis (mild to moderate in 17%; severe in 3%), kyphosis (mild to moderate in 18%; severe in 2%), hyperextensible joints (100%), wormian bones in cranial sutures, osteopenia.

Hearing. Impairment in 35%, secondary to otosclerosis, and usually first noted in third decade.

Other. Macrocephaly (18%), triangular facial appearance (30%), inguinal or umbilical hernia.

OCCASIONAL ABNORMALITIES.

Prenatal growth deficiency (7%), embryotoxon (opacity in the peripheral cornea), keratoconus, megalocornea, syndactyly, floppy mitral valve.

NATURAL HISTORY. Eight percent of patients have first fracture noted at birth, 23% in the first year, 45% in preschool, and 17% during school years. Bowing of the limbs is almost never noted in newborns. After adolescence, the likelihood of fracture diminishes, although inactivity, pregnancy, or lactation can apparently enhance the

likelihood of fracture. Scoliosis, usually not diagnosed before the end of the first decade, progresses during puberty and in some cases can be severe in adulthood. Loss of stature secondary to progressive platyspondyly and kyphosis caused by spinal osteoporosis occurs in adults. Hearing impairment is common in adults, who often require hearing aids or surgery for osteosclerosis. Virtually all patients are ambulatory. The cyclic administration of intravenous pamidronate has been effective in decreasing bone pain and increasing mobility as well as in reducing bone resorption and increasing bone density.

ETIOLOGY. This disorder has an autosomal dominant inheritance pattern with marked variability in expression. From the molecular standpoint, osteogenesis imperfecta type I results from mutations of COL1A1, the gene that encodes the pro-α-1(I) chain of type I collagen leading to a quantitative defect in the production of type I collagen.

COMMENT. Major features of types III through VI are summarized here.

Type III. Prenatal onset of growth deficiency. Macrocephaly with a triangular facial appearance. Multiple fractures usually present at birth. Progressive bone deformities from birth through childhood and adolescence. The sclera, although bluish in infancy, are usually normal in adults. Dentinogenesis imperfecta and hearing loss often occur. Severe kyphoscoliosis sometimes leads to respiratory compromise. Autosomal dominant, in most cases the result of dominant mutations in one of the two genes, COL1A1 and COL1A2 that encode the pro-α-1(I) and pro-α-2(I) chains of type I collagen. In some cases, type III presents prenatally with isolated femoral bowing. A rare autosomal recessive variety has also been described that may be the most common form of osteogenesis imperfecta in South African blacks.

Type IV. An autosomal dominant disorder associated with normal to moderately short stature with significant bone deformity, normal sclera, femoral bowing in the newborn period that straightens with time, and often dentinogenesis imperfecta. Mutations at both COL1A1 and COL1A2 loci can lead to type IV.

Type V. Moderate-to-severe tendency to fracture long bones and vertebrae. Hyperplastic callus formation. Decrease in pronation/supination at elbows associated with calcification of interosseous membrane and sometimes anterior dislocation of radial head. In growing patients, a radiodense metaphyseal band adjacent to the growth plate is common. Ligamentous laxity occurs, but blue sclera and dentinogenesis imperfecta are not features. Results of iliac biopsy reveals lamellae arranged in an irregular fashion or with a meshlike appearance. Autosomal dominant inheritance not associated with collagen type I mutations.

Type VI. Fractures first documented between 4 and 18 months. Sclera, white or faintly blue. Dentinogenesis imperfecta not a feature. Vertebral fractures occur uniformly. Iliac crest bone biopsy shows absence of the birefringent pattern of normal lamellar bone under polarized light. An accumulation of osteoid resulting from a mineralization defect in the absence of a disturbance in mineral metabolism is characteristic. The pattern of inheritance is unknown. Abnormalities in COL1A1 and COL1A2 have not been documented.

References

Freda VJ, Vosburgh GJ, Di Liberti C: Osteogenesis imperfecta congenital: A presentation of 16 cases and review of the literature. Obstet Gynecol 18:535, 1961.

Sillence DO, Senn A, Danks DH: Genetic heterogeneity in osteogenesis imperfecta. J Med Genet 16:101, 1979.

Sillence DO et al: Osteogenesis imperfecta type III. Delineation of the phenotype with reference to genetic heterogeneity. Am J Med Genet 23:821, 1986.

Byers PH: Osteogenesis imperfecta: An update. Growth Genet Horm 4:1, 1988.

Willing MC et al: Osteogenesis type I is commonly due to a COL1A1 null allele of type I collagen. Am J Hum Genet 51:508, 1992.

Molyneux K et al: A single amino acid deletion in the α-2(I) chain of type I collagen produces osteogenesis imperfecta type III. Hum Genet 90:621, 1993.

Glorieux FH et al: Cyclic administration of pamidronate in children with severe osteogenesis imperfecta. N Engl J Med 339:947, 1998.

Glorieux FH et al: Type V Osteogenesis Imperfecta: A new form of brittle bone disease. J Bone Miner Res 17:15, 1650, 2000.

Glorieux FH et al: Osteogenesis imperfecta type VI: A form of brittle bone disease with a mineralization defect. J Bone Miner Res 17:30, 2002.

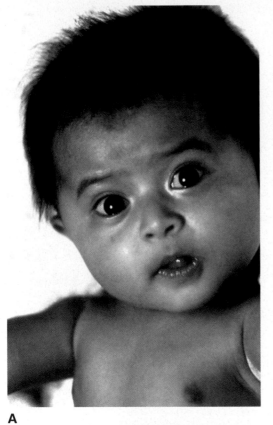

A

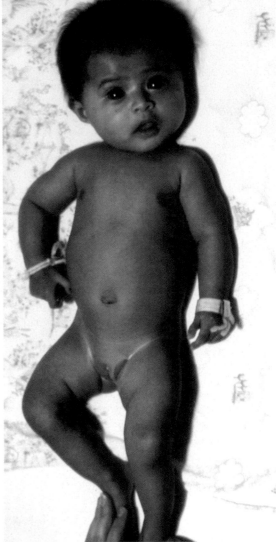

B

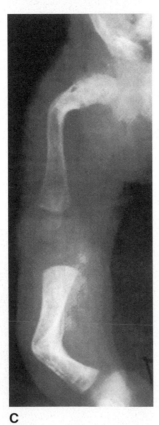

C

FIGURE 1. Osteogenesis imperfecta syndrome, type I.
A and **B,** A 6-month-old girl. Note the blue sclera.
C, Bowing of the femur and tibia of a 2-month-old child.
(**A** and **B,** Courtesy of Dr. Marilyn C. Jones, Children's
Hospital, San Diego.)

OSTEOGENESIS IMPERFECTA SYNDROME, TYPE II

(OSTEOGENESIS IMPERFECTA CONGENITA, VROLIK DISEASE)

Short, Broad Long Bones, Multiple Fractures, Blue Sclerae

A perinatally lethal variety of osteogenesis imperfecta, this disorder is characterized by short limbs; short, broad long bones; radiologic evidence of severe osseous fragility; and defective ossification. Based on subtle differences in radiographic features, Sillence and colleagues subdivided this disorder into three groups. Type A is characterized by short, broad crumpled femora and continuously beaded ribs; type B by short, broad crumpled femora but normal ribs or ribs with incomplete beading; and type C by long, thin, inadequately modeled, rectangular long bones with multiple fractures and thin, beaded ribs.

ABNORMALITIES

Growth. Prenatal short-limbed growth deficiency.
Craniofacial. Poorly mineralized, soft calvarium with large fontanels and multiple wormian bones; deep blue sclerae; shallow orbits; small nose; low nasal bridge.
Limbs. Short, thick, ribbon-like, poorly mineralized long bones with multiple fractures and callus formation, especially in lower limbs.
Other. Flattened vertebrae, hypotonia, inguinal hernias, variable hydrocephalus, hydrops.

NATURAL HISTORY. These patients usually are stillborn or die in early infancy of respiratory failure. However, in that the ribs are less affected in type B, affected babies may survive for months.

ETIOLOGY. In virtually all cases, this disorder is due to a dominant mutation in one of the two type I collagen genes (COL1A1 or COL1A2). The majority of cases of type II osteogenesis imperfecta are the result of sporadic mutations of an autosomal dominant gene. For these cases, a recurrence risk of approximately 6% has been observed and is thought to be the result of gonadal and usually somatic mosaicism in one parent.

References

Byers PH, Bonadio JF, Steinmann B: Invited editorial comment: Osteogenesis imperfecta. Update and perspective. Am J Med Genet 17:429, 1984.

Sillence DO et al: Osteogenesis imperfecta, type II. Delineation of the phenotype with reference to genetic heterogeneity. Am J Med Genet 17:407, 1984.

Spranger J: Invited editorial comment: Osteogenesis imperfecta: A pasture for splitters and lumpers. Am J Med Genet 17:425, 1984.

Horwitz AL, Lazda V, Byers PH: Recurrent type II (lethal) osteogenesis imperfecta: Apparent dominant inheritance. Am J Hum Genet 37:A59, 1985.

Tsipouras P et al: Osteogenesis imperfecta type II is usually due to new dominant gene. Am J Hum Genet 37:A79, 1985.

Byers PH et al: Perinatal lethal osteogenesis imperfecta (OI type II): A biochemically heterogeneous disorder usually due to new mutations in the gene for type I collagen. Am J Hum Genet 42:237, 1988.

Cole WG, Dalglcish R: Perinatal lethal osteogenesis imperfecta. J Med Genet 32:284, 1995.

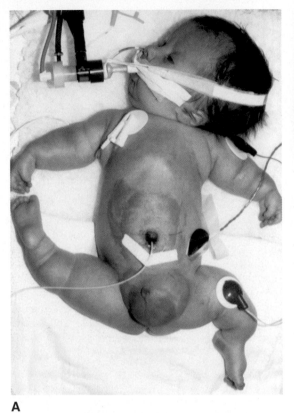

A

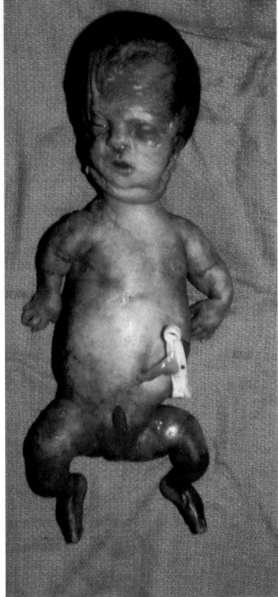

B

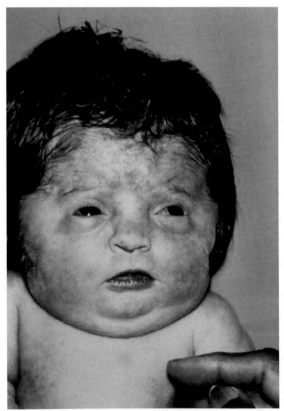

C

FIGURE 1. Osteogenesis imperfecta syndrome, type II.
A–C, Newborn infants. Note the short, bent limbs,
inguinal hernia, and blue sclera. (**C,** Courtesy of P. Baird,
University of British Columbia, Vancouver.)

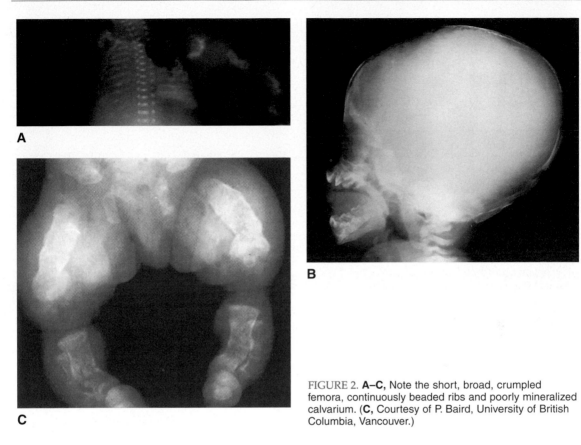

FIGURE 2. **A–C,** Note the short, broad, crumpled femora, continuously beaded ribs and poorly mineralized calvarium. (**C,** Courtesy of P. Baird, University of British Columbia, Vancouver.)

FIBRODYSPLASIA OSSIFICANS PROGRESSIVA SYNDROME

Short Hallux, Fibrous Dysplasia Leading to Ossification in Muscles and Subcutaneous Tissues

This condition, described in a letter by Guy Patin in 1692, was extensively reviewed by Rosenstirn in 1918. More than 500 cases have been reported.

ABNORMALITIES

Digits. Short hallux, often with synostosis; less frequently, short thumb.

Fibrous Tissues. Swellings, sometimes with pain and fever, in aponeuroses, fasciae, and tendons, leading to ossification in muscles and fibrous tissue; most prominent in neck, dorsal trunk, and proximal limbs, with sternocleidomastoid and masseters frequently involved.

Other. Progressive cervical vertebral spine fusion, scoliosis.

OCCASIONAL ABNORMALITIES.

Short phalanges other than hallux or thumb, clinodactyly of fifth finger, short femoral neck, flat broadened mandibular condyle, hip synovial osteochondromatosis, hernia, widely spaced teeth, hypogenitalism or delayed sexual development, easy bruising, hearing loss, cardiac conduction abnormalities.

NATURAL HISTORY.

Monophalangic great toes, the result of synostosis, are the earliest manifestations and are usually present at birth. Progressive heterotopic ossification of tendons, ligaments, fasciae, and striated muscles, heralded in most cases by large painful swelling, usually begins in the first decade. Restrictive heterotopic ossification develops in 85% of patients by 7 years of age, and severely restricted mobility of the arms develops by the age of 15 in more than 95%. Most patients are wheelchair-bound by the third decade and pulmonary complications often lead to death in the fifth and sixth decade. The most common locations for the initial heterotopic ossification are the neck, spine, and shoulder. Areas with lower risk include the wrists, ankles, and jaw. Diaphragm,

tongue, extraocular, facial, and cardiac muscles are usually spared. No effective treatment has been discovered, although symptomatic relief of pain may be achieved by salicylates or hydrocortisone analogue therapy. The natural history tends toward exacerbation and remission, and therefore, the results of therapy should be interpreted with caution. Another matter for caution is the interpretation of biopsies from affected tissues. The pathologic interpretation may be osteogenic sarcoma, although such a malignant growth is not a feature of this disease. Furthermore, any kind of trauma, including biopsy, surgery, or intramuscular injection, can be a focus for an area of ectopic ossification. Problems with anesthesia including difficulties with tracheal intubation, restrictive pulmonary disease, and abnormalities of cardiac conduction have occurred.

ETIOLOGY.

This disorder has an autosomal dominant inheritance pattern with almost full penetrance for short hallux and varying expression for the fibrodysplasia. Although the responsible gene has been mapped to 4q27-31, the molecular cause of this disorder is not yet known. Approximately 90% of patients represent fresh mutations, for which older paternal age has been noted.

COMMENT.

Because trauma uniformly exacerbates the condition, biopsy for the purpose of diagnosis is not appropriate and is usually unnecessary.

References

Rosenstirn J: A contribution to the study of myositis ossificans progressiva. Ann Surg 68:485, 1918.

Tünte W, Becker PE, Knorr G: Zur Genetik der Myositis ossificans progressiva. Humangenetik 4:320, 1967.

Rogers IG, Geho WB: Fibrodysplasia ossificans progressiva. J Bone Joint Surg [Am] 61:909, 1979.

Newton MC et al: Fibrodysplasia ossificans progressiva. Br J Anaesth 64:246, 1990.

Cohen RB et al: The natural history of heterotopic ossification in patients who have fibrodysplasia ossificans progressiva. J Bone Joint Surg [Am] 75:215, 1993.

Rocke DM et al: Age and joint-specific risk of initial heterotopic ossification in patients who have fibrodysplasia ossificans progressiva. Clin Orthop 301:243, 1994.

Kussmaul MG et al: Pulmonary and cardiac function in advanced fibrodysplasia ossificans progessiva. Clin Orthop 346:104, 1998.

Feldman G et al: Fibrodysplasia ossificans progessiva, a heritable disorder of severe heterotopic ossification, maps to human chromosome 4q27-31. Am J Hum Genet 66:128, 2000.

Mahboubi S, et al: Fibrodysplasia ossificans progressive. Pediatr Radiol 31:307, 2001.

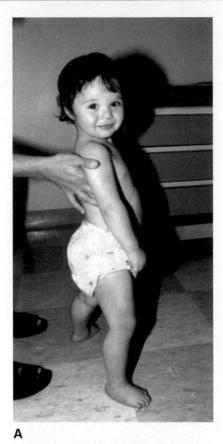

A

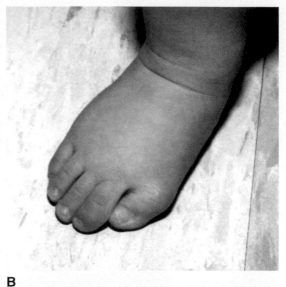

B

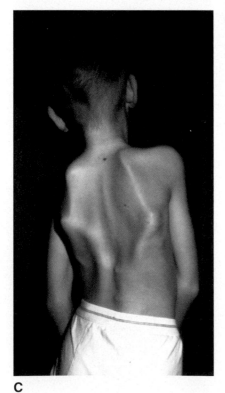

C

D

FIGURE 1. Fibrodysplasia ossificans progressiva syndrome. **A** and **B,** A 15-month-old child. Note the straight back, which is due to early ossification and the short hallux. (Courtesy of Dr. Marilyn C. Jones, Children's Hospital, San Diego.) **C** and **D,** A 13-year-old child showing progressive ossification in back musculature and short valgus hallux.

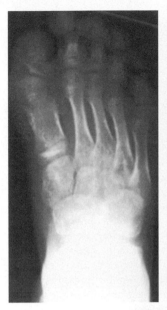
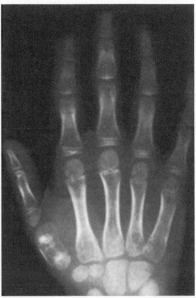
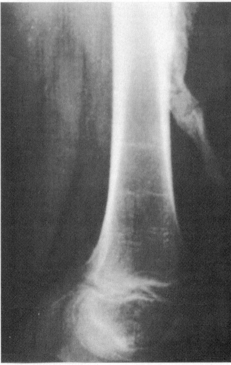

FIGURE 2. Note the short and deformed first metatarsal, hallux, and first metacarpal. Aberrant ossification is evident in the lower thigh. (From Herrmann J et al: Birth Defects 5(5), 1969. Courtesy of Dr. John M. Opitz, University of Utah, Salt Lake City.)

P Hamartoses

STURGE-WEBER SEQUENCE

Flat Facial Hemangiomata, Meningeal Hemangiomata with Seizures

The association and localization of aberrant vasculature in the facial skin, eyes, and meninges are compatible with a defect arising in a limited part of the cephalic neural crest, cells of which migrate to the supraocular dermis, choroid, and pia mater.

ABNORMALITIES

Facial. Port-wine capillary malformation, most commonly in a trigeminal facial distribution, sometimes involving the choroid of the eye with secondary buphthalmos or glaucoma as well as the conjunctiva or episcleral region; involvement usually unilateral, is sometimes bilateral; overgrowth of bony maxilla secondary to the vascular anomaly.

Meninges and Central Nervous System. Capillary malformation involving arachnoid and pia mater, especially in occipital and temporal areas with secondary cerebral cortical atrophy, sclerosis, and "double contour" convolutional calcification; seizures; paresis; mental deficiency.

OCCASIONAL ABNORMALITIES.
Capillary malformation in nonfacial areas; microgyria; macrocephaly; colobomata of iris, retinal vasculature tortuousity, iris heterochromia, retinal detachment, and strabismus; coarctation of aorta; enlargement of the ear when involved with capillary malformation; macrodactyly.

NATURAL HISTORY.
The surface capillary malformations are usually present at birth and seldom progress. Seizures most commonly begin between 2 and 7 months of age and are grand mal in type, often asymmetric. The degree of central nervous system (CNS) involvement is variable, with 30% having paresis and approximately 83% having seizures; 39% have normal intelligence. An increased risk for emotional and behavioral problems including attention deficit hyperactivity disorder in 22% of cases has been noted. Cerebral calcification is usually not evident by radiography until later infancy, the earliest occurring in a patient 13 months of age, first being noted in the occipital region.

Medical anticonvulsant treatment is often of limited value, and occasionally unihemispheric, hemispherectomy is advised as a measure to control seizures. Cognitive delay and mental deterioration are significantly correlated with seizure intensity in the first 18 months of life but not with age of seizure onset, degree of hemiparesis, or presence of ongoing seizures. Glaucoma presents before 2 years of age if tissues destined to form the anterior chamber angle are affected. If conjunctival and episcleral vascular tissues are involved, glaucoma frequently does not occur until after 5 years of age. Although pulsed dye laser therapy is the treatment of choice, complete clearance of the port-wine stain rarely occurs.

ETIOLOGY.
The cause of this disorder is unknown. It occurs sporadically, with rare exceptions. Occasionally, other family members may have hemangiomata of a lesser degree.

COMMENT.
Port-wine facial nevi occur frequently without eye or brain abnormalities. Only patients with lesions involving the opthalmic distribution of the trigeminal nerve are at risk for neuro-ocular complications. Rarely the leptomeninges are involved without the face or choroid.

References

Chaeo DH-C: Congenital neurocutaneous syndromes of childhood. III: Sturge-Weber disease. J Pediatr 55:635, 1959.

Butterworth T, Strean LP: Clinical Genodermatology. Baltimore: Williams & Wilkins, 1962.

Enolras O, Riche MC, Merland JJ: Facial port-wine stains and Sturge-Weber syndrome. Pediatrics 76:48, 1985.

Oakes WJ: The natural history of patients with the Sturge-Weber syndrome. Pediatr Neurosurg 18:287, 1992.

Sullivan TJ et al: The ocular manifestation of the Sturge-Weber syndrome. J Pediatr Ophthalmol Strabismus 29:349, 1992.

Chapieski L et al: Psychological functioning in children with Sturge-Weber syndrome. J Child Neurol 15:660, 2000.

Kramer U et al: Outcome of infants with unilateral Sturge-Weber syndrome and early onset seizures. Dev Med Child Neurol 42:756, 2000.

Kossof EM et al: Outcome of 32 hemispherectomies for Sturge-Weber syndrome worldwide. Neurology 59:1735, 2002.

Léaute-Labrèze C et al: Pulsed dye laser for Sturge-Weber syndrome. Arch Dis Child 87:434, 2002.

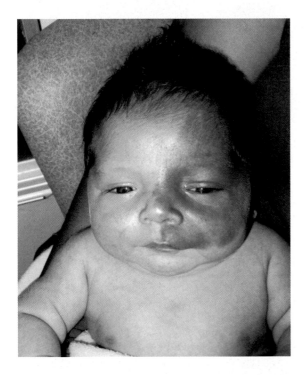

FIGURE 1. Sturge-Weber sequence. Note that the lesion involves the upper eyelid, which includes the ophthalmic distribution of the trigeminal nerve.

NEUROCUTANEOUS MELANOSIS SEQUENCE

Melanosis of Skin and Pia-Arachnoid, Central Nervous System Deterioration

This melanocytic hamartomatosis of the skin and pia-arachnoid was first described in 1861. More than 100 cases have been reported.

ABNORMALITIES

Skin. Giant pigmented nevi (66%) usually in a "bathing trunk" or lumbosacral distribution, less frequently in the occipital region or upper back; numerous congenital nevi without a prominent large lesion (34%); associated small or medium-sized congenital melanocytic nevi on the scalp, face, or neck occur in association with the larger lesions.

Pia-arachnoid. Thick and pigmented with nests and sheets of melanotic cells, 88% with cranial involvement and 88% with spinal involvement; leptomeningeal melanoma.

Central Nervous System. Liable to development of seizures and deterioration of CNS function; hydrocephalus secondary to blockage of cisternal pathways or obliteration of arachnoid villi by the tumor; involvement of spinal cord and its coverings; cranial nerve palsies, particularly VI and VII.

OCCASIONAL ABNORMALITIES.

Syringomyelia; Dandy-Walker malformation; psychosis; Meckel diverticulum; urinary tract anomalies, including renal pelvis and ureteral malformations, unilateral renal cysts, rhabdomyosarcoma; extracranial melanoma probably representing metastases from meningeal melanoma; liposarcoma; malignant peripheral nerve sheath tumor.

NATURAL HISTORY.

The cutaneous melanosis is grossly evident at birth. CNS function may be normal initially, but seizures and other signs of increased intracranial pressure often develop before the age of 2 years and mental deterioration may begin before 1 year of age, apparently related to the melanoblastic involvement of the pia-arachnoid and spinal cord compression.

Leptomeningeal melanoma occurs in 40% to 62% of patients, and CNS melanomas are found frequently.

The CNS consequences of the disorder often result in early demise. Three of the recognized patients were stillborn; the majority died before 2 years of age, and only 10% of the patients are known to have survived past the age of 25 years. The interval between the age at initial presentation and death ranges from immediate to 21 years, with more than one half occurring within 3 years of initial diagnosis.

In 25% of patients with neurologically asymptomatic, large congenital melanocytic nevi, focal magnetic resonance signals are present in the leptomeninges or adjacent brain parenchyma. Although the prognosis for these patients is unknown, the vast majority followed for 5 years have not developed symptomatic neurocutaneous melanosis. Patients with satellite nevi are of greatest risk for development of neurocutaneous melanosis. Patients without nevi on the head or neck or the posterior midline rarely develop neurologic complications.

The risk of malignant melanoma degeneration of the cutaneous melanosis is reported as 5% to 15%, with half becoming evident by 5 years of age. Thus, surgery to reduce the skin lesions is indicated in patients in whom careful evaluation has documented a lack of leptomeningeal involvement.

ETIOLOGY.

This disorder is sporadic; its cause unknown. The etiology is presumed to be an aberration in growth of early melanoblasts of neural crest origin, which contribute to the skin and pia-arachnoid. The sex incidence has been equal, and a family history of melanomata was noted in only one case.

References

Rokitansky J: Ein ausgezeichneter Fall von Pigmentmal mit ausgebreiteter Pigmentirung der inneren Hirn- und Rückenmarkshäute. Allg Wien Med Ztg 6:113, 1861.

Van Bogaert L: La Mélanose neurocutanée diffuse hérédofamiale. Bull Acad R Med Belg (6th series) 13:397, 1948.

Fox H et al: Neurocutaneous melanosis. Arch Dis Child 39:508, 1964.

Hoffman HJ, Freeman A: Primary malignant leptomeningeal melanoma in association with giant hairy nevus. J Neurosurg 26:62, 1967.

Kadonaga JH, Frieden IJ: Neurocutaneous melanosis: Definition and review of literature. J Am Acad Dermatol 24:747, 1991.

Frieden IJ et al: Giant congenital melanocytic nevi: Brain magnetic resonance findings in neurologically asymptomatic children. J Am Acad Dermatol 31:423, 1994.

Foster RD et al: Giant congenital melanocytic nevi: The significance of neurocutaneous melanosis in neurologically asymptomatic children. Plast Reconstr Surg 107:933, 2001.

Makkar HS, Frieden IJ: Congenital melanocytic nevi: An update for the pediatrician. Clin Opin Pediatr 14:397, 2002.

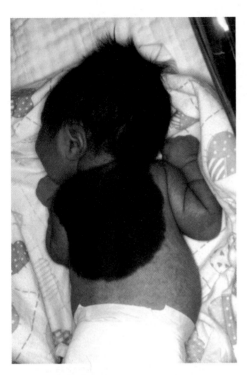

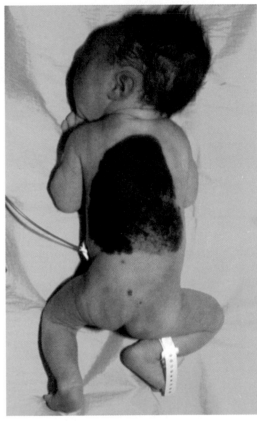

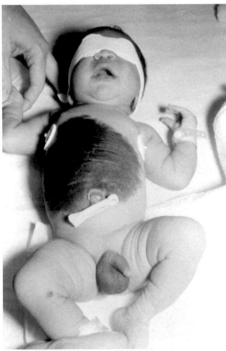

FIGURE 1. Neurocutaneous melanosis sequence.

LINEAR SEBACEOUS NEVUS SEQUENCE
(NEVUS SEBACEUS OF JADASSOHN, EPIDERMAL NEVUS SYNDROME)

Midfacial Nevus Sebaceus, Seizures, Mental Deficiency

Nevus sebaceous of Jadassohn is most commonly found in an otherwise normal individual. However, the association of this type of lesion in the midfacial area with seizures and mental deficiency has been reported in at least 100 cases.

ABNORMALITIES

Growth. Asymmetric overgrowth, advanced bone age.

Skin. Nevus sebaceous with hyperpigmentation and hyperkeratosis; lesions most commonly in the midfacial area, from the forehead down into the nasal area, tending to be linear in distribution; may also affect trunk and limbs.

Central Nervous System. Seizures of major motor, focal, or minor motor types; mental deficiency.

OCCASIONAL ABNORMALITIES

Skeletal. Cranial asymmetry or hemimacrocephaly; premature closure of sphenoid frontal sutures, sphenoid bone malformation, and abnormalities of sella turcica; scoliosis, kyphosis, abnormalities of ulna, head of radius, humerus, and fibula; polydactyly, syndactyly; vitamin D–resistant rickets.

Eyes. Esotropia, lipodermoid of conjunctiva, cloudy cornea, colobomata of eyelid, coloboma of iris and choroid, atrophy of optic nerve, subretinal neovascularization, microphthalmia.

Central Nervous System. Micro- and/or macrocephaly, cerebral and cerebellar hypoplasia, arachnoid cysts, hydrocephalus, hemiparesis, cranial nerve palsy, cortical blindness, hypertonia, cerebral vascular changes, intracerebral calcifications, cerebral neoplasia/hamartoma.

Other. Short palpebral fissures, pigmented nevi; spotty alopecia; coarctation of aorta, patent ductus arteriosus, hypoplastic left heart, ventricular septal defect; cardiac arrhythmias; hypoplasia of renal or pulmonary artery; cleft palate; hypoplastic teeth; renal hamartomata, nephroblastoma, double urinary collecting system, horseshoe kidneys; enlarged clitoris; undescended testes, cystic biliary adenoma of liver; dental anomalies.

NATURAL HISTORY. The nevus sebaceous is usually present at birth as a slightly yellow to orange to tan waxy appearing lesion containing deficiencies or papillomatous excesses of epidermal elements, especially sebaceous glands and immature hair follicles. With time, the lesions tend to become verrucous and unsightly. Early surgical removal should be considered, since there is a 15% to 20% risk of tumor, especially basal cell epithelioma. Furthermore, there may be unpredictable periods of rapid growth of the lesions. In the cases with associated CNS features, the onset of seizures has been from 2 months to 2 years, and they are difficult to control. The mental deficiency has been moderate to severe, although an occasional patient may have normal intelligence. The vitamin D–resistant rickets that sometimes occurs is a variant of tumor-induced osteomalacia. The associated ricketic lesions, muscle weakness, and bone pain, as well as the biochemical abnormalities reverse following surgical removal of the skin lesions.

ETIOLOGY. The cause of this disorder is unknown. Whether this disorder constitutes a single etiologic entity remains to be determined. Bianchine noted seizures or mental deficiency without skin lesions in several first-degree relatives of one patient. Hence, a cautious family evaluation is indicated in cases of this clinical disorder.

References
Mehregan AH, Pinkus H: Life history of organoid nevi: Special reference to nevus sebaceus of Jadassohn. Arch Dermatol 91:574, 1965.

Marden PM, Venters HD: A new neurocutaneous syndrome. Am J Dis Child 112:79, 1966.

Bianchine JW: The nevus sebaceous of Jadassohn: A neurocutaneous syndrome and a potentially premalignant lesion. Am J Dis Child 120:223, 1970.

Lansky LL et al: Linear sebaceous nevus syndrome. Am J Dis Child 123:587, 1972.

Leonidas JC et al: Radiographic features of the linear sebaceous syndrome. AJR 132:277, 1979.

Carey DE et al: Hypophosphatemic rickets/osteomalacia in linear sebaceous nevus syndrome: A variant of tumor-induced osteomalacia. J Pediatr 109:994, 1986.

Alfonso I et al: Linear nevus sebaceous syndrome: A review. J Clin Neuroophthalmol 7:170, 1987.

Grebe TA et al: Further delineation of the epidermal nevus syndrome: Two cases with new findings and literature review. Am J Med Genet 47:24, 1993.

Margulis A et al: Surgical management of the cutaneous manifestations of linear nevus sebaceous syndrome. Plast Reconstr Surg 111:1043, 2003.

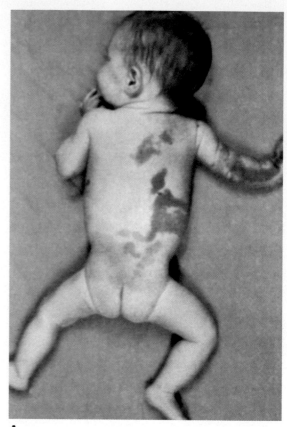

FIGURE 1. Linear sebaceous nevus sequence. **A,** A 2-week-old infant with facial and extensive body sebaceous nevi. Intractable seizures began at 5 months, and the patient died at 9 months with pneumonia. Necropsy revealed renal nodular nephronoblastomatosis. (**A,** From Lansky LL et al: Am J Dis Child 123:587, 1972, with permission.)   *Continued*   **A**

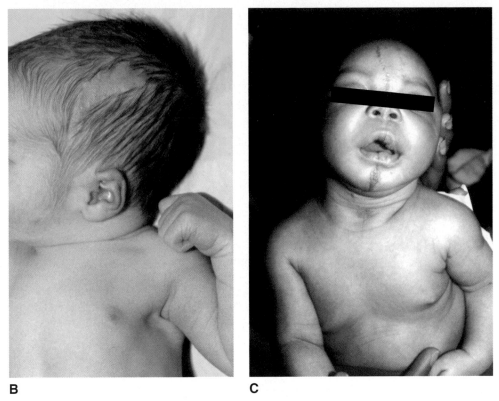

B **C**

Fig. 1, cont'd. Note the orange to tan waxy-appearing lesion (**B**) and verrucous change that has developed in older childhood (**C**).

INCONTINENTIA PIGMENTI SYNDROME
(BLOCH-SULZBERGER SYNDROME)

Irregular Pigmented Skin Lesions with or without Dental Anomaly, Patchy Alopecia

Bardach originally described the condition in twin sisters in 1925, and soon thereafter Bloch set forth the term incontinentia pigmenti to depict the unusual skin lesions. A major review of 635 cases by Carney includes only 16 affected males.

ABNORMALITIES

Skin. Most consistent feature; blisters, preceded by erythema, develop typically in a linear distribution along the limbs and around the trunk within the first few weeks of life; as the blisters begin to heal, hyperkeratotic lesions develop on the distal limbs and scalp and rarely on the trunk or face; hyperpigmentation, most apparent on the trunk distributed along lines of Blaschko, occur in streaks and whorls, usually developing after the blisters have disappeared; pale, hairless patches or streaks most evident on the lower legs develop usually at the time the hyperpigmentation disappears.

Dentition. Eighty percent have hypodontia, delayed eruption, or conical form.

Hair. Fifty percent have minor abnormalities; atrophic patchy alopecia, especially on the posterior scalp at the vertex, is common; lusterless, wiry, coarse hair as well as thin, sparse hair in early childhood.

Nails. Abnormalities in 40%, ranging from mild ridging or pitting to severe nail disruption.

Central Nervous System. Approximately one third have mental deficiency, microcephaly, spasticity, or seizures.

Eyes. Approximately 30% have strabismus, often with refractive errors; abnormalities of the retinal vessels and underlying pigment cells in 40% leading to retinal ischemia, new vessel proliferation, bleeding, and fibrosis; retinal detachment, uveitis, keratitis, cataract, microphthalmos, and optic atrophy occur infrequently.

Osseous. Approximately 20% have hemivertebrae, kyphoscoliosis, extra rib, syndactyly, hemiatrophy, or short arms and legs.

OCCASIONAL ABNORMALITIES.
Nail dystrophy, breast hypoplasia, abnormalities in nipple pigmentation, supernumerary nipple, nipple hypoplasia, dacryostenosis, eczema, short stature, hydrocephalus, subungual keratotic tumors.

NATURAL HISTORY. Bullous skin lesions are generally present in early infancy and tend to progress from inflammatory or vesicular to pigmented and may fade in childhood. General eosinophilia is often present in infancy and the vesicles contain eosinophils. Verrucous lichenoid lesions develop during infancy in approximately one third of cases, especially over the dorsum of the hands and feet. During the period when the blisters are present, the lesions should be kept dry and protected from trauma. The development of the irregular marble cake–like pigmentation may or may not coincide with the sites of bullous or verrucous lesions. The pigmented areas gradually fade in the second to third decades, and the adult may show only slightly atrophic depigmented "achromic stains," especially over the lower legs. Because the retinal vascular changes sometimes progress during the neonatal period, monthly ophthalmologic evaluations are recommended during the first 2 to 3 months of life. In approximately 10% of cases, this process progresses to severe scarring with significant visual loss. Approximately one half of the patients show other features, the most serious being the CNS abnormalities. Seizures in the neonatal period represent an ominous sign relative to future neurologic development. In their absence, prognosis, in most cases, is good.

ETIOLOGY. This disorder has an X-linked dominant inheritance pattern with male lethality in the vast majority of cases. Mutations in the nuclear factor-kappa B (NF-κB) essential modulator (NEMO) gene located at Xq28 are responsible. NF-κB is a transcription factor, which controls expression of many genes, including those for production of cytokines and chemokines, and protects against apoptosis. In females with IP, the functionally aberrant cell clone is eliminated by apoptosis, resulting in eradication of defective cells and healing of skin lesions soon after birth. In addition, because the functionally aberrant cell clone is for the most part eliminated, distribution of the normal and aberrant clones deviates from randomness, resulting in skewing of X inactivation that occurs in 98% of females with incontinentia pigmenti. Survival in males can be explained by a less deleterious mutation, a 47XXY karyotype, or somatic mosaicism.

References

Bardach M: Systematisierte Naevusbildungen bei einem cineiigen Zwillingspaar: Ein Beitrag zur Naevusätiologie. Z Kinderheilkd 39:542, 1925.

Bloch B: Eigentümliche bisher nicht beschriebene Pigmentaffektion (Incontinentia pigmenti). Schweiz Med Wochenschr 56:404, 1926.

Landy SJ, Donnai D: Incontinentia pigmenti (Bloch-Sulzberger syndrome). J Med Genet 30:53, 1993.

Sybert VP: Incontinentia pigmenti nomenclature. Am J Hum Genet 55:209, 1994.

International IP Consortium: Genomic rearrangement in NEMO impairs NF-κB activation and is a cause of incontinentia pigmenti. Nature 405:466, 2000.

Aradhya S et al: A recurrent deletion in the ubiquitously expressed NEMO (IKK-γ) gene accounts for the vast majority of incontinentia pigmenti mutations. Hum Mol Genet 10:2171, 2001.

International IP Consortium: Survival of male patients with incontinentia pigmenti carrying a lethal mutation can be explained by somatic mutation or Klinefelter syndrome. Am J Hum Genet 69:1210, 2001.

Happle R: A fresh look at incontinenti pigmenti. Arch Dermatol 139:1206, 2003.

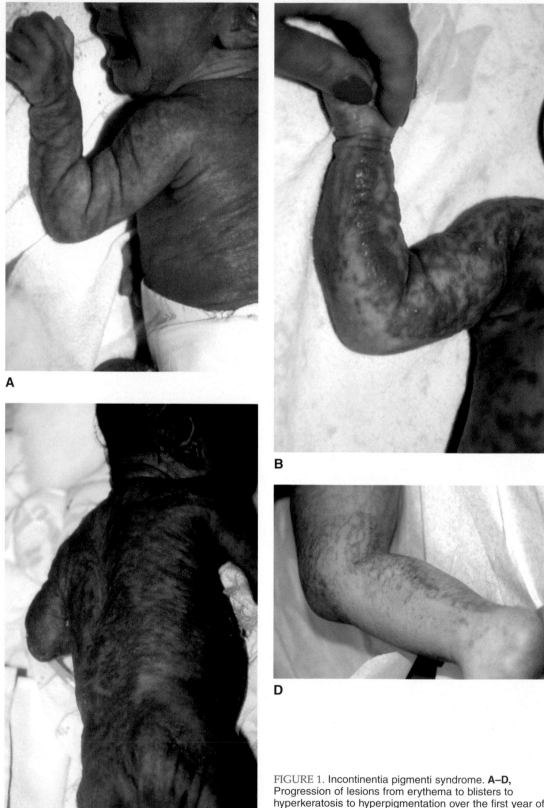

FIGURE 1. Incontinentia pigmenti syndrome. **A–D,**
Progression of lesions from erythema to blisters to
hyperkeratosis to hyperpigmentation over the first year of
life. (Courtesy of Dr. Marilyn C. Jones, Children's
Hospital, San Diego.)

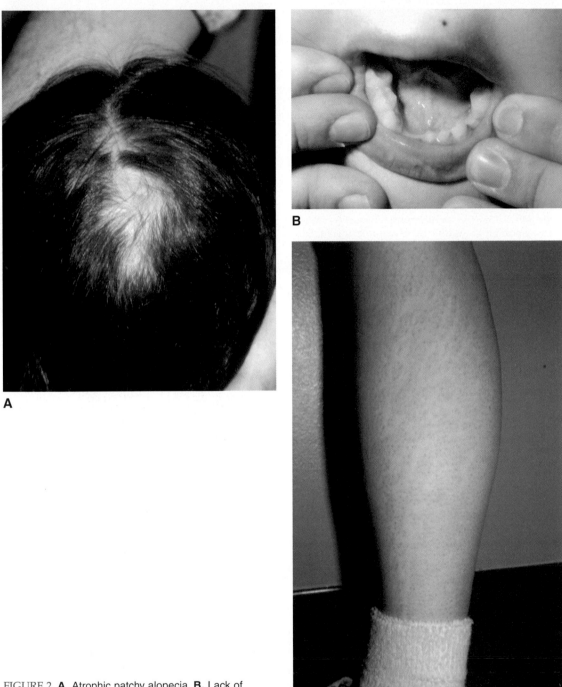

FIGURE 2. **A,** Atrophic patchy alopecia. **B,** Lack of alveolar ridge indicating anodontia. **C,** Pale hairless streaks on lower leg.

HYPOMELANOSIS OF ITO
(Incontinentia Pigmentosa Achromians)

Initially described by Ito in 1952, numerous affected individuals subsequently have been reported. The characteristic skin lesions involve streaked, whorled, or mottled areas of hypopigmentation on limbs or trunk usually evident in infancy. It is now clear that hypomelanosis of Ito is not a specific disorder, but is an etiologically heterogeneous physical finding that is frequently indicative of chromosomal or genetic mosaicism. Approximately 70% of reported cases have associated anomalies. With the exception of mental retardation (67%), seizures (35%), and cerebral atrophy (16%), all other associated abnormalities have occurred in less than 8% of patients.

ASSOCIATED ABNORMALITIES

Central Nervous System. Variable mental retardation, seizures, neurologic problems.

Craniofacial. Macrocephaly, coarse facies, hypertelorism, epicanthal folds, thick lips, cleft lip/palate, malformed auricles.

Eyes. Iridial heterochromia, abnormal retinal pigmentation, strabismus.

Hair and Teeth. Hypertrichosis, diffuse alopecia, dysplasia of teeth, irregularly spaced teeth.

Limbs. Clinodactyly, syndactyly, ectrodactyly, polydactyly, triphalangeal thumb, genu valga.

Skeletal. Kyphoscoliosis/lordosis, short stature.

NATURAL HISTORY. The skin lesions, which are best appreciated by a Wood lamp examination, do not go through a prodrome phase as in incontinentia pigmenti. The prognosis depends on the type and extent of associated abnormalities.

ETIOLOGY. Hypomelanosis of Ito is etiologically heterogeneous. Karyotyping of characteristic skin findings to rule out chromosomal mosaicism when developmental delay or structural anomalies are also present is indicated. Recurrence risk is low except in those chromosomally abnormal individuals in which a balanced parental translocation is present. A single-gene basis for hypomelanosis of Ito probably does not exist.

References

Ito M: Studies on melanin XI: Incontinentia pigmenti; achromians. Tohoku J Exp Med 55(Suppl):57, 1952.

Flannery DB: Pigmentary dysplasia: Hypomelanosis of Ito, and genetic mosaicism. Am J Med Genet 35:18, 1990.

Ritter CL et al: Chromosome mosaicism in hypomelanosis of Ito. Am J Med Genet 35:14, 1990.

Sybert VP et al: Pigmentary abnormalities and mosaicism for chromosomal aberration: Association with clinical features similar to hypomelanosis of Ito. J Pediatr 116:581, 1990.

Küster W, Künig A: Hypomelanosis of Ito: No entity, but a cutaneous sign of mosaicsm. Am J Med Genet 85:346, 1999.

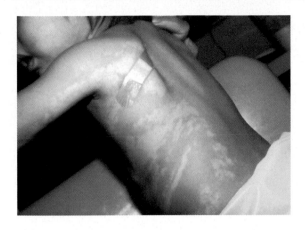

FIGURE 1. Hypomelanosis of Ito. A 14-month-old with developmental delay, hypotonia, and seizures. Note the irregular, streaky distribution of hypopigmentation. (Courtesy of Dr. Marilyn C. Jones, Children's Hospital, San Diego.)

TUBEROUS SCLEROSIS SYNDROME

Hamartomatous Skin Nodules,
Seizures, Phakomata, Bone Lesions

Von Recklinghausen is said to have described this disease, but Bourneville is usually given credit for its recognition in 1880. Hamartomatous lesions develop in many tissues, especially the skin and brain. Diagnostic criteria have been set forth by the National Tuberous Sclerosis Association.

ABNORMALITIES

Brain and Eyes. Glioma-angioma lesions in cortex and white matter, with seizures (93%) and mental deficiency (62%) as apparent consequences; behavioral problems and autism; radiologic evidence of intracranial mineralization (51%), most commonly in basal ganglia or periventricular region; however, early in the clinical course, the periventricular lesions may be noted as one of the most consistent features; hamartomas of retina or optic nerve in 53%; in half of these, the hamartomas are bilateral.

Skin. Fibrous-angiomatous lesions (83%), varying in color from flesh to pink to yellow to brown, develop in the nasolabial fold, cheeks, and elsewhere; white macules classified into three types: "thumb-print" macules, "lance-ovate" macules (one end rounded, the other with a sharp tip) or ash leaf macule, and the confetti macules (tiny 1- to 3-mm macules); café au lait spots; fibromatous plaques and nodules.

Bone. Cystlike areas in phalanges (66%) and elsewhere, with areas of periosteal thickening yielding radiologic evidence of "sclerosis."

Renal. Angiomyolipomata in 45% to 81%, usually multiple and benign; tubular enlargement and cyst formation with hyperplasia of tubular cells.

Dentition. Pit-shaped enamel defects, most evident by close inspection of labial premolar surfaces.

OCCASIONAL ABNORMALITIES.

Other hamartomata: fibromata (especially gingival and subungual), lipomata, angiomata, nevi, shagreen patches (goose flesh–like); rhabdomyomata and angiomata of heart, cystic changes in lung, hamartomata of liver and pancreas; renal cell carcinoma; hamartomatous rectal polyps; hypothyroidism; thyroid adenomata; sexual precocity; astrocytoma; lymphedema; hypertension.

NATURAL HISTORY. Hamartomata usually become evident in early childhood and may increase at adolescence. Facial nodular lesions are present in 50% of children by 5 years, whereas white macules are present at birth or in early infancy in almost all patients, and are easily visualized with help of the Wood lamp. Malignant transformation may occur, and brain tumors develop in approximately 6% of patients. However, malignant transformation of the periventricular nodules is rare. The seizures, which tend to develop in early childhood, may initially be myoclonic and later grand mal in type and are difficult to control. Electroencephalographic abnormality is found in 87% of patients and may be of the grossly disorganized hypsarrhythmic pattern. The seizures and mental defect seem to be related to the extent of hamartomatous change in the brain. For those with mental deficiency, 100% have seizures, 88% by 5 years of age; whereas of those without serious mental deficiency, 69% have seizures, 44% by 5 years of age. Mental deterioration is unusual, except in relation to frequent seizures of status epilepticus.

An unknown percentage of patients die before 20 years of age as the consequence of status epilepticus, general debility, pneumonia, or tumor. It should be appreciated that there is wide variability in expression of the disease—seizures, mental deficiency, or both do not develop in all patients with skin lesions, and the earlier noted pattern of abnormality is biased toward the more severe cases.

ETIOLOGY. This disorder has an autosomal dominant inheritance pattern. Approximately two thirds of cases represent fresh mutations. Mutations in TSC1, located at 9q34 and of TSC2 located at 16p13, encoding proteins referred to as hamartin and tuberin, respectively, are responsible. Although the pathways in which these two genes participate have not been elucidated, they most likely represent tumor suppressor genes. In general, when compared to patients with TSC2 mutations, those with mutations in TSC1 have a lower frequency of grade 2–4 kidney cysts or angiomyolipomas, forehead plaques, retinal hamartomas, and liver angiomyolipomas. In addition, sporadic cases with TSC1 mutations have milder disease manifest by lower frequency of seizures and moderate-to-severe mental retardation, fewer subependymal nodules and cortical tubers, less severe kidney involvement, no retinal hamartomas, and less severe facial angiofibromas. Affected individuals usually show some manifestations of the disorder by adulthood. A search for depigmented spots or hairs, enamel defects, and subungual hamartomas, as well as magnetic resonance imaging for periventricular lesions and renal ultrasound for angiomyolipomas should be considered in first-degree relatives of affected individuals before genetic counseling.

References

Bourneville D: Sclereuse tubereuse des circonvolutions cerebrales: Idiote et epilepsie hemiplegique. Arch Neurol (Paris) 1:81, 1880.

Lagos JC, Gomez MR: Tuberous sclerosis: Reappraisal of a clinical entity. Mayo Clin Proc 42:26, 1967.

Bundey S, Evans K: Tuberous sclerosis: A genetic study. J Neurol Neurosurg Psychiatry 32:591, 1969.

Hoff M et al: Enamel defects associated with tuberous sclerosis. Oral Surg 40:261, 1976.

Kenishi Y et al: Tuberous sclerosis: Early neurologic manifestations and CT features in 18 patients. Brain Dev 1:31, 1979.

Shepherd CW et al: Causes of death in patients with tuberous sclerosis. Mayo Clin Proc 66:792, 1991.

Roach ES et al: Diagnostic criteria: Tuberous sclerosis complex. Report of the diagnostic criteria committee of the National Tuberous Sclerosis Association. J Clin Neurol 7:221, 1992.

Janniger CK, Schwartz RA: Tuberous sclerosis: Recent advances for the clinician. Cutis 51:167, 1993.

Povey S et al: Two loci for tuberous sclerosis: One on 9q34 and one on 16p13. Ann Hum Genet 58:107, 1994.

Dabora SL et al: Mutational analysis in a cohort of 224 tuberous sclerosis patients indicates increased severity of TSC2, compared to TSC1 disease, in multiple organs. Am J Hum Genet 68:64, 2001.

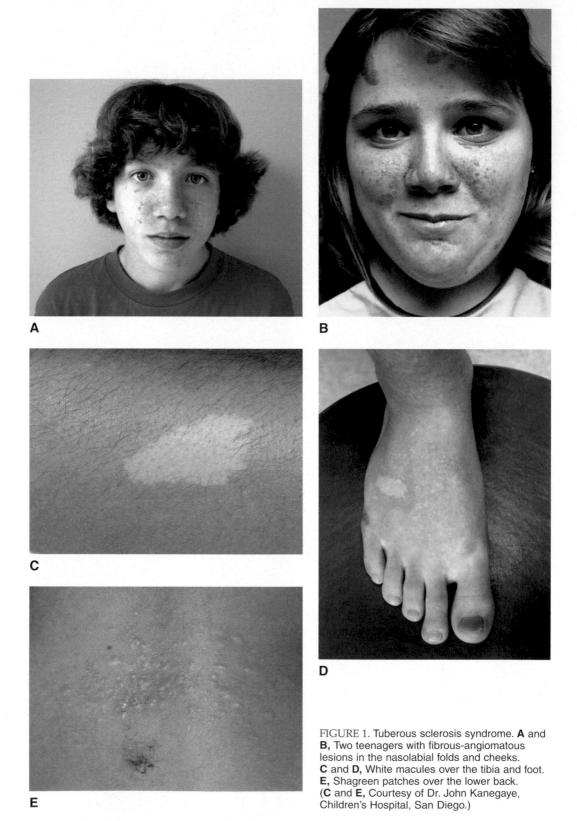

FIGURE 1. Tuberous sclerosis syndrome. **A** and
B, Two teenagers with fibrous-angiomatous
lesions in the nasolabial folds and cheeks.
C and **D,** White macules over the tibia and foot.
E, Shagreen patches over the lower back.
(**C** and **E,** Courtesy of Dr. John Kanegaye,
Children's Hospital, San Diego.)

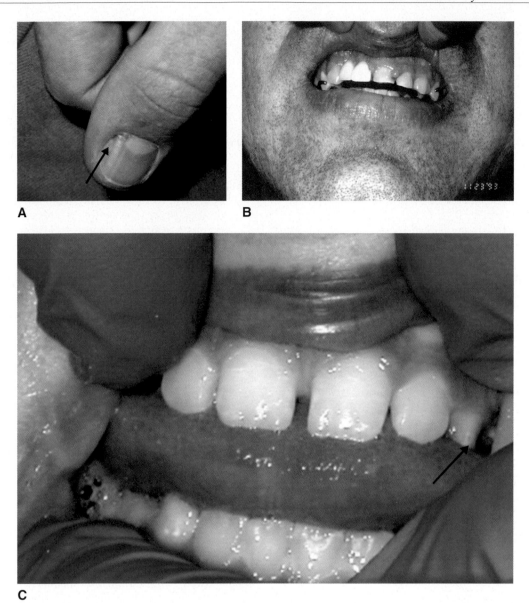

FIGURE 2. **A** and **B,** Gingival and subungal fibromata (*arrow* in **A** points to subungal fibroma). (**B,** Courtesy of Dr. Stephen Braddock, University of Missouri, Columbia.) **C,** Pit-shaped enamel defects. (**C,** Courtesy of Dr. John Kanegaye, Children's Hospital, San Diego.)

NEUROFIBROMATOSIS SYNDROME

Multiple Neurofibromata, Café au Lait Spots, with or without Bone Lesions

Von Recklinghausen described this disease in 1882. It is estimated to affect 1 in 3000 individuals.

ABNORMALITIES

Skin. Six or more café au lait macules over 5 mm in greatest diameter before puberty and over 15 mm following onset of puberty. Inguinal or axillary freckling (90% by 7 years). Ninety-nine percent have six or more macules greater than 5 mm in diameter by 1 year of age.

Tumors. Neurofibromas (a heterogeneous benign peripheral neural sheath tumor) occurring as discrete dermal masses, focal cutaneous or subcutaneous growths, dumbbell-shaped intraforaminal spinal tumors, or diffuse plexiform neurofibromas.

Other. Lisch nodules or pigmented iris hamartomata (70% by 10 years), macrocephaly of postnatal onset, mild short stature, unidentified bright objects of high signal density on T2-weighted magnetic resonance images of the brain (60%), mean IQ of 88.

OCCASIONAL ABNORMALITIES

Central Nervous System. Tumors, including optic pathway gliomas (1.5% to 7.5%, with median age of development 4.9 years) and other astrocytomas, neurilemomas, meningiomas, and neurofibromas. Seizures or electroencephalographic abnormalities in approximately 20%; mental deficiency in 2% to 5%, with learning disability, hyperactivity, or speech problems in 50%; cerebral vascular compromise; headaches; hydrocephalus.

Skeletal. Scoliosis; pectus excavatum; hypoplastic bowing of lower legs, with pseudoarthrosis at birth; osseous lesions with localized osteosclerosis, rib fusion, spina bifida, absence of patella, dislocation of radius and ulna, local overgrowth, and scalloping of vertebral bodies with deformed pedicles; sphenoid wing dysplasia.

Hamartomata. Cutaneous nevi, lipomata, angiomata, neurofibroma in kidney, stomach, heart, tongue, and bladder.

Other. Syndactyly, glaucoma, ptosis, corneal opacity, potentially malignant melanoma of iris, malignant peripheral nerve sheath tumors, precocious puberty, verrucous nevus, pheochromocytoma, pulmonic stenosis, vascular hyperplasia of the intima and media, pruritus. Hypertension.

NATURAL HISTORY. The majority of affected individuals have a benign course. Nearly all patients have enough features to allow diagnosis by 6 years. Neurofibromas rarely develop in children younger than 6 years of age, but are present in 48% of 10 year olds and 84% of 20 year olds. They may increase in size and number at puberty, during pregnancy, and between 50 and 70 years of age. The complications of neurofibromatosis can be divided into those that are structural (macrocephaly, segmental hypertrophy, scoliosis, pseudoarthrosis, cardiac defects), those that are functional (seizures, speech and learning disorders, hypertension, intellectual deficits), and those that relate to neoplasia. Screening for structural and functional complications can be done effectively through comprehensive physical evaluation every 6 months. Routine screening for CNS tumors is not warranted in the majority of cases. Rather, clinicians following affected individuals should maintain a high index of suspicion and evaluate specific signs and symptoms as they develop. Normal growth charts for affected children have been established. All newly diagnosed patients should have an ophthalmologic examination and then be followed yearly through 6 years of age to rule out an optic pathway glioma. Thereafter their occurrence is rare. Thirty-nine percent of children with an optic pathway glioma involving the optic chiasm develop precocious puberty. Malignant peripheral nerve sheath tumors, which arise almost exclusively in preexisting plexiform neurofibromas develop in approximately 2% to 5% of patients with NF1. The majority present in the second and third decade. The reproductive fitness of patients with NF1 is reduced by approximately one half. Survival is shortened, with mean age at death of 61.1 years.

ETIOLOGY.
This disorder has an autosomal dominant inheritance pattern with high penetrance but wide variability in expression. The neurofibromatosis type 1 (NF1) gene is located at chromosome 17q11.2. Approximately 50% of patients have a fresh gene mutation. The NF1 gene encodes a protein designated neurofibromin, which may function as a tumor suppressor.

COMMENT.
In addition to the classic form of neurofibromatosis, a second disorder exists, referred to as neurofibromatosis type 2 or acoustic neurofibromatosis. Also autosomal dominant, it is characterized by a later age of onset, the presence of bilateral acoustic neuromas, which generally develop over the second and third decades, as well as neurofibromas, meningiomas, gliomas, schwannomas, or juvenile posterior subcapsular cataracts. Usually only a few café au lait spots and cutaneous neurofibromas are present. NF2 is often more severe than NF1 in that multiple intracranial tumors can develop in childhood or early adulthood and schwannomas of the dorsal spinal roots occur. The NF2 gene is located at 22q11.2. Also, there exists a segmental form of neurofibromatosis characterized by café au lait spots, cutaneous neurofibromas, and intrathoracic or intra-abdominal neurofibromas limited to a circumscribed body segment. Unilateral Lisch nodules occur only when the involved

segment includes one of the eyes. Finally, based on molecular studies, it is now clear that the neurofibromatosis-Noonan syndrome, previously considered a separate entity, can in some cases represent a variant form of NF1.

References
Von Recklinghausen F: Ueber die multiplen Fibroma der Haut und ihre Beziehung zu den multiplen Neuromen. Berlin: Hirschwald, 1882.
Crowe FW, Schull WJ, Neel JV: Multiple Neurofibromatosis. American Lecture Series No. 281. Springfield, Ill: Charles C Thomas, 1952.
Miller RM, Sparkes RS: Segmental neurofibromatosis. Arch Dermatol 113:837, 1977.
Riccardi VM: Von Recklinghausen neurofibromatosis. N Engl J Med 305:1617, 1981.
Ragge NK: Clinical and genetic patterns of neurofibromatosis 1 and 2. Br J Ophthalmol 77:662, 1993.
Vickochil D et al: The neurofibromatosis type I gene. Annu Rev Neurosci 15:183, 1993.
The Consensus Developmental Panel: National Institutes of Health Consensus Developmental Conference Statement on Acoustic Neuroma, December 11–13, 1991. Arch Neurol 51:210, 1994.
Listernick R et al: Optic pathway gliomas in children with neurofibromatosis I: Consensus statement from the NF1 optic glioma task force. Ann Neurol 41:143, 1997.
DeBella K et al: Use of the National Institutes of Health criteria for diagnosis of neurofibromatosis 1 in children. Pediatrics 105:608, 2000.
Szudek J et al: Growth charts for young children with neurofibromatosis (NF1). Am J Med Genet 92:224, 2000.
Ferner RE, Gutman DH: International consensus statement on malignant peripheral nerve sheath tumors in neurofibromatosis 1. Cancer Res 62:1573, 2002.
Baralle D et al: Different mutations in the NF1 gene are associated with neurofibromatosis-Noonan syndrome (NFNS). Am J Med Genet 119:1, 2003.

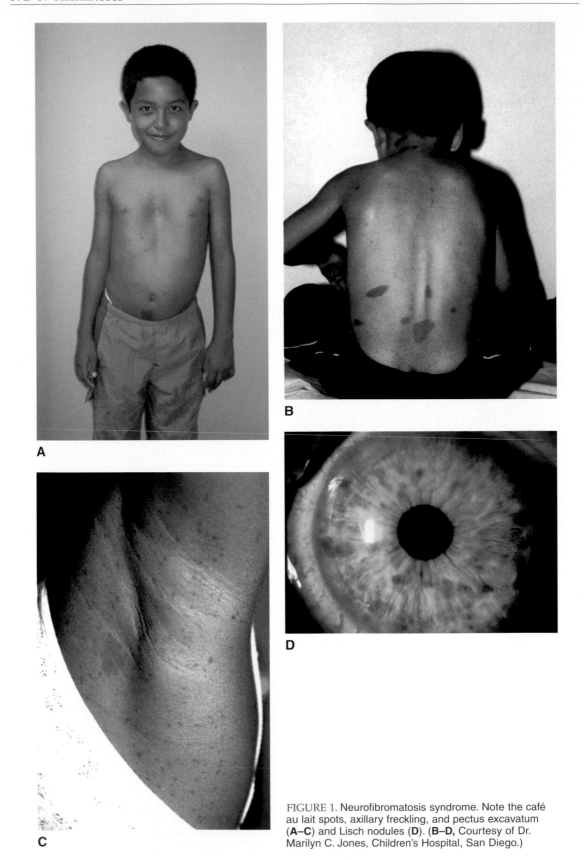

FIGURE 1. Neurofibromatosis syndrome. Note the café au lait spots, axillary freckling, and pectus excavatum (**A–C**) and Lisch nodules (**D**). (**B–D,** Courtesy of Dr. Marilyn C. Jones, Children's Hospital, San Diego.)

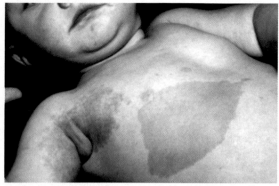

A

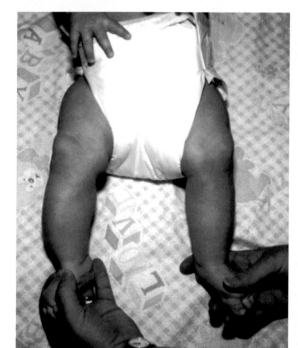

C

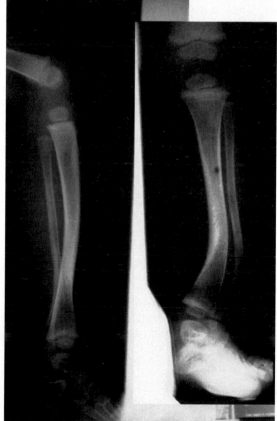

B

D

FIGURE 2. **A** and **B,** Plexiform neurofibromas on the upper trunk and orbit. **C** and **D,** Pseudoarthrosis of distal tibia. (**A–D,** Courtesy of Dr. Marilyn C. Jones, Children's Hospital, San Diego.)

McCUNE-ALBRIGHT SYNDROME

Polyostotic Fibrous Dysplasia, Irregular Skin Pigmentation, Sexual Precocity

McCune and Albright and colleagues described this condition in 1936 and 1937, respectively. More than 150 cases have been reported. The relative frequency of diagnosis in females versus males is 3:2.

ABNORMALITIES

Bone. Multiple areas of fibrous dysplasia, usually unilateral, most commonly in long bones and pelvis; may also include cranium, facial bones (causing facial asymmetry), ribs, and occasionally the spine; may result in deformity, increased thickness of bone, or both.

Skin. Irregular brown pigmentation, most commonly over sacrum, buttocks, upper spine; unilateral in approximately 50% of patients; the pattern of the pigmentary changes often follows the Blaschko lines.

Endocrine. Precocious puberty, hyperthyroidism, hyperparathyroidism, pituitary adenomas secreting growth hormone, acromegaly, Cushing syndrome, hyperprolactinemia; concentrations of tropic hormones are normal or reduced.

NATURAL HISTORY. The pigmentation is usually evident in infancy, and the bone dysplasia may progress during childhood, resulting in deformity, fracture, or both, most commonly in the upper femur. Malignant transformation into chondroblastic sarcoma occurs rarely. Thickening of bone in the calvarium can lead to cranial nerve compression with such serious consequences as blindness or deafness. The sexual precocity in the female is often unusual in character, with menstruation before development of breasts or pubic hair. The accelerated maturation coincident with sexual precocity may result in early attainment of full stature, so that adult height can be relatively short. Thyrotoxicosis occurs frequently, and postoperative thyroid storm has occurred on rare occasions. Although rare, when it occurs in infancy, the endocrine abnormalities can be life-threatening.

ETIOLOGY. A somatic activating mutation of the gene (GNAS1) encoding the α-subunit of the G protein is responsible for this disorder. G proteins are involved in signal transduction pathways that affect the production of cyclic adenosine monophosphate (cAMP). An overactive cyclic adenosine monophosphate pathway stimulates the growth and function of the gonads, adrenal cortex, specific pituitary-cell populations, osteoblasts, and melanocytes. This explains the observation that the endocrinologic abnormalities in McCune-Albright syndrome are the result of autonomous hyperfunction of the endocrine glands rather than being centrally mediated. The variable clinical expression is determined by the relative number of mutant cells as well as by the tissues and areas of the body involved.

References

McCune DJ: Osteitis fibrosa cystica. Am J Dis Child 52:745, 1936.

Albright F et al: Syndrome characterized by osteitis fibrosa disseminata, area of pigmentation and endocrine dysfunction, with precocious puberty in females: Report of five cases. N Engl J Med 216:727, 1937.

D'Armiento M et al: McCune-Albright syndrome: Evidence for autonomous multiendocrine hyper-function. J Pediatr 102:584, 1983.

Weinstein LS et al: Activating mutations of the stimulatory G protein in the McCune-Albright syndrome. N Engl J Med 325:1688, 1991.

Schwindinger WF et al: Identification of a mutation in the gene encoding the α subunit of the stimulatory G protein of adenyl cyclase in McCune-Albright syndrome. Proc Natl Acad Sci USA 89:5152, 1992.

Rieger E et al: Melanotic macules following Blaschko's lines in McCune-Albright syndrome. Br J Dermatol 130:215, 1994.

Ringle MD et al: Clinical implications of genetic defects in G proteins: The molecular basis of McCune-Albright syndrome and Albright hereditary osteodystrophy. Medicine 75:171, 1996.

Davies JH et al: Infantile McCune-Albright syndrome. Pediatr Dermatol 18:504, 2001.

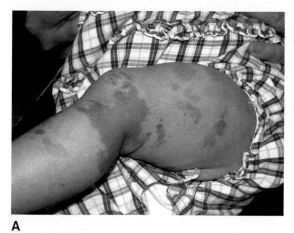

A

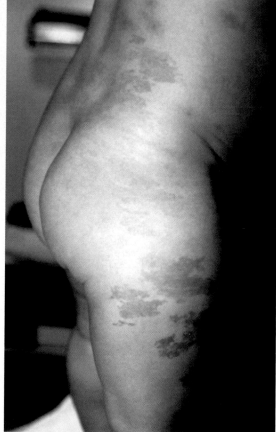

B

FIGURE 1. McCune-Albright syndrome. **A** and **B,** Irregular café au lait pigmentation over lower back and leg. (**A,** Courtesy of Dr. Lynne M. Bird, Children's Hospital, San Diego; **B,** courtesy of Dr. Marilyn C. Jones, Children's Hospital, San Diego.)

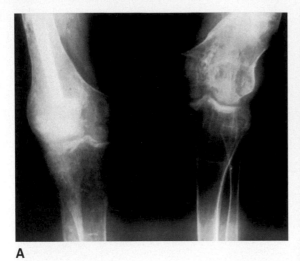

A

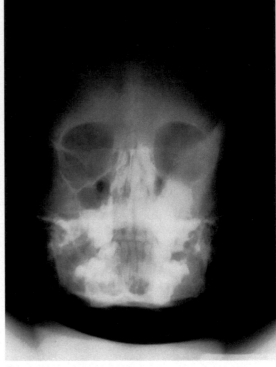

B

FIGURE 2. **A,** Multiple areas of fibrous dysplasia in long bones. (Courtesy of Dr. Michael Cohen, Dalhousie University, Halifax, Nova Scotia.) **B,** Left periocular fibrous dysplasia. *Continued*

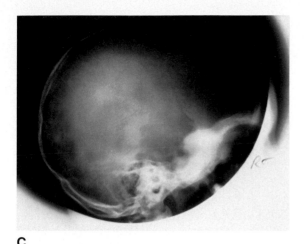

C

Fig. 2, cont'd. **C,** Dense thick bone at base of skull.

KLIPPEL-TRENAUNAY SYNDROME

Asymmetric Limb Hypertrophy, Vascular Malformation, Varicosities

This entity was originally reported by Klippel and Trenaunay in 1900. It has been confused with Park-Weber syndrome in which significant arteriovenous fistulas are a feature.

ABNORMALITIES

Limbs. Congenital or early childhood hypertrophy of usually one, but occasionally more than one, limb; the lower limb is involved in 95% of cases, the upper limb in 5%, and both are involved in 15%.

Skin. Vascular malformations of the capillary, venous, and lymphatic types occurring in any area, but more commonly on the legs, buttocks, abdomen, and lower trunk; unilateral distribution predominates, but bilateral involvement is not uncommon; varicosities of unusual distribution, particularly the lateral venous anomaly, which begins as a plexus of veins on the dorsum and lateral side of the foot and extends superiorly for various distances.

OCCASIONAL ABNORMALITIES

Limbs. Insignificant arteriovenous fistula, atrophy.

Skeletal. Macrodactyly, disproportionate growth of the digits whether large or small; syndactyly; polydactyly; oligodactyly; congenital hip dislocation.

Skin. Hyperpigmented nevi and streaks, neonatal and childhood ulcers and vesicles, cutis marmorata, telangiectasia.

Craniofacial. Asymmetric facial hypertrophy; microcephaly; macrocephaly caused by a large brain; intracranial calcifications; eye abnormalities such as glaucoma, cataracts, heterochromia, and a Marcus Gunn pupil.

Viscera. Visceromegaly; capillary malformation of the intestinal tract, urinary system, mesentery, and pleura; aberrant major blood vessel; lymphectasia.

Other. Enlargement of the genitalia, intravascular clotting problems, lipodystrophy, absence of inferior vena cava, hematochezia, hematuria, esophageal variceal bleeding, vaginal and vulvar bleeding.

NATURAL HISTORY. The usual patient with this syndrome does relatively well without any treatment or with elastic compression only. There may be disproportionate growth, which requires epiphyseal fusion or removal of the appropriate phalanx. Joint discomfort is not uncommon, and arthritic-type problems may develop. Leg swelling can be bothersome, and ulcers and other chronic skin difficulties may occur. Clinically significant arteriovenous shunting never occurs. Surgical intervention is almost never needed. However, in the rare situation in which the extremity reaches gigantic proportions or secondary clotting difficulties occur, amputation is necessary. Vascular malformations of the viscera, brain, eyes, urinary and gastrointestinal tracts, and other areas should always be looked for in this extremely variable disorder. Magnetic resonance imaging is the best noninvasive imaging technique to evaluate patients with vascular malformations.

ETIOLOGY. The cause of this disorder is unknown; it has a sporadic occurrence.

References

Klippel M, Trenaunay P: Du naevus variqueux osteohypertrophique. Arch Gen Med 185:641, 1900.

Kuffer FR et al: Klippel-Trenaunay syndrome, visceral angiomatosis, and thrombocytopenia. J Pediatr Surg 3:65, 1968.

Baskerville PA et al: The Klippel-Trenaunay syndrome: Clinical, radiological and haemodynamic features and management. Br J Surg 72:232, 1985.

Gloviczki P et al: Klippel-Trenaunay syndrome: The risks and benefits of vascular interventions. Surgery 110:469, 1991.

Cohen MM: Some neoplasms and some hamartomatous syndromes: Genetic considerations. Int J Oral Maxillofac Surg 27:363, 1998.

Cohen MM: Klippel-Trenaunay syndrome. Am J Med Genet 93:171, 2000.

Capraro PA et al: Klippel-Trenaunay syndrome. Plast Reconst Surg 109:2052, 2002.

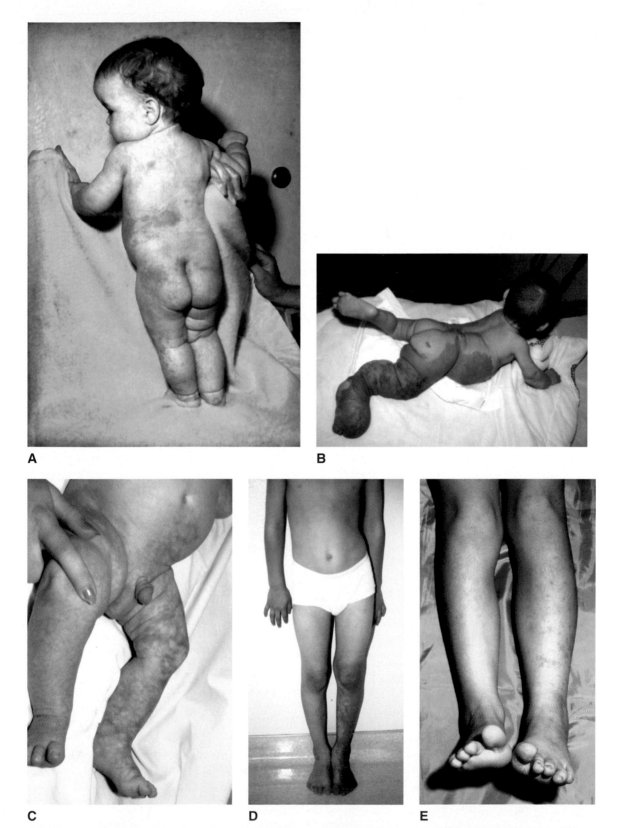

FIGURE 1. Klippel-Trenaunay. **A,** Mentally normal girl with macrocephaly and hemangiomata in left trunk and lower limb.
B, Child with severe involvement of right leg and trunk. (**B,** From Bird LM et al: Pediatrics 97:739, 1996. Reproduced with
permission from Pediatrics, vol. 97, pp. 739–741, copyright © 1996 by the AAP.) **C,** Less severely affected newborn boy.
D and **E,** A 14-year-old child showing asymmetric hypertrophy of legs with abnormal vasculature.

PROTEUS SYNDROME

Hemihypertrophy, Subcutaneous Tumors, Macrodactyly

Initially described in 1979 by Cohen and Hayden, this disorder was set forth as a clinical entity in 1983 by Wiedemann, who used the term "proteus" (after the Greek God Proteus, the polymorphous) to characterize the variable and changing phenotype of this condition. It has been suggested by Dr. Michael Cohen, Dalhousie University, Halifax, Nova Scotia, that John Merrick, the elephant man, most likely had the Proteus syndrome.

ABNORMALITIES

Growth. Asymmetric and disproportionate overgrowth of body parts, normal somatic growth during adolescence and normal final height attainment, tissue overgrowth plateaus after adolescence, macrocephaly.

Skin and Subcutaneous Tissue. Generalized thickening; epidermal nevi of the flat nonorganoid type; lipoma; regional absence of fat; vascular malformations of the venous, capillary, and lymphatic types with a predilection for the thorax and upper abdomen.

Skeletal. Hemihypertrophy, hyperostosis of skull, angulation defects of knees, scoliosis, kyphosis, hip dislocation, valgus deformities of halluces and feet, clinodactyly, dysplastic vertebrae, coarse ribs and scapula.

Hands and Feet. Macrodactyly; connective tissue nevi, most frequently on plantar surface of feet, but can be on hands.

OCCASIONAL ABNORMALITIES.

Elongation of neck and trunk; craniosynostosis; broad, depressed nasal bridge; gyriform hyperplasia over side of nose or in the other locations; ptosis; strabismus; epibulbar dermoid; enlarged eyes; microphthalmia; myopia; cataracts; nystagmus; submucous cleft palate; pectus excavatum; elbow ankylosis; mental deficiency; seizures; cyst-like alterations of lungs; muscle atrophy; abdominal and pelvic lipomatosis; café au lait spots; hyperostosis of external auditory canals, on alveolar ridges, and of nasal bridge; fibrocystic disease of breast; adenoma of parotid gland; ovarian cystadenoma; yolk sac tumor of testes; papillary adenoma of the epididymis; goiter; enlarged penis; macroorchidism; hypertrophic cardiomyopathy and cardiac conduction defects; renal abnormalities including enlarged kidneys with cysts, hemangiomas, and hydronephrosis; splenomegaly; enlarged thymus.

NATURAL HISTORY. The infants are frequently normal at birth, although birth weight is frequently increased and a few patients have had the characteristic features in the immediate newborn period. The characteristic features become obvious over the first year of life. Generally progressive throughout childhood, growth of the hamartomata and the generalized hypertrophy usually cease after puberty. Moderate mental deficiency in 20% of cases. Morbidity is significant. Spinal stenosis and neurologic sequelae may develop as a result of vertebral anomalies or tumor infiltration. Cystic emphysematous pulmonary disease, CNS tumors and abscesses, and pulmonary embolism related to vascular abnormalities are all associated with premature death. Affected individuals should be carefully monitored for the development of all types of neoplasms, because the full spectrum of this disorder is not known.

ETIOLOGY. The cause of this disorder is unknown. All cases have been sporadic events in otherwise normal families. This disorder is most likely caused by a somatic mutation of a gene that is lethal when occurring in the nonmosaic state.

COMMENT. A facial phenotype including dolichocephaly, long face, downslanting palpebral fissures, ptosis, anteverted nares, and an open mouth has been described in some children with Proteus syndrome who have mental retardation, seizures, and brain malformations.

References

Cohen MM, Hayden PW: A newly recognized hamartomatous syndrome. Birth Defects 15(5B):291, 1979.

Wiedemann HR et al: The proteus syndrome: Partial gigantism of the hands and/or feet, nevi, hemihypertrophy, subcutaneous tumors, macrocephaly or other skull anomalies and possible accelerated growth and visceral affections. Eur J Pediatr 140:5, 1983.

Burgio GR, Wiedemann HR: Further and new details on the proteus syndrome. Eur J Pediatr 143:71, 1984.

Clark RD et al: Proteus syndrome: An expanded phenotype. Am J Med Genet 27:99, 1987.

Cohen MM: Understanding proteus syndrome, unmasking the elephant man, and stemming elephant fever. Neurofibromatosis 1:260, 1988.

Cohen MM: Proteus syndrome: Clinical evidence for somatic mosaicism and selective review. Am J Med Genet 47:645, 1993.

Bieseckeer LG et al: Proteus syndrome: Diagnostic criteria, differential diagnosis and patient evaluation. Am J Med Genet 84:389, 1999.

Turner JT et al: Reassessment of the Proteus syndrome literature: Application of diagnostic criteria to published cases. Am J Med Genet 130:111, 2004.

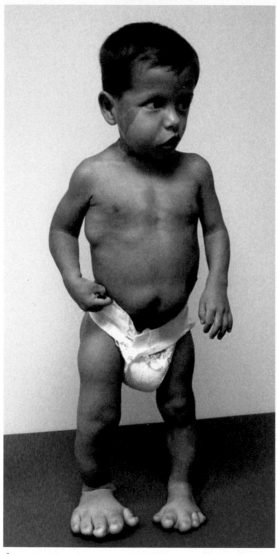

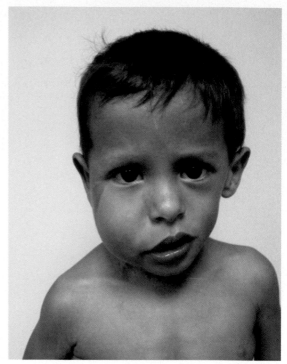

B   *Continued*

FIGURE 1. Proteus syndrome. A 2-year-old boy. Note
the large, soft tissue masses that have distorted the
abdomen and right leg (**A**); the asymmetry and
hyperpigmented areas over the face (**B**); the
hemangioma and lipoma over the abdomen (**C**); and
the splayed toes, macrodactyly, and thick, rugated
plantar surfaces of the feet (**D** and **E**).

A

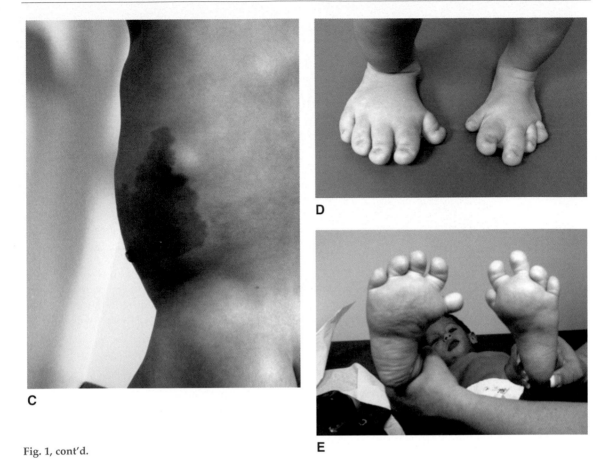

C

D

E

Fig. 1, cont'd.

ENCEPHALOCRANIOCUTANEOUS LIPOMATOSIS

Unilateral Craniofacial Lipomas, Ipsilateral Cerebral Atrophy, Focal Areas of Alopecia

This disorder was initially described by Haberland and Peron in 1970. Subsequently, more than 30 cases have been reported.

ABNORMALITIES

Performance. Marked developmental delay, mental retardation, seizures, spasticity.

Brain. Unilateral porencephalic cyst with cortical atrophy and calcification of the cerebral cortex overlying the cyst, ventricular dilatation, hemisphere atrophy, defective lamination of the cerebrum, micropolygyria, lipomas in the meninges covering the affected cerebral hemisphere.

Craniofacial. Unilateral hairless fatty tissue nevus of the scalp (nevus psiloliparus) with overlying alopecia, asymmetry of the skull and face, unilateral lipomatous involvement of the dermis of the skin covering the face on the same side as the brain defect, facial papules predominantly involving the periocular region, which histologically represent fibromas.

Eyes. Hard pedunculated outgrowths attached to margin of upper lid that are made up of connective tissue, unilateral epibulbar choristoma (lipodermoid).

OCCASIONAL ABNORMALITIES.

Microphthalmia, iris dysplasia including coloboma, cloudy cornea, areas of skin hypoplasia overlaying the craniofacial lipomas, café au lait spots, hydrocephalus, arachnoid cyst, spinal cord lipomatosis, skull defect overlaying the cerebral defect, lipomas of the heart, odontogenic tumor.

NATURAL HISTORY. Seizures develop during childhood in the majority of cases. Although motor delay is constant, the degree of mental retardation is variable and in some cases intellectual performance has been normal. Insufficient numbers of patients have been documented to provide adequate information regarding long-term follow-up. The localization of the CNS anomalies may be important relative to prognosis.

ETIOLOGY. Unknown. All affected patients have been sporadic. It is most likely that this disorder is the result of a somatic mutation that is lethal when occurring in the nonmosaic state.

References

Haberland C, Peron M: Encephalocranio-cutaneous lipomatosis. Arch Neurol 22:144, 1970.

Wiedemann HR, Burgio GR: Encephalocraniocutaneous lipomatosis and Proteus syndrome. Am J Med Genet 25:403, 1986.

Bamforth JSG et al: Encephalocraniocutaneous lipomatosis: Report of two cases and a review of the literature. Neurofibromatosis 2:166, 1989.

Kodsi SR et al: Ocular and systemic manifestations of encephalocraniocutaneous lipomatosis. Am J Ophthalmol 118:77, 1994.

Parazzini C et al: Encephalocraniocutaneous lipomatosis: Complete neuroradiologic evaluation and follow-up of two cases. Am J Neuroradiol 20:173, 1999.

Hauber K et al: Encephalocraniocutaneous lipomatosis: A case with unilateral odontomas and review of the literature. Eur J Pediatr 162:589, 2003.

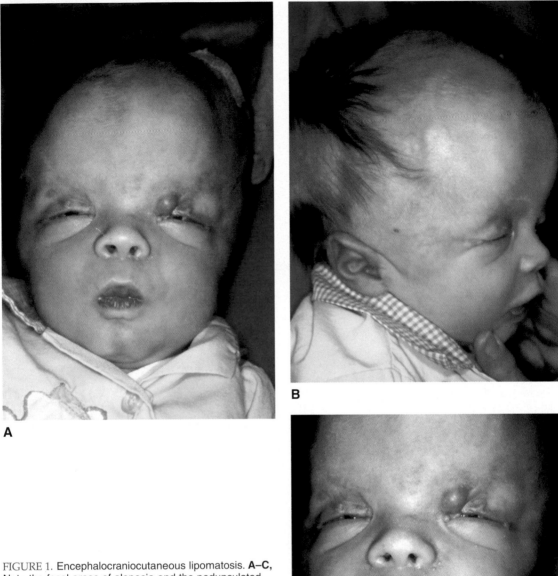

FIGURE 1. Encephalocraniocutaneous lipomatosis. **A–C,**
Note the focal areas of alopecia and the pedunculated
outgrowths attached to the margin of the eyelids.
(Courtesy of Dr. David Viskochil, University of Utah, Salt
Lake City.)

MAFFUCCI SYNDROME

Enchondromatosis, Vascular Malformations

Maffucci, in 1881, described a patient with dyschondroplasia and multiple cutaneous hemangiomata. More than 200 cases have been recorded subsequently.

ABNORMALITIES. Onset from the neonatal period to adolescence.

Skeletal. Variable early bowing of the long bones, with asymmetric retarded growth; enchondromata (40% unilateral) primarily in the hands, feet, and tubular long bones.

Vascular. Vascular malformations, most frequently located in the dermis and subcutaneous fat adjacent to the areas of enchondromatosis, but may occur anywhere; types of vascular malformations are capillary, venous, and especially phlebectasia, which often have a grape-like appearance; thrombosis of the dilated blood vessels with phlebolith formation occurs in 43% of cases.

OCCASIONAL ABNORMALITIES.

Lymphangiectasis; lymphangiomata; vascular malformations of the mucous membranes and gastrointestinal tract; other tumors, both malignant and benign and of mesodermal and nonmesodermal origin (approximately 15%), including intracranial tumors, goiter, parathyroid adenoma, pituitary adenoma, hemangioepithelioma, adrenal tumor, ovarian tumor, chondrosarcoma, breast cancer, and astrocytoma.

NATURAL HISTORY. The patients usually appear normal at birth, but within the first 4 years, vascular malformations appear, 25% during the first year. Subsequent enchondromata formation is noted by adolescence. The disorder can be mild, but it is often severe enough to require multiple surgical procedures and occasionally amputation. Approximately 26% have fractures related to enchondromata. The risk of chondrosarcomatous change is approximately 15%.

ETIOLOGY. The cause of this disorder is unknown. It has occurred sporadically in all cases.

References

Maffucci A: Di un caso di encondroma ed angioma multiplo: Contribuzione alla genesi embrionale dei tumor. Movimento Med Chir 3:399, 1881.

Bean WB: Dyschondroplasia and hemangiomata (Maffucci's syndrome) II. Arch Intern Med 102:544, 1958.

Lewis RJ, Ketcham AS: Maffucci's syndrome. J Bone Joint Surg [Am] 55:1465, 1973.

Sun Te-Ching et al: Chondrosarcoma in Maffucci's syndrome. J Bone Joint Surg [Am] 67-A:1214, 1985.

Kaplan RP et al: Maffucci's syndrome: Two case reports with a literature review. J Am Acad Dermatol 29:894, 1994.

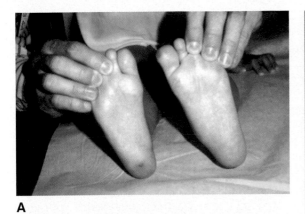

A

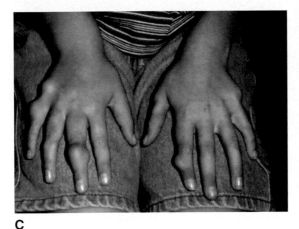

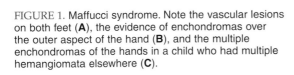

C

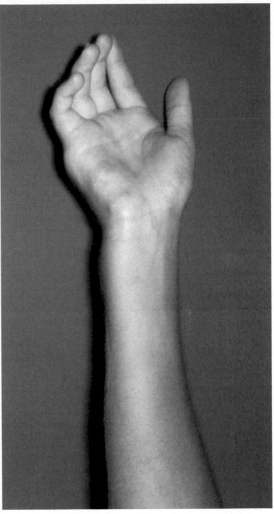

FIGURE 1. Maffucci syndrome. Note the vascular lesions on both feet (**A**), the evidence of enchondromas over the outer aspect of the hand (**B**), and the multiple enchondromas of the hands in a child who had multiple hemangiomata elsewhere (**C**).

B

PEUTZ-JEGHERS SYNDROME

Mucocutaneous Pigmentation, Intestinal Polyposis

In 1896, Hutchinson described the pigmentary changes in an individual who later died of intussusception. Peutz clearly set forth the disease in 1921, and Jeghers and colleagues further established this disease entity in 1949. Many cases have been documented.

ABNORMALITIES

Pigmentation. Vertical bands of epidermal pigment presenting as blue-gray or brownish spots on lips, buccal mucous membrane, perioral area, and sometimes digits and elsewhere.

Polyposis. Hamartomatous polyps in the stomach; small bowel (jejunum and duodenum more frequently than ileum) and colon; and occasionally in nasopharynx, bladder, biliary tract, and bronchial mucosa; polyps are usually multiple; adenomatous and malignant changes in the polyps as well as in any area of gastrointestinal tract lined by columnar epithelium have been documented.

Other Tumors. Approximately 35% of patients have extraintestinal malignancies including bronchogenic carcinomia, benign and malignant neoplasms of the thyroid, gallbladder, and biliary tract; breast cancer, usually ductal; pancreatic cancer; malignant tumors of the reproductive tract including malignant adenoma of the cervix, unique ovarian sex cord tumors leading to isosexual precocity, testicular sex cord and Sertoli cell tumors leading to sexual precocity and gynecomastia.

NATURAL HISTORY. The pigmentary spots appear from infancy through early childhood and tend to fade in the adult. Seventy percent of patients have some gastrointestinal problem by age 20 years, most commonly colicky abdominal pain (60%), intestinal bleeding (25%), or both. Intussusception, which may spontaneously recede, is the most serious complication. Iron deficiency anemia may result from chronic blood loss, and protein-losing enteropathy has been reported. An intestinal or extraintestinal cancer develops in approximately 50% of affected patients. Almost one half of the patients with malignancy are younger than 30 years of age. Clubbing of the fingers may occasionally occur in this disease. Screening of affected patients as well as potentially affected family members should include colonoscopy, an upper gastrointestinal series with small bowel follow-through, pelvic ultrasonography in females, and careful examination of testicles in males.

ETIOLOGY. This disorder has an autosomal dominant inheritance pattern. Mutations in the serine/threonine kinase gene (LKB1/STK11) on chromosome 19p13.3, which functions as a tumor suppressor gene, are responsible. Identification of LBK1/STK11 mutations in only 50% of clinically identified cases suggests that this condition is genetically heterogeneous.

References

Hutchinson J: Pigmentation of the lips and mouth. Arch Surg 7:290, 1896.

Peutz JLA: Very remarkable case of familial polyposis of mucous membrane of intestinal tract and nasopharynx accompanied by peculiar pigmentation of skin and mucous membrane. Ned Maanschr Geneesk 10:134, 1921.

Jeghers H, McKusick VA, Katz KH: Generalized intestinal polyposis and melanin spots of the oral mucosa, lips, and digits: A syndrome of diagnostic significance. N Engl J Med 241:993, 1949.

Bartholomew LG et al: Intestinal polyposis associated with mucocutaneous pigmentation. Surg Gynecol Obstet 115:1, 1962.

Tovar JA et al: Peutz-Jeghers syndrome in children: Report of two cases and review of the literature. J Pediatr Surg 18:1, 1983.

Buck JL: From the archives of AFIP: Peutz-Jeghers syndrome. Radiographics 12:365, 1992.

Rustgi AK: Hereditary gastrointestinal polyposis and nonpolyposis syndromes. N Engl J Med 331:1694, 1994.

Thomlinson IPM, Houlston RS: Peutz-Jeghers syndrome. J Med Genet 34:1007, 1997.

Hemminki A et al: A serine/threonine kinase gene defective in Peutz-Jeghers syndrome. Nature 391:184, 1998.

Dunlop MG: Guidance on gastrointestinal surveillance for hereditary non-polyposis colorectal cancer, familial adenomatous polyposis, juvenile polyposis, and Peutz-Jeghers syndrome. Gut 51(Suppl V):v21, 2002.

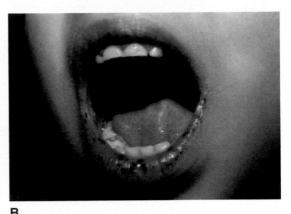

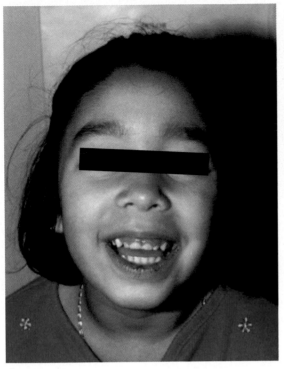

FIGURE 1. Peutz-Jeghers syndrome. **A** and **B,** Spotty pigmentation of lips and buccal mucous membrane in a 4-year-old girl. (Courtesy of Dr. Marilyn C. Jones, Children's Hospital, San Diego.)

A

B

BANNAYAN-RILEY-RUVALCABA SYNDROME

(RUVALCABA-MYHRE SYNDROME, RILEY-SMITH SYNDROME, BANNAYAN SYNDROME)

Macrocephaly, Polyposis of Colon, Pigmentary Changes of the Penis

In 1986, Saul and Stevenson proposed that Bannayan syndrome and Ruvalcaba-Myhre syndrome were the same disorder. Subsequently, Dvir and colleagues added Riley-Smith syndrome and suggested that all three of these conditions represent one etiologic entity, which Cohen referred to as Bannayan-Riley-Ruvalcaba syndrome.

ABNORMALITIES

Growth. Birth weight greater than 4 kg and birth length greater than 97th percentile, normal adult stature.

Performance. Hypotonia, gross motor and speech delay (50%), mild to severe mental deficiency (15% to 20%), seizures (25%).

Craniofacies. Macrocephaly, with ventricles of normal size; downslanting palpebral fissures (60%); high-arched palate; strabismus or amblyopia (15%); prominent Schwalbe lines and prominent corneal nerves (35%).

Intestines. Ileal and colonic hamartomatous polyps (45%).

Neoplasms. Hamartomas that are lipomas in 75%, hemangiomas in 10%, and mixed type in 20%. Most are subcutaneous, although they can be cranial (20%) or osseous (10%).

Penis. Tan, nonelevated spots on glans penis, and shaft, not always present at birth.

Other. Myopathic process in proximal muscles (60%). Cutaneous angiolipomas, encapsulated or diffusely infiltrating, in 50%. Joint hyperextensibility, pectus excavatum, and scoliosis in 50%.

OCCASIONAL ABNORMALITIES.

Frontal bossing, pseudopapilledema, diabetes, Hashimoto thyroiditis, acanthosis nigricans, lymphangiomyomas, angiokeratomas, verruca vulgaris–type facial skin changes, café au lait spots, tongue polyps, supernumerary nipples, enlarged testes, enlarged penis, broad thumbs/great toes, hypoglycemia, autistic behavior.

NATURAL HISTORY. Although overgrowth is usually present in the newborn period, final adult height is within the normal range. The ileal and colonic polyps often present in childhood with intussusception, rectal prolapse, and rectal bleeding; sometimes they do not become evident until middle age. Lipomas can be extremely large. Speckling of the penis more likely becomes evident in later childhood. Delays in performance frequently improve with age.

ETIOLOGY. This disorder has an autosomal dominant inheritance pattern. Mutations in the tumor suppressor PTEN (phosphatase and tensin homologue deleted from chromosome 10) gene located at 10q23.3 are responsible and have been found in approximately 60% of cases.

COMMENT. Cowden syndrome, characterized by trichilemmomas (small benign hair follicle tumors), oral papillomas, intestinal polyps, and an increased frequency of breast and thyroid cancer is also caused by mutations in PTEN. Therefore, this disorder and mutation positive Bannayan-Riley-Ruvalcaba syndrome (BRRS) are most likely different phenotypic presentations of the same syndrome. For this reason, individuals with PTEN-positive Bannayan-Riley-Ruvalcaba syndrome should be monitored for malignant tumors using a similar protocol as is used for Cowden syndrome. This should include periodic screening for breast, thyroid, renal, and endometrial cancers.

References

Riley HD, Smith WR: Macrocephaly, pseudopapilledema, and multiple hemangiomata. Pediatrics 26:293, 1960.

Bannayan GA: Lipomatosis, angiomatosis and macrocephaly: A previously undescribed congenital syndrome. Arch Pathol 92:1, 1971.

Ruvalcaba RHA, Myhre S, Smith DW: A syndrome with macrencephaly, intestinal polyposis and pigmentary penile lesions. Clin Genet 18:413, 1980.

Gorlin RJ et al: Bannayan-Riley-Ruvalcaba syndrome. Am J Med Genet 44:307, 1992.

Marsh DJ et al: PTEN mutation spectrum and genotype-phenotype correlations in Bannayan-Riley-Ruvalcaba syndrome suggest a single entity with Cowden syndrome. Hum Mol Genet 8:1461, 1999.

Parisi MA et al: The spectrum and evolution of phenotypic findings in PTEN mutation positive cases of Bannayan-Riley-Ruvalcaba syndrome. J Med Genet 38:52, 2001.

Hendriks YMC et al: Bannayan-Riley-Ruvalcaba syndrome: Further delineation and management of PTEN mutation-positive cases. Familial Cancer 2:79: 2003.

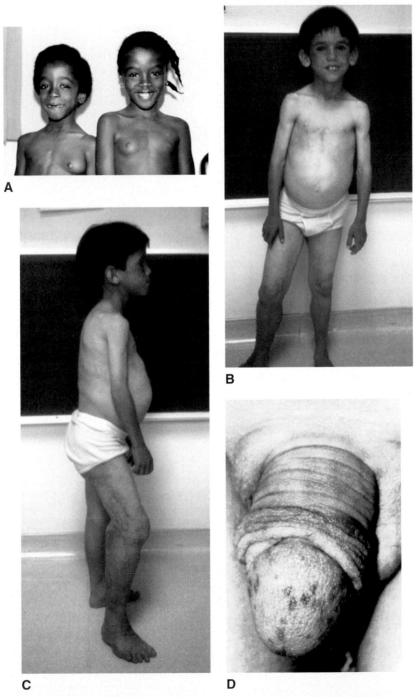

FIGURE 1. Bannayan-Riley-Ruvalcaba syndrome. **A,** Brother and sister with macrocephaly and lipomata. The boy is mentally retarded. (From Higginbottom MC et al: Pediatrics 69:632, 1982, with permission.) **B** and **C,** A boy with multiple subcutaneous hamartomas. The child had recurrent rectal prolapse. **D,** Pigmented spots on the penis. (**D,** Courtesy of Dr. Michael Cohen, Dalhousie University, Halifax, Nova Scotia.)

HEREDITARY HEMORRHAGIC TELANGIECTASIA
(Osler Hemorrhagic Telangiectasia)

Epistaxis, Multiple Telangiectases

This entity was set forth in 1901 by Osler. The telangiectases contain dilated vessels having only an endothelial wall with no elastic tissue and a tendency toward arteriovenous fistulae. Many affected families have been reported, and the incidence is approximately 1 in 50,000.

ABNORMALITIES

Vessels. Pinpoint, spider, or nodular telangiectases most commonly on tongue, mucosa of lips, face, conjunctiva, ears, fingertips, nail beds, and nasal mucous membrane; occasionally in gastrointestinal tract, bladder, vagina, uterus, lungs, liver, or brain; cutaneous telangiectases usually not evident until second or third decade.

OCCASIONAL ABNORMALITIES.
Arteriovenous fistulae in lungs (15%) and liver, mucosal and submucosal arteriovenous malformations of the gastrointestinal tract, arterial aneurysms, venous varicosities, and arteriovenous fistulas of celiac and mesenteric vessels, cirrhosis of liver, cavernous angiomata, port-wine stain, vascular anomalies in brain and spinal cord, duodenal ulcer.

NATURAL HISTORY.
Epistaxis, which often occurs in childhood, is the most common form of bleeding followed by gastrointestinal, genitourinary, pulmonary, and intracerebral. Intraocular hemorrhage is rare. Ten percent of patients never bleed, while approximately one third require hospitalization for bleeding. Neurologic complications occur at any age, with a peak incidence in the third decade, and result from pulmonary arteriovenous fistula (60%), vascular malformation of the brain (28%), and spinal cord (8%) and portosystemic encephalopathy (3%). Of major concern is the potential for brain abscess, cerebral embolism, and hypoxemia secondary to the pulmonary arteriovenous fistulas. Hepatic arteriovenous fistula can cause hepatomegaly, right upper quadrant pain, pulsatile mass, a thrill, or bruit. Left to right shunting through the fistula can lead to high-output congestive heart failure. Bleeding is generally aggravated by pregnancy. Fewer than 10% of patients die of associated complications. Oral iron supplementation is almost always necessary. Oral estrogen and septal dermoplasty have been used to successfully manage the epistaxis in some cases. Examinations for pulmonary arteriovenous fistulas and for retinal telangiectases should be performed periodically.

ETIOLOGY.
This disorder has an autosomal dominant inheritance pattern. Mutations in at least two genes have been identified; endoglin (ENG), a transforming growth factor β (TGF-β) binding protein located on chromosome 9q33-q34, and activin receptor-like kinase 1 gene (ACVRLK1 or ALK1), a member of the serine-threonine kinase receptor family expressed in endothelium and located in the pericentromeric region of chromosome 12. A higher frequency of pulmonary arteriovenous malformations has been associated with ENG mutations. At least one other, at present unidentified, locus must exist.

References

Osler W: On a family form of recurring epistaxis, associated with multiple telangiectases of skin and mucous membrane. Bull Hopkins Hosp 12:333, 1901.

Bird RM et al: Family reunion study of hereditary hemorrhagic telangiectasia. N Engl J Med 257:105, 1957.

Schaumann B, Alter M: Cerebrovascular malformations in hereditary hemorrhagic telangiectasia. Minn Med 56:951, 1973.

Peery WH: Clinical spectrum of hereditary hemorrhagic telangiectasia (Osler-Weber-Rendu disease). Am J Med 82:989, 1987.

McAllister KA et al: Endoglin, a TGF-β binding protein of endothelial cells is the gene for hereditary haemorragic telangiectasia type 1. Nat Genet 8:345, 1994.

Guttmacher AE et al: Hereditary hemorrhagic telangiectasia. N Engl J Med 333:918, 1995.

Johnson DW et al: Mutations in the activin receptor-like kinase 1 gene in hereditary haemorrhagic telangiectasia type 2. Nat Genet 13:189, 1996.

Abdalla SA et al: Visceral manifestations in hereditary haemorrhagic telangiectasia type 2. J Med Genet 40:494, 2002.

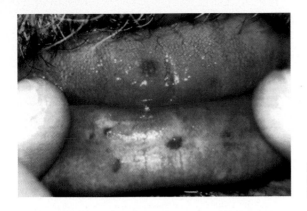

FIGURE 1. Osler hemorrhagic telangiectasia syndrome. Small telangiectases on mucosa of the lips. (Courtesy of Eric Rosenthal, University of California, San Diego.)

MULTIPLE ENDOCRINE NEOPLASIA, TYPE 2B
(MULTIPLE NEUROMA SYNDROME)

Multiple Neuromata of Tongue, Lips with or without Medullary Thyroid Carcinoma, with or without Pheochromocytoma

This disorder represents one of the three different forms of multiple endocrine neoplasia type 2 (MEN2). The other two forms, MEN2A and medullary thyroid cancer (MTC)–only are associated with normal physical appearance. MEN2A is characterized by medullary thyroid carcinoma, parathyroid hyperplasia, and pheochromocytoma, while the medullary thyroid cancer–only syndrome or FMTC represents familial medullary thyroid carcinoma without other components of MEN2A. MEN2B is the only one of these three disorders associated with a pattern of malformation.

ABNORMALITIES

Mucosa. Ganglioneuromatosis extending from lips to rectum and manifest by prominent lips, nodular tongue, involvement of nasal, laryngeal, and intestinal mucous membranes; thickened, anteverted eyelids caused by neuromatous involvement of the mucosal surface.

Other Tumors. Medullary thyroid carcinoma, pheochromocytoma.

Skeletal. Marfanoid habitus, pes cavus, slipped femoral capital epiphyses, pectus excavatum, kyphosis, lordosis, scoliosis, increased joint laxity, weakness of proximal extremity muscles.

Other. Tendency toward coarse-appearing facies.

OCCASIONAL ABNORMALITIES.
Slit-lamp examination may reveal medullated nerve fibers in the cornea; subconjunctival neuromas, cutaneous neuromata, or neurofibromata; parathyroid hyperplasia; hypotonia; developmental delay; deficient lacrimation.

NATURAL HISTORY.
Oral neuromata are usually evident in childhood, with medullary thyroid carcinoma or pheochromocytoma becoming serious risks after adolescence. When medullary thyroid carcinoma is implicated, a total thyroidec-tomy should usually be done because the lesion is often multicentric. When pheochromocytoma is implicated, a thorough exploration should be accomplished, since it is often bilateral and may also be extra-adrenal. Constipation with megacolon often severe enough to suggest Hirschsprung disease or diarrhea frequently develop before the endocrine neoplasms are detected. This is usually the result of gastrointestinal ganglioneuromatosis resulting in thickening of the myenteric plexi and hypertrophy of ganglion cells. An annual screening evaluation of all at-risk family members should be performed to identify and treat presymptomatic individuals.

ETIOLOGY. This disorder has an autosomal dominant inheritance pattern. The gene has been mapped to the long arm of chromosome 10 in band q11.2. Mutations in the RET proto-oncogene account for the clinical phenotype.

COMMENT. An abnormal response to histamine skin test possibly related to diffuse enlargement of cutaneous nerves has been reported in patients with this disorder.

References

Gorlin RJ et al: Multiple mucosal neuromas, pheochromocytoma and medullary carcinoma of the thyroid—a syndrome. Cancer 22:293, 1968.

Schimke RN et al: Syndrome of bilateral pheochromocytoma, medullary thyroid carcinoma and multiple neuromas. N Engl J Med 279:1, 1968.

Carney JA et al: Alimentary tract ganglioneuromatosis: A major component of the syndrome of multiple endocrine neoplasia, type 2b. N Engl J Med 295:1287, 1976.

Carney JA et al: Abnormal cutaneous innervation in multiple endocrine neoplasia, type 2b. Ann Intern Med 94:362, 1981.

Hofstra RMW et al: A mutation in the RET protooncogene associated with multiple endocrine neoplasia type 2b and sporadic medullary thyroid carcinoma. Nature 367:375, 1994.

Cohen MS et al: Gastrointestinal manifestations of multiple endocrine neoplasia type 2. Ann Surg 235:648, 2002.

Torre M et al: Diagnostic and therapeutic approach to multiple endocrine neoplasia type 2b in pediatric patients. Pediatr Surg Int 18:378, 2002.

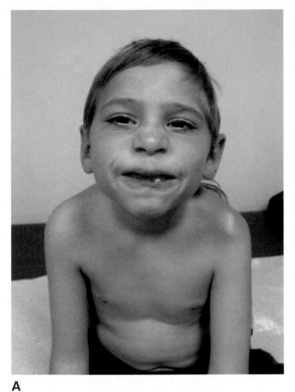

A

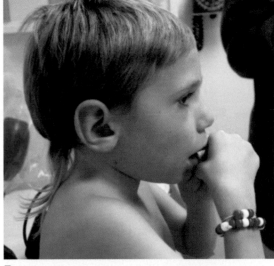

B

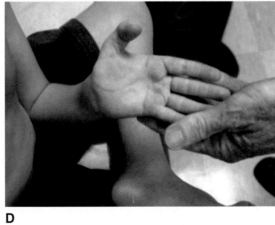

D

C

FIGURE 1. Multiple endocrine neoplasia type 2b. **A–D,** Note the multiple neuromata involving the conjunctiva and contributing to the prominent lips.

GORLIN SYNDROME
(NEVOID BASAL CELL CARCINOMA SYNDROME)

Basal Cell Carcinomas, Broad Facies, Rib Anomalies

Although this condition had been described, it was Gorlin and Goltz who recognized the full extent of this pattern of malformation in 1960. Its prevalence is approximately 1 per 60,000.

ABNORMALITIES

Craniofacial. Macrocephaly (80%); frontoparietal bossing (66%); broad nasal bridge (59%); well-developed supraorbital ridges; heavy, often fused eyebrows; mild hypertelorism; prognathism (33%); hyperpneumatization of paranasal sinuses; bony bridging of sella turcica (60% to 80%).

Dentition. Odontogenic keratocysts of jaws (75%), misshapen or carious teeth.

Hands. Short metacarpals, especially the fourth (29%).

Thorax. Bifid, synostotic, or partially missing ribs (60%); scoliosis; sloping, narrow shoulders (41%); thoracic or cervical vertebral anomalies (40%).

Skin. Nevoid basal cell carcinomas over neck, upper arms, trunk, and face; epidermal cysts; punctate dyskeratotic pits on palms (65%), soles (68%), or both (58%); milia, especially facial (52%).

Ectopic Calcification. Falx cerebri (85%), falx cerebelli (40%), petroclinoid ligament (20%), dura, pia, and choroid plexus.

Ovaries. Development of calcified ovarian fibromata (14%).

OCCASIONAL ABNORMALITIES.

Mental deficiency, agenesis of corpus callosum, vermian dysgenesis, anosmia, hydrocephalus, hypertelorism, telecanthus, inner canthal folds, highly arched eyebrows, cataract, coloboma of iris, prominent medullated retinal nerve fibers, retinal atrophy, glaucoma, chalazion, strabismus, cleft lip with or without cleft palate, mandibular coronoid process hyperplasia, low-pitched female voice, pectus excavatum/carinatum, Sprengel deformity, "marfanoid" build, arachnodactyly, pre- or postaxial polydactyly, immobile thumbs, pseudocystic lytic lesions of bones, lumbarization of sacrum, hypogonadism in males, subcutaneous calcifications of skin, renal anomalies, other neoplasms including medulloblastoma, meningioma, fibromata, lipomata, melanoma, neurofibromata of skin, cardiac fibromas, eyelid carcinomas, breast cancer, lung cancer, chronic lymphoid leukemia, non-Hodgkin lymphoma, ovarian dermoid, lymphomesenteric cysts that tend to calcify, hepatic mesenchymal tumor.

NATURAL HISTORY. Although nevoid basal cell carcinomas have occurred in 2-year-old children, they usually appear between puberty and 35 years of age with a mean age of about 20 years. Before puberty, the lesions are harmless. Thereafter, concern should be raised when the lesions begin to grow, ulcerate, bleed, or crust. The jaw cysts enlarge, especially in later childhood, and may recur following curettage. Mean age of onset is about 15 years. A constant vigil must be maintained to detect other tumors that are a common feature of this syndrome. In particular, medulloblastoma should be excluded with magnetic resonance imaging up to 8 years of age. Treatment with x-irradiation results in large numbers of invasive basal cell carcinomas appearing in the radiation field and should therefore be avoided. Palmar pitting can be made more obvious by immersion of the hands in water for 15 minutes.

ETIOLOGY. This disorder has an autosomal dominant inheritance pattern. Mutations in PCTH, a tumor suppressor gene that maps to 9q22.3-q31, are responsible. PCTH is a human homologue of the Drosophila segment polarity gene, *patch*. The PTCH protein is a receptor for Sonic hedgehog (Shh), a secreted molecule that is important in formation of embryonic structures and tumorigenesis.

References
Binkley GW, Johnson HH Jr: Epithelioma adenoides cysticum: Basal cell nevi, agenesis of the corpus callosum and dental cysts: A clinical and autopsy study. Arch Dermatol 63:73, 1951.

Gorlin RJ, Goltz RW: Multiple nevoid basal-cell epithelioma, jaw cysts, and bifid ribs: A syndrome. N Engl J Med 262:908, 1960.

Gorlin RJ et al: The multiple basal-cell nevi syndrome. Cancer 18:89, 1965.

Evans DGR et al: Complications of the naevoid basal cell carcinoma syndrome: Results of a population based study. J Med Genet 30:460, 1993.

Shanley S et al: Nevoid basal cell carcinoma syndrome: Review of 118 affected individuals. Am J Med Genet 50:282, 1994.

Gorlin RJ: Nevoid basal cell carcinoma syndrome. Dermatol Clin 13:113, 1995.

Hahn H et al: Mutations of the human homologue of Drosophila *patched* in the nevoid basal cell carcinoma syndrome. Cell 85:841, 1996.

Cohen MM: Nevoid basal cell carcinoma syndrome: molecular biology and new hypothesis. Int J Oral Maxillofac Surg 28:216, 1999.

Gorlin RJ: Nevoid basal cell carcinoma (Gorlin) syndrome: Unanswered issues. J Lab Clin Med 134:551, 1999.

GOLTZ SYNDROME

Poikiloderma with Focal Dermal Hypoplasia, Syndactyly, Dental Anomalies

This mesoectodermal disorder was recognized as a distinct entity by Goltz and colleagues in 1962, although well-described cases had been reported prior to that time. More than 175 cases have been documented.

ABNORMALITIES

Skin. Pink or red, atrophic macules that may be slightly raised or depressed and have a linear and asymmetric distribution; mainly on thighs, forearm, and cheeks; telangiectasis; lipomatous nodules projecting through localized areas of skin atrophy; angiofibromatous nodules around lips, in vulval and perianal areas, around the eyes, the ears (on pinnae and in middle ear), the fingers and toes, the groin and umbilicus, inside the mouth, and in esophagus; skin scarring.

Nails. Dystrophic nails, narrow or hypoplastic.

Hair. Sparse and brittle, localized areas of alopecia in head and pubic region.

Dentition. Hypoplasia of teeth, anodontia, enamel hypoplasia, late eruption, irregular placement, malocclusion, or notched incisors.

Skeletal. Asymmetric involvement of hands and feet in 60% including syndactyly, absence or hypoplasia of digits, ectrodactyly, polydactyly, and absence of an extremity; scoliosis (20%); longitudinal striations in the metaphyses of long bones; spina bifida occulta; clavicular dysplasia; failure of pubic bone fusion; skeletal asymmetry.

Face. Asymmetry with mild hemihypertrophy; narrow nasal bridge and broad tip sometimes with unilateral notch of ala nasi; thin, protruding, simple low-set ears; pointed chin.

Eyes. Strabismus, coloboma of the iris and aniridia, microphthalmos, anophthalmos, chorioretinal coloboma, involvement is frequently unilateral.

OCCASIONAL ABNORMALITIES.

Moderate short stature; microcephaly; aplasia cutis congenita; joint hypermotility; split sternum; vertebral anomalies; scoliosis; mental retardation (15%); hearing impairment; bulbar angiofibroma of eye; optic atrophy; ocular hypertelorism; alveolar irregularity; CNS malformation; congenital heart defects; expansile, tumor-like bone lesions; horseshoe kidney; cystic dysplasia of kidney; umbilical, inguinal, diaphragmatic, hiatus, or epigastric herniae; omphalocele; intestinal malrotation.

NATURAL HISTORY.

The skin lesions are usually present at birth, although the skin lipomata and the lip and anal papillomata may develop later. No effective therapy is known except plastic surgery for the syndactyly and removal of the papillomata when indicated. However, the latter may recur. Despite serious structural anomalies of the eyes, acuity may be surprisingly good.

ETIOLOGY.

The vast majority of cases have been sporadic and female. X-linked dominant inheritance with lethality in hemizygous males is the most likely mode of inheritance. Most cases represent fresh mutations.

References

Jessner M: Falldemonstration Breslauer dermatologische Vereinigung. Arch Dermatol Syph (Berlin) 133:48, 1921.

Wodniansky P: Über die Formen der congenitalen Poikilodermie. Arch Klin Exp Dermatol 205:331, 1957.

Goltz RW et al: Focal dermal hypoplasia. Arch Dermatol 86:708, 1962.

Gorlin RJ et al: Focal dermal hypoplasia syndrome. Acta Dermatovener (Stockholm) 43:421, 1963.

Holden JD, Akers WA: Goltz's syndrome: Focal dermal hypoplasia: A combined mesoectodermal dysplasia. Am J Dis Child 114:292, 1967.

Temple IK et al: Focal dermal hypoplasia (Goltz syndrome). J Med Genet 27:180, 1990.

Hancock S et al: Probable identity of Goltz syndrome and Van Allen-Myre syndrome: Evidence from phenotypic evolution. Am J Med Genet 110:370, 2002.

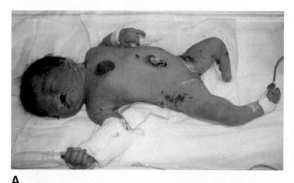

A

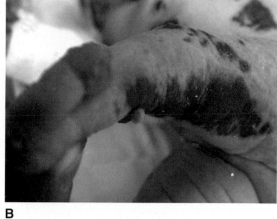

B

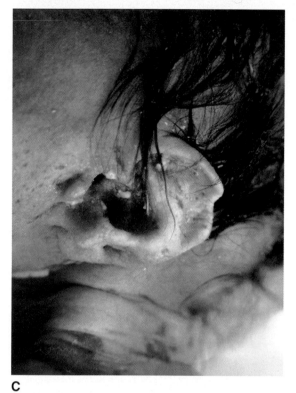

C

FIGURE 1. Goltz syndrome. A newborn girl. Red atrophic macules are depressed in **A** and raised in **B. C,** Note the angiofibromatous nodules around the ears. (From Loguercio Leite JC et al: Clin Dysmorphol 14:37, 2005, with permission.)

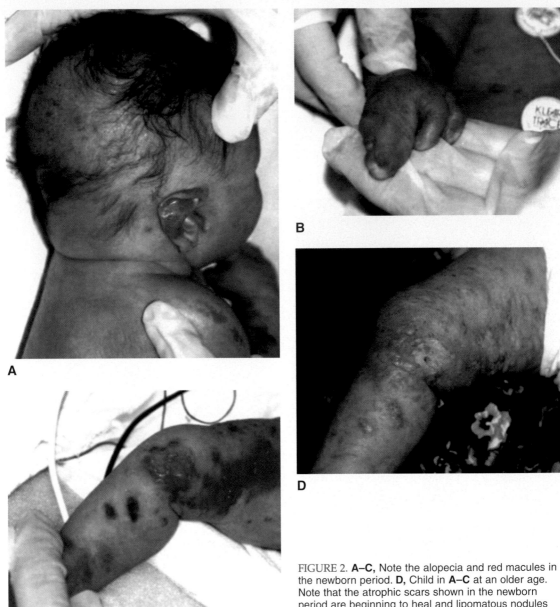

FIGURE 2. **A–C,** Note the alopecia and red macules in the newborn period. **D,** Child in **A–C** at an older age. Note that the atrophic scars shown in the newborn period are beginning to heal and lipomatous nodules now project through the localized areas of skin atrophy. (**A–D,** Courtesy of Dr. Marilyn C. Jones, Children's Hospital, San Diego.)

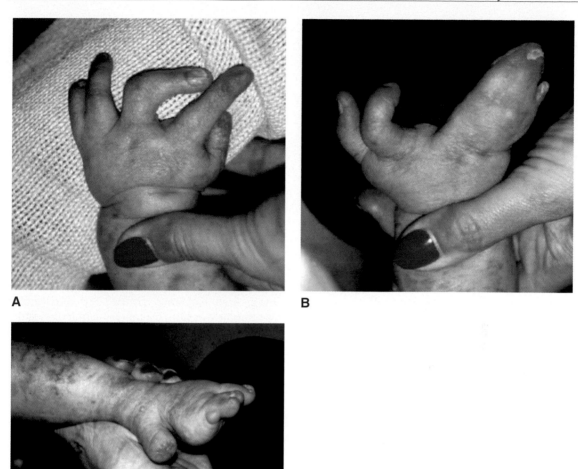

A

B

C

FIGURE 3. **A–C,** Note the severe defects of the hands and feet including syndactyly, ectrodactyly, and nail dystrophy. (Courtesy of Dr. Marilyn C. Jones, Children's Hospital, San Diego.)

MICROPHTHALMIA–LINEAR SKIN DEFECTS SYNDROME
(MIDAS Syndrome)

Al-Gazali and colleagues described two females with this disorder in 1988 and 1990. MIDAS (*Mi*crophthalmia, *D*ermal *A*plasia, and *S*clerocornea) has been suggested as a mnemonic designation. Approximately 24 cases have been reported.

ABNORMALITIES

Eyes. Microphthalmia, sclerocornea.
Skin. Dermal aplasia, without herniation of fatty tissue, usually involving face, scalp, and neck but occasionally upper part of the thorax that heal, leaving hyperpigmented areas.

OCCASIONAL ABNORMALITIES.

Microcephaly; CNS defects, including agenesis of corpus callosum, absence of septum pellucidum, and ventriculomegaly; mild to severe mental retardation (24%); infantile seizures; additional eye abnormalities, including anterior chamber defects, cataracts, iris coloboma, pigmentary retinopathy, and orbital cysts; structural cardiac defects (atrial septal defect, ventricular septal defect, overriding aorta); cardiac conduction defects; diaphragmatic hernia; nail dystrophy; rib/vertebral defects.

NATURAL HISTORY.

Developmental milestones are reached at an appropriate age in the majority of cases when the severe visual handicap is taken into consideration. Death occurred in the first year of life in two children, presumably secondary to cardiac arrhythmias.

ETIOLOGY.

The vast majority of patients have been females, indicative of an X-linked mutation lethal in males. All have had a gross deletion or a translocation involving the short arm of the X chromosome resulting in monosomy for Xp22.3. Three genes from this critical region have been characterized. Although none have been implicated as causing the clinical features of this disorder, loss of one of them, HCCS (holocytochrome c-type synthetase), has been demonstrated to cause the male lethality. Inactivation of mouse holocytochrome c-type synthetase, whose homologs in lower organisms are critical for function of cytochrome c or c1 in the mitochondrial respiratory chain lead to lethality of hemizygous, homozygous, and heterozygous embryos early in development.

References

Al-Gazali LI et al: An XX male and two t (X;Y) females with linear skin defects and congenital microphthalmia: A new syndrome at Xp22.3. J Med Genet 25:638, 1988.
Al-Gazali LI et al: Two 46XX, t (X;Y) females with linear skin defects and congenital microphthalmia: A new syndrome at Xp22.3. J Med Genet 27:59, 1990.
Linder NM et al: Xp22.3 Microdeletion syndrome with microphthalmia, sclerocornea, linear skin defects, and congenital heart defects. Am J Med Genet 44:61, 1992.
Happle R et al: MIDAS syndrome (microphthalmia, dermal aplasia, and sclerocornea): An X-linked phenotype distinct from Goltz syndrome. Am J Med Genet 47:710, 1993.
Kayserili H et al: Molecular characterization of a new case of microphthalmia with linear skin defects (MLS). J Med Genet 38:411, 2001.
Prakash SK et al: Loss of holocytochrome c-type synthetase causes the male lethality of x-linked dominant microphthalmia with linear skin defects (MLS) syndrome. Hum Mol Genet 11:3237, 2002.

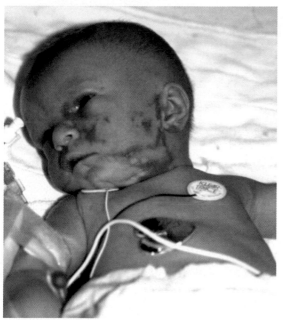

A

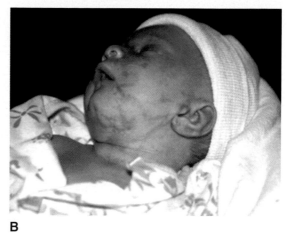

B

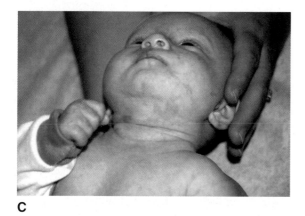

C

FIGURE 1. Microphthalmia-linear skin defects syndrome. Female infant: newborn (**A**), at 2 weeks (**B**), and at 2 months (**C**). Note the irregular areas of skin hypoplasia that have healed significantly by 2 months of age. (From Bird LM et al: Am J Med Genet 53:141, 1994. Copyright © 1994. Reprinted with permission of Wiley-Liss, Inc., a subsidiary of John Wiley & Sons, Inc.)

Q Ectodermal Dysplasias

HYPOHIDROTIC ECTODERMAL DYSPLASIA

Defect in Sweating, Alopecia, Hypodontia

There are a number of ectodermal dysplasia syndromes, only a few of which are represented in this text. The division into hypohidrotic and hidrotic categories based on the extent of the deficit of sweat glands is in no way absolute. Just as there is variable hypoplasia of hair follicles, there is variable hypoplasia of sweat glands.

Thurman described this entity in 1848. In 1875, Charles Darwin set forth the following concise commentary about this disease: "I may give an analogous case, communicated to me by Mr. W. Wedderhorn of a Hindoo family in Scinde, in which ten men, in the course of four generations, were furnished, in both jaws taken together, with only four small and weak incisor teeth and with eight posterior molars. The men thus affected have very little hair on the body, and became bald early in life. They also suffer much during hot weather from excessive dryness of the skin. It is remarkable that no instance has occurred of a daughter being thus affected." In 1929, Weech clearly separated this condition from other clinical problems having ectodermal dysplasia as a feature. At least 1 in 17,000 newborns is affected.

ABNORMALITIES

Skin. Thin and hypoplastic, with decreased pigment and tendency toward papular changes on face; periorbital wrinkling and hyperpigmentation; scaling or peeling of skin in immediate newborn period.

Skin Appendages. Hair: fine, dry, and hypochromic; sparse to absent; sweat glands: hypoplasia to absence of eccrine glands; apocrine glands more normally represented; sebaceous glands: hypoplasia to absence.

Mucous Membranes. Hypoplasia, with absence of mucous glands in oral and nasal membranes; mucous glands may also be absent from bronchial mucosa.

Dentition. Hypodontia to anodontia resulting in deficient alveolar ridge, anterior teeth tend to be conical in shape.

Craniofacial. Low nasal bridge, small nose with hypoplastic alae nasi, full forehead, prominent supraorbital ridges, prominent lips.

OCCASIONAL ABNORMALITIES.

Hoarse voice, hypoplasia to absence of mammary glands or nipples, absence of tears, failure to develop nasal turbinates, mild-to-moderate nail dystrophy, eczematous change in skin, asthmatic symptoms.

NATURAL HISTORY.

Hyperthermia as a consequence of inadequate sweating not only is a serious threat to life but may be the cause of mental deficiency, which is an occasional feature of this disorder. Living in a cool climate and cooling by water when overheated are important measures. The hypoplasia of mucous membranes plus thin nares may require frequent irrigation of the nares to limit the severity of purulent rhinitis. Otitis media and lung infection may also be consequences of the mucous membrane defect. Mucous glands have been hypoplastic to absent not only in the respiratory tract but in esophageal and colonic mucosa as well. Early radiologic evaluation may reveal the extent of dental deficit, and dentures are indicated. Although the patient is often hairless at birth, some hair may develop. Short stature is not considered a feature of this disorder. Therefore, affected males with growth deficiency should be evaluated for other causes of short stature, such as endocrine deficiencies.

ETIOLOGY.

This disorder has an X-linked recessive inheritance pattern. The gene (ED1) has been localized within the region Xq12-q13.1. It encodes a protein, ectodysplasin, which is important for normal development of ectodermal appendages. It has been estimated that approximately 90% of female carriers can be identified by dental examination and sweat testing. Sweat testing uses an iodine-in-alcohol followed by a cornstarch-in-castor-oil application to identify streaks devoid of sweat glands along the lines of Blaschko, forming a V-shape over the back of carrier females. Approximately 95% of patients with hypohidrotic ectodermal dysplasia have the X-linked form of disease.

COMMENT.

A clinically identical autosomal recessive form (ARHED) and a milder autosomal dominant form (ADHED) have been described. Mutations in the ectodysplasin anhidrotic receptor (EDAR) gene located at 2q11-q13 are responsible for both the autosomal recessive form and the autosomal dominant form. Mutations in the ectodysplasin anhidrotic receptor–associated death domain (EDARADD) gene located at 1q42.2-q43 also are responsible for the autosomal recessive form.

References

Thurman J: Two cases in which the skin, hair and teeth were very imperfectly developed. Medico-Chir Trans 31:71, 1848.

Darwin C: The Variations of Animals and Plants under Domestication, 2nd ed. London: John Murray, 1875.

Weech AA: Hereditary ectodermal dysplasia (congenital ectodermal defect): A report of two cases. Am J Dis Child 37:766, 1929.

Passarge E, Nuzum CT, Schubert WK: Anhidrotic ectodermal dysplasia as autosomal recessive trait in an inbred kindred. Humangenetik 3:181, 1966.

Gorlin RJ, Old T, Anderson VE: Hypohidrotic ectodermal dysplasia females: A critical analysis and argument for genetic heterogeneity. Z Kinderheilkd 108:1, 1970.

Clarke A: Hypohidrotic ectodermal dysplasia. J Med Genet 24:659, 1987.

Clarke A, Burn J: Sweat testing to identify female carriers of X-linked hypohidrotic ectodermal dysplasia. J Med Genet 28:330, 1991.

Crawford PJM et al: Clinical and radiographic dental findings in X-linked hypohidrotic ectodermal dysplasia. J Med Genet 28:181, 1991.

Zonana J et al: Detection of de novo mutations and analysis of their origin in families with X-linked hypohidrotic ectodermal dysplasia. J Med Genet 31:287, 1994.

Munoz F et al: Definitive evidence for an autosomal recessive form of hypohydrotic ectodermal dysplasia clinically indistinguishable from the more common X-linked disorder. Am J Hum Genet 61:94, 1997.

Ho L et al: A gene for autosomal dominant hypohydrotic ectodermal dysplasia (EDA3) maps to chromosome 2q11-q13. Am J Hum Genet 62:1102, 1998.

Monreal AW et al: Identification of a new splice form of the EDA1 gene permits detection of nearly all X-linked hypohydrotic ectodermal dysplasia mutations. Am J Hum Genet 63:380, 1998.

Headon DJ et al: Gene defect in ectodermal dysplasia implicates a death domain adapter in development. Nature 414:913, 2001.

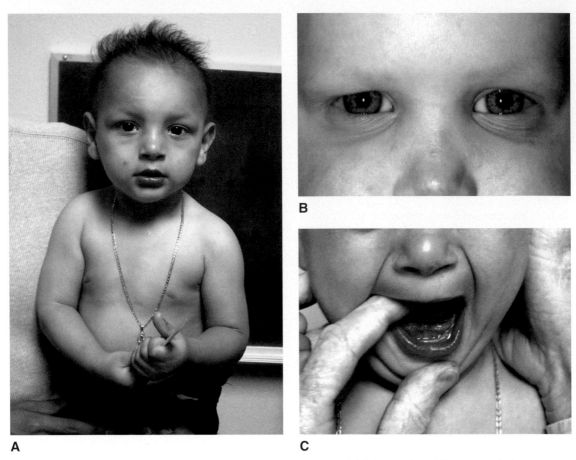

FIGURE 1. Hypohidrotic ectodermal dysplasia. **A,** Hypoplastic alae nasi; full forehead; and fine, sparse hair.
B, Periorbital skin wrinkling and sparse eyelashes and eyebrows. **C,** Hypoplasia of alveolar ridge in a 2-year-old child.
Continued

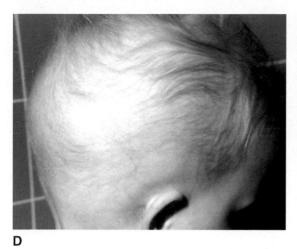

D

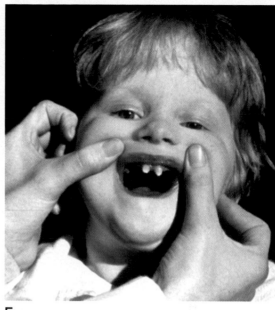

E

Fig. 1, cont'd. D, Fine, dry, hypochromic hair. **E,** Partial expression in a girl.

RAPP-HODGKIN ECTODERMAL DYSPLASIA

Hypohidrosis, Oral Clefts, Dysplastic Nails

Rapp and Hodgkin reported three affected individuals in 1968, and Summitt and Hiatt added one additional case. More than 40 cases have been reported.

ABNORMALITIES

Skin. Thin, with decreased number of sweat pores; sparse, fine hair; pili canaliculi.

Nails. Small.

Dentition. Hypodontia with small, conical teeth.

Face. Low nasal bridge, narrow nose with hypoplastic ala nasi, maxillary hypoplasia, high forehead.

Mouth. Small, cleft lip with or without cleft palate, cleft palate alone, cleft uvula, velopharyngeal incompetence.

Genitalia. Hypospadias.

OCCASIONAL ABNORMALITIES.

Short stature, ptosis, atretic ear canals, hearing loss, absent lacrimal puncta, labial anomalies, absent lingual frenulum and sublingual caruncles, glossy tongue, hypothelia, palmoplantar keratoderma, syndactyly.

NATURAL HISTORY.

These patients are liable to have hyperthermia in early childhood. Thereafter, although reduced sweating is described, heat intolerance is not usually a problem. There is frequent occurrence of purulent conjunctivitis and otitis media, the latter presumably related to palatal incompetence. Speech difficulties are common. Whereas the clefting seen in most genetic syndromes is consistent (i.e., either cleft lip with or without cleft palate [CLP] or cleft palate alone [CPA]), mixed clefting (the occurrence of CLP and cleft palate alone in the same family) occurs in this disorder. Deficient mucous coating of vocal cords can affect vocal quality.

ETIOLOGY.

This disorder has an autosomal dominant inheritance pattern. Mutations of the p63 gene located on 3q27 are responsible.

COMMENT.

Mutations of the p63 gene have been identified in certain other autosomal dominant disorders with some overlapping features including ectrodactyly-ectodermal dysplasia-clefting syndrome, Hay-Wells syndrome, and in some cases of nonsyndromic split-hand/foot syndrome.

References

Rapp RS, Hodgkin WE: Anhidrotic ectodermal dysplasia: Autosomal dominant inheritance with palate and lip anomalies. J Med Genet 5:269, 1968.

Summitt RL, Hiatt RL: Hypohidrotic ectodermal dysplasia with multiple associated anomalies. Birth Defects 7(8):121, 1971.

Wannarachue N, Hall BD, Smith DW: Ectodermal dysplasia and multiple defects (Rapp-Hodgkin type). J Pediatr 81:1217, 1972.

Schroeder HW, Sybert VP: Rapp-Hodgkin ectodermal dysplasia. J Pediatr 110:72, 1987.

Salinas CF, Montes GM: Rapp-Hodgkin syndrome: Observations on ten cases and characteristic hair changes (pili canaliculi). Birth Defects 24:149, 1988.

O'Donnell BP, James WD: Rapp-Hodgkin ectodermal dysplasia. J Am Acad Dermatol 27:323, 1992.

Neilson DE et al: Mixed clefting type in Rapp-Hodgkin syndrome. Am J Med Genet 108:281, 2002.

Bougeard G et al: The Rapp-Hodgkin syndrome results from mutations of the TP63 gene. Eur J Hum Genet 11:700, 2003.

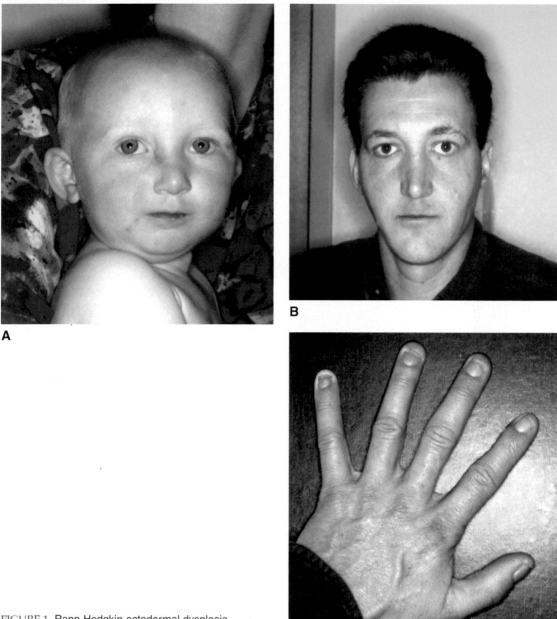

FIGURE 1. Rapp-Hodgkin ectodermal dysplasia.
A–C, Affected father and son. Note the narrow nose with hypoplastic ala nasi, small mouth, and hypoplastic fingernails.

TRICHO-DENTO-OSSEOUS SYNDROME
(TDO Syndrome)

Kinky Hair, Enamel Hypoplasia, Sclerotic Bone

Lichtenstein and colleagues defined this disorder in 107 individuals from one large kindred in 1972. Robinson and colleagues had previously described an autosomal dominant disorder with curly hair and enamel hypoplasia, with or without nail hypoplasia.

ABNORMALITIES

Hair. Kinky/curly present at birth.

Dentition. Small, widely spaced, pitted teeth with poor enamel, increased pulp chamber size (taurodontism), both primary and permanent dentition are affected.

Facies. Frontal bossing, dolichocephaly, square jaw.

Bone. Mild-to-moderate increased bone density, most evident in calvarium, which is thick, lacks visible pneumatization of the mastoid process, or visible obliteration of the cranial diploë; obtuse mandibular angles; short mandibular rami; long bones and spine also can be affected.

Nails. Brittle, with superficial peeling (approximately 50%).

Other. Delayed bone age.

OCCASIONAL ABNORMALITIES.
Partial craniosynostosis, congenitally missing teeth.

NATURAL HISTORY. The hair sometimes straightens with age. The teeth become eroded and discolored, are prone to periapical abscesses, and are lost by the second to third decade. The sclerotic bone appears to be secondary to closely compacted lamellae and is rarely associated with any clinical symptomatology.

ETIOLOGY. This disorder has an autosomal dominant inheritance pattern. A mutation in the DLX3 gene, a member of the distal-less homeobox gene family, located at 17q21 has been identified in affected members of six families. Murine studies have indicated the important role of DLX genes in the development of hair, teeth, and bone.

References

Robinson GC, Miller JR, Worth HM: Hereditary enamel hypoplasia, its association with characteristic hair structure. Pediatrics 37:489, 1966.

Lichtenstein J et al: The tricho-dento-osseous (TDO) syndrome. Am J Hum Genet 24:569, 1972.

Shapiro SD et al: Tricho-dento-osseous syndrome. Am J Med Genet 16:225, 1983.

Wright JR et al: Tricho-dento-osseous syndrome: Features of the hair and teeth. Oral Surg Oral Med Oral Pathol 77:487, 1994.

Wright JR et al: Analysis of the Tricho-dento-osseous syndrome geneotype and phenotype. Am J Med Genet 72:197, 1997.

Price JA et al: Identification of a mutation in DLX3 associated with tricho-dento-osseous (TDO) syndrome. Hum Mol Genet 7:563, 1998.

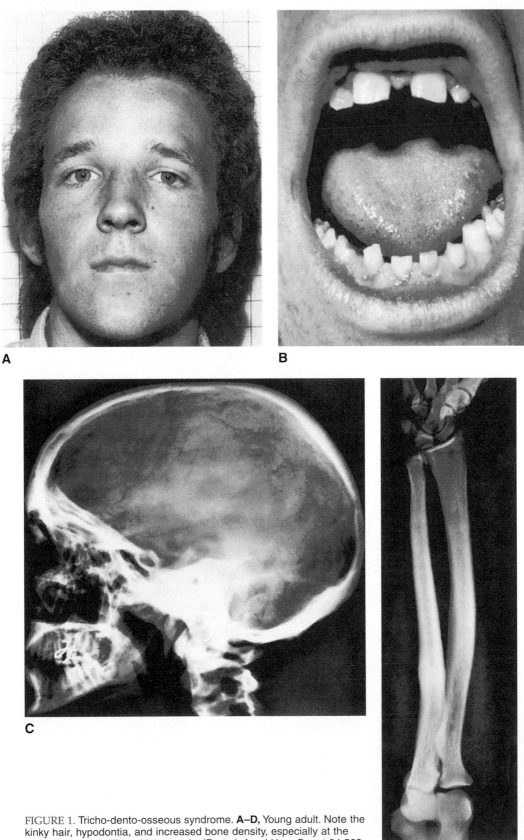

FIGURE 1. Tricho-dento-osseous syndrome. **A–D,** Young adult. Note the kinky hair, hypodontia, and increased bone density, especially at the base of the skull. (From Lichtenstein JR et al: Am J Hum Genet 24:569, 1972, with permission.)

CLOUSTON SYNDROME

Nail Dystrophy, Dyskeratotic Palms and Soles, Hair Hypoplasia

Clouston in 1939 reported 119 individuals in a French-Canadian family. Rajagopalan and Tay described an affected Chinese pedigree in 1977. Over 200 cases have been described.

ABNORMALITIES

Skin. Thick dyskeratotic palms and soles; hyperpigmentation over knuckles, elbows, axillae, areolae, and pubic area.

Hair. Hypoplasia to alopecia (61%), deficiency of eyelashes and eyebrows.

Nails. Hypoplasia to aplasia, dysplasia.

Eyes. Strabismus.

OCCASIONAL ABNORMALITIES.

Cataract, photophobia, hearing loss, dull mentality, short stature, thickened skull, tufting of terminal phalanges.

ETIOLOGY. This disorder has an autosomal dominant inheritance pattern. Mutations in the GJB6 gene located at chromosome 13q11-12.1, which encodes the gap junction protein connexin 30 are responsible. Connexin 30 is expressed in the epidermis, brain, and inner ear. Connexins are membrane proteins that are present in virtually all mammalian cells. Each connexon binds another connexin in an adjacent cell to form an intracellular communication channel known as a gap junction, which functions to allow rapid exchange of information between cells.

References

Joachim H: Hereditary dystrophy of the hair and nails in six generations. Ann Intern Med 10:400, 1936.

Clouston HR: The major forms of hereditary ectodermal dysplasia (with an autopsy and biopsies on the anhidrotic type). Can Med Assoc J 40:1, 1939.

Wilkey WD, Stevenson GH: A family with inherited ectodermal dystrophy. Can Med Assoc J 53:226, 1945.

Gold RJM, Scriver CR: Properties of hair keratin in an autosomal dominant form of ectodermal dysplasia. Am J Hum Genet 24:549, 1972.

Rajagopalan KV, Tay CH: Hydrotic ectodermal dysplasia: Study of a large Chinese pedigree. Arch Dermatol 113:481, 1977.

Kibar Z et al: The gene responsible for Clouston hidrotic ectodermal dysplasia maps to the pericentromeric region of chromosome 13q. Hum Mol Genet 5:543, 1996.

Lamartine J et al: Mutations in GJB6 cause hidrotic ectodermal dysplasia. Nat Genet 26:142, 2000.

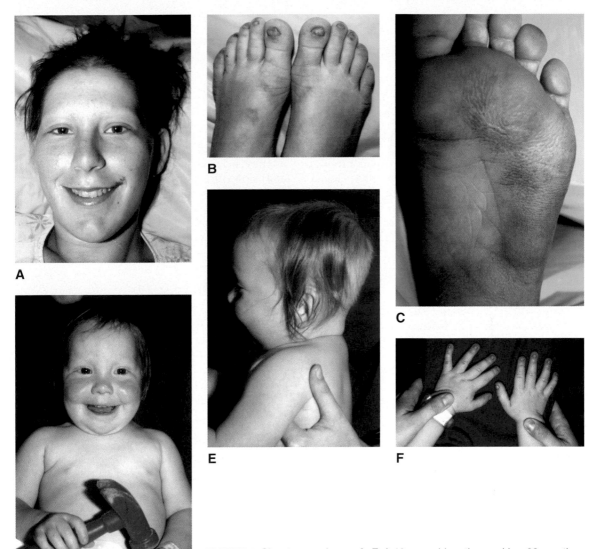

FIGURE 1. Clouston syndrome. **A–F,** A 19-year-old mother and her 22-month-old daughter. Note the sparse hair, dysplastic nails, and dyskeratotic soles.

GAPO SYNDROME

Growth Deficiency, Alopecia, Pseudoanodontia, Optic Atrophy

Initially reported in a Danish patient in 1947, this disorder was referred to as GAPO (*g*rowth deficiency, *a*lopecia, *p*seudoanodontia, *o*ptic atrophy) syndrome by Tipton and Gorlin in 1984. Ocular manifestations rather than optic atrophy is a more appropriate designation in that the latter has occurred in less than one half of cases. Approximately 25 patients have been reported.

ABNORMALITIES

Growth. Mildly decreased birth length, significant postnatal growth deficiency becomes obvious between 6 months and 1 year, delayed bone age.

Craniofacial. Frontal bossing, high forehead, prominent occiput, enlarged anterior fontanel with delayed closure, prominent scalp veins, periorbital swelling, drooping forehead skin, flat nasal bridge, anteverted nares, long philtrum, thick lips, large ears, micrognathia.

Ocular. Progressive optic atrophy, cataracts, exophthalmos, keratoconus, glaucoma, horizontal nystagmus.

Hair. Diminished scalp hair beginning between 2 and 3 months with total alopecia by 2 to 3 years, sparse eyelashes and eyebrows, the extent of body and facial hair are variable.

Teeth. Failure of tooth eruption (pseudo-anodontia) involving primary and permanent dentition.

Other. Mild skin laxity, umbilical hernia, hyperconvex nails, brachydactyly.

OCCASIONAL ABNORMALITIES.
Mild mental retardation, ptosis, alopecia at birth, craniosynostosis, absent pneumatization of maxillary sinuses, abnormal electroencephalograph, altered cerebral circulation with tortuousity of arteries and dilatation of basilar vertebral arteries and slow circulation time in one patient and occluded or absent right transverse and sigmoid sinus in another, hypoplastic middle and distal phalanges, wrinkled palms, scythe-like ribs, delayed menarche, hypogonadism, breast hypoplasia, hepatomegaly, hypospadias, polycystic kidney, nephrocalcinosis.

NATURAL HISTORY. Most patients are normal at birth with progressive changes beginning at approximately 6 months, including loss of hair, skin laxity, and optic atrophy. Two affected patients died at 35 and 39 years, respectively. Autopsy specimens from both showed interstitial fibrosis as well as atherosclerotic changes in multiple organs.

ETIOLOGY. This disorder has an autosomal recessive inheritance pattern.

References
Anderson TH et al: Et tilfaelde at total "pseudo-anodonti" I forbindelse med kraniedeformitet, dvaergvaekst og ektodermal displasi. Odont T 55:484–493, 1947.
Tipton RE, Gorlin RJ: Growth retardation, alopecia, pseudoanodontia, and optic atrophy—the GAPO syndrome: Report of a patient and review of the literature. Am J Med Genet 19:209–216, 1984.
Wajntal A et al: GAPO syndrome (McKusick 23074)—a connective tissue disorder: Report on two affected sibs and on the pathologic findings in the older. Am J Med Genet 37:213–223, 1990.
Bacon W et al: GAPO syndrome: A new case of this rare syndrome and a review of the relative importance of different phenotypic features in diagnosis. J Craniofac Genet Dev Biol 19:189–200, 1999.

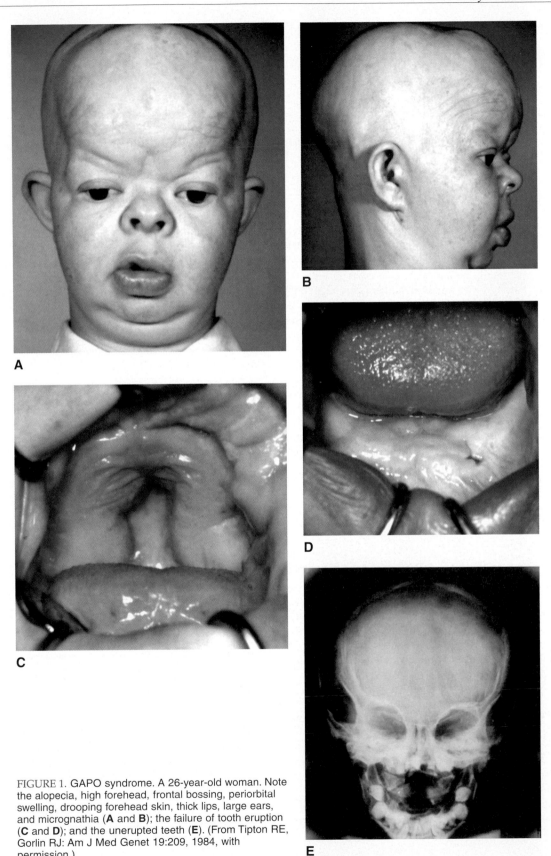

FIGURE 1. GAPO syndrome. A 26-year-old woman. Note the alopecia, high forehead, frontal bossing, periorbital swelling, drooping forehead skin, thick lips, large ears, and micrognathia (**A** and **B**); the failure of tooth eruption (**C** and **D**); and the unerupted teeth (**E**). (From Tipton RE, Gorlin RJ: Am J Med Genet 19:209, 1984, with permission.)

PACHYONYCHIA CONGENITA SYNDROME
Thick Nails, Hyperkeratosis, Foot Blisters

Pachyonychia congenita is an ectodermal dysplasia described by Jadassohn and Lewandowsky, in which there is hypertrophic dystrophy of the distal nails.

ABNORMALITIES

Nails. Progressive thickening, yellow-brown discoloration, pinched margins, and an upward angulation of distal tips; the nails may eventually be hypoplastic or even absent.

Skin. Patchy to complete hyperkeratosis of palms and soles, callosities of feet, palmar and plantar bullae formation in areas of pressure that are often painful; keratosis pilaris with tiny cutaneous horny excrescences, particularly on the extensor surfaces of the arms and legs and on the buttocks; epidermal cysts filled with loose keratin on face, neck, and upper chest; verrucous lesions on the elbows, knees, and lower legs.

Mucous Membranes. Leukokeratosis of mouth and tongue, especially in positions of increased trauma; scalloped tongue edge.

Dentition. Erupted teeth at birth, lost by 4 to 6 months; early eruption of primary teeth and early loss of secondary teeth as a result of severe caries.

OCCASIONAL ABNORMALITIES.
Mental deficiency; corneal thickening, cataracts, thickening of tympanic membrane, hyperhidrosis, particularly of palms and soles; dry and sparse hair; osteomata of frontal bones; intestinal diverticula; large joint arthritis; bushy eyebrows; hoarseness secondary to laryngeal leukokeratosis; malformed teeth and twinning of the incisors.

NATURAL HISTORY. Clinical manifestations are present at birth or by 6 months of age in approximately 80% of patients. Usually the nails are grossly thickened by 1 year of age. Complete surgical removal of the nails is sometimes merited, although any matrix left behind will reform abnormal nails. Severe recurrent upper respiratory symptoms have occurred in those with severe

laryngeal involvement. Areas of chronic bullous formation should be observed carefully for development of possible skin malignancy. An abnormality of cell-mediated immunity leading to a deficiency in the recognition and processing of *Candida* infection can result in recurrent oral and cutaneous candidiasis, which can compound the nail problems.

ETIOLOGY. This disorder has an autosomal dominant inheritance pattern. Mutations in two different keratin genes located at chromosome 17q12-q21 are responsible for the two major forms of pachyonychia congenita. The Jadassohn-Lewandowsky form is caused by mutations in keratin 16 and the Jackson-Lawler type by mutations in keratin 17.

COMMENT. Two forms have been described: the Jadossohn-Lewandowsky form is characterized by pachyonychia, palmoplantar hyperkeratosis, hyperhidrosis, occasional blistering, follicular keratosis, and oral leukokeratosis; and a rarer form defined by Jackson and Lawler is characterized by pachyonychia, multiple epidermal cysts, recurrent flexural infections, natal teeth, and straight bushy eyebrow hair. Oral leukokeratosis is not a feature of the form defined by Jackson and Lawler.

References

Jadassohn J, Lewandowsky F: Pachyonychia congenita, keratosis disseminata circumscripta (folliculosis): Tylomata; leukokeratosis linguae. Ikonographia Dermatologica Tab 629, 1906.

Soderquist NA, Reed WB: Pachyonychia congenita with epidermal cysts and other congenital dyskeratoses. Arch Dermatol 97:31, 1968.

Young LL, Lenox JA: Pachyonychia congenital: A long-term evaluation. Oral Surg 36:663, 1973.

Stieglitz JB, Centerwall WR: Pachyonychia congenita (Jadassohn-Lewandowsky syndrome): A seventeen-member, four-generation pedigree with unusual respiratory and dental involvement. Am J Med Genet 14:21, 1983.

Rohold AE, Brandrup F: Pachyonychia congenita: Therapeutic and immunologic aspects. Pediatr Dermatol 7:307, 1990.

Su WPD et al: Pachyonychia congenita: A clinical study of 12 cases and review of the literature. Pediatr Dermatol 7:32, 1990.

McLean WHI et al: Keratin 16 and keratin 17 mutations cause pachyonychia congenita. Nat Genet 9:273, 1995.

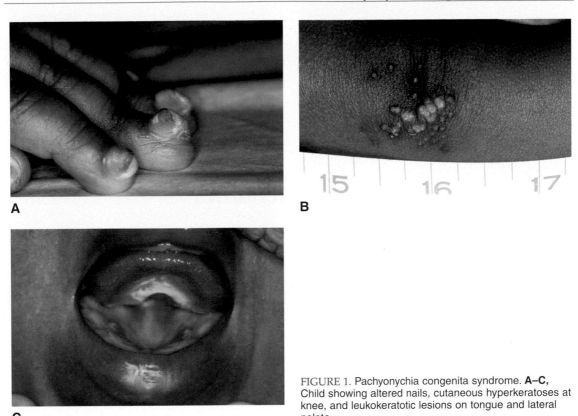

FIGURE 1. Pachyonychia congenita syndrome. **A–C,** Child showing altered nails, cutaneous hyperkeratoses at knee, and leukokeratotic lesions on tongue and lateral palate.

XERODERMA PIGMENTOSA SYNDROME

Undue Sunlight Sensitivity, Atrophic and Pigmentary Skin Changes, Actinic Skin Tumors

Xeroderma pigmentosa occurs in approximately 1 in 250,000 individuals. Nearly 1000 cases have been reported.

ABNORMALITIES

Skin. Sunlight sensitivity with first exposure; freckling; progressive skin atrophy with irregular pigmentation; cutaneous telangiectasia; angiomata; keratoses; development of basal cell and squamous cell carcinoma, and less often keratoacanthoma, adenocarcinoma, melanoma, neuroma, sarcoma, and angiosarcoma.

Eyes. Photophobia; recurrent conjunctival injection; corneal abnormalities consisting of exposure keratitis leading to corneal clouding or vascularization; neoplasms involving conjunctiva, cornea, and eyelids.

Oral. Atrophic skin of mouth sometimes leading to difficulty opening mouth; squamous cell carcinoma of tongue tip, gingiva, or palate.

Neurologic. Slowly progressive neurologic abnormalities sometimes associated with mental deterioration; microcephaly; cerebral atrophy; choreoathetosis, ataxia, and spasticity; impaired hearing; abnormal speech; abnormal electroencephalography.

OCCASIONAL ABNORMALITIES.

Primary internal neoplasms, including brain tumors, lung tumors, and leukemia; immune abnormalities; frequent infections.

NATURAL HISTORY.

Cutaneous symptoms have onset at median age of between 1 and 2 years. The mean age of first nonmelanoma skin cancer is 8 years. Ninety-seven percent of squamous cell and basal cell cancers occur on face, head, or neck, indicating the important role that sun exposure has in the induction of these neoplasms. Four percent of squamous cell carcinomas metastasize. Seventy percent probability of survival has been documented at age 40 years. Thirty-three percent of deaths are due to cancer and 11% to infection.

ETIOLOGY.

This disorder has an autosomal recessive inheritance pattern. The majority of affected patients have a defect in the excision repair of ultraviolet radiation–induced DNA damage. XP patients fall into one of ten complementation groups (A through I plus a variant). XPA, the gene for which is located on chromosome 9q34.1; XPC, the gene for which is located on chromosome 3p25.1; and XPD, the gene for which is located on chromosome 19q13.2, are most common. Neurologic problems are generally found in group A and D patients, who show the lowest level of DNA repair, whereas group C patients, who show the highest level of repair, are usually without overt neurologic disorders and have a longer life span. The severity of the skin and eye lesions relates more to the degree of sun exposure. The defect can be identified in cultured fibroblasts from amniocentesis.

COMMENT.

The DeSanctis-Cacchione syndrome is a subgroup of xeroderma pigmentosa with neurologic involvement that includes xeroderma pigmentosa, progressive mental deterioration, growth deficiency, microcephaly, and hypogonadism probably secondary to hypothalamic insufficiency. Natural history includes slow developmental progress and growth, with variable neurologic dysfunction, including seizures from early childhood, spasticity, ataxia, peripheral neuropathy, and sometimes sensorineural deafness. Progressive skin deterioration occurs especially related to exposure to the sun. Shortened life expectancy as a result of central nervous system deterioration or malignancy has been documented. The disorder is the result of a pair of autosomal recessive genes. Patients with DeSanctis-Cacchione syndrome usually belong to complementation group A or D.

References

DeSanctis C, Cacchione A: L'idiozia xerodermia. Riv Spec Freniatr 56:269, 1932.

Rook A, Wilkinson DS, Ebling FJG (eds): Textbook of Dermatology. Oxford: Blackwell Scientific Publications, 1968.

Regan JD et al: Xeroderma pigmentosa: A rapid sensitive method for prenatal diagnosis. Science 174:147, 1971.

Pawsey SA et al: Clinical, genetic and DNA repair studies on a consecutive series of patients with xeroderma pigmentosa. Q J Med 48:179, 1979.

Kraemer KH et al: Xeroderma pigmentosa: Cutaneous, ocular and neurologic abnormalities in 830 published cases. Arch Dermatol 123:241, 1987.

Greenhaw GA et al: Xeroderma pigmentosum and Cockayne syndrome: Overlapping clinical and bio-chemical phenotypes. Am J Hum Genet 50:677, 1992.

Cleaver JE et al: A summary of mutations in the UV-sensitive disorders: Xeroderma pigmentosum, Cockayne syndrome, and trichothiodystrophy. Hum Mutat 14:9, 1999.

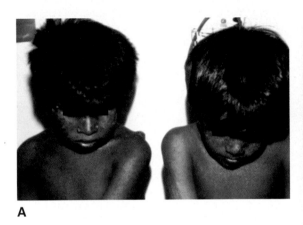

A

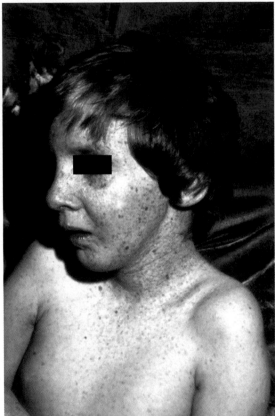

B

FIGURE 1. Xeroderma pigmentosa. **A,** Siblings with normal intelligence and light-sensitive xeroderma pigmentosa. **B,** Child with DeSanctis-Cacchione syndrome.

SENTER-KID SYNDROME

Ichthyosiform Erythroderma, Sensorineural Deafness

Initially reported by Burns in 1915, this disorder was further delineated by Senter and colleagues, who reported an affected child in 1978 and recognized 12 similar patients from the literature. Skinner and colleagues introduced the acronym KID (*k*eratitis, *i*chthyosis, *d*eafness) syndrome to highlight the principal features. However, controversy exists as to whether ichthyosis is actually a feature of this disorder.

ABNORMALITIES

Hearing. Sensorineural deafness with onset documented from birth to 7 years.

Skin. Changes occurring at birth in the majority of cases described variably as dry, red, rough skin, erythematous and scaly skin, erythrodermia, and most commonly as erythrokeratodermia; within the first 3 months, the skin becomes thicker with a leathery appearance; well-demarcated, erythrokeratodermic, non-scaling plaques with an erythematous border develop in 89% of cases; follicular keratosis commonly occurring over extensor surface of arms, scalp, and nose; palmoplantar hyperkeratosis.

Nails, Hair, Teeth. Variable nail dystrophy; variable malformations of teeth; sparse, fine hair involving scalp, eyebrows, and eyelashes.

Eyes. Corneal dystrophy manifest by progressive vascularization with photophobia and tearing leading to corneal destruction with the development of keratodermia (a pannus of vascular or fibrotic tissue) progressing to occlusion of vision.

Other. Cryptorchidism; variable flexion contractures; oral abnormalities including leukokeratosis, erythematous lesions, and scrotal tongue.

OCCASIONAL ABNORMALITIES.

Ichthyosis secondary to hyperkeratotic plaques; squamous cell carcinoma of skin and tongue; congenital alopecia; Hirschsprung disease; mental retardation; tight heel cords; growth deficiency; decreased sweating; breast hypoplasia; cochleosaccular abnormality of temporal bone.

NATURAL HISTORY. The corneal dystrophy, which occurs in 83% of patients, is the most serious aspect because it can lead to blindness. Lifelong ophthalmologic examinations are indicated. Early evaluation of hearing is necessary. Mycotic and bacterial skin infections as well as otitis media, conjunctivitis, and visceral infections (pneumonia, gastroenteritis, and sepsis) occur frequently.

ETIOLOGY. This disorder has an autosomal dominant inheritance pattern. Mutations in the GJB2 gene that encodes the gap junction protein connexin 26 are responsible. Most cases are sporadic and thus represent a fresh gene mutation. Connexins are membrane proteins that are present in virtually all mammalian cells. Each connexon binds another connexin in an adjacent cell to form an intracellular communication channel known as a gap junction, which functions to allow rapid exchange of information between cells.

References

Burns FS: A case of generalized congenital erythroderma. J Cutan Dis 33:255, 1915.

Senter TP et al: Atypical ichthyosiform erythroderma and congenital sensorineural deafness—a distinct syndrome. J Pediatr 92:68, 1978.

Cram DL, Resneck JS, Jackson WB: A congenital ichthyosiform syndrome with deafness and keratitis. Arch Dermatol 115:467, 1979.

Skinner BA et al: The keratitis, ichthyosis, and deafness (KID) syndrome. Arch Dermatol 117:285, 1981.

Langer K et al: Keratitis, ichthyosis and deafness (KID) syndrome: Report of three cases and a review of the literature. Br J Dermatol 122:689, 1990.

Nazzaro V et al: Familial occurrence of KID (keratitis, ichthyosis, deafness) syndrome. J Am Acad Dermatol 23:385, 1990.

Caceres-Rios H et al: Keratitis, ichthyosis, and deafness (KID syndrome): Review of the literature and proposal of a new terminology. Pediatr Derm 13:105, 1996.

van Steensel MA et al: A novel connexin 26 mutation in a patient diagnosed with keratitis-ichthyosis-deafness syndrome. J Invest Dermatol 118:724, 2002.

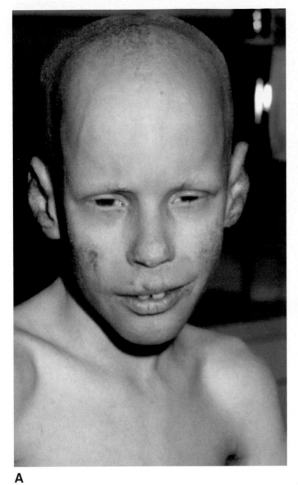

A

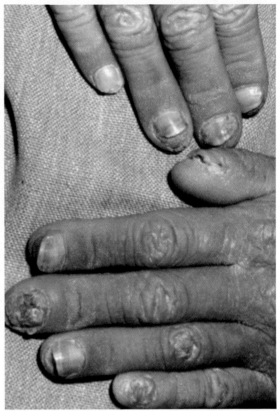

B

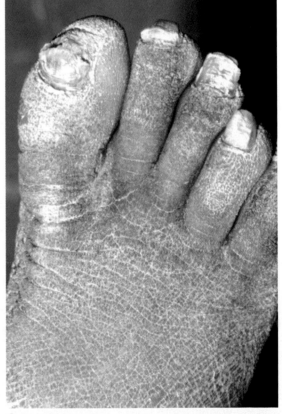

C

FIGURE 1. Senter syndrome. **A–C,** An 8-year-old child with alopecia, nail dystrophy, and lamellar ichthyosis. (From Senter TP et al: J Pediatr 92:68, 1978, with permission.)

645

R Environmental Agents

FETAL ALCOHOL SYNDROME

Prenatal Onset of Growth Deficiency, Microcephaly, Short Palpebral Fissures

In 1968, Lemoine of Nantes, France, recognized the multiple effects that alcohol can have on the developing fetus, including the more severe end of the spectrum, the fetal alcohol syndrome. Lemoine's report was not well accepted, and the disorder was independently rediscovered in 1973 by Jones and colleagues in the offspring of chronically alcoholic women. Alcohol is now appreciated as the most common major teratogen to which the fetus is liable to be exposed. The prevalence of this disorder across the United States is estimated to be 1 to 2 per 1000 live births. Hence, ethanol is of major public health concern as a teratogen.

In 1973, Jones and colleagues delineated this disorder in eight unrelated children, all born to women who were severe chronic alcoholics before and during their pregnancy. Additional studies have confirmed the initial observations.

ABNORMALITIES. Variable features from among the following:

Growth. Prenatal and postnatal onset of growth deficiency.

Performance. Average IQ of 65 with a range of 20 to 120; fine motor dysfunction manifested by weak grasp, poor eye-hand coordination, or tremulousness; irritability in infancy, hyperactivity in childhood.

Craniofacial. Mild-to-moderate microcephaly, short palpebral fissures, maxillary hypoplasia. Short nose, smooth philtrum with thin and smooth upper lip.

Skeletal. Joint anomalies including abnormal position or function, altered palmar crease patterns, small distal phalanges, small fifth fingernails.

Cardiac. Heart murmur, frequently disappearing by 1 year of age; ventricular septal defect most common, followed by atrial septal defect.

OCCASIONAL ABNORMALITIES.
Ptosis of eyelid, frank microphthalmia, cleft lip with or without cleft palate, micrognathia, pro-truding auricles, mildly webbed neck, short neck, cervical vertebral malformations (10% to 20%), rib anomalies, tetralogy of Fallot, coarctation of the aorta, strawberry hemangiomata, hypoplastic labia majora, short fourth and fifth metacarpal bones, meningomyelocele, hydrocephalus, characteristic neuropathologic features, including abnormalities of the corpus callosum and reduced size of the basal ganglia and cerebellar vermis.

NATURAL HISTORY. There may be tremulousness in the early neonatal period. Postnatal linear growth tends to remain retarded, and the adipose tissue is thin. This often creates an appearance of "failure to thrive." These individuals tend to be irritable as young infants, hyperactive as children, and more social as young adults. Problems with dental malalignment and malocclusion, eustachian tube dysfunction, and myopia develop with time. Specific abnormalities have been documented on tests of language, verbal learning and memory, academic skills, fine-motor speed, and visual-motor integration. Poor school performance is the rule even in children with IQ scores within the normal range.

ETIOLOGY. The cause of this disorder is ethanol. The least significant effect recognized at two drinks per day has been slightly smaller birth size (approximately 160 g smaller than average). It is not until four to six drinks per day are consumed that additional subtle clinical features are evident. Most of the children believed to have fetal alcohol syndrome have been born to frankly alcoholic women whose intake is eight to ten drinks or more per day. The risk of a serious problem in the offspring of a chronically alcoholic woman has been estimated to be 30% to 50%, the greatest risk being for varying degrees of mental retardation.

COMMENT. The most serious consequence of heavy prenatal alcohol exposure is the problem of brain development and function. Although the severity of the maternal alcoholism and the extent and severity of the pattern of malformation seem to be most predictive of ultimate prognosis, typical neurobehavioral abnormalities are often seen in children prenatally exposed to alcohol with completely normal physical examinations.

References

Lemoine P et al: Les enfants de parents alcooliques. Ovest Med 21:476, 1968.

Jones KL et al: Pattern of malformation in offspring of chronic alcoholic mothers. Lancet 1:1267, 1973.

Jones KL, Smith DW: Recognition of the fetal alcohol syndrome in early infancy. Lancet 2:999, 1973.

Jones KL et al: Outcome in offspring of chronic alcoholic women. Lancet 1:1076, 1974.

Majewski F et al: Zur Klinik und Pathogenese der Alkohol-Embryo: Bericht über 68 Fälle. Munch Med Wochenschr 118:1635, 1976.

Clarren SK, Smith DW: The fetal alcohol syndrome: A review of the world literature. N Engl J Med 198:1063, 1978.

Smith DW: The fetal alcohol syndrome. Hosp Pract 10:121, 1979.

Jones KL: Fetal alcohol syndrome. Pediatr Rev 8:122, 1986.

Streissguth AP et al: Fetal alcohol syndrome in adolescents and adults. JAMA 265:1961, 1991.

Jones KL: From recognition to responsibility: Josef Warkany, David Smith, and the fetal alcohol syndrome in the 21st century. Birth Defects Res (Part A) 67:13, 2003.

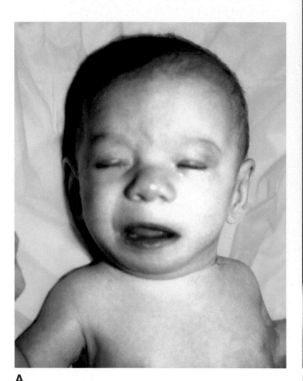
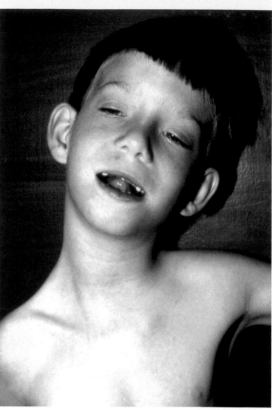

A

B

FIGURE 1. Fetal alcohol syndrome. Affected children of chronic alcoholic women. **A** and **B,** Same child at 4 months and 8 years of age. (**A** and **B,** From Jones KL: Birth Defects Res, Part A 67:13, 2003, with permission.)   *Continued*

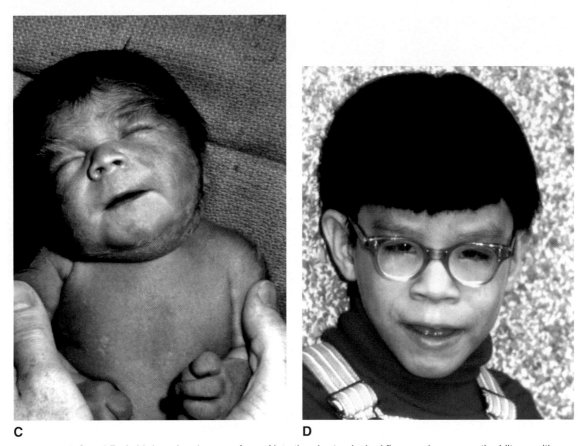

C   **D**

Fig. 1, cont'd. C and **D,** At birth and at 4 years of age. Note the short palpebral fissures; long, smooth philtrum with smooth vermilion border; and hirsutism in the newborn. (**C** and **D,** From Jones KL, Smith DW: Lancet 2:999, 1973.)

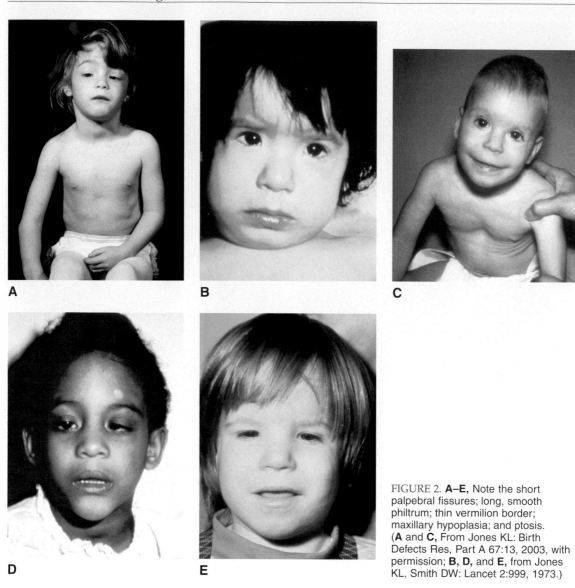

A

B

C

D

E

FIGURE 2. **A–E,** Note the short palpebral fissures; long, smooth philtrum; thin vermilion border; maxillary hypoplasia; and ptosis. (**A** and **C,** From Jones KL: Birth Defects Res, Part A 67:13, 2003, with permission; **B, D,** and **E,** from Jones KL, Smith DW: Lancet 2:999, 1973.)

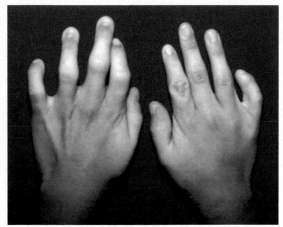

B

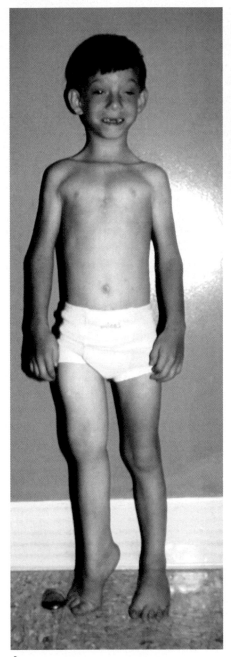

A

FIGURE 3. **A,** Short right leg secondary to congenital hip dislocation. (From Jones KL: Birth Defects Res, Part A 67:13, 2003.) **B,** Camptodactyly.

FETAL HYDANTOIN SYNDROME
(FETAL DILANTIN SYNDROME)

Although data suggesting the possible teratogenic effects of anticonvulsants were first presented by Meadow in 1968, convincing epidemiologic evidence of the association between hydantoins and congenital abnormalities awaited the studies of Fedrick and of Monson and colleagues. Further studies by Speidel and Meadow and by Hill and colleagues revealed a pattern of malformation that may include digit and nail hypoplasia, unusual facies, and growth and mental deficiencies.

ABNORMALITIES. Varying combinations of the following, with the fetal hydantoin syndrome representing the broader, more severe end of the spectrum.

Growth. Mild-to-moderate growth deficiency, usually of prenatal onset, but may be accentuated in the early postnatal months.

Performance. Occasional borderline to mild mental deficiency, performance in childhood may be better than that anticipated from progress in early infancy.

Craniofacial. Wide anterior fontanel; metopic ridging; ocular hypertelorism; broad, depressed nasal bridge; short nose with bowed upper lip; broad alveolar ridge; cleft lip and palate.

Limbs. Stiff, tapered fingers; hypoplasia of distal phalanges with small nails, especially postaxial digits; low-arch dermal ridge patterning of hypoplastic fingertips; digitalized thumb; shortened distal phalanges, metacarpals and coned epiphysis; dislocation of hip.

Other. Short neck, rib anomalies, widely spaced small nipples, umbilical and inguinal hernias, pilonidal sinus, coarse profuse scalp hair, hirsutism, low-set hairline, abnormal palmar crease, strabismus.

OCCASIONAL ABNORMALITIES.
Microcephaly, brachycephaly, positional foot deformities, strabismus, coloboma, ptosis, slanted palpebral fissures, webbed neck, pulmonary or aortic valvular stenosis, coarctation of aorta, patent ductus arteriosus, cardiac septal defects, single umbilical artery, pyloric stenosis, duodenal atresia, anal atresia, renal malformation, hypospadias, micropenis, ambiguous genitalia, cryptorchidism, symphalangism, syndactyly, terminal transverse limb defect, cleft hand, holoprosencephaly.

NATURAL HISTORY. The infants not uncommonly have relative failure to thrive during the early months for reasons unknown. Some improvement may be seen in the growth of nails and distal phalanges. The mild degrees of mental deficiency are the greatest concern. However, the degree and extent to which this occurs has not been adequately determined.

ETIOLOGY. The cause of this disorder is phenytoin (Dilantin) or one of its metabolites.

COMMENT. Similar craniofacial features referred to as the "anticonvulsant facies" are associated with prenatal exposure to carbamazepine, mysoline, and phenobarbital. In addition, a 1% risk for meningomyelocele has been associated with prenatal exposure to carbamazepine. Furthermore, there is evidence that exposure to a combination of the anticonvulsants may increase the risk to the fetus. The risk of the hydantoin-exposed fetus having the fetal hydantoin syndrome is approximately 10%, and the risk for having some effects of the disorder is an additional 33%. No dose-response curve has been demonstrated, nor has a "safe" dose been found below which there is no increased teratogenic risk. It has been suggested that susceptibility of the fetus to the teratogenic effects of hydantoins depends on the fetal genotype. Inherited defects of epoxide hydrolase (EPHX1), an enzyme that metabolizes phenytoin; production of free radicals by phenytoin; inhibition of potassium channel function that results in injury by hypoxia and reperfusion; and decreased maternal serum folate have all been suggested relative to etiology.

References

Meadow SR: Anticonvulsant drugs and congenital abnormalities. Lancet 2:1296, 1968.

Aase JM: Anticonvulsant drugs and congenital abnormalities. Am J Dis Child 127:758, 1970.

Speidel BD, Meadow SR: Maternal epilepsy and abnormalities of the fetus and newborn. Lancet 2:839, 1972.

Fedrick J: Epilepsy and pregnancy: A report from the Oxford Record Linkage Study. BMJ 2:442, 1973.

Monson RR et al: Diphenylhydantoin and selected congenital malformations. N Engl J Med 289:1049, 1973.

Hill RM et al: Infants exposed in utero to antiepileptic drugs. Am J Dis Child 127:645, 1974.

Hanson JW, Smith DW: The fetal hydantoin syndrome. J Pediatr 87:285, 1975.

Hanson JW et al: Risks to the offspring of women treated with hydantoin anticonvulsant, with emphasis on the fetal hydantoin syndrome. J Pediatr 89:662, 1976.

Phelen MC, Pellock JM, Nance WE: Discordant expression of fetal hydantoin syndrome in heteropaternal dizygotic twins. N Engl J Med 307:99, 1982.

Finnell RH, Chernoff GF: Editorial comment. Genetic background: The elusive component in the fetal hydantoin syndrome. Am J Med Genet 19:459, 1984.

Strickler SM et al: Genetic predisposition to phenytoin-induced birth defects. Lancet 2:746, 1985.

Jones KL et al: Pattern of malformation in the children of women treated with carbamazepine during pregnancy. N Engl J Med 320:1661, 1989.

Buehler BA et al: Prenatal prediction of risk of the fetal hydantoin syndrome. N Engl J Med 322:1567, 1990.

Holmes LB et al: The teratogenicity of anticonvulsant drugs. N Engl J Med 344:1132, 2001.

Holmes LB: The teratogenicity of anticonvulsant drugs: A progress report. J Med Genet 39:245, 2002.

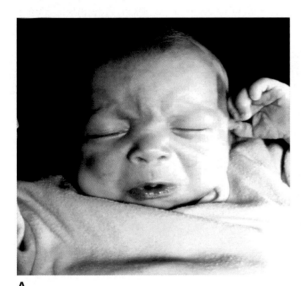
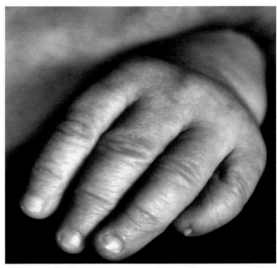

A   **B**

FIGURE 1. Fetal hydantoin syndrome. **A** and **B,** A 3-month-old infant with growth and mental deficiencies whose mother took diphenylhydantoin throughout pregnancy. Note the hypoplastic nails and phalanges, relatively low and broad nasal bridge.

FETAL VALPROATE SYNDROME

Concern was raised regarding prenatal valproic acid exposure in 1982 by Robert and Guiband, who documented an association between maternal ingestion of valproic acid and meningomyelocele in the offspring. DiLiberti and colleagues and Hanson and colleagues set forth a broader pattern of malformation in 1984.

ABNORMALITIES

Craniofacial. Narrow bifrontal diameter; high forehead; epicanthal folds connecting with an infraorbital crease or groove; telecanthus; broad, low nasal bridge with short nose and anteverted nostrils; midface hypoplasia; long philtrum with a thin vermilion border; relatively small mouth; micrognathia.

Cardiovascular. Aortic coarctation, hypoplastic left heart, aortic valve stenosis, interrupted aortic arch, secundum type atrial septal defect, pulmonary atresia without ventricular septal defect, perimembranous ventricular septal defect.

Limbs. Long, thin fingers and toes; small joint contractures; hyperconvex fingernails.

Other. Lumbosacral spina bifida, myopia.

OCCASIONAL ABNORMALITIES.

Growth and mental retardation, brain atrophy, cyst of septum pellucidum, septo-optic dysplasia, esotropia, nystagmus, tear duct anomalies, microphthalmia, iris defects, cataracts, corneal opacities, cleft palate, hearing loss, supernumerary nipples, hemangiomas, pigmentary abnormalities, hypospadias, inguinal and umbilical hernias, omphalocele, broad chest, bifid rib, postaxial polydactyly, radial ray reduction defects, nail hypoplasia, preaxial defects of feet, triphalangeal thumbs, tracheomalacia, lung hypoplasia, laryngeal hypoplasia, renal hypoplasia.

NATURAL HISTORY. Insufficient data are available to make any definitive conclusions regarding the long-term prognosis relative to intellectual performance in children prenatally exposed to valproic acid. However, concern has been raised regarding cognitive dysfunction as well as autism in prenatally exposed children. Among a group of fetuses exposed to valproic acid, 5 of 92 (5.4%) had an open (lumbo) sacral spina bifida.

ETIOLOGY. The cause of this disorder is prenatal valproic acid exposure.

References

Robert E, Guiband P: Maternal valproic acid and congenital neural tube defects. Lancet 2:934, 1982.

DiLiberti JH et al: The fetal valproate syndrome. Am J Med Genet 19:473, 1984.

Hanson JW et al: Effects of valproic acid on the fetus. Pediatr Res 18:306A, 1984.

Ardinger HH, Clark EB, Hanson JW: Cardiac malformations associated with fetal valproic acid exposure. Proc Greenwood Genet Center 5:162, 1986.

Jager-Roman E et al: Fetal growth, major malformations, and minor anomalies in infants born to women receiving valproic acid. J Pediatr 108:997, 1986.

Sharony R et al: Preaxial ray reduction defects as part of valproic acid embryofetopathy. Prenat Diagn 13:909, 1991.

Omtzigt JGC et al: The risk of spina bifida aperta after first-trimester exposure to valproate in a prenatal cohort. Neurology 42(Suppl 5):119, 1992.

Kozma C et al: Valproic acid embryopathy: Report of two siblings with further expansion of the phenotypic abnormalities and a review of the literature. Am J Med Genet 98:168, 2001.

Shepard TH et al: Update on new developments in the study of human teratogens. Teratology 65:153, 2002.

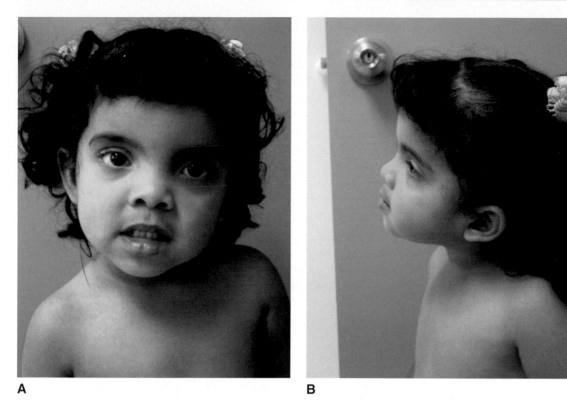

A   **B**

FIGURE 1. Fetal valproate syndrome. **A** and **B,** A 3-year-old girl with high forehead, broad nasal bridge, short nose, anteverted nares, and long philtrum.

FETAL WARFARIN SYNDROME
(WARFARIN EMBRYOPATHY, FETAL COUMARIN SYNDROME)

Nasal Hypoplasia, Stippled Epiphyses, Coumarin Derivative Exposure in First Trimester

Isolated reports of infants who, in retrospect, were affected by warfarin were followed in 1975 by simultaneous recognition of this association in five infants. A number of infants are known to have been affected.

ABNORMALITIES

Facies. Nasal hypoplasia and depressed nasal bridge, often with a deep groove between the alae nasi and nasal tip.

Skeletal. Stippling of uncalcified epiphyses, particularly of axial skeleton (vertebrae and pelvis), at the proximal femora and in the calcanei; stippling disappears after the first year.

Limbs. Hypoplastic distal phalanges that are shaped like inverted triangles with the apices pointing proximally.

Growth. Low birth weight; most demonstrate catch-up growth.

OCCASIONAL ABNORMALITIES.
Central nervous system (CNS) and eye abnormalities, including microcephaly, hydrocephalus, Dandy-Walker malformation, agenesis of corpus callosum; optic atrophy, cataracts, microphthalmia, Peter anomaly of eye, mental retardation; severe rhizomelia; scoliosis; congenital heart defect; vertebral anomalies.

NATURAL HISTORY.
Infants often present with upper airway obstruction, which is relieved by the placement of an oral airway. Cervical spine abnormalities with resultant instability has led to severe neurological dysfunction and even sudden death in some cases. The majority of affected children have done well except for persistent cosmetic malformation of the nose. The stippling is incorporated into the calcifying epiphyses and has resulted in few problems.

ETIOLOGY.
This disorder is caused by prenatal exposure to the vitamin K antagonist anticoagulant warfarin (Coumarin, Coumadin). Although the critical period of coumarin exposure is between 6 and 9 weeks' gestation, controversy exists regarding second- and third-trimester exposure. An estimate of the overall risk in pregnancies in which coumarin derivatives are used is that approximately two thirds will have a normal outcome, with the others ending in the birth of infants with fetal warfarin syndrome or CNS effects or in spontaneous abortion. Previous studies have suggested that the CNS abnormalities and mental retardation are associated with exposure limited to the second or third trimester and are related to secondary disruption of CNS architecture most likely due to hemorrhage. However, a case report suggests that prenatal coumarin exposure between the 8th and 12th weeks of gestation can lead to CNS abnormalities, indicating a direct teratogenic effect on CNS morphogenesis. Furthermore, three prospective studies of children exposed during the second and third trimesters revealed no evidence of CNS or eye abnormalities, suggesting that the incidence of CNS problems in babies born to women receiving coumarin limited to the later two trimesters must be exceedingly low.

COMMENT.
Two additional disorders with similar clinical features have been associated with disturbances of vitamin K metabolism. Pseudowarfarin embryopathy is the result of a defect of vitamin K epoxide reductase and severe maternal malabsorption resulting in fetal vitamin K deficiency are both associated with a similar phenotype. In addition, identical clinical features are seen in X-linked recessive chondrodysplasia punctata (CDPX). In vitro studies have shown that warfarin inhibits arylsulfatase E (ARSE) activity, a deficiency of which is responsible for the clinical phenotype of X-linked recessive chondrodysplasia punctata, thus explaining the phenotypic similarity.

References

DiSaia PJ: Pregnancy and delivery of a patient with a Starr-Edwards mitral valve prosthesis: Report of a case. Obstet Gynecol 28:469, 1966.

Kerber IJ, Warr OS, Richardson C: Pregnancy in a patient with a prosthetic mitral valve. JAMA 203:223, 1968.

Becker MH et al: Chondrodysplasia punctata: Is maternal warfarin a factor? Am J Dis Child 129:356, 1975.

Pettifor JM, Benson R: Congenital malformations associated with the administration of oral anticoagulants during pregnancy. J Pediatr 86:459, 1975.

Shaul WL, Emergy H, Hall JG: Chondrodysplasia punctata and maternal warfarin use during pregnancy. Am J Dis Child 129:360, 1975.

Hall JG, Pauli RM, Wilson KM: Maternal and fetal sequelae of anticoagulation during pregnancy. Am J Med 68:122, 1980.

Kaplan LC: Congenital Dandy Walker malformation associated with first trimester warfarin: A case report and literature review. Teratology 32:333, 1985.

Iturbe-Alessio I et al: Risks of anticoagulant therapy in women with artificial heart valves. N Engl J Med 315:1390, 1986.

Francho B et al: A cluster of sulfatase genes on Xp22.3: Mutations in chondrodysplasia punctata (CDPX) and implications for warfarin embryopathy. Cell 81:15, 1995.

Howe AM et al: Severe cervical dysplasia and nasal cartilage calcification following prenatal warfarin exposure. Am J Med Genet 71:391, 1997.

Menger H et al: Vitamin K deficiency embryopathy: A phenocopy of the warfarin embryopathy due to a disorder of embryonic vitamin K metabolism. Am J Med Genet 72:129, 1997.

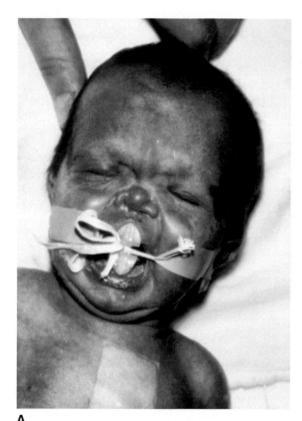

A

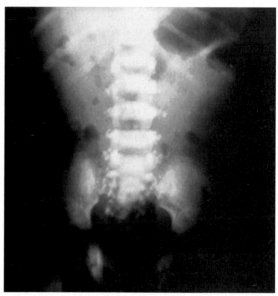

B

FIGURE 1. Fetal warfarin syndrome. Patient at 5 days of age. **A,** Note hypoplastic nose with low nasal bridge and broad, flat face. **B**, Radiograph at 1 day of age showing stippling along the vertebral column, in the sacral area, and in the proximal femurs. Stippling was also noted in the cervical vertebrae, acromion process, and tarsal bones. (**A** and **B**, From Shaul WL, Emery H, Hall JG: Am J Dis Child 129:360, 1975, with permission.)

FETAL AMINOPTERIN / METHOTREXATE SYNDROME

Cranial Dysplasia, Broad Nasal Bridge, Low-Set Ears

The folic acid antagonist aminopterin has occasionally been used as an abortifacient during the first trimester of pregnancy. Thiersch first noted abnormal morphogenesis in three abortuses and one full-term offspring of mothers who received aminopterin from 4 to 9 weeks following the presumed time of conception. Subsequently, other cases have been published, including an account of teratogenicity secondary to methotrexate, the methyl derivative of aminopterin that is frequently used for the treatment of rheumatoid arthritis and psoriasis as well as being an abortifacient.

ABNORMALITIES

Growth. Prenatal onset of growth deficiency, microcephaly.

Craniofacial. Severe hypoplasia of frontal bone, parietal bones, temporal or occipital bones, wide fontanels, and synostosis of lambdoid or coronal sutures; upsweep of frontal scalp hair; broad nasal bridge, shallow supraorbital ridges, prominent eyes, micrognathia, low-set ears, maxillary hypoplasia, epicanthal folds.

Limbs. Relative shortness, especially of forearm (mesomelia), talipes equinovarus, hypodactyly, syndactyly.

OCCASIONAL ABNORMALITIES.

Cleft palate, neural tube closure defect, mental retardation, dislocation of hip, retarded ossification of pubis and ischium, rib anomalies, short thumbs, single crease on fifth finger, dextroposition of the heart, hypotonia.

NATURAL HISTORY. Although fetal or early postnatal death does occur, a number of patients have survived beyond the first year of age. Postnatal growth deficiency occurs frequently. However, mental and motor performance usually has been described as normal.

ETIOLOGY. The cause of this disorder is aminopterin or methotrexate, its methyl derivative. Both are folic acid antagonists that inhibit dihydrofolate reductase, resulting in decreased production of purines and interference with normal DNA methylation. It has been suggested that a critical period for exposure exists at 6 through 8 weeks after conception and that a maternal methotrexate dose above 10 mg/week is necessary to produce defects in the fetus.

References

Thiersch JB: Therapeutic abortions with a folic acid antagonist, 4-aminopteroylglutamic acid (4-amino P.G.A.) administered by the oral route. Am J Obstet Gynecol 63:1298, 1952.

Milunsky A, Graef JW, Gaynor MF Jr: Methotrexate induced congenital malformations with a review of the literature. J Pediatr 72:790, 1968.

Shaw EB, Steinbach HL: Aminopterin-induced fetal malformation. Am J Dis Child 115:477, 1968.

Feldkamp M, Carey JC: Clinical teratology counseling and consultation case report: Low dose methotrexate exposure in the early weeks of pregnancy. Teratology 47:533, 1993.

Del Campo M et al: Developmental delay in fetal aminopterin/methotrexate syndrome. Teratology 60:10, 1999.

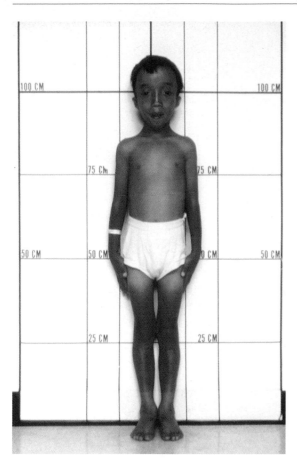

FIGURE 1. Fetal aminopterin syndrome.

RETINOIC ACID EMBRYOPATHY
(ACCUTANE EMBRYOPATHY)

Central Nervous System Defects, Microtia, Cardiac Defects

First licensed in the United States in September 1982, with the brand name Accutane, isotretinoin (13-*cis*-retinoic acid) was initially recognized to be a human teratogen 1 year later. In 1985, Lammer and colleagues set forth the spectrum of structural defects. Of 21 affected infants, 17 had defects of the craniofacial area, 12 had cardiac defects, 18 had altered morphogenesis of the CNS, and 7 had anomalies of thymic development.

ABNORMALITIES

Craniofacial. Mild facial asymmetry, bilateral microtia or anotia with stenosis of the external ear canal, posterior helical pits, facial nerve paralysis ipsilateral to malformed ear, accessory parietal sutures, a narrow sloping forehead, micrognathia, hair pattern abnormalities, flat depressed nasal bridge and ocular hypertelorism, abnormal mottling of teeth.

Cardiovascular. Conotruncal malformations, including transposition of the great vessels, tetralogy of Fallot, double-outlet right ventricle, truncus arteriosus communis, and supracristal ventricular septal defect; aortic arch interruption (type b); retroesophageal right subclavian artery; aortic arch hypoplasia; hypoplastic left ventricle.

Central Nervous System. Hydrocephalus; microcephaly; structural errors of cortical and cerebellar neuronal migration and gross malformations of posterior fossa structures, including cerebellar hypoplasia, agenesis of the vermis, cerebellar microdysgenesis, and megacisterna.

Performance. Subnormal range of intelligence.

Other. Thymic and parathyroid abnormalities.

OCCASIONAL ABNORMALITIES.
Cleft palate, vestibular dysfunction.

NATURAL HISTORY. Among the 21 affected infants evaluated by Lammer and colleagues, three were stillborn and nine were live-born infants who died secondary to cardiac defects, brain malformations, or combinations of the two. Information regarding the nine affected infants who survived the neonatal period is unknown. However, in a study designed to determine natural history, 19% of 31 prospectively ascertained 5-year-old children prenatally exposed to isotretinoin had a full-scale IQ less than 70 and an additional 28% had IQs between 71 and 85. Although each of the five patients whose IQ was less than 70 had major malformations, 6 of the 10 patients with an IQ in the borderline range did not have major malformations, indicating that the lack of major structural abnormalities does not necessarily predict normal intellectual performance. Of further potential significance, when evaluated at 10 years of age, reduced general mental ability remained with the effect more pronounced in males than females.

ETIOLOGY. The cause of this disorder is isotretinoin (Accutane). A 35% risk for the isotretinoin embryopathy exists in the offspring of women who continue to take isotretinoin beyond the 15th day following conception. There have been no affected babies born to women who stopped taking isotretinoin before the 15th day following conception. Furthermore, there is no evidence to suggest that maternal use of the drug before conception is teratogenic. Daily dosage of isotretinoin from 0.5 to 1.5 mg/kg of maternal body weight is thought to be teratogenic.

References

Rosa FW: Teratogenicity of isotretinoin. Lancet 2:513, 1983.

Fernoff PM, Lammer EJ: Craniofacial features of isotretinoin embryopathy. J Pediatr 105:595, 1984.

Lott IT et al: Fetal hydrocephalus and ear anomalies associated with maternal use of isotretinoin. J Pediatr 105:597, 1984.

Lammer EJ et al: Retinoic acid embryopathy. N Engl J Med 313:837, 1985.

Lammer EJ et al: Risk for major malformations among human fetuses exposed to isotretinoin (13-*cis*-retinoic acid). Teratology 35:68A, 1987.

Teratology Society: Recommendations for isotretinoin use in women of childbearing potential. Teratology 44:1, 1991.

Adams J, Lammer EJ: Neurobehavioral teratology of isotretinoins. Reprod Toxicol 7:175, 1993.

Adams J et al: Neuropsychological characteristics of children embryologically exposed to isotretinoin (Accutane): Outcome at age 10. Neurotoxicol Teratol 23:297, 2001.

McCaffery PJ et al: Too much of a good thing: Retinoic acid as an endogenous regulator of neural differentiation and exogenous teratogen. Eur J Neurosci 18:457, 2003.

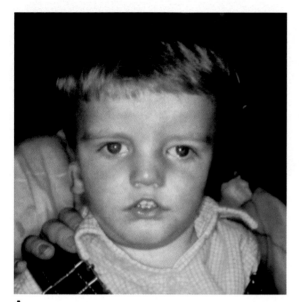

A

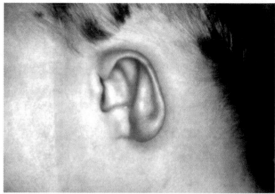

B

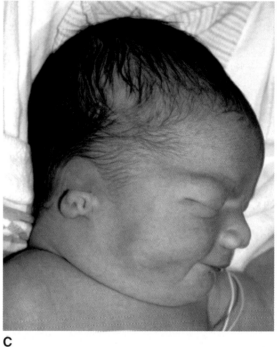

C

FIGURE 1. Retinoic acid embryopathy. **A** and **B,** A 2½-year-old boy showing triangular facies, ocular hypertelorism, downslanting palpebral fissures, and malformed external ear. (Courtesy of Dr. Edward Lammer, Children's Hospital, Oakland, Calif.) **C,** More severely affected neonate with hydrocephalus and microtia. (**C,** Courtesy of Dr. Cynthia Curry, University of California, San Francisco.)

FETAL VARICELLA SYNDROME

Cicatricial Skin, Limb Hypoplasia, Mental Deficiency with Seizures

LaForet and Lynch first described defects in the child of a woman who had varicella during early gestation. Strabstein and colleagues summarized five cases, and Dudgeon has personally evaluated at least eight additional cases. Many additional cases have been reported.

ABNORMALITIES

Performance. Mental deficiency with or without seizures.
Growth. Variable prenatal growth deficiency, microcephaly.
Eyes. Chorioretinitis.
Limbs. Hypoplasia of limb, with or without rudimentary digits, with or without paralysis with atrophy of limb; clubfoot.
Skin. Cutaneous scars.

OCCASIONAL ABNORMALITIES.
Cataracts; microphthalmia; atrophy and hypoplasia of optic disk; nystagmus; Horner syndrome; underdeveloped clavicle, scapula, and rib; anal/vesicle sphincter dysfunction; scoliosis.

NATURAL HISTORY. Fifty percent of affected babies have died in early infancy. Although it has previously been suggested that the majority of the survivors have had mental deficiency with seizures, prospective studies indicate that a wide spectrum of severity exists for this disorder. One of the two affected patients reported by Jones and colleagues had mild cutaneous scars on the face, arms, and legs, a left Horner syndrome, a retinal scar, and normal IQ.

ETIOLOGY. Most cases have occurred in the wake of maternal varicella during the period of 8 to 20 weeks' gestation. The incidence of problems in the offspring of women infected with varicella before the 20th week of pregnancy is between 1% and 2%. Only a small proportion (8.4%) of fetuses whose mothers are infected with varicella are themselves infected with the virus.

COMMENT. Children born to women infected with varicella-zoster virus during pregnancy and who do not have the structural features characteristic of the fetal varicella syndrome are not neurodevelopmentally different from unexposed, uninfected control children.

References

LaForet EG, Lynch CL Jr: Multiple congenital defects following maternal varicella. N Engl J Med 236:534, 1947.

Strabstein JC et al: Is there a congenital varicella syndrome? J Pediatr 64:239, 1974.

Higa K et al: Varicella-zoster virus infections during pregnancy: Hypothesis concerning the mechanisms of congenital malformations. Obstet Gynecol 69:214, 1987.

Lambert SR et al: Ocular manifestations of the congenital varicella syndrome. Arch Ophthalmol 107:52, 1989.

Jones KL et al: Offspring of women infected with varicella during pregnancy: A prospective study. Teratology 49:29, 1994.

Mouly F et al: Prenatal diagnosis of fetal varicella-zoster virus infection with polymerase chain reaction of amniotic fluid in 107 cases. Am J Obstet Gynecol 177:894, 1997.

Mattson SN et al: Neurodevelopmental follow-up of children of women infected with varicella during pregnancy: A prospective study. Pediatr Infect Dis J 22:819, 2003.

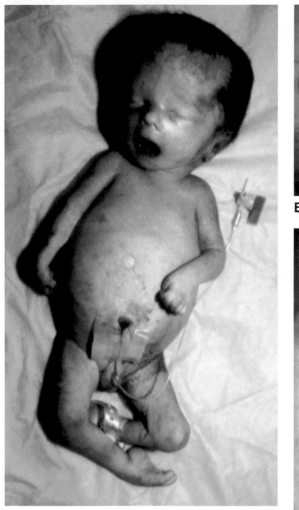

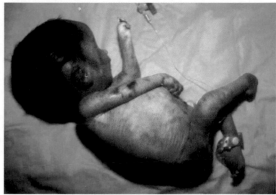

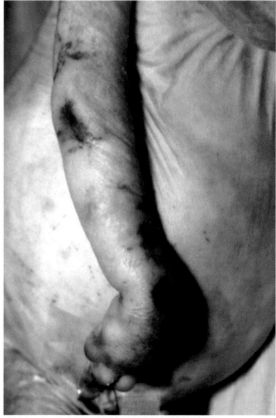

FIGURE 1. Fetal varicella effects. **A–C,** Note the hydrocephalus, short limbs with severe neurologic compromise, and cicatricial skin changes in limbs.

HYPERTHERMIA-INDUCED SPECTRUM OF DEFECTS

A number of animal studies, the most extensive of which have been those of Edwards on the guinea pig, have shown severe maternal hyperthermia during the first one third to one half of gestation to be teratogenic.

Although studies in the human are limited, problems of growth, development, and dysfunction of the brain similar to those seen in the animal studies have been documented. The nature of the defects relates to the timing and extent of the hyperthermia rather than to its cause. Most of the relevant cases have been tentatively related to febrile illness, with the patient having a temperature of 38.9°C or higher, most commonly 40°C or above. The duration of the high fever has been 1 day or more, usually several days, which is unusual in the first third of gestation. The illness has varied, with influenza, pyelonephritis, and streptococcal pharyngitis being the most common. Two cases were considered secondary to severe hyperthermia induced by prolonged sauna bathing (30 to 45 minutes), and one case was thought to be related to very prolonged hot tub bathing. These three cases are extraordinary in the duration of heat exposure.

Retrospective human studies of more than 170 cases of neural tube defect, including anencephaly, meningomyelocele, and occipital encephalocele, have disclosed an overall history of maternal hyperthermia during the week of neural tube closure (21 to 28 days) in approximately 10% of the cases, whereas no such history was determined in the controls. These findings are compatible with the hypothesis that hyperthermia is one cause for neural tube defects in the human.

A 14% incidence of "febrile" illness during early pregnancy in the mothers of 113 embryos with neural tube defects who were aborted therapeutically was documented. The embryos were obtained through the Congenital Anomaly Research Center of Kyoto University. The history of maternal fever was documented before or immediately after the fetal loss, before the neural tube defect was documented.

In addition, a number of craniofacial anomalies including microcephaly, small midface, microphthalmia, micrognathia, and occasionally cleft lip with or without palate, cleft palate alone, conotruncal heart defects, and ear anomalies as well as mental deficiency and hypotonia have been seen.

A single prospective study involving 115 pregnant women who reported a fever of 38.9°C or greater lasting for at least 24 hours (group 1), 147 pregnant women who reported fever of either less than 38.9°C or lasting less than 24 hours (group 2), and 289 pregnant women who reported no fever (group 3) has been reported. The combined prevalence of all major structural malformations was increased but not significantly so in those women in group 1. However, 2 of 34, or 5.9%, of women in group 1 who had a high fever during the critical period for neural tube closure carried fetuses with anencephaly, compared to none in group 2 or 3. In addition, the specific craniofacial anomalies previously documented in retrospective studies were found more frequently in the offspring of pregnant women in group 1.

In addition to potential dysmorphogenesis in early gestation, maternal hyperthermia has been associated with an increase in spontaneous abortion, stillbirth, and prematurity.

References

Edwards MJ: Congenital defects in guinea pigs following induced hyperthermia during gestation. Arch Pathol 84:42, 1967.

Edwards MJ: Congenital defects in guinea pigs: Prenatal retardation of brain growth of guinea pigs following hyperthermia during gestation. Teratology 2:239, 1969.

Edwards MJ: The experimental production of arthrogryposis multiplex congenita in guinea pigs by maternal hyperthermia during gestation. J Pathol 104:221, 1971.

Chance PI, Smith DW: Hyperthermia and meningomyelocele and anencephaly. Lancet 1:769, 1978.

Halperin LR, Wilroy RS: Maternal hyperthermia and neural tube defects. Lancet 2:212, 1978.

Miller P, Smith DW, Shepard T: Maternal hyperthermia as a possible cause of anencephaly. Lancet 1:519, 1978.

Smith DW, Clarren SK, Harvey MA: Hyperthermia as a possible teratogenic agent. J Pediatr 92:878, 1978.

Clarren SK et al: Hyperthermia—a prospective evaluation of a possible teratogenic agent in man. J Pediatr 95:81, 1979.

Shiota K: Neural tube defects and maternal hyperthermia in early pregnancy: Epidemiology in a human embryo population. Am J Med Genet 12:281, 1982.

Milunsky A et al: Maternal heat exposure and neural tube defects. JAMA 268:882, 1992.

Lynberg MC: Maternal flu, fever and the risk of neural tube defects: A population based case-control study. Am J Epidemiol 140:244, 1994.

Chambers CD et al: Maternal fever and birth outcome: A prospective study. Teratology 58:251, 1998.

Shaw GM et al: Maternal periconceptional vitamins: Interactions with selected factors and congenital anomalies? Epidemiology 13:625, 2002.

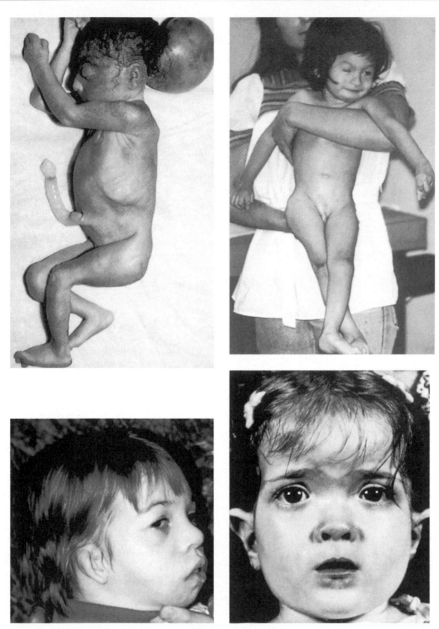

FIGURE 1. Hyperthermia-induced defects. *Upper left*, Encephalocele; maternal history of high fever between days 23 and 25 of gestation. *Upper right*, An 18-month-old severely retarded boy with hypotonic diplegia, micropenis, unilateral microphthalmia, cleft palate, and micrognathia. Maternal fever of 40°C to 41°C between the fourth and fifth weeks of gestation. *Lower left*, A 12-year-old severely retarded girl with hypotonic diplegia, midface hypoplasia, micrognathia, incomplete ear morphogenesis, and a cardiac defect. Maternal "flu" with high fever between the sixth and eighth weeks of gestation. *Lower right*, A 14-month-old infant with moderate hypotonic diplegia and developmental deficiency, who has a hypoplastic midface with mild ocular hypertelorism, low nasal bridge, and prominent auricles. Maternal fever of 40°C between the seventh and eighth weeks of gestation. (*Lower right,* from Pleet H, Graham JM Jr, Smith DW: J Pediatr 67:785, 1981, with permission.)

S Miscellaneous Syndromes

COFFIN-SIRIS SYNDROME

Hypoplastic to Absent Fifth Finger and Toenails, Coarse Facies

Coffin and Siris reported three patients with this disorder in 1970, and Weiswasser and colleagues reported an additional case in 1973. Also, several of the patients described by Senior might represent examples of this syndrome. More than 70 cases have been reported.

ABNORMALITIES

Growth. Prenatal onset of mild-to-moderate growth deficiency, delayed bone age.
Performance. Mild-to-moderate mental retardation, moderate-to-severe hypotonia, seizures.
Craniofacial. Mild microcephaly, coarse facies, a wide mouth with full lips, flat nasal bridge, broad nasal tip, long philtrum, abnormal ears, bushy eyebrows, long eyelashes.
Limbs. Hypoplastic to absent fifth finger and toenails, with lesser hypoplasia in other digits; absence of terminal phalanges (particularly of the fifth digit); lax joints with radial dislocation at elbow; coxa valga; small patellae.
Hair. General hirsutism with tendency to have sparse scalp hair.
Other. Visual problems, hearing loss, abnormal/delayed dentition.

OCCASIONAL ABNORMALITIES.

Ptosis of eyelids, hypotelorism, macroglossia, absent tear ducts, preauricular skin tag, choanal atresia, cleft palate, hemangioma, cryptorchidism, umbilical or inguinal hernias, short sternum, cardiac defect (patent ductus arteriosus, ventricular septal defect, atrial septal defect, tetralogy of Fallot, patent foramen ovale with aberrant pulmonary vein), gastrointestinal anomalies (gastric and duodenal ulcer, neonatal intussusception, intestinal malrotation, gastric outlet obstruction secondary to redundant gastric mucosa), short forearm, vertebral anomalies, kyphosis, scoliosis, diaphragmatic hernia, Dandy-Walker anomaly of brain, hypoplasia or partial agenesis of corpus callosum, small cerebellum, and in one patient abnormal olivae and arcuate nuclei and cerebellar heterotopias, renal anomalies (hydronephrosis, microureters with stenosis of the vesicoureteral junction, ectopic kidney), genital anomalies including cryptorchidism, hypospadias, and absent uterus, hypoglycemia, premature thelarche.

NATURAL HISTORY. Feeding problems and recurrent upper and lower respiratory tract infections are frequent during early life. Onset of speech is severely delayed. The coarse facies may not be present at birth. The sparse scalp hair improves with age.

ETIOLOGY. The majority of cases have been sporadic. Both an autosomal recessive inheritance pattern, based on four sibling pairs born to unaffected parents, and autosomal dominant inheritance, based on two siblings with a mildly affected father, have been suggested. A similar 7q breakpoint in two affected patients with balanced translocations suggests that 7q32-q34 is a candidate region for the gene responsible for Coffin-Siris syndrome.

References
Coffin GS, Siris E: Mental retardation with absent fifth fingernail and terminal phalanx. Am J Dis Child 119:433, 1970.
Senior B: Impaired growth and onychodysplasia: Short children with tiny toenails. Am J Dis Child 122:7, 1971.
Carey JC, Hall BD: The Coffin-Siris syndrome. Am J Dis Child 132:667, 1978.
DeBassio WA, Kemper TL, Knoelel JE: Coffin-Siris syndrome: Neuropathologic findings. Arch Neurol 42:350, 1985.
Bodurtha J et al: Distinctive gastrointestinal anomaly associated with Coffin-Siris syndrome. J Pediatr 109:1015, 1986.
Levy P, Baraitser M: Coffin-Siris syndrome. J Med Genet 28:338, 1991.
Swillen A et al: The Coffin-Siris syndrome: Data on mental development, language, behavior and social skills in 12 children. Clin Genet 48:177, 1995.
McGhee EM et al: Candidate region for Coffin-Siris syndrome at 7q32-34. Am J Med Genet 93:241, 2000.
Fleck BJ et al: Coffin-Siris syndrome: Review and presentation of new cases from a questionnaire study. Am J Med Genet 99:1, 2001.

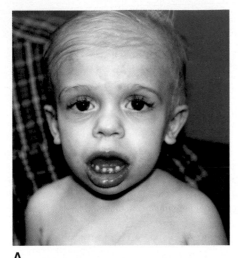

A

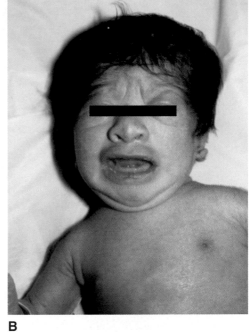

B

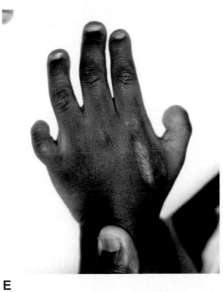

C

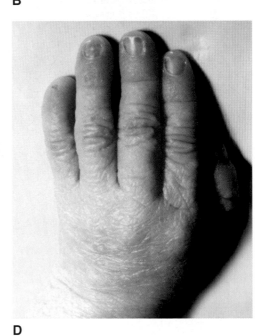

D

E

FIGURE 1. Coffin-Siris syndrome. **A–E,** Note the course face, wide mouth with full lips, long eyelashes, and hypoplastic fifth fingernails. (**A, C,** and **E,** Courtesy of Dr. D. Bryan Hall, University of Kentucky, Lexington.)

667

BÖRJESON-FORSSMAN-LEHMANN SYNDROME

Large Ears, Hypogonadism, Severe Mental Deficiency

In 1961, Börjeson and colleagues described an entity of X-linked mental deficiency, epilepsy, hypogonadism, obesity, and dysmorphic facies seen in three related males and three of their less severely affected female relatives.

ABNORMALITIES

Growth. Height usually less than 50th percentile, moderate obesity may decrease in later life.

Performance. Severe mental deficiency, with an IQ of 10 to 40; supraspinal hypotonia; markedly abnormal electroencephalograph, with very poor alpha rhythms; seizures may be present.

Craniofacial. Microcephaly, coarse facies with prominent supraorbital ridges and deep-set eyes, large (7.5 to 9 cm) but normally formed ears.

Eyes. Nystagmus, ptosis, and poor vision, with a variety of retinal or optic nerve abnormalities.

Genitalia. Small penis with small and soft or undescended testes and delayed secondary sexual characteristics; hypogonadism appears to be hypogonadotropic.

Skeletal. Variable radiographic abnormalities: thick calvarium, small cervical spinal canal, mild scoliosis, kyphosis, Scheuermann-like vertebral changes, metaphyseal widening of the long bones and hands, hypoplastic distal and middle phalanges, thin cortices.

Other. Central nervous system anomalies are due to a primary abnormality of neuronal migration, soft and fleshy hands with tapering fingers.

NATURAL HISTORY.
From birth, these patients are hypotonic, with severe developmental delay. Walking may begin as late as 4 to 6 years and remains awkward. Speech is limited to a few phrases at most. There is no known unusual susceptibility to health problems, although broncho-pneumonia was responsible for the demise of two of the original patients at the ages of 20 and 44 years. Life span is presumed to be normal. A sheltered environment is necessary because of severe limitations of neurodevelopmental performance.

ETIOLOGY.
This disorder has an X-linked recessive inheritance pattern. Mutations of plant homeodomain (PHD)-like finger gene (PHF6) located at Xq26-27 are responsible. PHF6 is a zinc-finger gene of unknown function. Heterozygotes fall into a spectrum of those without any observable features to those with the abnormalities of growth and craniofacial, ocular, and skeletal features characteristic of this syndrome. Performance ranges from moderate mental retardation (IQ of 56 to 70) to above-average intelligence in heterozygous females.

References

Börjeson M, Forssman H, Lehmann O: Combination of idiocy, epilepsy, hypogonadism, dwarfism, hypometabolism, and morphologic peculiarities inherited as an X-linked recessive syndrome. Proceedings of the Second International Congress on Mental Retardation, Vienna (1961), Part I. Basel: Karger Publishers, 1963, p 188.

Börjeson M, Forssman H, Lehmann O: An X-linked, recessively inherited syndrome characterized by grave mental deficiency, epilepsy, and endocrine disorder. Acta Med Scand 171:13, 1962.

Brun A, Börjeson M, Forssman H: An inherited syndrome with mental deficiency and endocrine disorder: A pathoanatomical study. J Ment Defic Res 18:317, 1974.

Robinson LK et al: The Börjeson-Forssman-Lehmann syndrome. Am J Med Genet 15:457, 1983.

Ardinger HH, Hanson JW, Zellweger HU: Börjeson-Forssman-Lehmann syndrome: Further delineation in five cases. Am J Med Genet 19:653, 1984.

Matthews KD et al: Linkage localization of Börjeson-Forssman-Lehmann syndrome. Am J Med Genet 34:470, 1989.

Turner G et al: Börjeson-Forssman-Lehmann syndrome: Clinical manifestations and gene localization to Xq26-27. Am J Med Genet 34:463, 1989.

Lower KM et al: Mutations in PHF6 are associated with Börjeson-Forssman- Lehmann syndrome. Nat Genet 32:661, 2002.

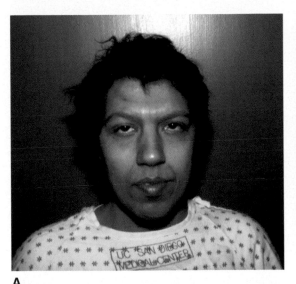
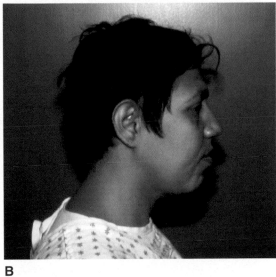

A   **B**

FIGURE 1. Börjeson-Forssman-Lehmann syndrome. **A** and **B,** A man with coarse face, prominent supraorbital ridges, ptosis, and large ears. (From Robinson LK et al: Am J Med Genet 15:487, 1983.)

ALAGILLE SYNDROME
(Arteriohepatic Dysplasia)

Cholestasis, Peripheral Pulmonic Stenosis, Peculiar Facies

Initially described by Alagille and colleagues in 1969, this disorder was more completely delineated in 1973 by Watson and Miller, who reported five families with 21 affected individuals. Since then, more than 200 cases have been described. Males and females are affected equally.

ABNORMALITIES

General. Growth retardation (50%).
Craniofacial. Typical facies (95%) consisting of deep-set eyes, broad forehead, long straight nose with flattened tip, prominent chin, small, low-set or malformed ears.
Eyes. Posterior embryotoxon (abnormal prominence of the Schwalbe line, the line formed by the junction of the Descement membrane with the uvea at the anterior chamber angle causing the margin of the cornea to be opaque) in 88%, Axenfeld anomaly (iris strands).
Cardiac. Right-sided defects or pulmonary circulation defects; 67% have peripheral pulmonary artery stenosis with or without associated complex cardiovascular abnormalities.
Skeletal. Butterfly-like vertebral arch defects (87%); other vertebral defects, including hemivertebrae and spina bifida occulta; rib anomalies.
Hepatic. Paucity of intrahepatic interlobular bile ducts (85%); chronic cholestasis (96%); hypercholesterolemia.

OCCASIONAL ABNORMALITIES

General. Mild mental retardation (16%).
Eyes. Retinal degeneration including chorioretinal involvement and pigmentary clumping, strabismus, ectopic pupils, choroidal folds, anomalous optic disk or vessels and refractive errors.
Cardiac. Atrial septal defect, ventricular septal defect, patent ductus arteriosus, coarctation of the aorta.
Hands. Short distal phalanges, fifth finger clinodactyly.

Liver. Extrahepatic biliary duct involvement (20%), primary hepatocellular cancer.
Renal. Structural and parenchymal abnormalities (10%), decreased creatinine clearance, increased blood urea nitrogen, histologic abnormalities consisting of mesangiolipidosis.
Genitalia. Hypogonadism.
Endocrine. Decreased growth hormone, increased testosterone, hypothyroidism, delayed puberty.
Other. Cleft palate, shortened ulna, spina bifida occulta, lack of normal increase in interpedicular distance from L1–L5, abnormalities of inner ear structures, clubfeet, craniosynostosis, thyroid cancer, high-pitched voice, hypodontia, palatal and gingival xanthomas, radioulnar synostosis.

NATURAL HISTORY. Most patients present with neonatal jaundice. Cholestasis (elevated serum bile acids), which develops within the first 3 months in 44% and between 4 months and 3 years in the remainder, is manifested by pruritus, acholic stools, xanthomata, or hepatomegaly. Intrahepatic bile duct paucity is often progressive but may not be evident in newborns. Progression to cirrhosis and liver failure occurs in many. Transplantation is required in 15%. Long-term prognosis depends on severity and duration of early cholestasis, severity of cardiovascular defects, liver status as it relates to liver failure or portal hypertension, and occurrence of intracranial bleed. The 20-year predicted life expectancy is 75% for all patients, 80% for those not requiring liver transplantation, and 60% for those who require liver transplantation.

ETIOLOGY. This disorder has an autosomal dominant inheritance pattern with highly variable expressivity. Mutations in JAG1 located within chromosome band 20p12 are responsible in 70% of cases. Less than 7% have a chromosomal deletion or rearrangement involving 20p12. JAG1 is a cell surface protein that is a ligand for the Notch transmembrane receptor. JAG1 and Notch are parts of the Notch signaling pathway, which is critical for the regulation of cell fate decisions. The name

Notch comes from the characteristic notched wing found in fruit flies carrying only one functional copy of the gene.

References

Alagille D et al: L'atrésie des voies biliaires intrahépatiques avec voies biliaires extrahépatiques perméables chez l'enfant. J Par Pediatr 301, 1969.

Watson GH, Miller V: Arteriohepatic dysplasia: Familial pulmonary arterial stenosis with neonatal liver disease. Arch Dis Child 48:459, 1973.

Alagille D et al: Hepatic ductular hypoplasia associated with characteristic facies, vertebral malformations, retarded physical, mental and sexual development, and cardiac murmur. J Pediatr 86:63, 1975.

Bryne JLB et al: Del(20p) with manifestations of arteriohepatic dysplasia. Am J Med Genet 24:673, 1986.

Alagille D et al: Syndromic paucity of interlobular bile ducts (Alagille syndrome or arteriohepatic dysplasia): Review of 80 cases. J Pediatr 110:195, 1987.

Spinner NB et al: Cytogenetically balanced t(2;20) in a two-generation family with Alagille syndrome: Cytogenetic and molecular studies. Am J Hum Genet 55:238, 1994.

Emerick KM et al: Features of Alagille syndrome in 92 patients: Frequency and relation to prognosis. Hepatology 29:822, 1999.

Krantz I et al: Clinical and molecular genetics of Alagille syndrome. Curr Opin Pediatr 11:558, 1999.

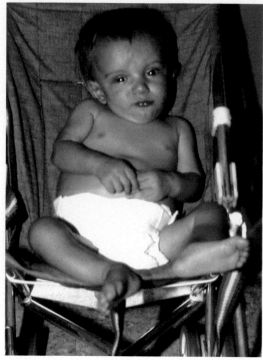

A

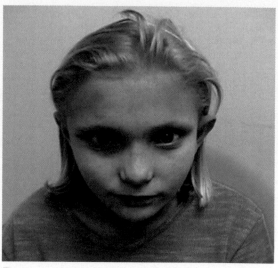

B

FIGURE 1. Arteriohepatic dysplasia. **A,** A 1½-year-old with broad forehead and prominent chin. **B–E,** Note the deep-set eyes; broad forehead; long, straight nose with flattened tip and prominent chin. (**B–F,** Courtesy of Dr. Ian Krantz, University of Pennsylvania.)

Continued

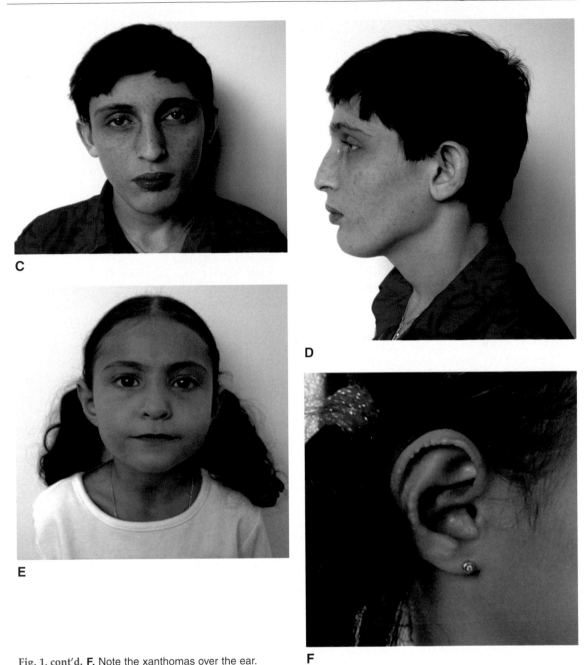

Fig. 1, cont'd. **F,** Note the xanthomas over the ear.

MELNICK-NEEDLES SYNDROME

Prominent Eyes, Bowing of Long Bones, Ribbon-Like Ribs

This disorder was reported by Melnick and Needles in 1966, and subsequently approximately 50 cases have been documented.

ABNORMALITIES

Craniofacial. Small facies with prominent hirsute forehead and exophthalmos, mild hypertelorism, full cheeks, small mandible with an obtuse angle and hypoplastic coronoid process, late closure of fontanels, dense base of skull, lag in paranasal sinus development, micrognathia, malaligned teeth.

Limbs. Short upper arms and distal phalanges; bowing of humerus, radius, ulna, and tibia; metaphyseal flaring of long bones; coxa valga; genu valgum; short distal phalanges with cone-shaped epiphyses.

Other Skeletal. Relatively small thoracic cage with irregular ribbon-like ribs and short clavicles with wide medial ends and narrow shoulders, short scapulae, and pectus excavatum; tall vertebrae with anterior concavity in thoracic region; iliac flaring; kyphoscoliosis.

OCCASIONAL ABNORMALITIES.

Strabismus, coarse hair, cleft palate, large ears, hoarse voice, ureteral stenosis leading to hydronephrosis, hip dislocation, clubfeet, pes planus, delayed motor development, short stature, muscle hypotonia, limitations of elbow extension, acroosteolysis, mitral and tricuspid valve prolapse, hyperlaxity of skin in males.

NATURAL HISTORY.

Small face with prominent and hyperteloric-appearing eyes. Abnormal gait and bowing may be the first evident signs of the disorder. Dental malocclusion is frequent, and with time, osteoarthritis of the back or hip may become a problem. A contracted pelvis in the female may make vaginal delivery difficult. Stature is usually normal. Frequent respiratory infections may be due to the small thoracic cage. Pulmonary hypertension has occurred.

ETIOLOGY.

This disorder has an X-linked dominant inheritance pattern. The vast majority of cases have been female. Mutations in the gene, FLNA which encodes filamin A, a protein that regulates reorganization of the actin cytoskeleton, are responsible. Males with characteristic features of this disorder have been born to unaffected mothers and thus represent fresh gene mutations. However, early lethality, as well as a much more severe phenotype, has been documented in all males that have been born to affected mothers. Characteristic features in those cases include widely spaced, prominent eyes; severe micrognathia; omphalocele; hypoplastic kidneys; positional deformities of the hands and feet; cervicothoracic kyphosis; thoracolumbar lordosis; bowing of the long bones; and pseudoarthrosis of the clavicles.

COMMENT.

In addition to Melnick-Needles syndrome, mutations in FLNA are responsible for oto-palato-digital syndrome, types 1 (OPD1) and 2 (OPD2), and frontometaphyseal dysplasia, disorders with overlapping clinical phenotypes, which have been referred to as the OPD-spectrum disorders.

References

Melnick JC, Needles CF: An undiagnosed bone dysplasia. Am J Roentgenol Radium Ther Nucl Med 97:39, 1966.

Coste F, Maroteaux P, Chouraki L: Osteoplasty (Melnick-Needles syndrome). Ann Rheum Dis 27:360, 1968.

von Oeyen P et al: Omphalocele and multiple severe congenital anomalies associated with osteodysplasty (Melnick-Needles syndrome). Am J Med Genet 13:453, 1982.

Krajewska-Walasek M et al: Melnick-Needles syndrome in males. Am J Med Genet 27:153, 1987.

Eggli K et al: Melnick-Needles syndrome: Four new cases. Pediatr Radiol 22:257, 1992.

Robertson S et al: Are Melnick-Needles syndrome and oto-palato-digital syndrome type II allelic? Observations in a four-generation kindred. Am J Med Genet 71:341, 1997.

Verloes A et al: Fronto-otopalatodigital osteodysplasia: Clinical evidence for a single entity encompassing Melnick-Needles syndrome, otopalatodigital syndrome types 1 and 2, and frontometaphyseal dysplasia. Am J Med Genet 90:407, 2000.

Robertson SP et al: Localized mutations in the gene encoding the cytoskeletal protein filamin A cause diverse malformations in humans. Nat Genet 33:487, 2003.

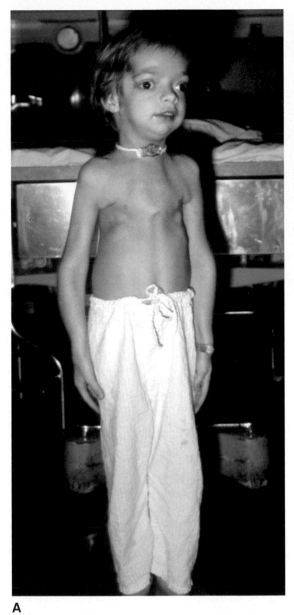

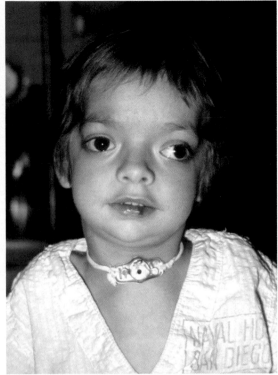

FIGURE 1. Melnick-Needles syndrome. **A** and **B,** Note the exophthalmos, hypertelorism, full cheeks, small mandible, and relatively small thorax. (Courtesy of Dr. William Nyhan, University of California, San Diego.)

BARDET-BIEDL SYNDROME

Retinal Pigmentation, Obesity, Polydactyly

The variable manifestations of this syndrome were initially described by Bardet and Biedl in the 1920s. Subsequently, more than 300 cases have been reported. This disorder is clearly different from the condition described in 1865 by Laurence and Moon, although it was referred to as the Laurence-Moon-Biedl syndrome in the third edition of this book.

ABNORMALITIES

Growth. Obesity (83%) with the majority below the 50th percentile for height.

Performance. Mental deficiency with verbal IQ of 79 or below in 77% and performance IQ of 79 or below in 44%, inappropriate mannerisms and shallow affect are common, IQ correlates with visual handicap.

Ocular. Retinal dystrophy (100%), myopia (75%), astigmatism (63%), nystagmus (52%), glaucoma (22%), posterior capsular cataracts (44%), mature cataracts or aphakia (30%), typical retinitis pigmentosa (8%).

Limbs. Postaxial polydactyly (58%); syndactyly; brachydactyly of hands (50%); broad, short feet.

Kidney. Abnormal calyces (95%), communicating cysts or diverticulae (62%), fetal lobulations (95%), diffuse cortical loss (29%), focal scarring (24%).

Hypogonadism. Small penis and testes (88%).

OTHER ABNORMALITIES.

Cardiac defects, macrocephaly, dental anomalies, urologic anomalies, diabetes mellitus, diabetes insipidus, clinodactyly of the fifth finger, cystic dilatation of the intrahepatic and common bile ducts, hepatic fibrosis, hirsutism, ovarian stromal hyperplasia, vaginal atresia, hearing loss.

NATURAL HISTORY.

The average age at diagnosis is 9 years. Obesity begins to develop at approximately 2 to 3 years of age. The mental deficiency is usually mild to moderate. However, significant behavioral problems occur in 33% including immaturity, frustration, disinhibition, and poor concentration/hyperactivity. Schizophrenia has been described occasionally. Ataxia, poor coordination, and imbalance are common. The retinal dystrophy generally results in problems with night vision during childhood, constricted visual fields, abnormalities of color vision, and extinguished or minimal rod-and-cone responses on electroretinography. Visual acuity deteriorates with age. Only approximately 15% of patients show an atypical retinal pigmentation by 5 to 10 years of age. However, by age 20, 73% of patients are blind. Most patients have mild problems in renal function with partial defects in urine concentration and renal tubular acidosis. Renal failure occurs, although infrequently requiring transplant in 4%. Hypertension is present in 60%. The hypogonadism has been described as primary germinal hypoplasia and also as hypogonadotropic in type. Although no affected male has fathered a child, women have given birth to children. Normal development of secondary sexual characteristics is the rule in women. Irregular menstrual periods are common. Asthma has occurred in 25% of cases. An increased prevalence of renal malformations and renal cell carcinoma has been described in unaffected relatives of affected individuals.

ETIOLOGY.

Eight independent BBS loci have been mapped, and each of them has been cloned. BBS is thought to result primarily from ciliary dysfunction. The previously held concept that Bardet-Biedel syndrome is a Mendelian recessive disorder may be too simplistic because, in at least some cases, two mutations in one BBS gene and a third mutation in another BBS gene are required for manifestation of the clinical phenotype (triallelic inheritance). From a practical standpoint, recurrence risk for unaffected parents who have had one affected child is 25%.

COMMENT.

The gene for BBS6 (MKKS), located on chromosome 20p12, encodes chaperonins and is also responsible for McKusick-Kaufman syndrome, a disorder with striking phenotypic overlap.

References

Bardet G: Sur un syndrome d'obesité infantile avec polydactylie et rétinite pigmentaire. (Contribution à l'étude des formes cliniques de l'obesité hypophysaire.) Faculté de Medicine de Paris, Thesis, 470, 1920.

Biedl A: Ein Geschwisterpaar mit adiposo-genitaler Dystropie. Dtsch Med Wochenschr 48:1630, 1922.

Klein D, Ammann F: The syndrome of Laurence-Moon-Bardet-Biedl and allied diseases in Switzerland: Clinical, genetic and epidemiological studies. J Neurol Sci 9:479, 1969.

Hurley RM et al: The renal lesion of the Laurence-Moon-Beidl syndrome. J Pediatr 87:206, 1975.

Green JS et al: The cardinal manifestations of Bardet-Biedl syndrome: A form of Laurence-Moon-Biedl syndrome. N Engl J Med 321:1002, 1989.

Kwitek-Black AE et al: Linkage of Bardet-Biedl syndrome to chromosome 16q and evidence for non-allelic genetic heterogeneity. Nat Genet 5:392, 1993.

Elbedour K et al: Cardiac abnormalities in the Bardet-Biedl syndrome: Echocardiographic studies of 22 patients. Am J Med Genet 52:164, 1994.

Beales PL et al: New criteria for improved diagnosis of Bardet-Biedl syndrome: Results of a population survey. J Med Genet 36:437, 1999.

Slavotinek AM et al: Mutations in MKKS cause Bardet-Biedl syndrome. Nat Genet 26:15, 2000.

Beales PL et al: Genetic interaction of BBS1 mutations with other alleles at other BBS loci can result in non-mendelian Bardet-Biedel syndrome. Am J Hum Genet 72:1187, 2003.

Mykytyn K et al: Evaluation of complex inheritance involving the most common Bardet-Biedel syndrome locus (BBS1). Am J Hum Genet 72:429, 2003.

Fan Y et al: Mutations in a member of the Ras superfamily of small GTP-binding proteins causes Bardet-Biedl syndrome. Nat Genet 36:989, 2004.

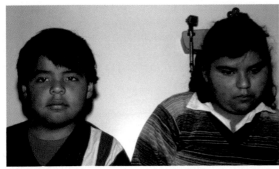

A

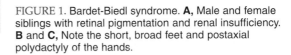

B

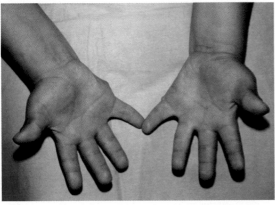

C

FIGURE 1. Bardet-Biedl syndrome. **A,** Male and female siblings with retinal pigmentation and renal insufficiency. **B** and **C,** Note the short, broad feet and postaxial polydactyly of the hands.

McKUSICK-KAUFMAN SYNDROME

Hydrometrocolpos, Postaxial Polydactyly, Congenital Heart Defects

Initially described by McKusick and colleagues in the Older Order Amish of Lancaster County, Pennsylvania, this disorder was further delineated by Kaufman and colleagues. More than 60 cases have been reported.

ABNORMALITIES

Genital. Hydrometrocolpos secondary to vaginal atresia, transverse vaginal stenosis and, in one case, cervical atresia.
Urinary Tract. Hydronephrosis, hydroureters.
Limbs. Postaxial polydactyly of hands or feet.
Gastrointestinal. Imperforate anus, rectovaginal or vesicovaginal fistula.
Other. Cardiac defects.

OCCASIONAL ABNORMALITIES.
Esophageal atresia with T-E fistula, Hirschsprung disease, intestinal malrotation, vaginal duplication, high urethral opening, hypospadias, cryptorchidism, polycystic kidneys, congenital hip dislocation, bilateral cervical ribs, syndactyly, nonimmune hydrops.

NATURAL HISTORY. Compression by the distended uterus can result in multiple secondary complications. These include obstruction of the bladder leading to dilatation of the proximal urinary tract with renal destruction, oligohydramnios, and secondary pulmonary hypoplasia; intestinal tract obstruction leading to perforation and intrauterine peritonitis; compression of the inferior vena cava resulting in hydrops fetalis and edema of the legs; and anterior displacement of the bladder leading to difficulty with urination. Vaginal patency should be documented periodically to avoid re-stenosis and recurrence of the hydrometrocolpos.

ETIOLOGY. This disorder has an autosomal recessive inheritance pattern. Postaxial polydactyly is usually the only manifestation in males, although cryptorchidism and hypospadias have occurred infrequently and one male had an associated cardiac defect. The gene that encodes a putative chaperonin molecule, has been mapped to 20p12. It has been suggested that mutation of this gene interfered with ATP hydrolysis, which in other chaperonins leads to reduced function.

COMMENT. Because vaginal atresia and postaxial polydactyly occur in both McKusick-Kaufman and Bardet-Biedl syndromes, significant difficulty exists differentiating between the two prior to 3 years of age. At that age, obesity and retinal dystrophy develop in Bardet-Biedl syndrome allowing for a definitive diagnosis of that disorder.

References

McKusick VA et al: Hydrometrocolpos as a simply inherited malformation. JAMA 189:813, 1964.

Kaufman RL et al: Family studies in congenital heart disease II: A syndrome of hydrometrocolpos, postaxial polydactyly and congenital heart disease. Birth Defects Orig Artic Ser 8(5):85, 1972.

Chitayata D et al: Further delineation of the McKusick-Kaufman hydrometrocolpos polydactyly syndrome. Am J Dis Child 141:1133, 1987.

David A et al: Hydrometrocolpos and polydactyly: A common neonatal presentation of Bardet-Biedl and McKusick-Kaufman syndromes. J Med Genet 36:599, 1999.

Stone DL et al: Mutation of a gene encoding a putative chaperonin cause McKusick-Kaufman syndrome. Nat Genet 25:79, 2000.

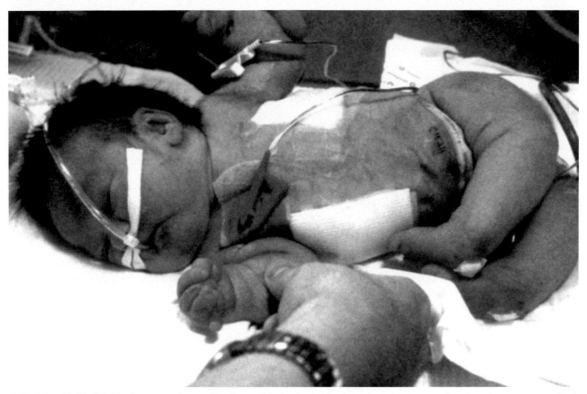

FIGURE 1. McKusick-Kaufman syndrome. Newborn girl who had a hydrometrocolpos secondary to a transverse vaginal septum. Note the postaxial polydactyly and hyperextension of the hip and knee with genu recurvatum. (From Jabs EW et al: Birth Defects 18:161,1982. Permission granted by the March of Dimes.)

RIEGER SYNDROME
Iris Dysplasia, Hypodontia

In 1935, Rieger described the malformation of the anterior segment of the eye that now bears his name, the Rieger eye malformation. Subsequently, dental anomalies were observed in individuals with this defect and the combination has come to be known as the Rieger syndrome.

ABNORMALITIES

Ocular. Dysplasia of the iris (goniodysgenesis) including iris hypoplasia, strands of tissue connecting the iris to the posterior cornea, prominent Schwalbe line (posterior embryotoxon), glaucoma, abnormal placement of pupil.

Facial. Broad nasal bridge, maxillary hypoplasia, thin upper lip, short philtrum.

Dentition. Hypodontia usually of upper incisors.

Other. Failure of involution of the periumbilical skin.

OTHER ABNORMALITIES. Cleft palate, pectus anomalies, hypospadias, imperforate anus, Meckel's diverticulum, growth hormone deficiency.

ETIOLOGY. This disorder has an autosomal dominant inheritance pattern with marked clinical and genetic heterogeneity. Loci at 4q25, 6p25, 13q14, and chromosome 11 have been identified. The affected locus at 4q25 encodes the homeodomain transcription factor PITX2. Mutations in PITX2 are responsible for 40% of cases of Rieger syndrome. The affected locus at 6p25 encodes a fork-like transcription factor FOX-C1, while the affected locus at chromosome 11 encodes the paired-like transcription factor PAX6. The affected gene at 13q14 has not yet been identified.

COMMENT. The Rieger eye malformation, also known as the Axenfeld-Rieger anomaly or mesodermal dysgenesis of the iris, is a defect that can occur as an isolated manifestation or as one component of several distinct syndromes. These include the Rieger syndrome, several other Mendelian conditions, and various chromosomal abnormalities including dup(3p), del(4p), del(4q), and del(13q). Regardless of the etiology, glaucoma will develop during childhood or adolescence in approximately 50% of patients with the Rieger eye malformation.

References

Rieger H: Beiträge zur Kenntnis schener Missbildungen der Iris. Arch Ophthalmol 133:602, 1935.

Fitch N, Kaback M: The Axenfeld syndrome and the Rieger syndrome. J Med Genet 15:30, 1978.

Jorgensen RJ et al: The Rieger syndrome. Am J Med Genet 2:307, 1978.

Shields MB et al: Axenfeld-Rieger syndrome: A spectrum of developmental disorders. Ophthalmology 29:387, 1985.

Semina EV et al: Cloning and characterization of a novel bicoid-related homeobox gene, RIEG, involved in Reiger syndrome. Nat Genet 14:392, 1996.

Craig JE, Mackey DA: Glaucoma genetics: Where are we? Where will we go? Curr Opin Ophthalmol 10:126, 1999.

Amendt BA et al: Rieger syndrome: A clinical, molecular, and biochemical analysis. Cell Mol Life Sci 57:1652, 2000.

Espinoza HM et al: A molecular basis for differential developmental anomalies in Axenfeld-Rieger syndrome. Hum Mol Genet 11:743, 2002.

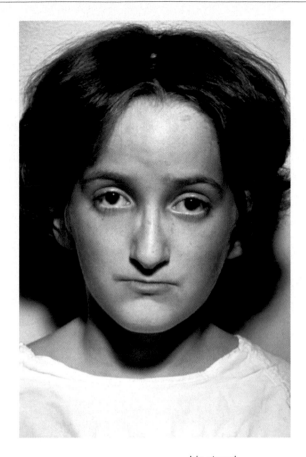

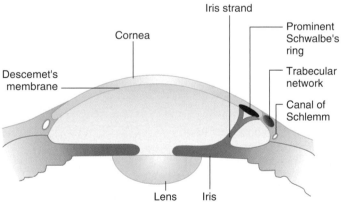

FIGURE 1. Rieger syndrome. This female patient has irregular pupils, hypodontia, maxillary hypoplasia with malocclusion, and a short philtrum. The diagram depicts the transverse section of the ocular anterior chamber with a normal angle on the left and the Rieger eye malformation on the right. Note the hypoplasia of the iris and the iris strands.

PETERS'-PLUS SYNDROME

Peters' Anomaly, Short Limb Dwarfism, Mental Retardation

This disorder was initially set forth in 1984 by Van Schooneveld, who described 11 affected individuals and introduced the term Peters'-Plus syndrome. Greater than 50 cases have now been reported.

ABNORMALITIES

Performance. Mental retardation (83%) varying from mild (34%) to moderate (20%) to severe (26%).

Growth. Prenatal onset of growth deficiency; birth length less than third percentile for gestational age in 82%; postnatal short limb growth deficiency in 100%, with adult height in females ranging from 128 to 151 cm and in males ranging from 141 to 155 cm.

Craniofacial. Round face in childhood; prominent forehead; hypertelorism; long philtrum; cupid-bow shape of upper lip; thin vermilion border; small, mildly malformed ears; preauricular pits; micrognathia; broad neck.

Eyes. Peters' anomaly or other anterior chamber cleavage disorder, narrow palpebral fissures, nystagmus, glaucoma.

Limb. Short limbs, primarily rhizomelic; decreased range of motion at elbows; hypermobility of other joints; broad, short hands and feet; fifth finger clinodactyly.

Other. Cardiac defects, including atrial and ventricular septal defects and pulmonary stenosis; hydronephrosis; duplication of kidneys; cryptorchidism.

OCCASIONAL ABNORMALITIES.

Cleft lip and palate, short lingular frenulum, microcephaly, macrocephaly, dilated lateral ventricles, abnormal ossification of the skull, upslanting palpebral fissures, cataract, mild cutaneous syndactyly, simian crease, pes cavus, seizures, spastic diplegia, hypoplastic labia majora, hypoplastic clitoris, hypospadias, abnormal foreskin, vertebral anomaly, pectus excavatum, agenesis of corpus callosum.

NATURAL HISTORY. Feeding problems often requiring prolonged gavage are common. All patients learn to speak and acquire simple skills, although developmental milestones are significantly delayed. The corneal opacities may diminish during the first 6 months of life, but they never clear enough to permit normal vision.

ETIOLOGY. This disorder has an autosomal recessive inheritance pattern.

COMMENT. Peters' anomaly, a defect of the anterior chamber, includes central corneal opacity (leukoma), thinning of the posterior aspect of the cornea, and iridocorneal adhesions attached to the edges of the leukoma. Peters' anomaly usually occurs as an isolated defect in an otherwise normal individual. However, it can occur as one feature of a multiple malformation syndrome such as Peters'-Plus syndrome.

References

Van Schooneveld MJ et al: Peters'-Plus: A new syndrome. Ophthal Paediatr Genet 4:141, 1984.

Saal HM et al: Autosomal recessive Robinow-like syndrome with anterior chamber cleavage anomalies. Am J Med Genet 30:709, 1988.

Hennekam RCM et al: The Peters'-Plus syndrome: Description of 16 patients and review of the literature. Clin Dysmorphol 2:283, 1993.

Thompson EM et al: Kivlin syndrome and Peters'-Plus syndrome: Are they the same disorder? Clin Dysmorphol 2:301, 1993.

Liesbeth JJM et al: The Peters' Plus syndrome: A review. Annales de Génétique 45:97, 2003.

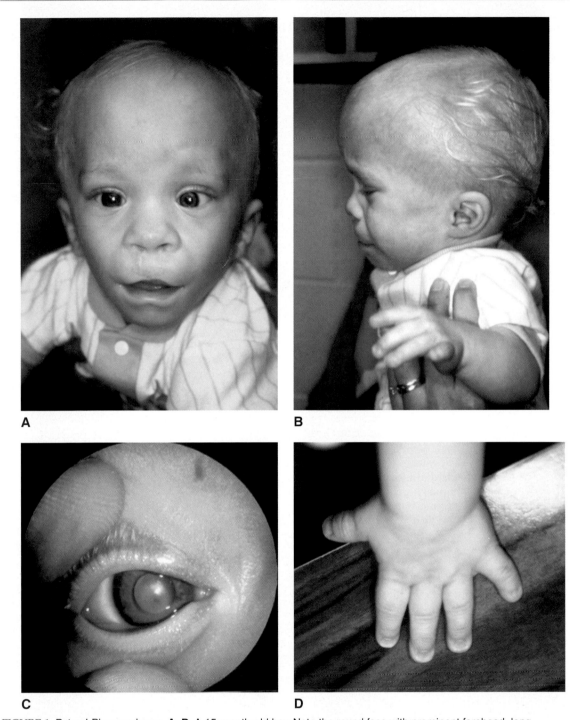

A

B

C

D

FIGURE 1. Peters'-Plus syndrome. **A–D,** A 15-month-old boy. Note the round face with prominent forehead, long philtrum with cupid-bow shape of upper lip, and thin vermilion border. The corneal opacity noted in the right eye at 4 months (**C**) was markedly decreased by 15 months. (From Hennekam RCM et al: Clin Dysmorphol 2:283, 1993, with permission.)

TORIELLO-CAREY SYNDROME

Agenesis/Hypoplasia of Corpus Callosum, Robin Sequence, Short Palpebral Fissures

Initially described in 1988 by Toriello and Carey, approximately 15 cases of this disorder now have been reported.

ABNORMALITIES

Growth. Postnatal growth deficiency with respect to length and weight.

Performance. Hypotonia, mental retardation.

Craniofacial. Microcephaly of postnatal onset, large fontanels, telecanthus (lateral displacement of medial canthi), short palpebral fissures, small nose, anteverted nares, depressed nasal bridge, cleft palate, submucous cleft palate, micrognathia, malformed ears, excess nuchal skin.

Cardiovascular. Defects in approximately 90% including atrial septal defect, ventricular septal defect, patent ductus arteriosus, pulmonary valve stenosis, hypoplastic left heart, atretic mitral valve, double outlet right heart with type-B interrupted aortic arch, cardiomyopathy, endocardial fibroelastosis.

Other. Agenesis/hypoplasia of corpus callosum, laryngeal/hypopharyngeal defects, brachydactyly, cryptorchidism.

OCCASIONAL ABNORMALITIES.

Ventricular dilatation, Dandy-Walker malformation, cerebellar hypoplasia, hydrocephalus, electroencephalograph abnormalities, speech delay, conductive and sensorineural hearing loss, sparse, thin hair, hyperkeratosis on dorsum of hands, downslanting palpebral fissures, 13 pairs of ribs, vertebral defects, clavicular defects, hypoplastic/dysplastic nails, pes varus, pes calcaneovalgus, metatarsus adductus, hypermobile joints, increased gap between first and second toes, narrow chest, pectus carinatum, uretero-pelvic junction obstruction, omphalocele, Hirschsprung disease, micropenis, anteriorly placed anus.

NATURAL HISTORY. Obstructive apnea associated with the Robin sequence as well as the laryngeal/hypopharyngeal anomalies lead frequently to serious airway compromise. Death before 3 months has occurred in approximately 60% of cases. The survivors, who range from 2 months to 6 years, are all developmentally delayed. The three children older than 3 years of age have developmental quotients of 43, 50, and 70, respectively.

ETIOLOGY. An autosomal recessive inheritance pattern is most likely.

References

Toriello HV, Carey JC: Corpus callosum agenesis, facial anomalies, Robin sequence, and other anomalies: A new autosomal recessive syndrome. Am J Med Genet 31:17, 1988.

Czarnecki P et al: Toriello-Carey syndrome: Evidence for X-linked inheritance. Am J Med Genet 65:291, 1996.

Chinen Y et al: Two sisters with Toriello-Carey syndrome. Am J Med Genet 87:262, 1999.

Wegner KJ, Hersh JA: Toriello-Carey syndrome: An additional case and summary of previously reported cases. Clin Dysmorphol 10:145, 2001.

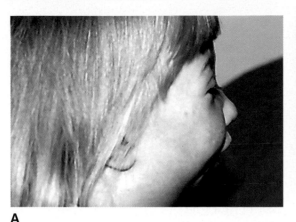 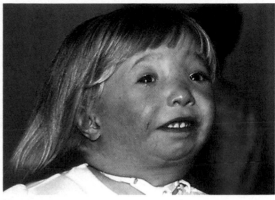

A **B**

FIGURE 1. Torriello-Carey syndrome. **A** and **B,** A 3-year-old girl. Note the small chin, telecanthus, and thickened helix of the ear. (From Toriello HG, Carey JC: Am J Med Genet 31:17, 1988, with permission.)

MOWAT-WILSON SYNDROME

Microcephaly, Distinctive Facies, Hirschsprung Disease

This disorder was initially described in six patients, with a distinctive facies, mental retardation, and microcephaly, five of whom had Hirschsprung disease. Forty-five affected individuals have been reported.

ABNORMALITIES

Growth. Postnatal onset of short stature.

Performance. Moderate-to-severe mental retardation, speech disproportionately delayed relative to comprehension, happy demeanor with frequent smiling.

Neurologic. Microcephaly, hypotonia, wide-based gait, elbows held in flexed position with hands up, seizures or abnormal electroencephalograph, total or partial agenesis of corpus callosum.

Facies. High forehead; square face; sparse hair; low nasal bridge; prominent nasal tip; prominent vertical philtral ridges; full or everted lower lip; upper lip full centrally and thin laterally; posteriorly rotated ears; large, uplifted ear lobes; in childhood, the face lengthens, prognathism develops, and the columella becomes more prominent.

Cardiac. Defects in 45%, including patent ductus arteriosus, atrial septal defect, ventricular septal defect, tetralogy of Fallot, pulmonary atresia, aortic coarctation, bicuspid aortic valve, and aortic valve stenosis.

Genitourinary. Hypospadias; cryptorchidism; hooding of penis; webbed penis; renal anomalies in boys including vesico-ureteral reflux, hydronephrosis, pelvic kidney, duplex kidney.

Other. Hirschsprung disease (62%), tapered fingers, long toes, calcaneovalgus.

OCCASIONAL ABNORMALITIES.

Nystagmus, strabismus, ptosis, irregular patches of dark iris pigmentation, bifid uvula, submucous cleft palate, cerebral atrophy, poor hippocampal formation, prominent interphalangeal joints developing in adolescence, broad hallux, duplicated hallux.

NATURAL HISTORY. Mean age of walking is 4 years, and those who walk are ataxic. Some remain nonambulatory. Most children develop only limited speech, although some communicate successfully with signing. The age of onset of seizures has varied from several months to over 10 years and some have been difficult to control.

ETIOLOGY. All cases have been sporadic resulting from a de-novo deletion or heterozygous mutation of the ZFHX1B (SIP1) gene located on chromosome 2q22. Sibling recurrence is thus likely to be very low.

COMMENT. Because of the wide-based gait, typical stance with arms held flexed at the elbows and hands up, smiling face and lack of speech, this disorder should be considered in patients thought to have Angelman syndrome for whom the diagnosis is not confirmed.

References

Mowat DR et al: Hirschsprung disease, microcephaly, mental retardation and characteristic facial features: Delineation of a new syndrome and identification of a locus of chromosome 2q22-q23. J Med Genet 35:617–623, 1998.

Wakamatsu N et al: Mutations in SIP1, encoding Smad interacting protein-1, cause a form of Hirschsprung disease. Nat Genet 27:369–370, 2001.

Zweier C et al: "Mowat-Wilson" syndrome with and without Hirschsprung disease is a distinct, recognizable multiple congenital anomalies-mental retardation syndrome caused by mutations in the zinc finger homeo box 1B gene. Am J Med Genet 108:177–181, 2002.

Mowat DR et al: Mowat-Wilson syndrome. J Med Genet 40:305, 2003.

Wilson MJ et al: Further delineation of the phenotype associated with heterozygous mutations in ZFHX1B. Am J Med Genet 119:257, 2003.

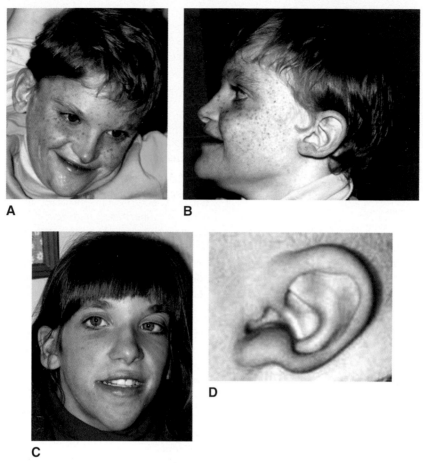

FIGURE 1. Mowat-Wilson syndrome. **A–D,** Note the prominent nasal tip; upper lip, which is full centrally and thin laterally; posteriorly rotated ears and large uplifted ear lobes; and prognathism, which develops in adolescence. (Courtesy of Dr. David Mowat, Sydney Children's Hospital, New South Wales, Australia.)

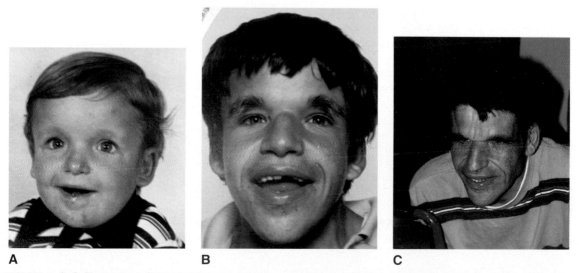

FIGURE 2. **A–C,** The same individual at 3 years, 14 years, and 31 years of age, respectively. Note the high forehead, square face, prominent nasal tip, and prognathism. (Courtesy of Dr. David Mowat, Sydney Children's Hospital, New South Wales, Australia.)

CEREBRO-COSTO-MANDIBULAR SYNDROME

Rib-Gap Defect with Small Thorax, Severe Micrognathia

This disorder was initially described by Smith and colleagues in 1966, and approximately 60 cases have been reported.

ABNORMALITIES

Performance. Mental deficiency and speech difficulties are frequent among the survivors.

Growth. Postnatal growth deficiency.

Facies. Severe micrognathia with glossoptosis (the Robin sequence) and short to cleft soft palate.

Thorax. Bell-shaped small thorax with gaps between posterior ossified rib and anterior cartilaginous rib, especially fourth to tenth ribs; rudimentary ribs; anomalous rib insertion to vertebrae; missing 12th rib; vertebral anomalies.

OCCASIONAL ABNORMALITIES.

Microcephaly, short neck, redundant skin including pterygium colli, choanal atresia, dental abnormalities (no tooth buds), indistinct speech, conductive hearing loss, absence of auditory canals, fifth finger clinodactyly, malformed tracheal cartilages, hypoplastic humerus, elbow hypoplasia, renal cyst or ectopia, clubfoot, scoliosis, congenital hip dislocation, sacral fusion, flask-shaped configuration of pelvis, hypoplastic sternum, clavicles, and pubic rami, epiphyseal stippling of calcaneus, ventricular septal defect, porencephaly, corpus callosal agenesis, dilated lateral ventricles, hydranencephaly, meningomyelocele, omphalocele.

NATURAL HISTORY.
Approximately 32% have died in the neonatal period and approximately 56% by 1 year of age, the majority as a result of severe respiratory insufficiency. Of those who survive, feeding and speech difficulties are common, as well as mental deficiency in one third to one half of cases. The rib-gap defects resolve into pseudoarthroses with time.

ETIOLOGY. This disorder has an autosomal recessive inheritance pattern, which is implied by the occurrence of offspring from normal parentage as well as consanguinity. However, parent-to-child transmission has been reported, suggesting autosomal dominant inheritance for some cases of this disorder.

COMMENT. The clinical manifestations of this disorder in the newborn period are extremely variable and can be limited to the Robin sequence. Thus, cerebro-costo-mandibular syndrome should be considered in newborns with the Robin sequence who show more serious respiratory problems.

References

Smith DW, Theiler K, Schachenmann G: Rib-gap defect with micrognathia, malformed tracheal cartilages, and redundant skin: A new pattern of defective development. J Pediatr 69:799, 1966.

Doyle JF: The skeletal defects of the cerebro-costo-mandibular syndrome. Irish J Med Sci (7th Ser) 2:595, 1969.

McNicholl B et al: Cerebro-costo-mandibular syndrome: A new familial developmental disorder. Arch Dis Child 45:421, 1970.

Silverman FN et al: Cerebro-costo-mandibular syndrome. J Pediatr 97:406, 1980.

Tachibina K et al: Cerebro-costo-mandibular syndrome. Hum Genet 54:283, 1980.

Leroy JG et al: Cerebro-costo-mandibular syndrome with autosomal dominant inheritance. J Pediatr 99:441, 1981.

Hennekam RCM et al: The cerebro-costo-mandibular syndrome: Third report of familial occurrence. Clin Genet 28:118, 1985.

Burton EM, Oestreich AE: Cerebro-costo-mandibular syndrome with stipped epiphysis and cystic fibrosis. Pediatr Radiol 18:365, 1988.

Plötz FB et al: Cerebro-costo-mandibular syndrome. Am J Med Genet 62:286, 1996.

Van den Ende JJ et al: The cerbro-costo-mandiblar syndrome: Seven patients and review of the literature. Clin Dysmorphol 7:87, 1998.

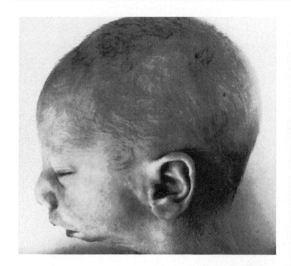

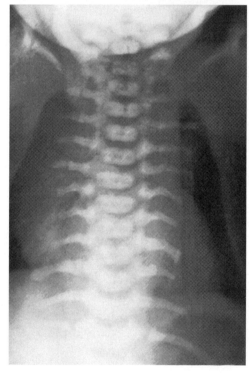

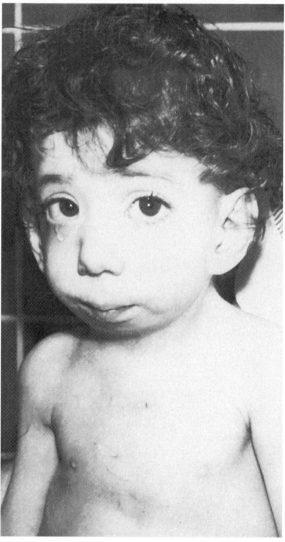

FIGURE 1. Cerebro-costo-mandibular syndrome. *Left*, Newborn showing severe micrognathia and incompletely ossified aberrant ribs. (From Smith DW et al: J Pediatr 69:799, 1966, with permission.) *Right*, A 4-year-old child. (*Right*, From McNicholl B et al: Arch Dis Child 45:421, 1970, with permission.)

JARCHO-LEVIN SYNDROME

Jarcho and Levin described this disorder in 1938. It is now clear that Jarcho-Levin syndrome (JLS) represents one of at least three disorders characterized by multiple vertebral segmentation defects. Most reported cases of Jarcho-Levin syndrome have occurred in Puerto Rican individuals.

ABNORMALITIES

Growth. Short trunk dwarfism of prenatal onset.
Craniofacial. Prominent occiput; tendency to have broad forehead, wide nasal bridge, anteverted nares, and upslant to palpebral fissures.
Thorax and Spine. Short thorax with "crab-like" rib cage associated with multiple vertebral segmentation defects and ribs that flare in a fan-like pattern; posterior fusion and absence of ribs; short neck and low posterior hairline; pectus carinatum; increased anteroposterior chest diameter; lordosis; kyphoscoliosis.
Limbs. Normal with impression of being long.
Other. Protuberant abdomen.

OCCASIONAL ABNORMALITIES.

Cleft palate, cryptorchidism, hernias, hydronephrosis with ureteral obstruction, bilobed bladder, absent external genitalia, anal and urethral atresia, uterus didelphys, cerebral polygyria, neural tube defects, single umbilical artery.

NATURAL HISTORY. The vast majority of affected individuals die in early infancy as a result of recurrent pulmonary infection and respiratory insufficiency secondary to the small thoracic volume.

ETIOLOGY. This disorder has an autosomal recessive inheritance pattern.

COMMENT. Based on clinical and radiologic evaluation of infants with multiple vertebral segmentation defects, three distinct entities have been identified: Jarcho-Levin syndrome is characterized by symmetric "crab-like" thoracic spine and ribs with short-trunk short stature, radiographic features of multiple hemivertebrae and rib fusion, and early lethality in virtually all cases. Spondylothoracic dysostosis is also an autosomal recessive disorder. Intrafamilial variability in clinical severity is striking. Despite multiple vertebral segmentation defects, a "crab-like" thoracic spine is not evident. Spondylocostal dysostosis is an autosomal dominant disorder that usually presents after infancy with problems related to kyphoscoliosis, low back pain, or decreased mobility of the spine. Although the vertebral segmentation defects tend to be milder, they frequently occur throughout the entire spine. A normal life span is the rule.

References

Jarcho S, Levin PM: Hereditary malformations of the vertebral bodies. Johns Hopkins Med J 62:216, 1938.
Pérez-Comas A, Garcia-Castro JM: Occipitofacial-cervico-thoracic-abdomino-digital dysplasia: Jarcho-Levin syndrome of vertebral anomalies. J Pediatr 85:388, 1974.
Poor MA et al: Nonskeletal malformations in one of three siblings with Jarcho-Levin syndrome of vertebral anomalies. J Pediatr 103:270, 1983.
Karnes PS et al: Jarcho-Levin syndrome: Four new cases and classification of subtypes. Am J Med Genet 40:264, 1991.
Mortier GR et al: Multiple vertebral segmentation defects: Analysis of 26 new patients and review of the literature. Am J Med Genet 61:310, 1996.
Bannykh S et al: Abberant Pax1 and Pax9 in Jarcho-Levin syndrome: Report of two Caucasian siblings and literature review. Am J Med Genet 120A:241, 2003.

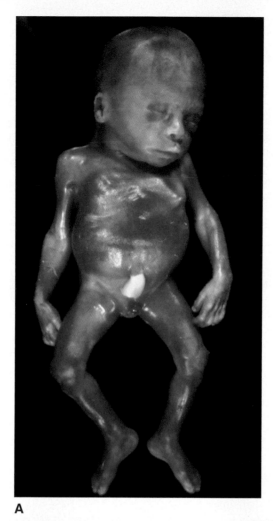

A

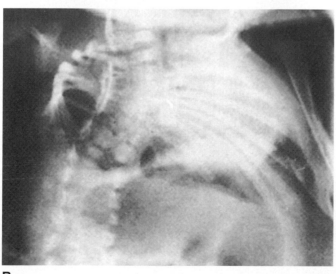

B

FIGURE 1. Jarcho-Levin syndrome. **A** and **B,** Affected neonate with radiograph. (**A,** From Bannykh SI et al: Am J Med Genet 120:241, 2003, with permission; **B,** from Pérez-Comas A, Garcia-Castro JM: J Pediatr 85:388, 1974.)

MANDIBULOACRAL DYSPLASIA

Short Stature, Mandibular Hypoplasia, Acro-Osteolysis

Described initially by Cavallazzi and colleagues as an atypical from of cleido-cranial dysostosis, this disorder has now been reported in more than 30 patients. Onset of phenotype occurs between 3 and 14 years.

ABNORMALITIES

Growth. Postnatal onset of growth deficiency.

Craniofacial. Prominent scalp veins, thin beak-like nose with alar hypoplasia, hypoplastic facial bones with prominent eyes, mandibular hypoplasia, difficulty opening mouth.

Limbs. Short, contracted fingers with hypoplastic distal phalanges and broad interphalangeal joints; dystrophic nails; generalized joint limitations.

Skin, Hair, Teeth. Thin, mottled, hyperpigmented skin; loss of subcutaneous fat in extremities and fat accumulation in trunk, face, submental and occipital regions; premature loss of teeth; dental crowding.

Skeletal. Wormian bones, widened cranial sutures, clavicular hypoplasia, acro-osteolysis, hypoplastic distal phalanges, bell-shaped chest.

OCCASIONAL ABNORMALITIES.

Cataracts, soft tissue calcification, scoliosis, acanthosis nigricans, hypospadias, delayed puberty, hypogonadism, partial lipodystrophy, insulin-resistant diabetes mellitus, hepatomegaly, renal failure secondary to focal scleroses.

NATURAL HISTORY. Affected children are normal at birth. Characteristic features develop between 3 and 14 years of age with onset of growth deficiency, premature aging, and progressive skeletal changes involving primarily the chin, clavicles, and digits.

ETIOLOGY. This disorder has an autosomal recessive inheritance pattern. A mutation in the lamin A/C gene (LMNA), which maps to chromosome 1q21 was identified in all individuals affected with this disorder in five consanguineous Italian females.

References

Cavallazzi C et al: Si du caso di disostosi cleido-cranica. Rev Clin Pediatr 65:313–326, 1960.

Teuconi R et al: Another Italian family with mandibuloacral dysplasia: Why does it seem more frequent in Italy? Am J Med Genet 24:357–364, 1986.

Toriello HV: Mandibulo-acral dysplasia: Heterogeneity versus variability. Clin Dysmorphol 4:12–24, 1995.

Novelli G: Mandibuloacral dysplasia is caused by a mutation in LMNA-Encoding Lamin A/C. Am J Hum Genet 71:426–431, 2002.

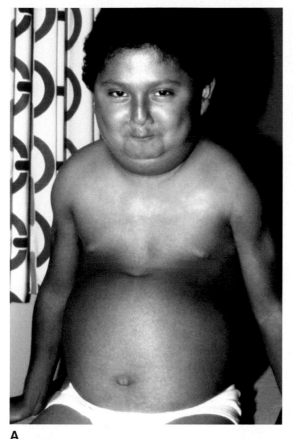

A

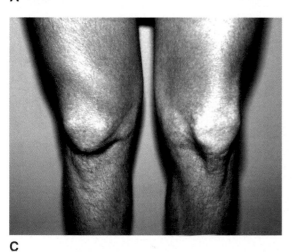

C

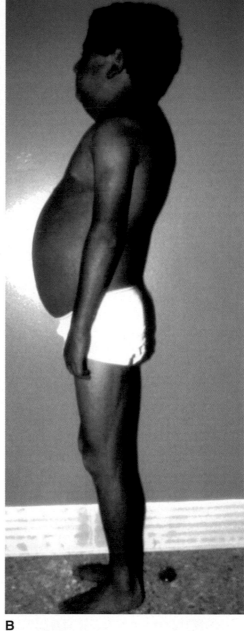

B

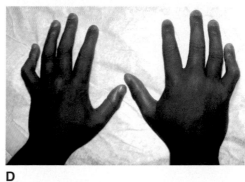

D

FIGURE 1. Mandibuloacral dysplasia. **A–D,** A 10-year-old boy with a thin, beaked nose with alar hypoplasia; hyperpigmented skin; loss of subcutaneous fat in the extremities; fat accumulation in the trunk, face, and submental region; bell-shaped chest; and camptodactyly. (Courtesy of Dr. Marilyn C. Jones, Children's Hospital, San Diego.)

BERARDINELLI LIPODYSTROPHY SYNDROME
(Congenital Generalized Lipodystrophy)

Lipoatrophy, Phallic Hypertrophy, Hepatomegaly, Hyperlipemia

Berardinelli reported this unusual lipodystrophic syndrome in 1954. Although many cases have been recorded subsequently, the metabolic defect responsible for this inborn error of metabolism has not been determined.

ABNORMALITIES

Performance. Mental deficiency as a variable feature.

Growth. Accelerated growth and maturation during early childhood, final height is normal or slightly above normal, slight enlargement of hands and feet, phallic enlargement, muscle hyperplasia, lack of metabolically active adipose from early life with sparing of mechanical adipose tissue (i.e., in orbits, palms and soles, crista galli, buccal region, tongue, scalp, breasts, perineum, periarticular regions, and epidural areas).

Skin. Coarse with hyperpigmentation, especially in axillae; variable acanthosis nigricans.

Hair. Hirsutism with curly scalp hair.

Vascular. Large superficial veins.

Liver. Hepatomegaly with excess neutral fat and glycogen and eventual cirrhosis.

Plasma. Hyperlipidemia, hypertriglyceridemia, insulin-resistant diabetes mellitus.

Other. Umbilical hernia.

OCCASIONAL ABNORMALITIES.
Hypertrophic cardiomyopathy, corneal opacities, hyperproteinemia, hyperinsulinemia, polycystic ovarian disease, percussion myxedema, hyperhidrosis, clitoromegaly, amenorrhea, polycystic ovaries.

NATURAL HISTORY. Accelerated growth, voracious appetite, and increased metabolic rate are most prominent in early childhood. Hyperinsulinemia and elevated serum triglycerides occur even in infancy resulting in chylomicronemia, eruptive xanthomas, and acute pancreatitis. Low levels of high-density lipoprotein cholesterol occur. Abnormal glucose tolerance and diabetes appear during puberty. Fatty infiltration of the liver may lead to cirrhosis and esophageal varices may become a fatal complication. Early onset of diabetes mellitus and dyslipidemia may result in atherosclerosis. Diabetic nephropathy and retinopathy occur.

ETIOLOGY. This disorder has an autosomal recessive inheritance pattern. Mutations in the AGPAT2 gene encoding 1-acylglycerol-3-phosphate O-acyltransferase 2, located at 9q34 and in BSCL2, located at 11q13, are responsible. Whether there are other loci has yet to be established. Individuals with BSCL2 mutations have lower serum leptin levels, a higher prevalence of mild mental retardation and an earlier onset of diabetes.

COMMENT. Although the accelerated growth and maturation plus the muscle hypertrophy and enlargement of the phallus are suggestive of androgen effect, neither androgens nor gonadotropins are elevated, and the hirsutism does not include pubic and axillary hair. Oserd and colleagues found that mononuclear leukocytes from affected patients bound less insulin than cells from controls, suggesting that altered insulin receptors are responsible for the insulin resistance and decreased synthesis of triglycerides.

References

Berardinelli W: An undiagnosed endocrinometabolic syndrome: Report of two cases. J Clin Endocrinol Metab 14:193, 1954.

Scip M, Trygstad O: Generalized lipodystrophy. Arch Dis Child 38:447, 1963.

Senior B, Gellis SS: The syndromes of total lipodystrophy and of partial lipodystrophy. Pediatrics 33:593, 1964.

Oserd S et al: Decreased binding of insulin to its receptor in patients with congenital generalized lipodystrophy. N Engl J Med 296:245, 1977.

Garg A et al: Peculiar distribution of adipose tissue in patients with congenital generalized lipodystrophy. J Clin Endocrinol Metab 75:358, 1991.

Klein S et al: Generalized lipodystrophy: In vivo evidence of hypermetabolism and insulin-resistant lipid, glucose and amino acid kinetic. Metabolism 41:893, 1992.

Garg A et al: Lipodystropies. Am J Med 108:143, 2000.

Agarwal AA et al: Phenotypic and genetic heterogeneity in congenital generalized lipodystrophy. J Clin Endocrinol Metab 88:4840, 2003.

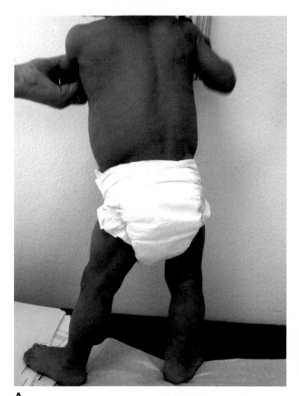
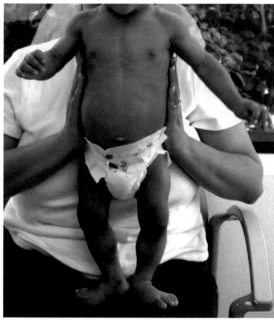

A   **B**

FIGURE 1. Berardinelli lipodystrophy syndrome. **A** and **B,** A 2-year-old boy showing hypertrophied muscle and relative lack of subcutaneous fat. (Courtesy of Dr. Lynne M. Bird, Children's Hospital, San Diego.)

DISTICHIASIS-LYMPHEDEMA SYNDROME

Double Row of Eyelashes, Lymphedema

ABNORMALITIES

Eyes. Distichiasis, an extra row of eyelashes, replacing meibomian glands (100%).
Limbs. Lymphedema, predominantly from knee downward (66%).
Other. Vertebral anomalies (62%), epidural cysts (46%), cardiac defects (38%).

OCCASIONAL ABNORMALITIES.

Short stature, ptosis, microphthalmia, strabismus, partial ectropion of lower lid, epicanthal folds, pterygium colli, chylothorax, cleft palate, bifid uvula, micrognathia, scoliosis/kyphosis, cryptorchidism, double uterus.

NATURAL HISTORY. The extra eyelashes

may cause irritative ocular problems and often require surgical removal. The lymphedema usually becomes evident between the ages of 5 and 20 years, especially at the time of adolescence and sometimes for the first time during pregnancy. The possibility of epidural cysts with secondary neurologic or other complications must always be considered in this disorder. Eyelash removal or surgery for the lymphedema is difficult to accomplish with good results; hence, treatment is generally withheld unless grossly indicated.

ETIOLOGY. This disorder has an autosomal dominant inheritance pattern with marked variability of expression. Mutations in the Forkhead family gene FOXC2 located on chromosome 16q23 have been identified in members of a number of families. Diagnosis in sporadic cases is often difficult, because affected individuals might have only one of the characteristic features.

References

Falls HF, Kertesz ED: A new syndrome combining pterygium colli with developmental anomalies of the eyelids and lymphatics of the lower extremities. Trans Am Ophthalmol Soc 62:248, 1964.

Robinow M, Johnson GF, Verhagen AD: Distichiasis-lymphedema: A hereditary syndrome of multiple congenital defects. Am J Dis Child 119:343, 1970.

Hoover RE, Kelley JS: Distichiasis and lymphedema: A hereditary syndrome with possible multiple defects—a report of a family. Trans Ophthalmol Soc 69:293, 1971.

Holmes LB, Fields JP, Zabriskiek JB: Hereditary late onset lymphedema. Pediatrics 61:575, 1978.

Schwartz JF, O'Brien MS, Hoffman JC: Hereditary spinal arachnoid cysts, distichiasis, and lymphedema. Ann Neurol 7:340, 1980.

Temple IK, Collin JRO: Distichiasis-lymphoedema syndrome: A family report. Clin Dysmorphol 3:139, 1994.

Fang J et al: Mutations in FOXC2 (MFH-1), a forkhead family transcription factor, are responsible for the hereditary lymphedemia-distichiasis syndrome. Am J Hum Genet 67:1382, 2000.

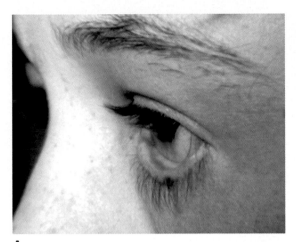

A

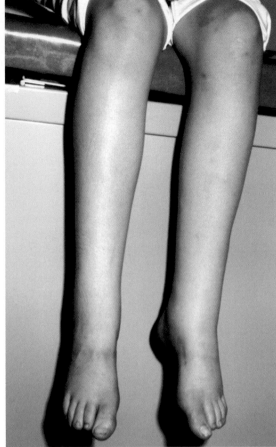

FIGURE 1. Distichiasis-lymphedema syndrome. Distichiasis in the eye of this teenage girl (**A**) and lymphedema in her leg (**B**).

B

T Miscellaneous Sequences

LATERALITY SEQUENCES

In addition to reversal of the sides, with partial to complete situs inversus, there can be bilateral left- or right-sidedness. The primary defect in both is a failure of normal asymmetry in morphogenesis. The basic problem would presumably be present before 30 days of development. The accompanying chart sets forth the differences as well as the similarities between the patterns predominantly caused by left-sided bilaterality and by right-sided bilaterality. Among other differences, the spleen dramatically reflects the variant laterality in the two. With left-sided bilaterality, there is polysplenia (usually bilateral spleens plus rudimentary extra splenic tissue), and with right-sided bilaterality there is asplenia or a hypoplastic spleen. The defect in lateralization leading to the failure of normal asymmetry in morphogenesis is most likely etiologically heterogeneous. As such, although usually sporadic, autosomal dominant, autosomal recessive, and X-linked recessive inheritance have all been documented. A gene for X-linked laterality sequence has been mapped to Xq24-27.1. Mutations in ZIC3, an X-linked zinc-finger transcription factor located at Xq26.2, are responsible for a small number of cases. In addition, mutations of LEFTY A, located on chromosome 1q42, have been implicated in two sporadic cases.

Left-right axis malformations are usually isolated but can occur as one feature of a multiple malformation syndrome, the most common of which is the immotile cilia syndrome. As a result of defective cilia and flagella, chronic respiratory tract infections occur commonly and infertility in males, chronic ear infections and decreased or absent smell occur variably. The cilia are functionally abnormal and have absent or abnormal dynein arms connecting the nine pairs of microtubules on electron microscopy. A subgroup of the immotile cilia syndrome is Kartagener syndrome, an autosomal recessive disorder associated with situs inversus, partial to complete, with gross defects in cardiac septation in 50%, in addition to the other features of immotile cilia syndrome.

BILATERAL LEFT-SIDEDNESS SEQUENCE. Bilateral left-sidedness sequence is also known as *polysplenia syndrome*. The gender incidence is about equal. The cardiac anomalies are usually not as severe as those with bilateral right-sidedness.

BILATERAL RIGHT-SIDEDNESS SEQUENCE. Bilateral right-sidedness sequence is also known as *asplenia syndrome, Ivemark syndrome, triad of spleen agenesis, defects of heart and vessels, and situs inversus*. The sequence is two to three times more common in males than in females. The complex cardiac anomalies, usually giving rise to cyanosis and early cardiac failure, are the major cause of early death. The possibility of gastrointestinal problems must also be considered, especially as related to the aberrant mesenteric attachments. Renal anomalies are also more frequent (25%). Survivors have had an increased frequency of cutaneous, respiratory, and other infections, possibly related to the asplenia. Tests to detect asplenia include evaluation of red blood cells for Howell-Jolly bodies and Heinz bodies.

OCCASIONAL ABNORMALITIES. Intestinal malrotation, biliary atresia, anomalous portal and hepatic vessels, intestinal obstruction, meningomyelocele, cerebellar hypoplasia, arrhinencephaly.

COMMENT. Both bilateral left-sidedness (polysplenia) and bilateral right-sidedness (asplenia) have been documented in different persons in the same family, indicating that the two conditions represent different manifestations of a primary defect in lateralization leading to failure of normal body asymmetry.

The molecular determinants of normal body asymmetry are beginning to emerge. In the mouse, motile embryonic cilia generate directional flow of extraembryonic fluid surrounding the node located at the tip of the embryo in the midline. This flow concentrates left-right determinants to one side of the node activating asymmetric gene expression at the node and beyond. In the chick, activin on the right side of the primitive streak, represses expression of the gene Sonic hedgehog (*Shh*). The remaining expression of *Shh* on the left induces nodal on the left, leading to the normal looping of the heart tube to the right.

References

Freedom RM: The asplenia syndrome. J Pediatr 81:1130, 1972.

Van Mierop LHS, Gessner IH, Schiebler GL: Asplenia and polysplenia syndromes. Birth Defects 8:74, 1972.

Afzelius AB: Kartagener's syndrome and abnormal cilia. N Engl J Med 297:1011, 1977.

Arnold GL, Bixler D, Gerod D: Probable autosomal recessive inheritance of polysplenia, situs inversus and cardiac defects in an Amish family. Am J Med Genet 16:35, 1983.

Mathias RS et al: X-linked laterality sequence: Situs inversus, complex cardiac defects, splenic defects. Am J Med Genet 28:111, 1987.

Casey B et al: Mapping a gene for familial situs abnormalities to human chromosome Xq24-q27.1. Nat Genet 5:403, 1993.

Mikkila SP et al: X-linked laterality sequence in a family with carrier manifestations. Am J Med Genet 49:435, 1994.

Levin M et al: A molecular pathway determining left-right asymmetry in chick embryogenesis. Cell 82:803, 1995.

Casey B: Two rights make a wrong: human left-right malformations. Hum Mol Genet 7:1565, 1998.

McGrath J, Brueckner M: Cilia are at the heart of vertebrate left-right asymmetry. Curr Opinion Genet Devel 13:385, 2003.

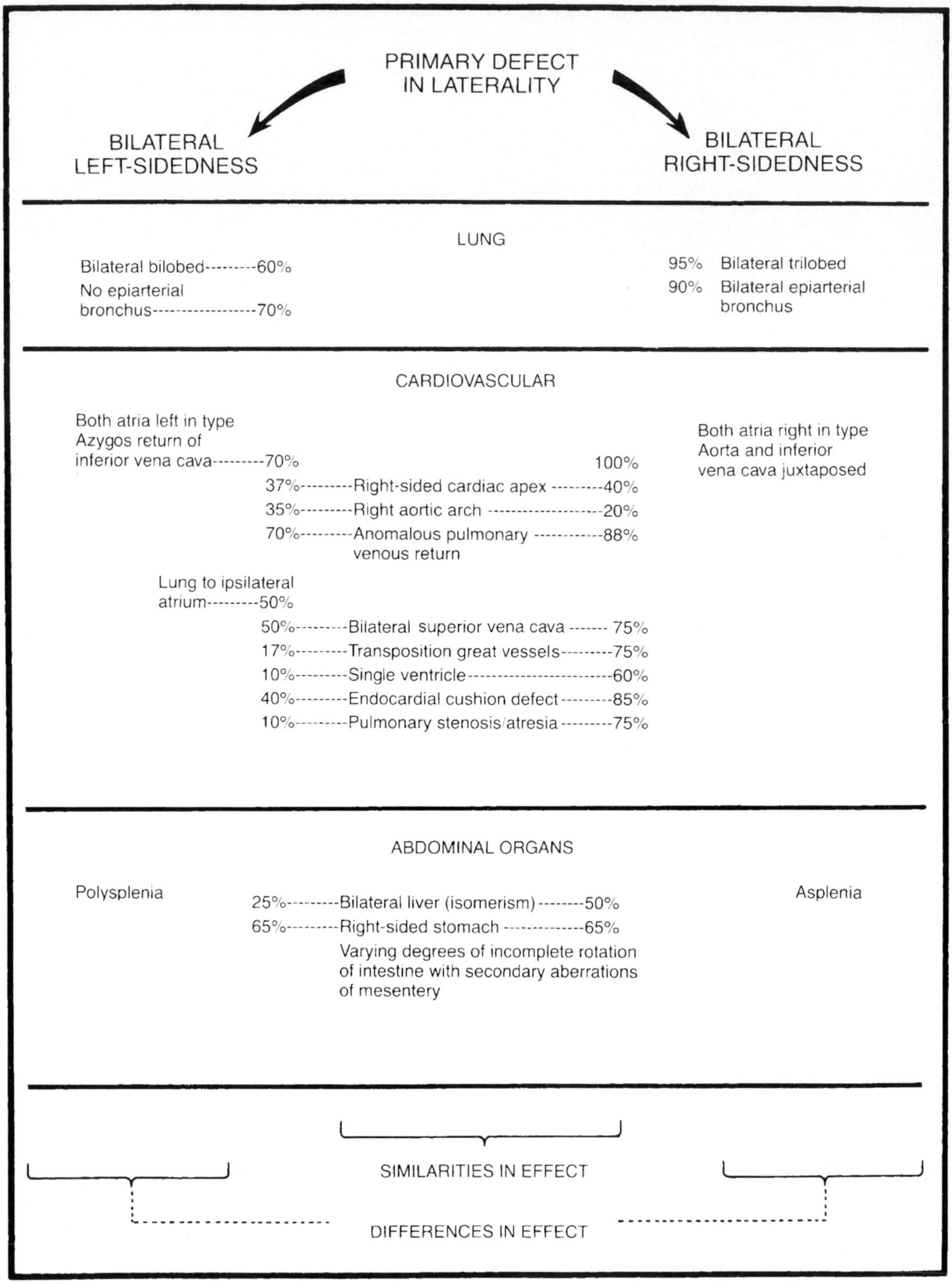

PRIMARY DEFECT
IN LATERALITY

BILATERAL
LEFT-SIDEDNESS

BILATERAL
RIGHT-SIDEDNESS

LUNG

Bilateral bilobed---------60%

No epiarterial
bronchus------------------70%

95%   Bilateral trilobed
90%   Bilateral epiarterial
          bronchus

CARDIOVASCULAR

Both atria left in type
Azygos return of
inferior vena cava---------70%

Both atria right in type
Aorta and inferior
vena cava juxtaposed

100%

37%---------Right-sided cardiac apex ---------40%

35%---------Right aortic arch -------------------20%

70%---------Anomalous pulmonary ------------88%
                  venous return

Lung to ipsilateral
atrium---------50%

50%---------Bilateral superior vena cava ------- 75%

17%---------Transposition great vessels---------75%

10%---------Single ventricle------------------------60%

40%---------Endocardial cushion defect---------85%

10%---------Pulmonary stenosis/atresia---------75%

ABDOMINAL ORGANS

Polysplenia

25%---------Bilateral liver (isomerism)--------50%

65%---------Right-sided stomach --------------65%

Varying degrees of incomplete rotation
of intestine with secondary aberrations
of mesentery

Asplenia

SIMILARITIES IN EFFECT

DIFFERENCES IN EFFECT

FIGURE 1. Laterality. Primary defects of bilateral left-sidedness and bilateral right-sidedness.

HOLOPROSENCEPHALY SEQUENCE

Arrhinencephaly-Cebocephaly-Cyclopia: Primary Defect in Prechordal Mesoderm

During the third week of fetal development, the prechordal mesoderm migrates forward into the area anterior to the notochord and is necessary for the development of the midface as well as having an inductive role in the morphogenesis of the forebrain. The consequences of prechordal mesoderm defect are varying degrees of deficit of midline facial development, especially the median nasal process (premaxilla), and incomplete morphogenesis of the forebrain. Cyclopia represents a severe deficit in early midline facial development, and the eyes become fused, the olfactory placodes consolidate into a single tube-like proboscis above the eye, and the ethmoid and other midline bony structures are missing. With cyclopia, there is failure in the cleavage of the prosencephalon, with grossly incomplete morphogenesis of the forebrain. Less severe deficits result in hypotelorism and varying degrees of inadequate midfacial and incomplete forebrain development that are more common than cyclopia and frequently include cleft lip and palate. The important clinical point is that incomplete midline facial development, such as hypotelorism, absence of the philtrum or nasal septum, a single central incisor, congenital nasal pyriform aperture stenosis, and a missing frenulum of the upper lip, suggests the possibility of a serious anomaly in brain development and function.

Although the cause is unknown and the defects are isolated in the vast majority of cases, holoprosencephaly is etiologically heterogeneous with both genetic and environmental causes identified. Aneuploidy syndromes including trisomies 13 and 18 as well as several structural chromosome aberrations including del2p21, dup3pter, del7q36, del13q, del18p, and del21q22.3 should be considered. In addition, mutations in a number of genes have been identified, the most common of which, *Shh* at 7q36, is responsible for an autosomal dominant form of holoprosencephaly in which wide variability of expression is the rule. Mutations in other genes that have been identified in both sporadic and familial cases include *ZIC2* at 13q32, *SIX3* at 2p21, *tgif* at 18p11.3, as well as a number of genes involved in signaling pathways important for brain development including PATCHED1 (*ptch*) and *GLI2*, which are involved in *Shh* signaling and *TDGF1* and *FAST1*, which are involved in the Nodal/transforming growth factor β (TGF-β) pathway. Parents of an affected child should be checked for mild manifestations such as a single central incisor, a missing upper lip frenulum and absence of the nasal cartilage. Finally, holoprosencephaly has been seen in the offspring of diabetic mothers and in the Meckel-Gruber syndrome. The prognosis for central nervous system (CNS) function in individuals with this type of defect is very poor, and the author recommends serious consideration of limiting extraordinary medical assistance toward survival in patients in whom the forebrain is obviously severely affected.

References

Adelmann HB: The problem of cyclopia. Part II. Q Rev Biol 11:284, 1936.

DeMeyer W, Zeman W, Palmer CG: The face predicts the brain: Diagnostic significance of median facial anomalies for holoprosencephaly (arrhinencephaly). Pediatrics 34:256, 1964.

Cohen MM: An update on the holoprosencephalic disorders. J Pediatr 101:865, 1982.

Siebert JR, Cohen MM, Sulik KK, et al: Holoprosencephaly: An Overview and Atlas of Cases. New York: Wiley-Liss, 1990.

Gurrieri F et al: Physical mapping of the holoprosencephaly critical region on chromosome 7q36. Nat Genet 3:247, 1993.

Muenke M et al: Linkage of a human brain malformation, familial holoprosencephaly, to chromosome 7 and evidence for genetic heterogeneity. Proc Natl Acad Sci USA 91:8102, 1994.

Ming JE, Muenke M: Multiple hits during early embryonic development: Digenic diseases and holoprosencephaly. Am J Hum Genet 71:1017, 2002.

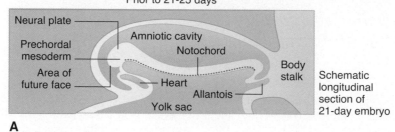

Primary Defect in Prechordal Mesoderm
Prior to 21-25 days

A

FIGURE 1. Holoprosencephaly sequence. **A,** Schematic longitudinal section of 21-day embryo.
Continued

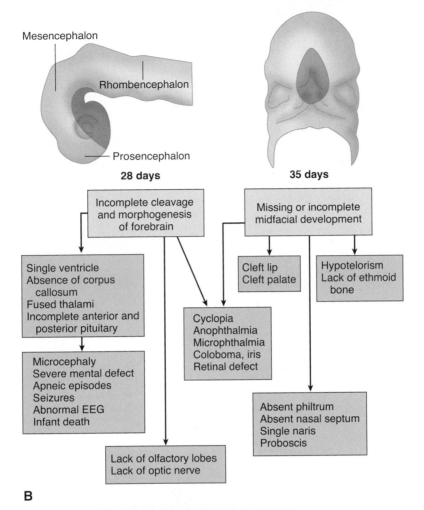

28 days

35 days

Incomplete cleavage
and morphogenesis
of forebrain

Missing or incomplete
midfacial development

Single ventricle
Absence of corpus
  callosum
Fused thalami
Incomplete anterior and
  posterior pituitary

Cleft lip
Cleft palate

Hypotelorism
Lack of ethmoid
  bone

Microcephaly
Severe mental defect
Apneic episodes
Seizures
Abnormal EEG
Infant death

Cyclopia
Anophthalmia
Microphthalmia
Coloboma, iris
Retinal defect

Absent philtrum
Absent nasal septum
Single naris
Proboscis

Lack of olfactory lobes
Lack of optic nerve

B

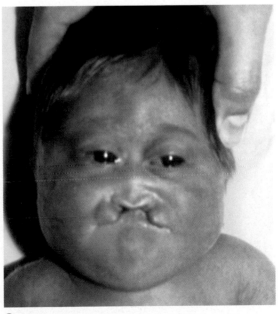

C

Fig. 1, cont'd. **B,** Developmental pathogenesis of the sequence. **C,** Affected individual.

MENINGOMYELOCELE, ANENCEPHALY, INIENCEPHALY SEQUENCES

Primary Defect in Neural Tube Closure

The initiating malformation appears to be a defect in closure of the neural groove to form an intact neural tube, which is normally completely fused by 28 days. Anencephaly represents a defect in closure at the anterior portion of the neural groove. The secondary consequences are these: (1) The unfused forebrain develops partially and then tends to degenerate; (2) the calvarium is incompletely developed; and (3) the facial features and auricular development are secondarily altered to a variable degree, including cleft palate, and frequent abnormality of the cervical vertebrae.

Defects of closure at the mid- or caudal neural groove can give rise to meningomyelocele and other secondary defects, as depicted. Of greatest concern relative to outcome for independence and survival is the hydrocephalus and other manifestations of the Chiari II malformation that is present in virtually all cases.

Defects of closure in the cervical and upper thoracic region can culminate in the iniencephaly sequence, in which secondary features may include retroflexion of the upper spine with short neck and trunk, cervical and upper thoracic vertebral anomalies, defects of thoracic cage, anterior spina bifida, diaphragmatic defects with or without hernia, and hypoplasia of lung and/or heart. Recent evidence suggesting that there are four sites of anterior neural tube closure explains the variations observed in their location, recurrence risk, and etiology. Most commonly no mode of etiology is appreciated, and the recurrence risk is 1.9% for parents who have had one affected child. Liberation of alpha-fetoprotein into the amniotic fluid from the anencephaly or meningomyelocele that is not skin-covered allows for early amniocentesis detection, which may be augmented by sonography or radiography.

The U.S. Public Health Service has recommended that women of childbearing age should consume 0.4 mg of folic acid daily to reduce their risk of conceiving a child with a neural tube defect. For women who previously have had an affected infant, it has been recommended that 4.0 mg daily of folic acid should be consumed from 1 month before conception through 3 months of pregnancy.

References

Giroud A: Causes and morphogenesis of anencephaly. Ciba Foundation Symposium on Congenital Malformations, 1960, pp 199–218.

Lemire RJ, Shepard TH, Alvord EC Jr: Caudal myeloschisis (lumbo-sacral spina bifida cystica) in a five millimeter (horizon XIV) human embryo. Anat Rec 152:9, 1965.

Lemire RJ, Beckwith JB, Shepard TH: Iniencephaly and anencephaly with spinal retroflexion. Teratology 6:27, 1972.

Centers for Disease Control and Prevention: Recommendations for use of folic acid to reduce number of spina bifida cases and other neural tube defects. JAMA 269:1233, 1993.

Van Allen MI et al: Evidence for multi-site closure of the neural tube in humans. Am J Med Genet 47:723, 1993.

Golden JA, Chernoff GF: Multiple sites of anterior neural tube closure in humans: Evidence from anterior neural tube defects (anencephaly). Pediatrics 95:506, 1995.

McLone DG, Dias MS: The Chiari II malformation: Cause and impact. Childs Nerv Syst 19:540, 2003.

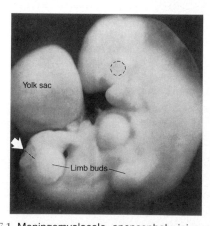 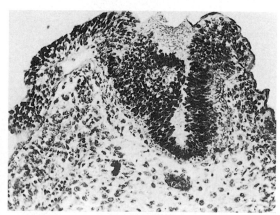

FIGURE 1. Meningomyelocele, anencephaly, iniencephaly sequences. Otherwise normal 28-day embryo with incomplete closure of the posterior neural groove (*arrow*), which shows aberrant growth of cells to the side in a transverse section (*right*). Had this embryo survived, it would presumably have developed a meningomyelocele. (From Lemire R: Anat Rec 152:9, 1965. Copyright © 1965. Reprinted with permission of Wiley-Liss, Inc., a subsidiary of John Wiley & Sons, Inc.)

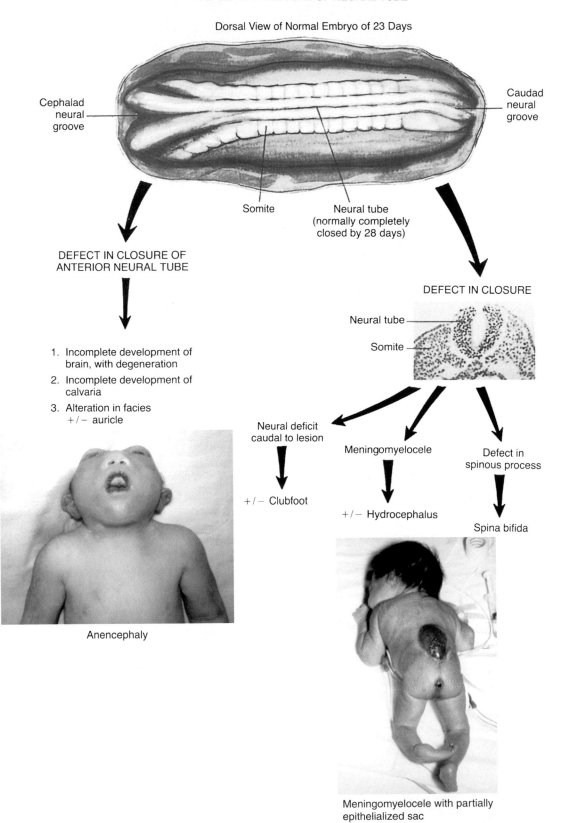

DEFECTS IN CLOSURE OF NEURAL TUBE

Dorsal View of Normal Embryo of 23 Days

Cephalad neural groove

Caudad neural groove

Somite

Neural tube (normally completely closed by 28 days)

DEFECT IN CLOSURE OF ANTERIOR NEURAL TUBE

1. Incomplete development of brain, with degeneration
2. Incomplete development of calvaria
3. Alteration in facies +/− auricle

Anencephaly

DEFECT IN CLOSURE

Neural tube

Somite

Neural deficit caudal to lesion

+/− Clubfoot

Meningomyelocele

+/− Hydrocephalus

Defect in spinous process

Spina bifida

Meningomyelocele with partially epithelialized sac

FIGURE 2. Developmental pathogenesis of anencephaly and meningomyelocele.

705

OCCULT SPINAL DYSRAPHISM SEQUENCE
(Tethered Cord Malformation Sequence)

Following closure of the neural groove at approximately 28 days, the cell mass caudal to the posterior neuropore tunnels downward and forms a canal in a process that gives rise to the most distal portions of the spinal cord—the filum terminale and conus medullaris. Failure of normal morphogenesis in this region leads to a spectrum of structural defects that cause orthopedic or urologic symptoms through tethering or compression of the sacral nerve roots, with restriction of the normal cephalic migration of the conus medullaris. Defects involve structures derived from both mesodermal and ectodermal tissue and include mesodermal hamartomas, sacral vertebral anomalies, hyperplasia of the filum terminale, and structural alterations of the distal cord itself. In most situations, there is a cutaneous marker at the presumed junction between the caudal cell mass and the posterior neuropore in the region of L2-L3. Markers consist of tufts of hair, skin tags, dimples, lipomata, and aplasia cutis congenita. Cutaneous markers such as a pit at the tip of the coccyx are extremely common and are not usually associated with a tethered cord.

The recognition of the surface manifestations of such a malformation sequence at birth should ideally lead to further evaluation and management. Roentgenograms of the spine may or may not show any abnormality. Ultrasound to document normal movement of the spinal cord with respiration followed by magnetic resonance imaging in questionable cases is usually sufficient to document the defect. Early management will prevent neuromuscular lower limb or urologic problems such as retention, incontinence, or infection secondary to continued tractional tethering of the cord and nerve roots. If the physician waits for signs of such serious complications, the neurologic damage may not be reversible. A 4% incidence of open neural tube defects has been documented in first-degree relatives of probands.

References

Anderson FM: Occult spinal dysraphism: Diagnosis and management. J Pediatr 73:163, 1968.

Carter CO, Evans KA, Till K: Spinal dysraphism: Genetic relation to neural tube malformations. J Med Genet 13:343, 1976.

Tavafoghi V et al: Cutaneous signs of spinal dysraphism. Arch Dermatol 114:573, 1978.

Higginbottom MC et al: Aplasia cutis congenita: Cutaneous marker of occult spinal dysraphism. J Pediatr 96:687, 1980.

Soonawala N et al: Early clinical signs and symptoms in occult spinal dysraphism: A retrospective case study of 47 patients. Clin Neuro Neurosurg 101:11, 1999.

Hughes JA et al: Evaluation of spinal ultrasound in spinal dysraphism. Clin Radiol 58:227, 2003.

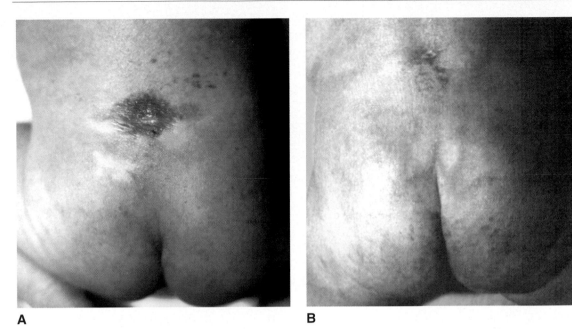

A   **B**

FIGURE 1. Occult spinal dysraphism sequence. Note the location of these lesions, which were the clues that resulted in surgical correction of tethered cord in early infancy. In addition to the flat hemangioma (**A**), the mound of connective tissue (**B**), and the localized absence of skin (**A** and **B**), surface anomalies may consist of lipomas, deep dimples, hair tufts, and skin tags. (From Higginbottom MC et al: J Pediatr 96:687, 1980, with permission.)

SEPTO-OPTIC DYSPLASIA SEQUENCE

De Morsier recognized the association between the absence of the septum pellucidum and hypoplasia of the optic nerves and called it septo-optic dysplasia. The clinical spectrum of altered development and function arising from this defect has been reported by Hoyt and others to include hypopituitary dwarfism. The presumed developmental pathogenesis is depicted to the right.

ABNORMALITIES

Eyes. Hypoplastic optic nerves, chiasm, and infundibulum with pendular nystagmus and visual impairment, occasionally including field defects.

Endocrine. Low levels of growth hormone, thyroid-stimulating hormone, luteinizing hormone, follicle-stimulating hormone, and antidiuretic hormone; hypoglycemia.

Other. Agenesis of septum pellucidum in approximately half of cases, microcephaly, schizencephaly.

OCCASIONAL ABNORMALITIES.

Trophic hormone hypersecretion, including growth hormone, corticotropin, and prolactin; sexual precocity; hemiplegia; spasticity; athetosis; epilepsy; autism; cranial nerve palsy; mental retardation; learning disabilities; attention deficit disorders; neonatal intrahepatic cholestasis.

NATURAL HISTORY.

Visual impairment, including partial to complete amblyopia, is frequent, and funduscopic evaluation discloses hypoplastic optic disks. Hypopituitarism of hypothalamic origin is a frequent feature and merits hormone replacement therapy. Affected newborns can develop hypoglycemia, apnea, hypotonia, or seizures. In an affected child with absence of the septum pellucidum and hypoplasia of the optic nerves who has no other associated defects of central nervous system development, prognosis relative to intellectual performance is good. However, mental retardation does occur, particularly when associated central nervous system defects are present. Onset of puberty is variable.

Features of the septo-optic dysplasia sequence may occur as a part of a broader pattern of early brain defect, such as the holoprosencephaly type of defect, in which case the prognosis for brain function and survival is poor.

ETIOLOGY.

This disorder is etiologically heterogeneous. Although most cases are sporadic, with several etiologies suggested including intrauterine viral infection, teratogens, and vascular disruption, autosomal recessive inheritance has been suggested in some cases. Mutations in HESX1, located at chromosome 3p21.1-21.2, are responsible for some sporadic as well as familial cases. HESX1 is a paired-like homeodomain transcription factor with repressing domains located in the N terminus and homeodomain. Expression of *Hesx1* in the developing mouse initially occurs during gastrulation, and later becomes restricted to Rathke's pouch, the precursor of the pituitary gland. Although the exact function of HESX1 is unknown, its repressing function appears to be critical, at least with respect to pituitary development.

References

de Morsier G: Études sur les dysraphies crânioencéphaliques. III. Agénésie du septum lucidum avec malformation du tractus optique: La dysplasie septo-optique. Schweiz Arch Neurol Neurochir Psychiatry 77:267, 1956.

Hoyt WF et al: Septo-optic dysplasia and pituitary dwarfism. Lancet 1:893, 1970.

Brook CGD et al: Septo-optic dysplasia. BMJ 3:811, 1972.

Haseman CA et al: Sexual precocity in association with septo-optic dysplasia and hypothalamic hypopituitarism. J Pediatr 92:748, 1978.

Blethen SL, Weldon VV: Hypopituitarism and septo-optic "dysplasia" in first cousins. Am J Med Genet 21:123, 1985.

Margalith D, Tze WJ, Jan JE: Congenital optic nerve hypoplasia with hypothalamic-pituitary dysplasia. Am J Dis Child 139:361, 1985.

Morgan SA et al: Absence of the septum pallucidum: Overlapping clinical syndromes. Arch Neurol 42:769, 1985.

Hanna CE et al: Puberty in the syndrome of septo-optic dysplasia. Am J Dis Child 143:186, 1989.

Dattani MT et al: Mutations in the homeobox gene HESX1/Hesx1 associated with septo-optic dysplasia in human and mouse. Nat Genet 19:125, 1998.

Dattani MT, Robinson IC: HESX1 and septo-optic dysplasia. Rev Endocr Metab Disord 3:289, 2002.

Cohen RN et al: Enhanced repression by HESX1 as a cause of hypopituitarism and septooptic dysplasia. J Clin Endocrinol Metab 88:4832, 2003.

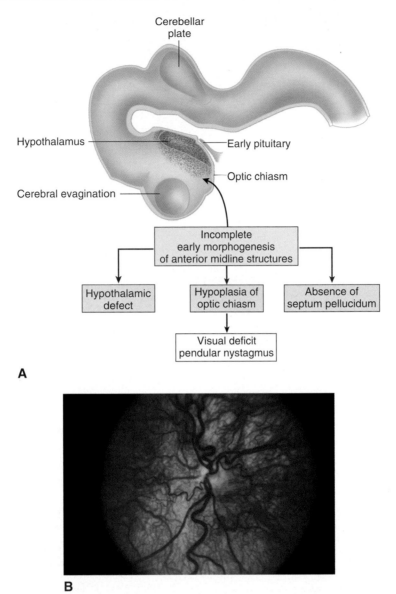

FIGURE 1. Septo-optic dysplasia. **A,** Presumed localization of early single defect (*stippled area*) as shown in sagittal view of 38-day brain. **B,** Photo of retina of 4-year-old patient with the septo-optic dysplasia sequence who had reduced vision, pendular nystagmus, and growth deficiency secondary to pituitary growth hormone deficiency. Note the hypoplastic optic nerve heads and aberrant vascular arrangement.

ATHYROTIC HYPOTHYROIDISM SEQUENCE
(HYPOTHYROIDISM SEQUENCE)

Primary Defect in Development of Thyroid Gland

Athyrotic hypothyroidism is usually a sporadic occurrence in an otherwise normal child. Severe hypothyroidism does not give rise to growth deficiency until after birth. Postnatally, morphogenesis and function are grossly impaired as a metabolic consequence of the lack of thyroid hormone. Adequate thyroid hormone replacement therapy, at least ¾ grain of U.S.P. desiccated thyroid per day for the affected infant, will allow for a complete return to physical normality for age. However, the detrimental effect of the hypothyroid state on morphogenesis and function of the brain is irreparable. Therefore, the earlier a diagnosis is made and adequate thyroid hormone therapy instituted, the better the prognosis for mental function.

ABNORMALITIES. The following are some of the early signs that may allow for detection of the hypothyroid baby early in life.

General

Feeding problems	39%
Decreased activity	56%
Constipation	11%
Neonatal jaundice	50%
Prolonged gestation	—

Cutaneous-Vascular

Cold to touch	33%
Dry skin	45%
Mottling	17%

Myxedema

Enlarged tongue	17%
Hoarse cry	39%
Periorbital edema	88%

Other

Umbilical hernia	58%
Enlarged anterior fontanel	71%
Enlarged posterior fontanel	65%
Cardiac defect	—

NATURAL HISTORY. When treatment is delayed until after 3 months, poor neurologic outcome is the rule. For those infants detected by neonatal screening and treated appropriately, growth and development have been demonstrated to be normal.

References

Wilkins L: The Diagnosis and Treatment of Endocrine Disorders in Childhood and Adolescence. Springfield, Ill: Charles C Thomas, 1965.

Klein AH et al: Improved prognosis in congenital hypothyroidism treated before age three months. J Pediatr 81:912, 1972.

Smith DW, Popich G: Large fontanels in congenital hypothyroidism. J Pediatr 80:753, 1972.

Virtanen M et al: Congenital hypothyroidism: Age at start of treatment versus outcome. Acta Paediatr Scand 72:197, 1983.

New England Congenital Hypothyroidism Collaborative: Characteristics of infantile hypothyroidism discovered on neonatal screening. J Pediatr 104:539, 1984.

Thompson GN et al: Management and outcome of children with congenital hypothyroidism detected on neonatal screening in South Australia. Med J Aust 145:18, 1986.

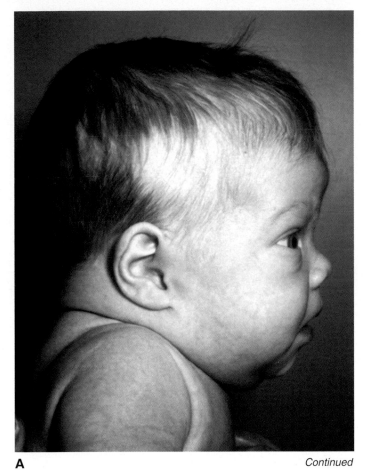

A   *Continued*

FIGURE 1. Athyrotic hypothyroidism. **A** and **B,** Evidence of osseous immaturity in a 3-month-old infant with athyrotic hypothyroidism. Note the immature facies with low nasal bridge and full subcutaneous tissues. (**A,** From Smith DW, Popich G: J Pediatr 80:753, 1972, with permission.)

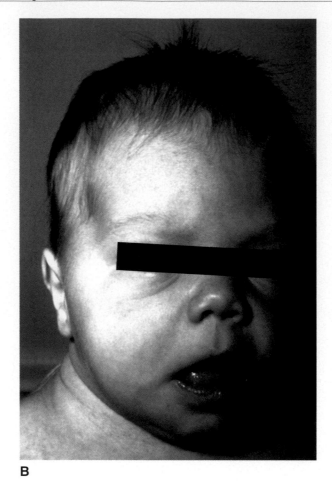

B

Fig. 1, cont'd.

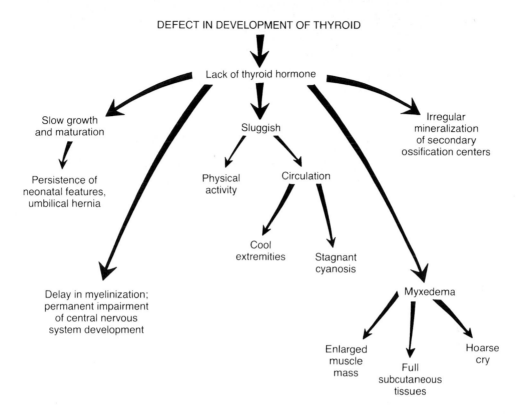

DEFECT IN DEVELOPMENT OF THYROID

Lack of thyroid hormone

Slow growth and maturation

Persistence of neonatal features, umbilical hernia

Sluggish

Physical activity

Circulation

Cool extremities

Stagnant cyanosis

Irregular mineralization of secondary ossification centers

Delay in myelinization; permanent impairment of central nervous system development

Myxedema

Enlarged muscle mass

Full subcutaneous tissues

Hoarse cry

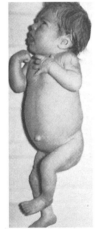
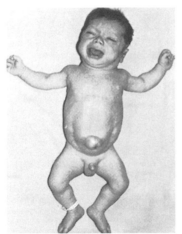
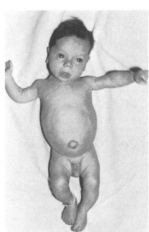
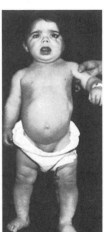

Age: 2 months
Height age: 1 month
Bone age: birth

Age: 9 months
Height age: 2 months
Bone age: birth

After 3 weeks of thyroid replacement

Age: 3 years, untreated
Height age: 12 months
Bone age: 3 months

FIGURE 2. Diagram showing developmental pathogenesis of athyrotic hypothyroidism. Photographs of athyrotic patients.

DiGEORGE SEQUENCE

Primary Defect—Fourth Branchial Arch and Derivatives of Third and Fourth Pharyngeal Pouches

This pattern of malformation was emphasized by DiGeorge and variably includes defects of development of the thymus, parathyroids, and great vessels. Conley and colleagues observed 19 cases at necropsy. The illustration shows the presumed developmental pathogenesis.

ABNORMALITIES. Varying features from among the following:

Thymus. Hypoplasia to aplasia, with deficit of cellular immunity allowing for severe infectious disease.

Parathyroids. Hypoplasia to absence, allowing for severe hypocalcemia and seizures in early infancy.

Cardiovascular. Aortic arch anomalies, including right aortic arch, interrupted aorta, conotruncal anomalies such as truncus arteriosus and ventricular septal defect, patent ductus arteriosus, and tetralogy of Fallot.

Facial. (Specific to partial monosomy 22q; see later.) Lateral displacement of inner canthi with short palpebral fissures, short philtrum, micrognathia, ear anomalies.

OCCASIONAL ABNORMALITIES.

Mental deficiency of mild to moderate degree, esophageal atresia, choanal atresia, velopharyngeal insufficiency, imperforate anus, diaphragmatic hernia.

NATURAL HISTORY. There is a significant neonatal morbidity and mortality associated with the cardiac defects, sequelae of the immunodeficiency, and seizures relative to hypocalcemia. The natural history is dependent on the etiology of the DiGeorge sequence. For those children with partial monosomy of the long arm of chromosome 22, the natural history is the same as that of the Shprintzen syndrome.

ETIOLOGY. This pattern is etiologically heterogeneous. It has been associated with prenatal exposure to alcohol and Accutane and a variety of chromosome abnormalities. The majority of cases, however, are a result of partial monosomy of the proximal long arm of chromosome 22 caused by a microdeletion of 22q11.2 (see Deletion 22q11.2 syndrome).

References

Lobdell DH: Congenital absence of the parathyroid glands. Arch Pathol 67:412, 1959.

Kretschmer R, Say B, Brown D, Rosen FS: Congenital aplasia of the thymus gland (DiGeorge's syndrome). N Engl J Med 279:1295, 1968.

Freedom RM, Rosen FS, Nadas AS: Congenital cardiovascular disease and anomalies of the third and fourth pharyngeal pouch. Circulation 46:165, 1972.

Conley ME et al: The spectrum of the DiGeorge syndrome. J Pediatr 94:883, 1979.

Greenberg F et al: Familial DiGeorge syndrome and associated partial monosomy of chromosome 22. Hum Genet 65:317, 1984.

Stevens CA et al: DiGeorge anomaly and velocardiofacial syndrome. Pediatrics 85:526, 1990.

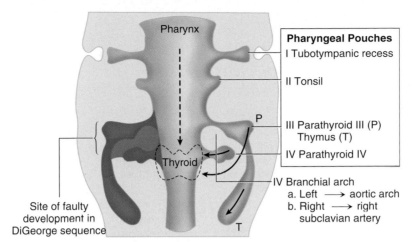

FIGURE 1. DiGeorge sequence. Schematic appearance of anterior foregut and its derivatives at around the fifth week of development, showing the presumed site of defect.

KLIPPEL-FEIL SEQUENCE

Short Neck with Low Hairline and Limited Movement of Head: Primary Defect—Early Development of Cervical Vertebrae

In this malformation sequence, originally described by Klippel and Feil in 1912, the cervical vertebrae are usually fused, although hemivertebrae and other defects may also be found. There may also be secondary webbed neck, torticollis, and/or facial asymmetry. The frequency is approximately 1 in 42,000 births, and 65% of patients are female. The sequence may be a part of a serious problem in early neural tube development, as is found in iniencephaly, cervical meningomyelocele, syringomyelia, or syringobulbia. Primary or secondary neurologic deficits may occur, such as paraplegia, hemiplegia, cranial or cervical nerve palsies, and synkinesia (mirror movements). A strong association exists between mirror movements and cervicomedullary neuroschisis.

The following defects have occurred in a nonrandom association in patients with the Klippel-Feil sequence: deafness, either conductive or neural, noted in as many as 30%; congenital heart defects, the most common being a ventricular septal defect; mental deficiency; cleft palate; rib defects; the Sprengel anomaly; posterior fossa dermoid cysts; scoliosis; renal abnormalities.

Lateral flexion-extension radiographs of the cervical spine should be performed on all patients to determine the motion of each open interspace. Clinically, flexion-extension is often maintained if a single functioning open interspace is maintained. Those with hypermobility of the upper cervical segment are at risk of developing neurologic impairment. They should be evaluated at least annually and should avoid violent activities. Affected individuals with hypermobility of the lower cervical segment are at increased risk for degenerative disk disease and should be treated symptomatically. Usually a sporadic occurrence of unknown etiology, this sequence has rarely been found in siblings. A close evaluation of the immediate family is indicated, because autosomal dominant inheritance with variable expression in affected individuals has been noted, although this is presumably rare.

References

Klippel M, Feil A: Un cas d'absence des vertébres cervicales, avec cage thoracique remontant jusqu'à la base du crâne (cage thoracique cervicale). Mouv Inconogr Salpêt 25:223, 1912.

Morrison SG, Perry LW, Scott LP III: Congenital brevicollis (Klippel-Feil syndrome) and cardiovascular anomalies. Am J Dis Child 115:614, 1968.

Palant DJ, Carter BL: Klippel-Feil syndrome and deafness. Am J Dis Child 123:218, 1972.

Hensinger RW, Lang JE, MacEwen GD: Klippel-Feil syndrome. J Bone Joint Surg 56-A:1246, 1974.

Dickey W et al: Posterior fossa dermoid cysts and the Klippel-Feil syndrome. J Neurol Neurosurg Psychiatry 54:1016, 1991.

Pizzutillo PD et al: Risk factors in Klippel-Feil syndrome. Spine 19:2110, 1994.

Royal SA et al: Investigations into the association between cervicomedullary neuroschisis and mirror movements in patients with Klippel-Feil syndrome. AJNR 23:724, 2002.

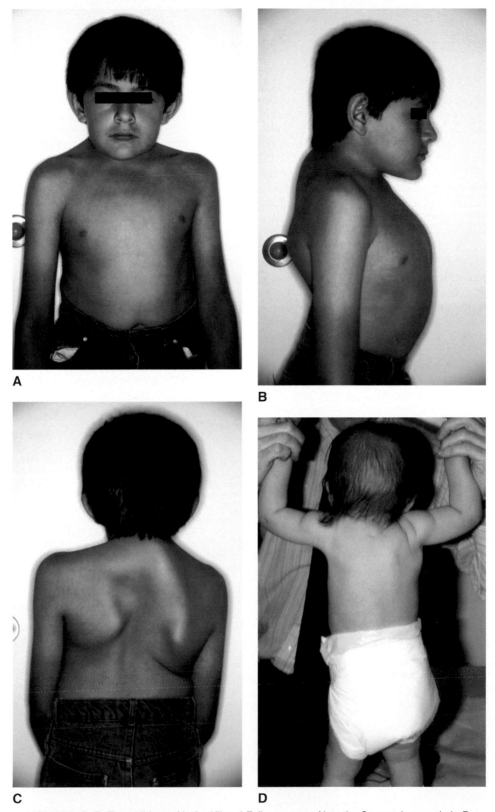

FIGURE 1. **A–D,** Two children with the Klippel-Feil sequence. Note the Sprengel anomaly in **D**.

EARLY URETHRAL OBSTRUCTION SEQUENCE

Early urethral obstruction is most commonly the consequence of urethral valve formation during the development of the prostatic urethra. Less commonly, it is due to urethral atresia, bladder neck obstruction, or distal urethral obstruction. With urine formation occurring, by 7 to 8 weeks of fetal life, there is a progressive back-up of urine flow, leading to the consequences shown in the flow diagram. The male-to-female ratio of 20:1 in this disorder is a result of the predominant malformations being in the development of the prostatic urethra. Cryptorchidism occurs secondary to the bulk of the distended bladder, preventing full descent of the testes. The back-pressure usually limits full renal morphogenesis and may result in dilatation of the renal tubules, which in all cases show mixed cystic and dysplastic changes. Hypoplasia of the prostate is an essential feature of the disorder and is most likely a primary event in the pathogenesis of the urethral obstruction. The compressive mass of the bladder may limit full rotation of the colon and may even compress the iliac vessels to the point of causing partial defects or vascular disruption of the lower limb(s). The oligohydramnios will give rise to all the secondary phenomena of the oligohydramnios deformation sequence.

Severe early urethral obstruction is often lethal by mid- to late fetal life unless the bladder ruptures and is thereby decompressed. The bladder rupture may occur through a patent urachus, an obstructing urethral "valve," or the wall of the bladder or ureter. Following decompression, the fetus will be left with a "prune belly."

Unfortunately, most of those who survive to term have incurred severe renal damage and are unable to live long after birth. Those who do survive may be assisted by urologic procedures to aid urinary drainage and control urinary tract infection. Respiration and bowel movements may be eased by wrapping the abdomen with a "belly binder." With advancing age, the hypoplastic abdominal musculature will usually improve in volume and strength to the point of being no serious problem.

The recurrence risk for the disorder is dependent on the specific cause of the urethral obstruction, and these data have not yet been determined. This defect most commonly occurs in an otherwise normal individual, but may be but one feature of a broader pattern of malformation, such as the VATERR association. Early fetal diagnosis is possible, because sonography will show the distended bladder by 10 weeks from conception.

In some cases, this sequence may be the result of an intrauterine vascular accident. Support for this is based on its occurrence in one member of a monozygotic twin pair as well as its association with single umbilical artery, prenatal exposure to cocaine, and with younger maternal age.

References

Stumme EG: Ueber die symmetrischen kongenitalen Bauchmuskel defeckte und über die Kombination derselben mit anderen Bildunganomalien des Rumfes. Mitt Grenzigebeite Med Chir 6:548, 1903.

Silverman FN, Huang N: Congenital absence of the abdominal muscles. Am J Dis Child 80:91, 1950.

Lattimer JK: Congenital deficiency of abdominal musculature and associated genitourinary anomalies. J Urol 79:343, 1958.

Pagon RA, Smith DW, Shepard TH: Urethral obstruction malformation complex: A cause of abdominal muscle deficiency and the "prune belly." J Pediatr 94:900, 1979.

Popek EJ et al: Prostate development in prune belly syndrome (PBS) and posterior urethral valves (PUV): Etiology of PBS lower urinary tract obstruction or primary mesenchymal defect? Pediatr Pathol 11:1, 1991.

Jones KL et al: Vascular steal associated with single umbilical artery: A mechanism responsible for the urethral obstruction malformation sequence. Proc Greenwood Genet Clinic 19:85, 2000.

Poucell-Hatton S et al: Fetal obstructive uropathy: Patterns of renal pathology. Pediatr Devel Pathol 3:223, 2000.

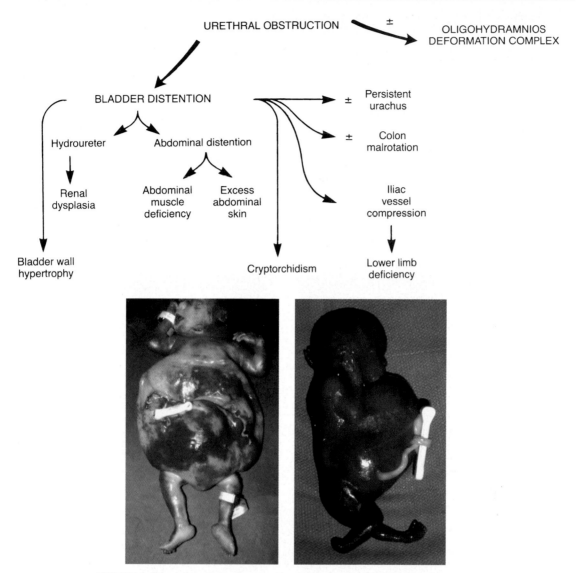

FIGURE 1. Developmental pathogenesis of early urethral obstruction sequence.

EXSTROPHY OF BLADDER SEQUENCE
Primary Defect in Infraumbilical Mesoderm

Normally the bladder portion of the cloaca and the overlying ectoderm are in direct contact (the cloacal membrane) until the infraumbilical mesenchyme migrates into the area at approximately the sixth to seventh week of fetal development, giving rise to the lower abdominal wall, genital tubercles, and pubic rami. A failure of the infraumbilical mesenchyme to invade the area allows for a breakdown in the cloacal membrane, in similar fashion to that which normally occurs at the oral, anal, and urogenital areas, where mesoderm does not intercede between ectoderm and endoderm. Thus, the posterior bladder wall is exposed, in conjunction with defects in structures derived from the infraumbilical mesenchyme.

This malformation sequence is estimated to occur in approximately 1 in 30,000 births and is more likely to occur in the male than in the female. In most cases, the defect can be closed within the first few days of life, genital function can be expected to be satisfactory, and urinary control will be achieved. Of 13 affected individuals older than 17 years of age, 12 reported sexual experiences, 6 were married, 13 attended college, and 7 were employed. All were considered well adjusted. However, for both the parents and affected child, intervention from a multidisciplinary team during different stages of childhood is advised.

The recurrence risk for unaffected parents who have had a child with bladder extrophy or epispadias is less than 1% (1 in 275). For the offspring of a parent with bladder extrophy or epispadias, recurrence risk is approximately 1 in 70 live births.

References

Wyburn GM: The development of the infraumbilical portion of the abdominal wall, with remarks on the aetiology of ectopia vesicae. J Anat 71:201, 1937.

Muecke EC: The role of the cloacal membrane in exstrophy: The first successful experimental study. J Urol 92:659, 1964.

Shapiro E et al: The inheritance of the exstrophy-epispadias complex. J Urol 132:308, 1984.

Jeffs RD: Exstrophy, epispadias, and cloacal and urogenital sinus abnormalities. Pediatr Clin North Am 34:1233, 1987.

Stjernqvist K, Kockum CC: Bladder exstrophy: Psychological impact during childhood. J Urol 162:2125, 1999.

Reutter H et al: Seven new cases of familial isolated bladder exstrophy and epispadias complex (BEEC) and review of the literature. Am J Med Genet 120A:215, 2003.

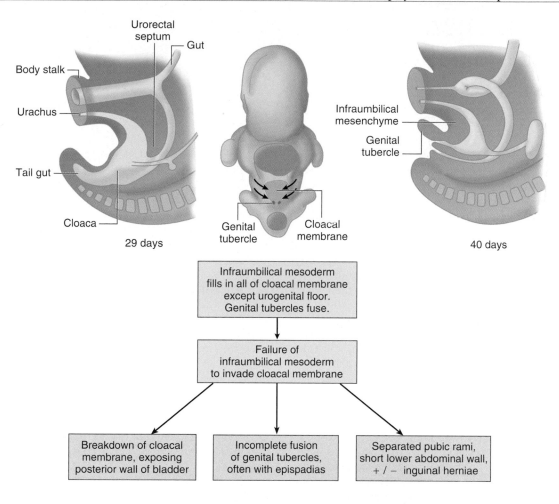

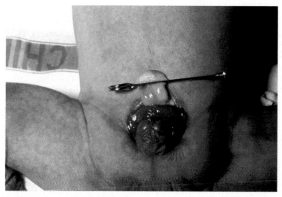

FIGURE 1. Developmental pathogenesis of exstrophy of bladder sequence.

EXSTROPHY OF CLOACA SEQUENCE

*Primary Defect—Early Mesoderm That Will
Contribute to Infraumbilical Mesenchyme,
Cloacal Septum, and Lumbosacral Vertebrae*

Occurring in approximately 1 in 400,000 births, the remarkable similarity among otherwise normal individuals with this bizarre type of defect suggests a similar mode of developmental pathology having its inception as a single localized defect—theoretically in the early development of the mesoderm, which will later contribute to the infraumbilical mesenchyme, cloacal septum, and caudal vertebrae. The consequences are (1) failure of cloacal septation, with the persistence of a common cloaca into which the ureters, ileum, and a rudimentary hindgut open; (2) complete breakdown of the cloacal membrane with exstrophy of the cloaca, failure of fusion of the genital tubercles and pubic rami, and often omphalocele; and (3) incomplete development of the lumbosacral vertebrae with herniation of a grossly dilated central canal of the spinal cord (hydromyelia), yielding a soft, cystic, skin-covered mass over the sacral area, sometimes asymmetric in its positioning. Tethering of the cord is frequently recognized and scoliosis is common. Bladder function, bladder neck continence, lower extremity function, and erectile capacity all relate, at least partially, to neurologic function. The rudimentary hindgut may contain two appendices, and there is no anal opening. The small intestine may be relatively short. Cryptorchidism is a usual finding in the male. Urinary tract anomalies including pelvic kidneys, renal agenesis, multicystic kidney, and ureteral duplication occur commonly. Affected females have unfused müllerian elements with completely bifid uterine horns and short, duplicated, or atretic vaginas. Most patients have a single umbilical artery, and anomalies of the lower limbs occasionally occur and include congenital hip dislocation, talipes equinovarus, and agenesis of a limb.

Excellent survival rates following surgical repair is now the rule. Although the "short bowel syndrome" is a significant problem in early years, the bowel usually adapts and nutritional status stabilizes. Continence of urine, mainly by catheterization, and of stool, mainly by enema washouts, is achievable in most patients. Gender assignment and psychological aspects relating to gender have become a major issue. Previously, many affected children with a 46XY karyotype have undergone gender reassignment. Recent evidence indicates that this may not necessarily be the correct approach. Although quality of life is described as similar among those who have been raised female whether they have an XY or XX karyotype, those with XY chromosomes who have been raised female consistently scored lower on measurements of social adjustment and relationships with family and peers as well as on overall body appearance.

References

Spencer R: Exstrophia splanchnica (exstrophy of the cloaca). Surgery 57:751, 1965.

Beckwith JB: The congenitally malformed. VII. Exstrophy of the bladder and cloacal exstrophy. Northwest Med 65:407, 1966.

Hurwitz RS et al: Cloacal exstrophy: A report of 34 cases. J Urol 138:1060, 1987.

Jeffs RD: Exstrophy, epispadius and cloacal and urogenital sinus abnormalities. Pediatr Clin North Am 34:1233, 1987.

Lund DP et al: Coacal exstrophy: A 25-year experience with 50 cases. J Pediatr 36:68, 2001.

Schober JM et al: The ultimate challenge of cloacal exstrophy. J Urol 167:300, 2002.

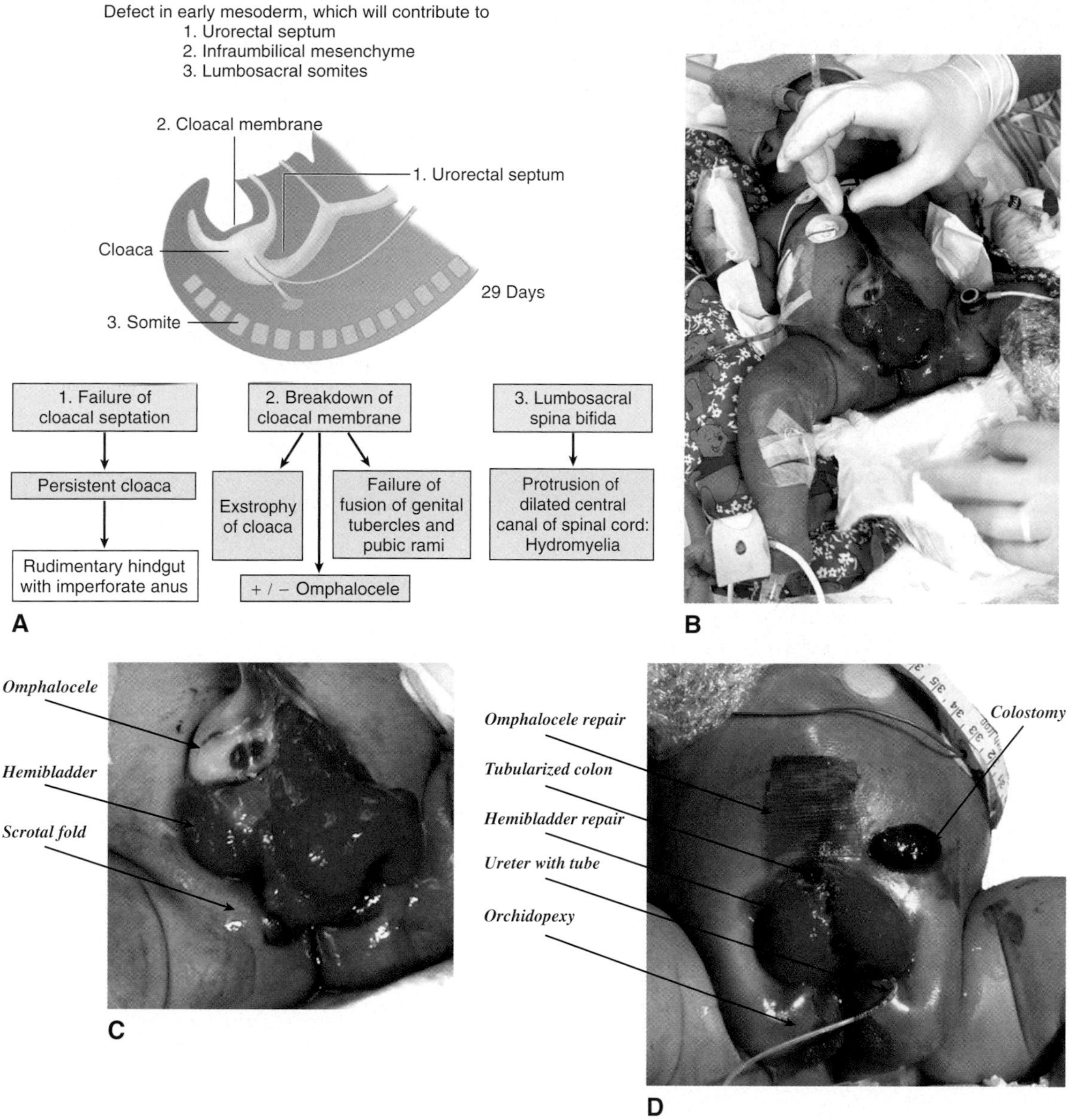

FIGURE 1. **A,** Developmental pathogenesis of exstrophy of cloaca sequence. **B** and **C,** Before surgery. **D,** Following first stage of surgical repair. (**B–D,** Courtesy of Dr. Kurt Benirschke, University of California, San Diego.)

URORECTAL SEPTUM MALFORMATION SEQUENCE

In 1987, Escobar and colleagues reported six patients with this disorder and reviewed a number of previously reported cases, many of whom had been diagnosed as female pseudohermaphrodites. The principal features include the following: striking ambiguity of the external genitalia with a short phallus-like structure that lacks corpora cavernosa and absent urethra and vaginal openings; imperforate anus; bladder, vaginal, and rectal fistulas; and müllerian duct defects. Other common associated findings include cystic dysplasia/agenesis of kidneys, vertebral anomalies, cardiac defects, tracheoesophageal fistula, talipes equinovarus, and single umbilical artery.

It has been suggested that this pattern of malformation is due to two related events in the development of the urorectal septum. Normally, by the sixth week of development, the urorectal septum divides the cloacal cavity into a urogenital sinus anteriorly and a rectum posteriorly and fuses with the cloacal membrane. At the same time that the urorectal septum fuses with the cloacal membrane, the membrane breaks down, leaving an open urogenital sinus and rectum. Failure of the urorectal septum to divide the cloaca or fuse with the cloacal membrane leads in a cascading fashion to the urorectal septum malformation sequence. Because the cloacal membrane has failed to breakdown, the median raphe, which represents fusion of the labioscrotal folds in an XY fetus, is not present.

Long-term survival of affected individuals is extremely rare. Virtually all patients are stillborn or die in the neonatal period secondary to respiratory complications of oligohydramnios or renal failure.

Recurrence risk for isolated cases of the urorectal septum malformation sequence is negligible. However, when it occurs as one feature in a multiple malformation syndrome, recurrence risk is for that disorder.

References

Escobar LF et al: Urorectal septum malformation sequence: Report of six cases and embryological analysis. Am J Dis Child 141:1021, 1987.

Wheeler PG et al: Urorectal septum malformation sequence: Report of thirteen additional cases and review of the literature. Am J Med Genet 73:456, 1997.

Qi BQ et al: Clarification of the process of separation of the cloaca into rectum and urognital sinus in the rat embryo. J Pediatr Surg 35:1810, 2000.

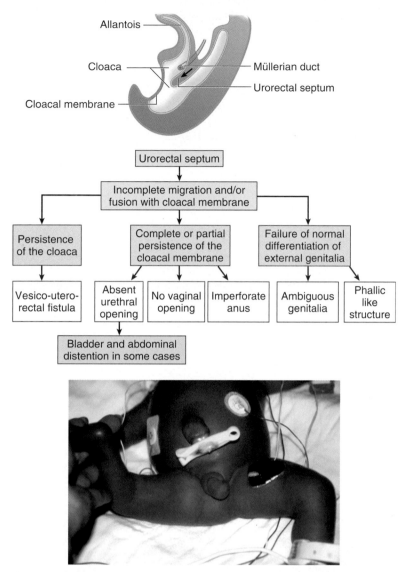

FIGURE 1. *Top*, Developmental pathogenesis of the urorectal septum malformation sequence. (From Escobar LF et al: Am J Dis Child 141:1021, 1987, with permission. Copyright 1987, American Medical Association.) *Bottom*, 46XX individual with urorectal septum malformation sequence. Note the phallus-like structure, absent urethral and vaginal opening, and imperforate anus.

OLIGOHYDRAMNIOS SEQUENCE
(POTTER SYNDROME)

Primary Defect—Development of Oligohydramnios

Renal agenesis, which must occur before 31 days of fetal development, will secondarily limit the amount of amniotic fluid and thereby result in further anomalies during prenatal life. The renal agenesis may be the only primary defect, or it may be one feature of a more extensive caudal axis anomaly. Other types of urinary tract defects such as polycystic kidneys or obstruction may also be responsible for oligohydramnios and its consequences. Another cause is chronic leakage of amniotic fluid from the time of midgestation. Regardless of the cause, the secondary effects of oligohydramnios are the same and would appear to be the result of compression of the fetus, as depicted subsequently. The cause of death is respiratory insufficiency, with a lack of the late development of alveolar sacs. A similar lag in late development of the lung is observed with diaphragmatic hernia or asphyxiating thoracic dystrophy. In both of these situations, there is external compression of the developing lung; this is considered the most likely cause in oligohydramnios, as shown in the figure.

When the oligohydramnios is secondary to agenesis or dysgenesis of both kidneys or agenesis of one kidney and dysgenesis of the other, renal ultrasonographic evaluation of both parents and siblings of affected infants should be performed, because 9% of first-degree relatives had asymptomatic renal malformations in a study by Roodhooft and colleagues.

References

Potter EL: Bilateral renal agenesis. J Pediatr 29:68, 1946.

Bain AD, Scott JS: Renal agenesis and severe urinary tract dysplasia: A review of 50 cases with particular reference to the associated anomalies. BMJ 1:841, 1960.

Thomas IT, Smith DW: Oligohydramnios, cause of the nonrenal features of Potter's syndrome, including pulmonary hypoplasia. J Pediatr 84:811, 1974.

Roodhooft AM, Birnholz JC, Holmes LB: Familial nature of congenital absence and severe dysgenesis of both kidneys. N Engl J Med 310:1341, 1984.

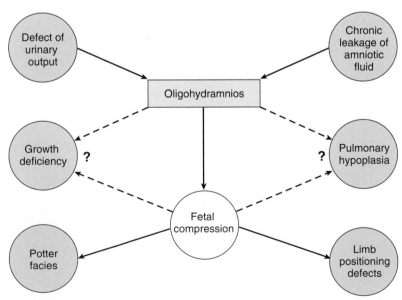

FIGURE 1. Depiction of the origin and effects of oligohydramnios. The oligohydramnios sequence is implied to be secondary to fetal compression.

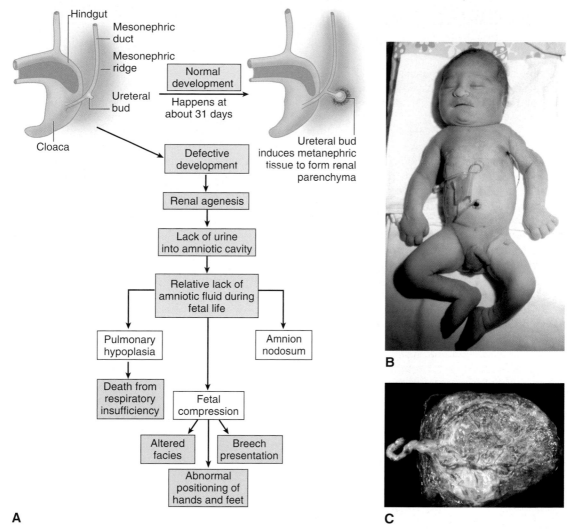

A

B

C

FIGURE 2. **A–C,** The consequences of renal agenesis. Note the multiple deformational defects in **B** and the amnion nodosum (brown-yellow granules from vernix that have been rubbed into defects of the amnionic surface) in **C**.

SIRENOMELIA SEQUENCE

This defect has previously been thought to be the consequence of a wedge-shaped early deficit of the posterior axis caudal blastema, allowing for fusion of the early limb buds at their fibular margins with absence or incomplete development of the intervening caudal structures. However, Stevenson and colleagues showed that sirenomelia and its commonly associated defects are produced by an alteration in early vascular development. Rather than blood returning to the placenta through the usual paired umbilical arteries arising from the iliac arteries, blood returns to the placenta through a single large vessel, a derivative of the vitelline artery complex, which arises from the aorta just below the diaphragm. The abdominal aorta distal to the origin of this major vessel is always subordinate and usually gives off no tributaries, especially renal or inferior mesenteric arteries, before it bifurcates into iliac arteries. This vascular alteration leads to a "vitelline artery steal" in which blood flow and thus nutrients are diverted from the caudal structures of the embryo to the placenta. Resultant defects include a single lower extremity with posterior alignment of knees and feet, arising from failure of the lower limb bud field to be cleaved into two lateral masses by an intervening allantois; absence of sacrum and other defects of vertebrae; imperforate anus and absence of rectum; absence of external and internal genitalia; renal agenesis; and absence of the bladder. Based on the variable alterations that could exist in blood flow, a variable spectrum of abnormalities occurs in structures dependent on the distal aorta for nutrients. Thus, as with other disruptive vascular defects, no two cases of sirenomelia are ever the same.

References

Wolff E: Les bases de la tératogénèse expérimentale des vertèbres amniotes, d'après les résultats de méthodes directes. Arch Anat Histol Embryol (Strasb) 22:1, 1936.

Stevenson RE et al: Vascular steal: The pathogenic mechanism producing sirenomelia and associated defects of the viscera and soft tissues. Pediatrics 78:451, 1986.

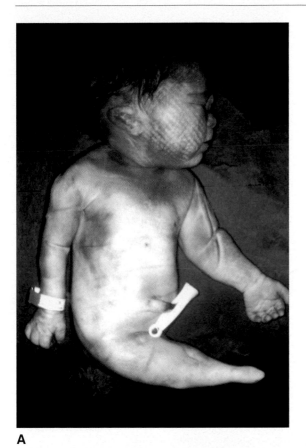

A

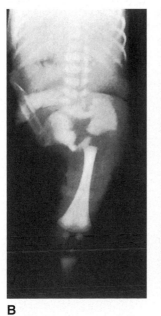

B

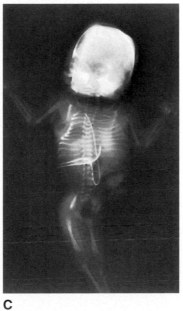

C

FIGURE 1. **A,** Stillborn infant with sirenomelia. **B** and **C,** The bones in the single leg vary from completely separate to a single broad femur with two distal ossification centers and a broad tibia with two ossification centers.

CAUDAL DYSPLASIA SEQUENCE
(CAUDAL REGRESSION SYNDROME)

This disorder has previously been grouped with sirenomelia, which was thought to represent its most severe form. Recent evidence suggests that the two are pathogenetically unrelated. Whereas sirenomelia and its associated defects are produced by an early vascular alteration leading to a "vitelline artery steal," the caudal dysplasia sequence is most likely heterogenous with respect to its etiology and developmental pathogenesis.

Structural defects of the caudal region observed in this pattern of malformation include the following to variable degrees: incomplete development of the sacrum and, to a lesser extent, the lumbar vertebrae; absence of the body of the sacrum, leading to flattening of the buttocks, shortening of the intergluteal cleft, and dimpling of the buttocks; disruption of the distal spinal cord leading secondarily to neurologic impairment, varying from incontinence of urine and feces to complete neurologic loss; and extreme lack of growth in the caudal region resulting from decreased movement of the legs secondary to neurologic impairment. The most severely affected infants have flexion and abduction at the hips and popliteal webs secondary to lack of movement. Talipes equinovarus and calcaneovalgus deformities are common.

Occasional abnormalities include renal agenesis, imperforate anus, cleft lip, cleft palate, microcephaly, and meningomyelocele.

NATURAL HISTORY. In the most severely affected individuals, prognosis is poor. Urologic and orthopedic management is required in the vast majority of those who survive.

ETIOLOGY. The cause of this disorder is unknown. Sixteen percent have occurred in offspring of diabetic mothers. Although usually sporadic, a few instances of affected siblings born to unaffected parents have been described.

References

Rusnak SL, Driscoll SG: Congenital spinal anomalies in infants of diabetic mothers. Pediatrics 35:989, 1965.

Passarge E, Lenz W: Syndrome of caudal regression in infants of diabetic mothers: Observations of further cases. Pediatrics 37:672, 1966.

Gellis SS, Feingold M: Picture of the month: Caudal dysplasia syndrome. Am J Dis Child 116:407, 1968.

Price DL, Dooling EC, Richardson EP: Caudal dysplasia (caudal regression syndrome). Arch Neurol 23:212, 1970.

Finer NN, Bowen P, Dunbar LG: Caudal regression anomalad (sacral agenesis in siblings). Clin Genet 13:353, 1978.

Stewart JM, Stoll S: Familial caudal regression anomalad and maternal diabetes. J Med Genet 16:17, 1979.

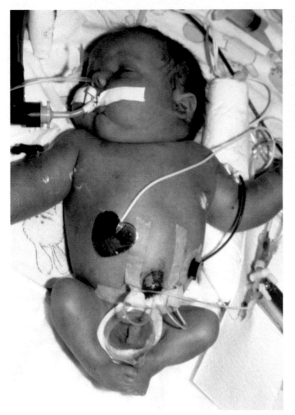

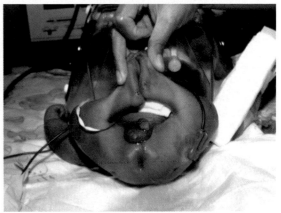

FIGURE 1. Caudal dysplasia sequence. **A,** Newborn male infant with a normal upper body and a short lower segment. **B,** Note the pterygia in the popliteal region, which are secondary to neurologically related flexion contractures at the knees.

A

AMNION RUPTURE SEQUENCE

Although the structural defects consequent to amnion rupture were reported by Portal in 1685, it was not until more recent times that the full spectrum of defects that can occur was delineated by Torpin as well as by others. Secondary to amnion rupture, small strands of amnion can encircle developing structures (usually the limbs) leading to annular constrictions, pseudosyndactyly, intrauterine amputations, and umbilical cord constriction. In addition to these disruptive defects, deformational defects can occur secondary to decreased fetal movement, the result of tethering of a limb by an amniotic band; or constraint, the result of decreased amniotic fluid. The decreased fetal activity may result in scoliosis or foot deformities. It may also cause edema, hemorrhage, and resorptive necrosis. As is the case with all disruptive defects, no two affected fetuses will have exactly the same features, and there is no single feature that consistently occurs. Examination of the placenta and membranes is diagnostic. Aberrant bands or strands of amnion are noted, or there may be the rolled-up remnants of the amnion at the placental base of the umbilical cord.

Incorrectly, thoraco- or abdominoschisis, exencephaly/encephalocele, and facial clefts usually associated with amnion adhesions and sometimes complicated by rupture of the amnion with amputation defects have been considered part of the amnion rupture sequence. This pattern of defects, now referred to as the limb–body wall complex, is due to a different pathogenetic mechanism.

NATURAL HISTORY AND MANAGEMENT. The natural history varies with the severity of the problem. Amnion constrictive bands or amputations of the limb in an otherwise normal child occur most commonly. Occasionally, plastic surgery may be indicated, especially for the partially constrictive, deep residual groove that encircles a limb and is associated with partial limitation of vascular or lymphatic return from the distal limb. In such instances, a Z-plasty of the skin may be done to relieve the partial constriction. If there has been chronic amnion leakage, the neonate may show features of the oligohydramnios deformation sequence, including incomplete development of the lung, with respiratory insufficiency. Every attempt should be made to oxygenate and support such an infant, since with continued lung morphogenesis, the prognosis can be excellent. Because the result of amnion rupture is external compression or disruption, internal anomalies do not occur. Hence, the features evident by surface examination are usually the only abnormalities.

ETIOLOGY. The etiology of this disorder has been, with rare exceptions, idiopathic. Those rare exceptions are known or presumed to be caused by trauma and include two examples of attempted early termination of pregnancy by using a coat hanger and one incident of a woman falling from a horse while pregnant. It has generally been a sporadic event in an otherwise normal family, and hence the recurrence risk is usually stated as being negligible. Although the disruptive defect resulting from amniotic bands may occur at any time during gestation, amnion rupture most likely occurs before 12 weeks' gestation. Before that time, the amnion and chorion are completely separate membranes and as such it has been suggested that the amnion is vulnerable to rupture.

References

Portal P: La Pratique des Accouchements. Paris, 1685.

Torpin R: Amniochorionic mesoblastic fibrous strings and amniotic bands: Associated constricting fetal malformations of fetal death. Am J Obstet Gynecol 91:65, 1965.

Torpin R: Fetal Malformations Caused by Amnion Rupture during Gestation. Springfield, Ill: Charles C Thomas, 1968.

Kalousek DK, Bamforth S: Amnion rupture sequence in previable fetuses. Am J Med Genet 31:63, 1988.

Moerman P et al: Constrictive amniotic bands, amniotic adhesions, and limb-body wall complex: Discrete disruption sequences with pathogenetic overlap. Am J Med Genet 42:470, 1992.

Martinez-Frias ML et al: Epidemiological characteristics of amniotic band sequence (ABS) and body wall complex (BWC): Are they different entities? Am J Med Genet 73:176, 1997.

Werler MM et al: Epidemiologic analysis of maternal factors and amniotic band defects. Birth Defects Res A Clin Mol Teratol 67:68, 2003.

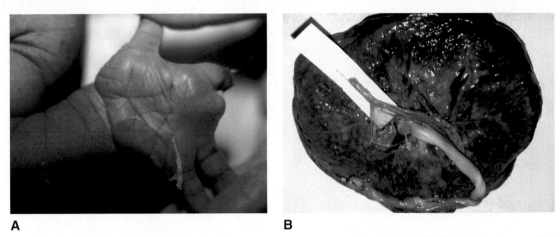

A   **B**

FIGURE 1. Amnion rupture sequence. **A,** Amputation of the fingers by strands of amnion. **B,** The child's placenta. Note the amnion that has stripped off the left side of the fetal surface of the placenta and is rolled up at the base of the umbilical cord.

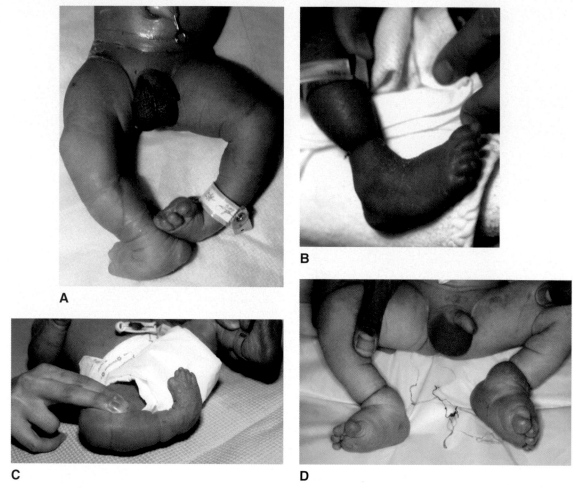

A

B

C

D

FIGURE 2. Variable limb anomalies secondary to aberrant bands. **A–D,** Bands constricting the ankle leading to deformational defects and amputation. (**A–F,** From Jones KL et al: J Pediatr 84:90, 1974, with permission.)

Continued

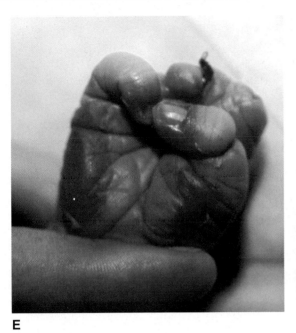

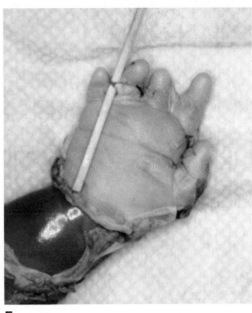

E

F

Fig. 2, cont'd. **E** and **F**, Pseudosyndactyly, amputation, and disruption of finger morphogenesis.

LIMB–BODY WALL COMPLEX

The limb–body wall complex consists of thoraco- or abdominoschisis and limb defects frequently associated with exencephaly/encephalocele and facial clefts. The vast majority of cases are spontaneously aborted; the remainder are stillborn.

The thoraco-abdominoschisis involves an anterolateral body wall defect with evisceration of thoracic or abdominal organs into a persistent extraembryonic coelom. The extraembryonic coelom, the space between the amnion and chorion, is obliterated normally by 60 days' gestation. Failure of the ventral body wall to fuse because of damage to part of the body wall or failure of normal ventral folding of the embryo leads to a persistence of the extraembryonic coelom. The amnion is continuous with the skin at the edge of the defect and the umbilical cord is short and partially devoid of its normal amniotic membrane covering. Limb defects similar to those seen in the amnion rupture sequence such as amputations secondary to ring constrictions and pseudosyndactyly occur occasionally. However, other limb defects such as single forearm or lower leg bones, ectrodactyly, radioulnar synostosis, and polydactyly (defects that cannot be explained on the basis of constriction or tethering by amniotic bands) occur more frequently. The encephaloceles are usually anterior, often multiple, and are occasionally attached to the amnion. The facial clefts do not conform to the usual lines of closure of the facial processes and are frequently associated with disruption of the frontonasal processes.

In addition, there is a high incidence of associated anomalies of the internal organs including the heart, lungs (lobation defects), diaphragm (absent), intestine (nonrotation, atresia, shortened), gallbladder, kidney (absent, hydronephrotic, dysplastic), and genitourinary tract (abnormal external genitalia or uterus, absent gonad, streak ovaries, bladder extrophy).

The developmental pathogenesis as well as the etiology of limb–body wall complex is controversial. Incorrectly it has been included in the past as part of the spectrum of the amnion rupture sequence, a concept that is clearly untenable based on the observation that the amniotic membrane is intact in some cases.

Van Allen and colleagues suggested that an early systemic alteration of embryonic blood supply between 4 and 6 weeks' gestation leads to disruptive vascular defects to the developing embryo including facial clefts, damage to the calvaria or brain resulting in neural tube–like defects, many of the limb reduction defects, and the internal visceral anomalies. Adhesion of the amnion to these necrotic areas could lead secondarily to amniotic adhesive bands. Failure of the ventral body wall to close because of vascular compromise could lead to persistence of the extraembryonic coelom. Features typical of the amnion band rupture sequence such as constriction bands are secondary to rupture of the amnion that is not adequately supported because the extraembryonic coelom has not been obliterated.

Others have suggested that the limb–body wall complex is secondary to early intrauterine constraint leading to the myriad of defects including the persistence of the extraembryonic coelom that is secondary to lack of ventral folding of the body wall.

It is most likely that the limb–body wall complex is heterogeneous from the standpoint of etiology and developmental pathogenesis. However, recognition that the associated defects are disruptive in nature suggests that recurrence risk is negligible.

References

Graham JM et al: Limb reduction anomalies and early in-utero limb compression. J Pediatr 96:1052, 1980.

Miller ME et al: Compression-related defects from early amnion rupture: Evidence for mechanical teratogenesis. J Pediatr 98:292, 1981.

Van Allen ME et al: Limb–body wall complex: I. Pathogenesis. Am J Med Genet 28:529, 1987.

Van Allen ME et al: Limb–body wall complex II. Limb and spine defects. Am J Med Genet 28:549, 1987.

Luebke HJ et al: Fetal disruptions: Assessment of frequency, heterogeneity, and embryologic mechanisms in a population referred to a community-based stillbirth assessment program. Am J Med Genet 36:56, 1990.

Moerman P et al: Constrictive amniotic bands, amniotic adhesions, and limb–body wall complex: Discrete disruption sequences with pathogenetic overlap. Am J Med Genet 42:470, 1992.

Russo R et al: Limb body wall complex: A critical review and a nosological proposal. Am J Med Genet 47:893, 1993.

Martinez-Frias ML: Clinical and epidemiological characteristics of infants with body wall complex with and without limb deficiency. Am J Med Genet 73:170, 1997.

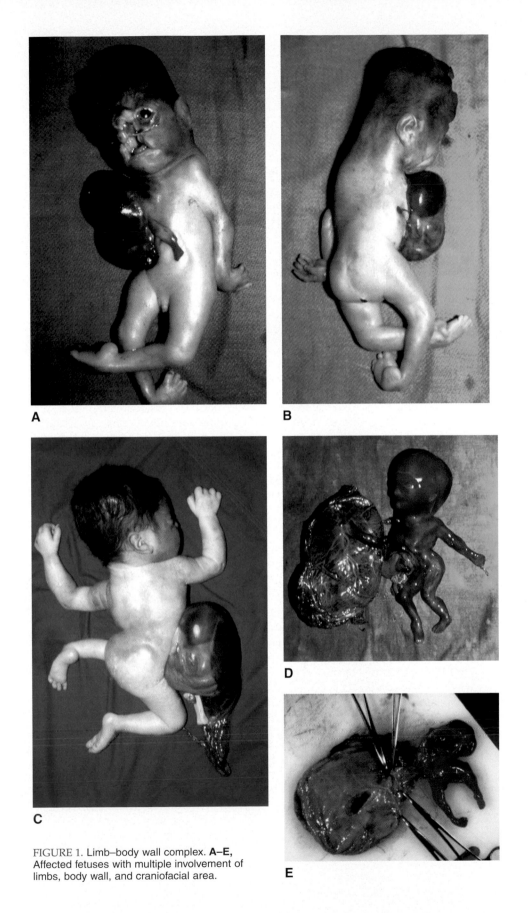

FIGURE 1. Limb–body wall complex. **A–E,** Affected fetuses with multiple involvement of limbs, body wall, and craniofacial area.

Spectra of Defects

OCULO-AURICULO-VERTEBRAL SPECTRUM

(First and Second Branchial Arch Syndrome, Facio-Auriculo-Vertebral Spectrum, Hemifacial Microsomia, Goldenhar Syndrome)

The predominant defects in this spectrum represent problems in morphogenesis of the first and second branchial arches, sometimes accompanied by vertebral anomalies, renal defects, or ocular anomalies. The occurrence of epibulbar dermoid with this pattern of anomaly, especially when accompanied by vertebral anomalies, was designated as the Goldenhar syndrome, and the predominantly unilateral occurrence was designated as hemifacial microsomia. However, the occurrence of various combinations and gradations of this pattern of anomalies, both unilateral and bilateral, with or without epibulbar dermoid, and with or without vertebral anomalies, has suggested that hemifacial microsomia and the Goldenhar syndrome may simply represent variable manifestations of a similar error in morphogenesis. The frequency of occurrence is estimated to be 1 in 3000 to 1 in 5000, and there is a slight (3:2) male predominance.

ABNORMALITIES. Variable combinations of the following, tending to be *asymmetric* and 70% unilateral.

Facial. Hypoplasia of malar, maxillary, or mandibular region, especially ramus and condyle of mandible and temporomandibular joint; lateral cleft-like extension of the corner of the mouth (macrostomia); hypoplasia of facial musculature; hypoplasia of depressor anguli oris.

Ear. Microtia, accessory preauricular tags or pits, most commonly in a line from the tragus to the corner of the mouth; middle ear anomaly with variable deafness.

Oral. Diminished to absent parotid secretion, anomalies in function or structure of tongue, malfunction of soft palate.

Vertebral. Hemivertebrae or hypoplasia of vertebrae, most commonly cervical but may also be thoracic or lumbar.

OCCASIONAL ABNORMALITIES

Eye. Epibulbar dermoid, lipodermoid, notch in upper lid, strabismus, microphthalmia.

Ear. Inner ear defect with deafness.

Oral. Cleft lip, cleft palate.

Cardiac. Ventricular septal defect, patent ductus arteriosus, tetralogy of Fallot, and coarctation of aorta, in decreasing order.

Genitourinary. Ectopic or fused kidneys, renal agenesis, vesicoureteral reflux, ureteropelvic junction obstruction, ureteral duplication, and multicystic dysplastic kidney.

Other. Mental deficiency (IQ below 85 in 13%), abnormal caruncles, branchial cleft remnants in anterior-lateral neck, laryngeal anomaly, hypoplasia to aplasia of lung, esophageal atresia, tracheomalacia caused by extrinsic vascular compression, hydrocephalus, Arnold-Chiari malformation, occipital encephalocele, agenesis of corpus callosum, calcification of falx cerebri, hypoplasia of septum pellucidum, intracranial dermoid cyst, lipoma in corpus callosum, radial and/or rib anomalies, prenatal growth deficiency, low scalp hairline.

NATURAL HISTORY. Cosmetic surgery is strongly indicated. Most of these patients are of normal intelligence. Mental deficiency is more common in association with microphthalmia. Deafness should be tested for at an early age.

ETIOLOGY. The cause of this disorder is unknown; cases are usually sporadic. Estimated recurrence in first-degree relatives is approximately 2%, although minor features of this disorder may be more commonly noted in relatives. When unilateral it tends to be right-sided. Maternal diabetes has been associated in some cases.

References

Goldenhar M: Associations malformatives de l'oeil et de l'oreille. J Genet Hum 1:243, 1952.

Summitt RL: Familial Goldenhar syndrome. Birth Defects 5:106, 1969.

Pashayan H, Pinsky L, Fraser FD: Hemifacial microsomia-oculo-auriculo-vertebral dysplasia: A patient with overlapping features. J Med Genet 7:185, 1970.

Baum JL, Feingold M: Ocular aspects of Goldenhar's syndrome. Am J Ophthalmol 75:250, 1973.

Rollnick BR et al: Oculoauriculovertebral dysplasia and variants: Phenotypic characteristics of 294 patients. Am J Med Genet 26:631, 1987.

Cohen MM Jr et al: Oculoauriculovertebral spectrum: An updated critique. Cleft Palate J 26:276, 1989.

Kumar A et al: Pattern of cardiac malformation in oculo-auriculovertebral spectrum. Am J Med Genet 46:423, 1993.

Ritchey ML et al: Urologic manifestations of Goldenhar syndrome. Urology 43:88, 1994.

Nijhawan N et al: Caruncle abnormalities in the oculo-auriculo-vertebral spectrum Am J Med Genet 113:320, 2002.

Wang R et al: Infants of diabetic mothers are at increased risk for the oculo-auriculo-vertebral sequence: A case-based and case-control approach. J Pediatr 141:611, 2002.

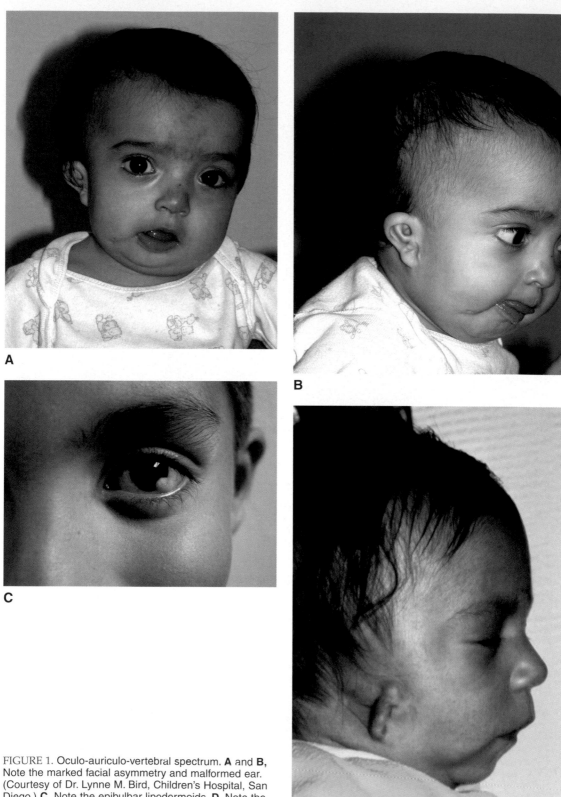

FIGURE 1. Oculo-auriculo-vertebral spectrum. **A** and **B,** Note the marked facial asymmetry and malformed ear. (Courtesy of Dr. Lynne M. Bird, Children's Hospital, San Diego.) **C,** Note the epibulbar lipodermoids. **D,** Note the micotia and micrognathia. (**D,** Courtesy of Dr. Michael Cohen, Dalhousie University, Halifax, Nova Scotia.)

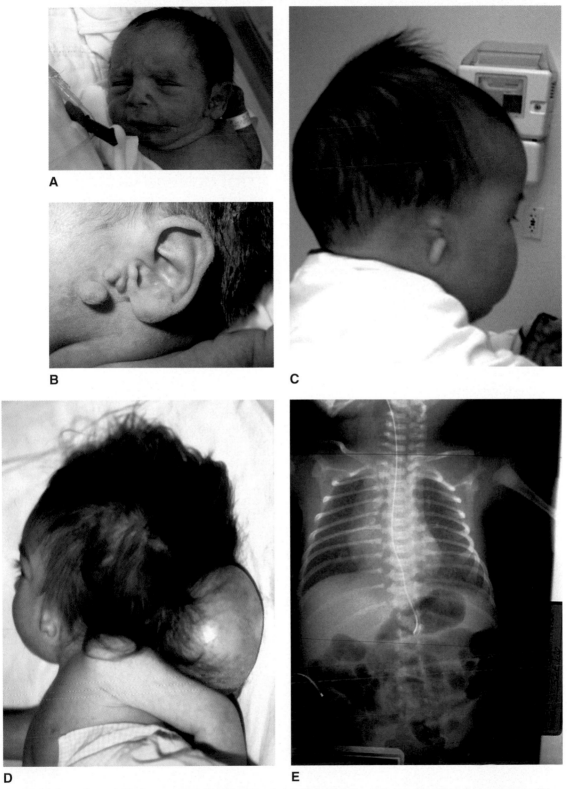

FIGURE 2. Note the variable features including the lateral cleft-like extension of the mouth (**A**), preauricular tags (**B**), and microtia (**C**). (Courtesy of Dr. Lynne Bird, Children's Hospital, San Diego.) **D,** Encephalocele. (Courtesy of Dr. Michael Cohen, Dalhousie University, Halifax, Nova Scotia.) **E,** Vertebral anomalies.

OROMANDIBULAR-LIMB HYPOGENESIS SPECTRUM
(Hypoglossia-Hypodactyly Syndrome, Aglossia-Adactyly Syndrome, Glossopalatine Ankylosis Syndrome, Facial-Limb Disruptive Spectrum)

Limb Deficiency, Hypoglossia, Micrognathia

In 1932, Rosenthal described aglossia and associated malformations. More recently, Kaplan and colleagues emphasized a "community" or spectrum of disorders and have suggested some common elements in modes of developmental pathology.

ABNORMALITIES. Various combinations from among the following features:

Craniofacial. Small mouth, micrognathia, hypoglossia, variable clefting or aberrant attachments of tongue; mandibular hypodontia; cleft palate; cranial nerve palsies including Moebius sequence; broad nose; telecanthus; lower eyelid defect; facial asymmetry.

Limbs. Hypoplasia of varying degrees, to point of adactyly; syndactyly.

Other. Brain defect, especially of cranial nerve nuclei, causing Moebius sequence; splenogonadal fusion.

NATURAL HISTORY. Early feeding and speech difficulties may occur. Orthopedic and/or plastic surgery may be indicated for the limb problems. Intelligence and stature are generally normal. Serious problems with hyperthermia can occur in children with four-limb amputation.

ETIOLOGY. The cause of this disorder is unknown; cases are usually sporadic. The hypothesis that the abnormalities are the disruptive consequence of hemorrhagic lesions has experimental backing from the studies of Poswillo. The presumed vascular problem is more likely to occur in distal regions, such as the distal limbs, tongue, and occasionally parts of the brain. Chorionic villus sampling, particularly when performed between 56 and 66 days of gestation, has been associated with this disorder, as has the use of misoprostol as an abortifacient, giving further credence to a disruptive vascular hypothesis.

References

Rosenthal R: Aglossia congenital: A report of the condition combined with other congenital malformations. Am J Dis Child 44:383, 1932.

Poswillo D: The pathogenesis of the first and second branchial arch syndrome. Oral Surg 35:302, 1973.

Kaplan P, Cummings C, Fraser FC: A "community" of face-limb malformation syndromes. J Pediatr 89:241, 1976.

Pauli RM, Greenlaw A: Limb deficiency and splenogonadal fusion. Am J Med Genet 13:81, 1982.

Lipson AH, Webster WS: Transverse limb deficiency, oromandibular limb hypogenesis sequences, and chorionic villus biopsy: Human and animal experimental evidence for a uterine vascular pathogenesis. Am J Med Genet 47:1141, 1993.

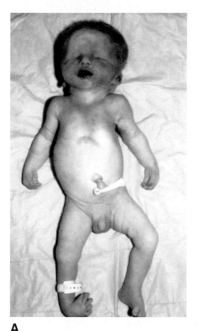

A

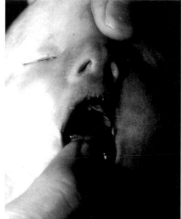

B

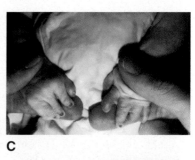

C

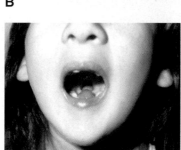

E

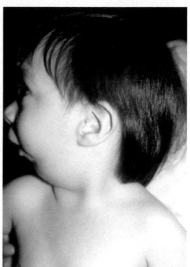

F

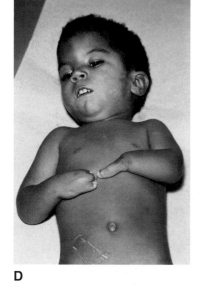

D

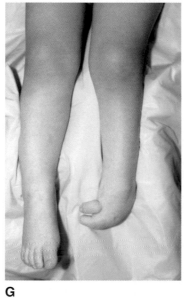

G

FIGURE 1. Oromandibular-limb hypogenesis spectrum. No one instance is the same as the next. There are varying degrees of limb deficiency, hypoglossia, or micrognathia. **A–C,** Necropsy photograph of a newborn. **D,** Note that the child has Moebius sequence as an associated feature. **E–G,** This child has splenogonadal fusion as an associated feature.

CONGENITAL MICROGASTRIA–LIMB REDUCTION COMPLEX

Microgastria, Limb Defects, Splenic Abnormalities

Robert described the first patient with this disorder in 1842. Subsequently, 16 additional cases have been described.

ABNORMALITIES

Gastrointestinal. Microgastria, intestinal malrotation.

Limb. Varying degrees of radial and ulnar hypoplasia, bilateral in 40% of cases; isolated absence of thumbs (20%); terminal transverse defects of humerus (10%); phocomelia (10%); oligodactyly.

Spleen. Abnormalities in 70% including asplenia, hyposplenia, or splenogonadal fusion.

Other. Renal anomalies in 50%, including pelvic kidney in two cases, and unilateral renal agenesis and bilateral cystic dysplasia in one patient each; defects in laterality; cardiac defects in 20% (secundum atrial septal defect and type I truncus arteriosus); central nervous system defects in 20% (arrhinencephaly, fused thalami, polymicrogyria, agenesis of corpus callosum, and hydrocephalus).

OCCASIONAL ABNORMALITIES.
Congenital megacolon, esophageal atresia, anal atresia, abnormal lung lobation, anophthalmia and porencephalic cyst, Amelia, cryptorchidism, bicornuate uterus, horseshoe kidney, and absent gallbladder.

NATURAL HISTORY. Microgastria usually presents with gastroesophageal reflux and failure to thrive. Death before 6 months of age has occurred in almost 50% of cases. Surgical intervention to create a gastric reservoir improves the ability of patients to tolerate normal feeding volumes.

ETIOLOGY. The cause of this disorder is unknown. All cases have represented sporadic events in otherwise normal families. The occurrence of three cases in which discordance for this disorder has occurred in twins is noteworthy.

References
Robert HLF: Hummungsbildung des magens, mangel der milz und des netzes. Arch Anat Physiol Wissenschaftliche Med 57, 1842.

Lueder GT et al: Congenital microgastria and hypoplastic upper limb anomalies. Am J Med Genet 32:368, 1989.

Meinecke P et al: Microgastria–hypoplastic upper limb association: A severe expression including microphthalmia, single nostril and arrhinencephaly. Clin Dysmorphol 1:43, 1992.

Cunniff C et al: Congenital microgastria and limb reduction defects. Pediatrics 91:1192, 1993.

Lurie IW et al: Microgastria–limb reduction complex with congenital heart disease and twinning. Clin Dysmorphol 4:150, 1995.

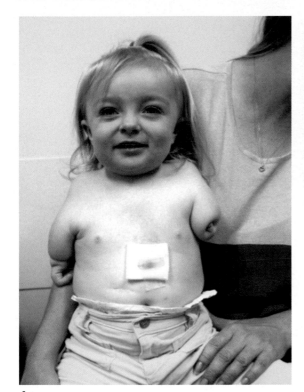

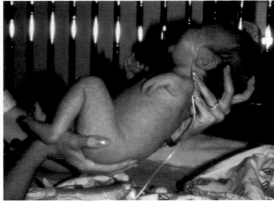

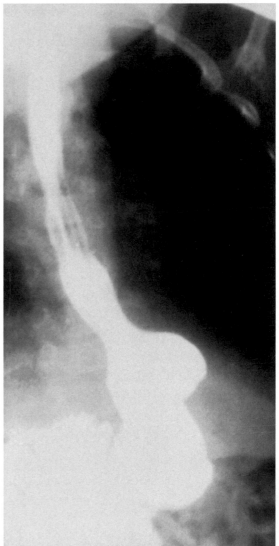

FIGURE 1. Congenital microgastria-limb reduction complex. **A–C,** Note the limb reduction anomalies and, on the barium-contrast roentgenogram, microgastria and intestinal malrotation.

STERNAL MALFORMATION–VASCULAR DYSPLASIA SPECTRUM

In 1985, Hersh and colleagues described two patients with this disorder and summarized the findings in 13 previously reported cases. The principal features include cleft of the sternum that is covered with atrophic skin; a median abdominal raphe extending from the sternal defect to the umbilicus; and cutaneous craniofacial hemangiomata.

In 13 of the cases, the hemangiomata were localized to cutaneous structures, while in one the upper respiratory tract was involved and in another there were multiple hemangiomata in the mucosa of the small bowel, mesentery, and pancreas. The sternal defect varies from a complete cleft to a partial cleft involving the upper one third of the sternum.

Occasional abnormalities have included absent pericardium anteriorly, unilateral cleft lip, micrognathia, and glossoptosis.

A significant morbidity is related to respiratory compromise, gastrointestinal bleeding, and infection, as rapid expansion of the vascular lesion leads to tissue hypoxia and necrosis.

All reported cases of this disorder have been sporadic events in otherwise normal families with the exception of a male with asternia and a facial hemangioma who had a sister with isolated asternia. The etiology of this condition is unknown.

An overlap exists between this disorder and the PHACE syndrome, a term applied to the association of *p*osterior fossa brain abnormalities, *h*emangiomas, *a*rterial anomalies in the cranial vasculature, *c*oarctation of the aorta/cardiac defects, and *e*ye abnormalities. Sternal clefting and supraumbilical raphe can also be present. Thus all children with the sternal malformation–vascular dysplasia spectrum should undergo a complete neurologic examination, four limb blood pressures, echocardiography, magnetic resonance imaging of the brain, and ophthalmologic evaluation.

References

Hersh JH et al: Sternal malformation–vascular dysplasia association. Am J Med Genet 21:177, 1985.

James PA, McGaughran J: Complete overlap of PHACE syndrome and sternal malformation–vascular dysplasia association. Am J Med Genet 110:78, 2002.

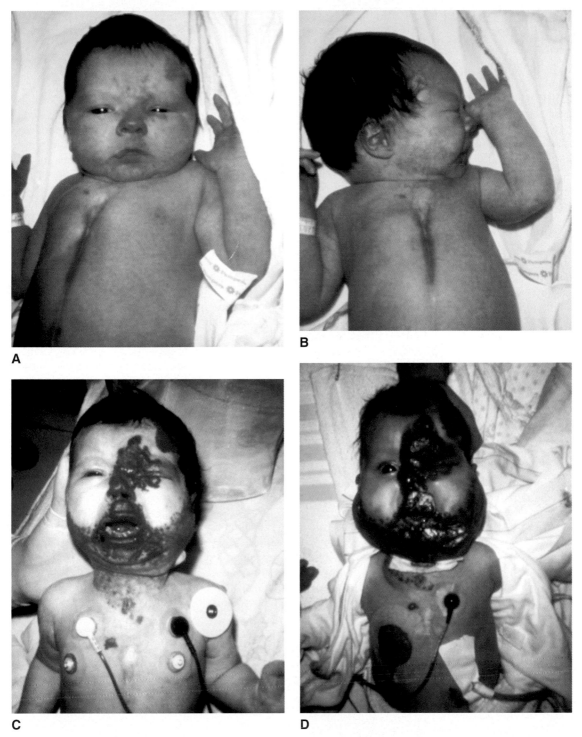

FIGURE 1. Sternal malformation-vascular dysplasia spectrum. **A** and **B,** Affected child in newborn period. **C,** At 6 weeks. **D,** At 4 months. Note the capillary hemangiomata over the face and the cleft of the upper one third of the sternum, which is covered with atrophic skin. (From Hersh JH: Am J Med Genet 21:177, 1985, with permission from Wiley-Liss, a division of John Wiley & Sons.)

MONOZYGOTIC TWINNING AND STRUCTURAL DEFECTS—GENERAL

Monozygotic (MZ) twinning occurs in approximately 1 in 200 births and, as such, represents the most common aberration of morphogenesis noted in the human. The frequency of MZ twin conceptuses is probably appreciably higher than 1 in 200. Livingston and Poland found a threefold excess of MZ twins among spontaneous abortuses versus live-born twins, with the ratio of MZ to dizygotic (DZ) being 17:1 in the abortuses versus 0.8:1 in the live-born twins. Most of these MZ aborted twins had structural defects and may represent the early lethal effect of the types of structural defects that have been noted to occur with excess frequency in MZ twins.

Structural defects occur two to three times more commonly in live-born MZ twins than in dizygotic twins or singletons. The origin and nature of these defects are summarized in Table 1-1, and the first three categories are individually set forth in the following subsections. The fourth category of deformation caused by in utero crowding, which is not increased in MZ versus dizygotic twins, is set forth in *Smith's Recognizable Patterns of Human Deformation* by John M. Graham, Jr. (2nd ed. Philadelphia: Saunders, 1988) and will not be detailed here.

MZ twinning may occur soon after conception, and this type may even have separate placentas with dichorionic-diamnionic membranes. The development of two embryonic centers in the blastocyst by 4 to 5 days of gestation yields twins with monochorionic-diamnionic membranes, the most common type of MZ twinning. The final potential timing for the induction of MZ twinning is by 15 to 16 days of development, with the formation of more than one Hensen node and primitive streak in the embryonic plate. This will result in monochorionic-monoamnionic twins, who account for approximately 4% of MZ twins.

In addition to the problems that were alluded to concerning MZ twins, there appears to be an increased likelihood of fetal death in one or more of MZ twins who develop in a monoamnionic sac, at least partially because of cord entanglements leading to vascular problems. There is also an overall excess of perinatal mortality in MZ twins. The primary cause is prematurity, but the excess of structural defects also contributes to this high mortality.

The value and importance of examining the placenta for the condition of the membranes, vascular interconnections between the twins, and evidence of a deceased twin should be obvious.

The etiologies for MZ twining are largely unknown. A single-gene, dominant type of inheritance has been implicated in an occasional family. Experimental studies have implied environmental factors, such as late fertilization of the ovum in the rabbit and vincristine administration in the rat.

MONOZYGOTIC TWINS AND EARLY MALFORMATIONS

The excess of early types of malformation among MZ twins may be the consequence of the same etiology that gave rise to the MZ twinning aberration of morphogenesis. For example, Stockard was able to produce both MZ twinning *and* early malformation such as cyclopia by early environmental insults (alterations of oxygen level and temperature) to the developing Atlantic minnow

TABLE 1-1   ORIGIN AND TYPES OF STRUCTURAL DEFECTS IN MONOZYGOTIC TWINS

ORIGIN	TYPES OF DEFECTS
A. ? The same causative factor that gave rise to MZ twinning	Early malformations or malformation sequences
B. Incomplete twinning	Conjoined twins
C. Consequence of vascular placental shunts	
1. Artery-artery	Disruptions, including acardiac and amorphous twins
2. Artery-vein	Twin-twin transfusion, causing unequal size, unequal hematocrit, or other problems
3. Death of one twin leading to decreased blood flow and hypoxia	
D. Constraint in fetal life	Deformations caused by uterine constraint

(*Fundulus*). The findings of Schinzel and colleagues confirm this hypothesis. They found that the malformations in MZ twins were predominantly early defects, presumably engendered at the same time as the MZ twinning. The incidence of associated early malformations was greatest in the monochorionic-monoamnionic cases, which would usually have been induced at the time of embryonic plate development and hence would theoretically be more likely to have associated early malformations. The early types of defects that have been considered to be of excess frequency in MZ twins are the following:

1. Sacrococcygeal teratoma.
2. Sirenomelia (see Subchapter 1T).
3. The VATERR association (see Subchapter 1V).
4. Exstrophy of the cloaca malformation sequence (see Subchapter 1T).
5. Holoprosencephaly malformation sequence (see Subchapter 1T).
6. Anencephaly (see Subchapter 1T).

Approximately 5% to 20% of such cases are concordant; thus, the majority of cases are discordant. When one twin has the more severe degree of a malformation sequence, the other twin may show lesser degrees of the same type of initiating defect.

These early defects are individually presented in this text. Most are early lethals and cause spontaneous abortion. This is probably a partial explanation of the excess of MZ twins among spontaneous abortuses.

Recurrence risk counseling should involve the total problem, namely, the MZ twinning plus the associated malformation sequence. To our knowledge, this risk is of low to negligible magnitude, although the specific etiologies for this type of problem are unknown.

CONJOINED TWINS

Conjoined twins may be viewed as examples of incomplete twinning and occur in approximately 1% of MZ twins. Although it is feasible that two closely placed embryonic centers in the 4- to 5-day-old blastocyst could result in conjoined twins, it seems more likely that they originate at the primitive streak stage of the embryonic plate (15 to 17 days). Current experimental techniques in animals have not been successful in producing conjoined twins.

The most common type of conjoined twins is termed thoracopagus, in which the twins are joined at the thorax. Juncture at the head, buttocks, and less commonly, other anatomic sites also occurs. Partial to complete duplication of only the upper or lower body parts may also take place.

As with MZ twins in general, there is a higher incidence of early malformations in conjoined twins. Disregarding the incidence of anomalies related to the sites of juncture, there is a 10% to 20% occurrence of major early defects. As with separate MZ twins, the malformations in conjoined twins are often not concordant. The high frequency of associated malformations in conjoined twins may relate to the timing of the defect, which is presumed to be at the embryonic plate-primitive streak stage of development.

The likelihood of particular types of early malformation occurring in certain kinds of conjoined twins is increased very nonrandomly. For example, the dicephalic-conjoined twin frequently has anencephaly, most commonly affecting only one of the heads. Whether this relates to differences in early blood flow to the respective heads remains to be determined. Furthermore, the right-sided twin of a dicephalic conjoined twin pair virtually always has situs inversus. The recurrence risk for conjoined twins appears to be negligible.

PLACENTAL VASCULAR SHUNTS IN MONOZYGOTIC TWINS—GENERAL

Benirschke has indicated that the great majority of monochorionic (single placenta) twins have a conjoined placenta with vascular interconnections. These develop on a chance basis and are usually evident on the fetal surface of the placenta where the major vessels course between the fetuses and the major cotyledons. The magnitude of intertwin vascular shunts may be judged by the caliber of the connecting vessels, which relates to the amount of flow they have carried. Much of the early in utero mortality and excess of structural defects in MZ twins may well relate to the secondary consequences of these vascular connections between the twins. Some of the types of shunts and their adverse effects on one or both of the MZ twins are set forth subsequently.

Artery-Artery Twin Disruption Sequence

Benirschke emphasized the dire consequences that could result from a sizable artery-artery placental shunt, usually accompanied by a vein-vein shunt. The tendency will be for the arterial pressure of one twin to overpower that of the other, usually early in morphogenesis. The "defeated" recipient then has reverse flow from the co-twin. This sends "used" arterial blood from the donor into the iliac vessels of the recipient, perfusing the lower part of the body more than the upper part. The results are a host of disruptions, with deterioration of previously existing tissues as well as incomplete morphogenesis (malformation) of tissues that are in the process of formation. The variably missing tissues include the head, heart, upper limbs, lungs, pancreas, and upper intestine. Rudiments of early disrupted tissues may be found in the residuum. The extent of disruption may be even broader, leaving as the residuum an "amorphous" twin. There is every gradation, from amorphia to acardia to less severe degrees of disruption, with no one case being identical to another. Examples of some of the gradations of severity are shown in the accompanying figure.

The donor twin may have an excessive cardiac load resulting in cardiomegaly and even cardiac decompensation, with secondary liver dysfunction, hypoalbuminemia, and edema. Sometimes this may progress to the level of hydrops.

Artery-Vein Twin Transfusion Sequence

Artery-vein transfusion may result in problems such as those summarized in Table 1-2. The excessive volume in the recipient twin not only tends to lead to increased growth and an enlarged heart but also causes increased kidney size and excess urine output, with resultant polyhydramnios. The high hematocrit may constitute a serious risk of vascular problems and merits early postnatal management. The donor twin, being hypovolemic, tends to have diminished renal blood flow, smaller kidneys, and oligohydramnios (when the twins are diamnionic).

There may even be evidence of transient renal insufficiency in the smaller twin during the first days after birth, as the kidneys have been hypofunctional since before birth.

Tan and colleagues have found that 18% of MZ twins are discrepant in size and hematocrit at birth; hence, this is not a rare occurrence. Treatment may be warranted soon after birth to provide each affected twin with a more normal hematocrit.

Complications in a Monozygotic Twin from the in utero Death of the Co-twin

Benirschke first implicated death of an MZ co-twin (stillborn or fetus papyraceus) as a potential cause for problems in the surviving twin. Decreased blood flow caused by hemodynamic changes with consequent hypoxia is the most likely mechanism. The resultant areas of ischemia and disruption, with subsequent loss of tissue, lead to disruptive vascular defects in the co-twin of the deceased MZ twin, some of which are the following:

1. Disseminated intravascular coagulation.
2. Aplasia cutis.
3. Porencephalic cyst to hydranencephaly.
4. Limb amputation.
5. Intestinal atresia.
6. Gastroschisis.

Melnick has concluded from the Collaborative Perinatal Project (50,000 deliveries) that approximately 3% of near-term MZ twins have a deceased co-twin, and about one third of the survivors, or 1% of MZ twin births, have severe brain defects as a consequence of the foregoing mechanisms. The surviving infants with porencephalic cysts or hydranencephaly are usually severely mentally deficient with microcephaly, spastic diplegia, and seizures.

TABLE 1-2 PROBLEMS SECONDARY TO ARTERIOVENOUS TWIN-TWIN TRANSFUSION

FEATURE	DONOR TWIN	RECIPIENT TWIN
Growth	Smaller size	Larger size
Hematocrit	Low	High
Blood volume	Hypovolemia	Hypervolemia
Renal blood flow and renal size	Diminished	Increased
Amnionic fluid	Oligohydramnios	Polyhydramnios
Heart size	Diminished	Increased

References

General

Stockard CR: Developmental rate and structural expression: An experimental study of twins, "double monsters," and single deformities and the interaction among embryonic organs during their origin and development. Am J Anat 28:115, 1921.

Benirschke K: Twin placenta in perinatal mortality. NY State J Med 61:1499, 1961.

Benirschke K, Driscoll SG: The placenta in multiple pregnancy. Handbuch Pathol Histol 7:187, 1967.

Bomsel-Helmreich O: Delayed ovulation and monozygotic twinning in the rabbit. Acta Genet Med Gemellol 23:19, 1974.

Myrianthopoulos NC: Congenital malformations in twins. Acta Genet Med Gemellol 24:331, 1976.

Harvey MAS, Huntley RM, Smith DW: Familial monozygotic twinning. J Pediatr 90:246, 1977.

Kaufman MH, O'Shea KS: Induction of monozygotic twinning in the mouse. Nature 276:707, 1978.

Schinzel AAGL, Smith DW, Miller JR: Monozygotic twinning and structural defects. J Pediatr 95:921, 1979.

Livingston JE, Poland BJ: A study of spontaneously aborted twins. Teratology 21:139, 1980.

Early Malformations in Monozygotic Twins

Stockard CR: Developmental rate and structural expression: An experimental study of twins, "double monsters," and single deformities and the interaction among embryonic organs during their origin and development. Am J Anat 28:115, 1921.

Gross RE, Clatworthy HW, Mecker JA: Sacrococcygeal teratomas in infants and children. Surg Gynecol Obstet 92:341, 1951.

Mohr HP: Misibilundugen bei Zwillingen. Ergeb Inn Med Kinderheilkd 33:1, 1972.

Davies J, Chazen E, Nance WE: Symmelia in one of monozygotic twins. Teratology 4:367, 1976.

Smith DW, Bartlett C, Harrah LM: Monozygotic twinning and the Duhamel anomalad (imperforate anus to sirenomelia): A nonrandom association between two aberrations in morphogenesis. Birth Defects 12:53, 1976.

Schinzel AAGL, Smith DW, Miller JR: Monozygotic twinning and structural defects. J Pediatr 95:921, 1979.

Livingston JE, Poland BJ: A study of spontaneously aborted twins. Teratology 21:139, 1980.

Conjoined Twins

Riccardi VM, Bergmann CA: Anencephaly with incomplete twinning (diprosopus). Teratology 16:137, 1977.

Schinzel AAGL, Smith DW, Miller JR: Monozygotic twinning and structural defects. J Pediatr 95:921, 1979.

Vascular Shunts between Monozygotic Twins

Confalonieri C: Gravidanza gemellare monocoriale biamniotica con feto papiraceo ed atresia inestinale congenita nell'altro feto. Riv Ost Ginec Prat 33:199, 1951.

Naeye RL: Human intrauterine parabiotic syndrome and its complications. N Engl J Med 268:804, 1963.

Hague IU, Glassauer FE: Hydranencephaly in twins. NY State J Med 69:1210, 1969.

Moore CM, McAdams AJ, Sutherland J: Intrauterine disseminated intravascular coagulation: A syndrome of multiple pregnancy with a dead twin fetus. J Pediatr 74:523, 1969.

Saier F, Burden L, Cavanagh D: Fetus papyraceus: An unusual case with congenital anomaly of the surviving fetus. Obstet Gynecol 45:271, 1975.

Balvour RP: Fetus papyraceus. Obstet Gynecol 47:507, 1976.

Weiss DB, Aboulafia Y, Isackson M: Gastroschisis and fetus papyraceus in double ovum twins. Harefuah 91:392, 1976.

Benirschke K, Harper V: The acardiac anomaly. Teratology 15:311, 1977.

Mannino FL, Jones KL, Benirschke K: Congenital skin defects and fetus papyraceus. J Pediatr 91:599, 1977.

Melnick M: Brain damage in survivor after death of monozygotic co-twin. Lancet 2:1287, 1977.

Schinzel AAGL, Smith DW, Miller JR: Monozygotic twinning and structural defects. J Pediatr 95:921, 1979.

Tan KL et al: The twin transfusion syndrome. Clin Pediatr 18:111, 1979.

Jones KL, Benirschke K: The developmental pathogenesis of structural defects: The contribution of monozygotic twins. Semin Perinatol 7:239, 1983.

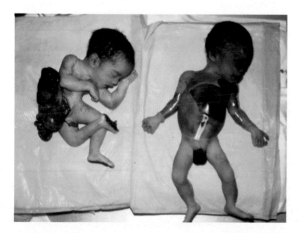

FIGURE 1. MZ twins discordant for limb–body wall complex. (Courtesy of Dr. Kurt Benirschke, University of California, San Diego.)

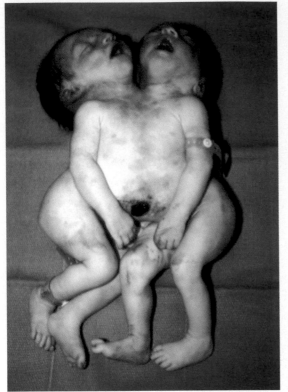

A

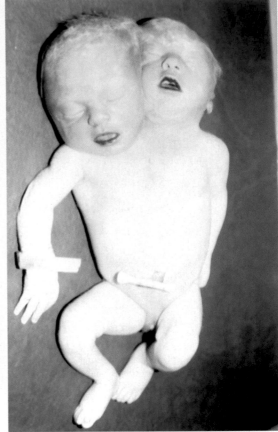

B

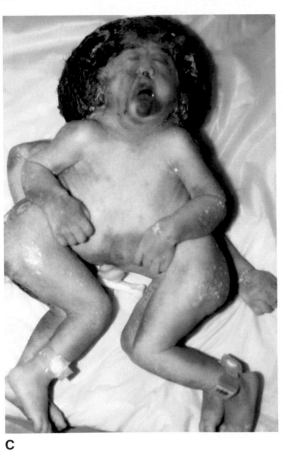

C

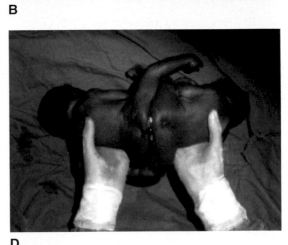

D

FIGURE 2. Varying degrees of conjoined twins.
A, Attached at the chest (thoracopagus), which is the most common type. **B,** Dicephalus (two heads).
C, Cephalothoracopagus. **D,** Joined at the buttocks. (Courtesy of Dr. Kurt Benirschke, University of California, San Diego.)

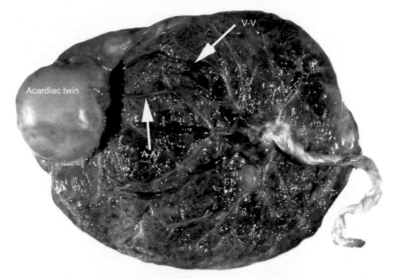

A

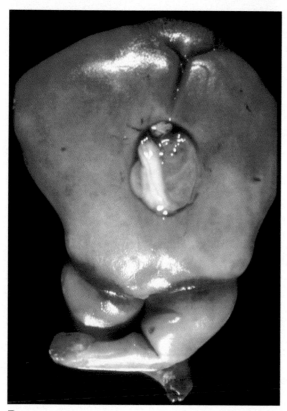

B

C

FIGURE 3. Artery-artery twin disruption sequence. **A,** Amorphous acardiac twin partially embedded in the placenta. Note the artery-artery vascular anastomosis (*left arrow*) and the vein-vein vascular anastomosis (*right arrow*), which have led to the reversal of blood flow. **B** and **C,** Acardiac twin with upper limb deficiency, marked disruption of the craniofacial area and upper body, and relative sparing of the lower body caused by artery-artery shunt and reverse circulation from co-twin. (Courtesy of Dr. Kurt Benirschke, University of California, San Diego.)

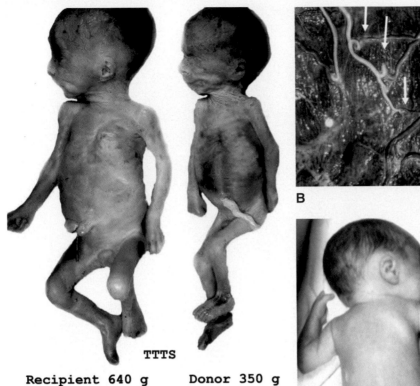

TTTS

Recipient 640 g   **Donor 350 g**

A

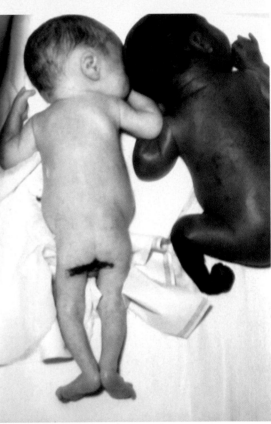

B

C

FIGURE 4. Artery-vein twin transfusion sequence. **A** and **B,** Discrepant size of MZ twins as the result of an arteriovenous shunt (*arrows*) in the monochorionic-diamnionic placenta. The direction of the flow is from the smaller donor on the right to the overgrown recipient on the left. **C,** Note that the plethoric, overgrown, recipient twin has necrosis of the left leg most likely related to decreased blood flow secondary to polycythemia. (Courtesy of Dr. Kurt Benirschke, University of California, San Diego.)

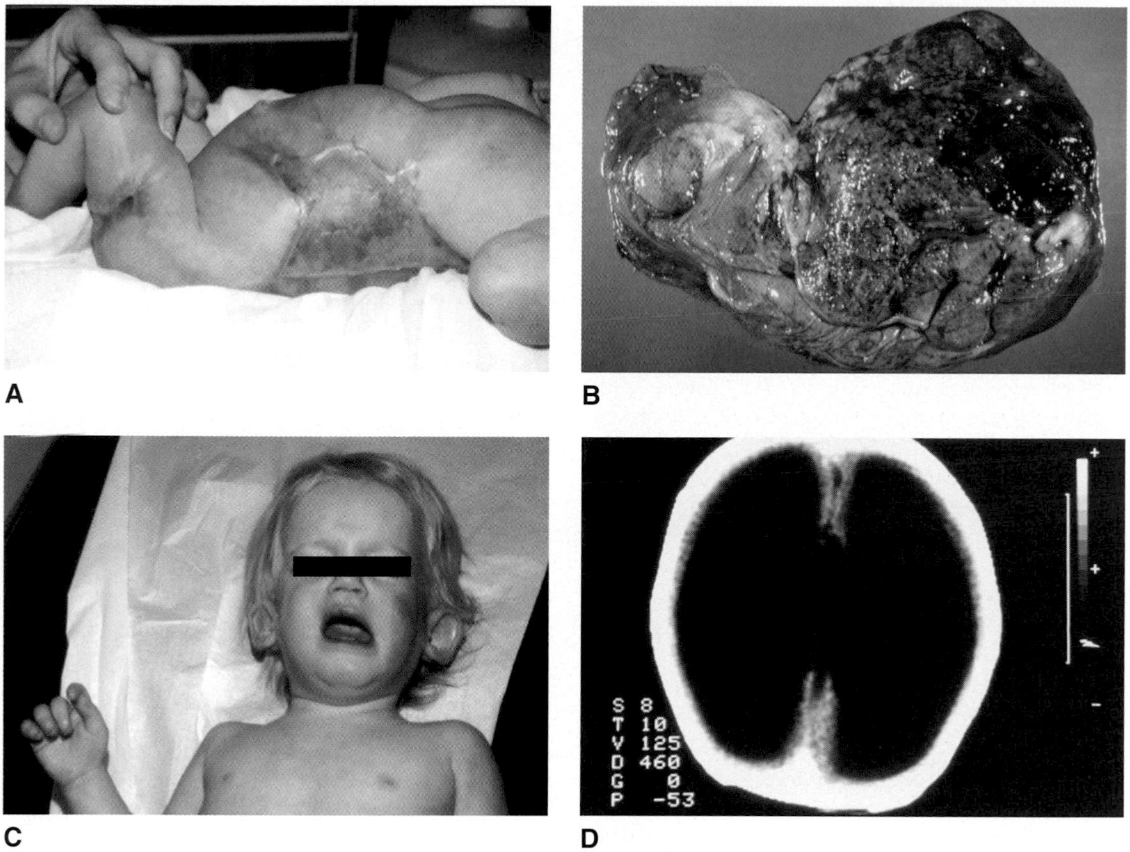

FIGURE 5. Impact of death of MZ twin on surviving co-twin. **A** and **B,** A newborn infant with aplasia cutis congenita related to the in utero death of his MZ co-twin, who can be seen embedded in the left of the placental membranes. **C** and **D,** Child with hypertonic diplegia, seizures, and developmental deficiency, who had hydranencephaly. At birth, there was a macerated 30-cm co-twin of the same sex.

VATERR ASSOCIATION

An association is a term used to designate the nonrandom tendency of some malformations to occur together more commonly than would be expected by chance, without being components of a syndrome. VATERR is an acronym that includes *v*ertebral defects, *a*nal atresia, *T-E* fistula with esophageal atresia, and *r*adial and *r*enal dysplasia. Cardiac defects and a single umbilical artery as well as prenatal growth deficiency are also nonrandom features of this pattern of anomalies. The general spectrum of the pattern in 34 cases is presented subsequently, as summarized by Temtamy and Miller.

ABNORMALITIES. Thirty-four cases with three or more VATERR association defects.

Vertebral anomalies	70%
Ventricular septal defects and other cardiac defects	53%
Anal atresia with or without fistula	80%
T-E fistula with esophageal atresia	70%
Radial dysplasia, including thumb or radial hypoplasia, preaxial polydactyly, syndactyly	65%
Renal anomaly	53%
Single umbilical artery	35%

OTHER LESS FREQUENT DEFECTS. Prenatal growth deficiency, postnatal growth deficiency, laryngeal stenosis, ear anomaly, large fontanels, defect of lower limb (23%), rib anomaly, defects of external genitalia, spinal dysraphia with tethered cord.

NATURAL HISTORY. Though many of these patients may fail to thrive and have slow developmental progress in early infancy related to their defects, the majority of them have normal brain function and thus merit vigorous attempts toward rehabilitation, surgical and otherwise.

ETIOLOGY. This pattern of malformation has generally been a sporadic occurrence in an other-wise normal family. The etiology is unknown. It has been more frequently seen in the offspring of diabetic mothers.

COMMENT. Features of this association may occur in an otherwise normal child or as a part of a broader pattern, such as the trisomy 18 or del(13q) syndromes, in which case the prognosis is not favorable. It is also important to recognize that VATERR association is not in and of itself a diagnosis, but rather a nonrandom association of defects. As such, when one of the associated features is identified, careful evaluation for other VATERR association defects should be undertaken, and particularly in the cases in which a malformation not usually encountered with VATERR association defects is identified, karyotypic analysis is warranted. A distinct, genetically determined disorder referred to as VATERR with hydrocephalus has been reported. Both autosomal and X-linked recessive inheritance have been documented for that disorder. The hydrocephalus is due to aqueductal stenosis. Although a poor prognosis is the rule, survival with a relatively good outcome has been noted in some cases.

References

Say B, Gerald PS: A new polydactyly, imperforate anus, vertebral anomalies syndrome. Lancet 2:688, 1968.

Say D et al: A new syndrome of dysmorphogenesis–imperforate anus associated with poly-oligodactyly and skeletal (mainly vertebral) anomalies. Acta Paediatr Scand 60:197, 1971.

Silver W et al: The Holt-Oram syndrome with previously undescribed associated anomalies. Am J Dis Child 124:911, 1972.

Quan L, Smith DW: The VATER association, *V*ertebral defects, *A*nal atresia, *T-E* fistula with esophageal atresia, *R*adial and *R*enal dysplasia: A spectrum of associated defects. J Pediatr 82:104, 1973.

Temtamy SA, Miller JD: Extending the scope of the VATER association: Definition of a VATER syndrome. J Pediatr 85:345, 1974.

Evans JA et al: VACTERL with hydrocephalus: Further delineation of the syndrome(s). Am J Med Genet 34:177, 1989.

Wang H et al: VACTERL with hydrocephalus: Spontaneous chromosome breakage and rearrangement in a family showing apparent sex-linked recessive inheritance. Am J Med Genet 47:114, 1993.

James HE et al: Distal spinal cord pathology in the VATER association. J Pediatr Surg 29:1501, 1994.

Botto L et al: The spectrum of congenital anomalies of the VATER association: An international study. Am J Med Genet 71:8, 1997.

Källén K et al: VATER non-random association of congenital malformations: Study based on data from four malformation registers. Am J Med Genet 101:26, 2001.

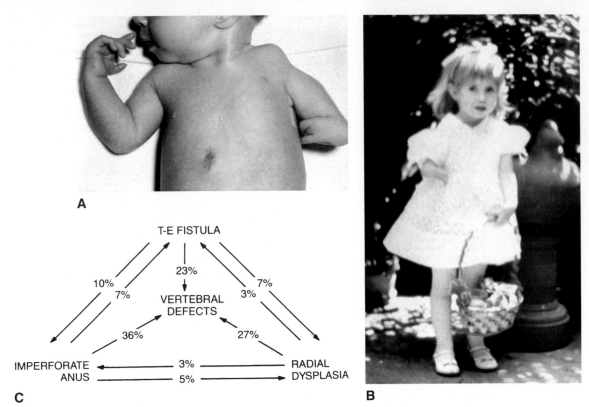

FIGURE 1. VATERR association. **A,** Young infant with vertebral anomalies, anal atresia, esophageal atresia with T-E fistula, radial aplasia on the left, and thumb hypoplasia on the right. **B,** Same patient at 2 years of age, with normal intelligence. **C,** Relative frequencies of some of the other VATERR association defects when the patient is ascertained by virtue of having one of the defects. (From Quan L, Smith DW: J Pediatr 82:104, 1973, with permission.)

TRACHEO-ESOPHAGEAL
FISTULA

CARDIAC
DEFECT

RADIAL LIMB
DEFECT

SINGLE
UMBILICAL
ARTERY

VERTEBRAL
DEFECT

ANAL
ATRESIA

RENAL
DEFECT

GENITAL DEFECT

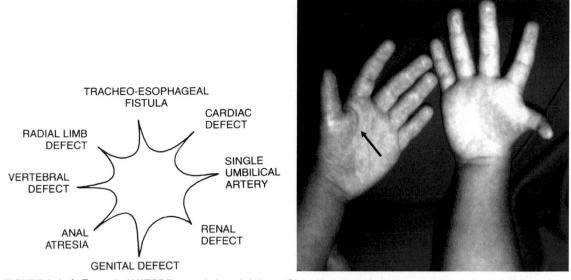

FIGURE 2. *Left*, Expanded VATERR association of defects. *Right,* Note the relatively severe thumb (radial) defect of the right hand and the much more subtle "radial" defect of the left hand (*arrow*). The *arrow* depicts a hypoplastic thenar eminence and crease.

MURCS ASSOCIATION

Müllerian Duct, Renal and Cervical Vertebral Defects

The MURCS association, as described in 30 patients by Duncan and colleagues in 1979, consists of a nonrandom association of *m*üllerian duct aplasia, *r*enal aplasia, and *c*ervicothoracic *s*omite dysplasia.

ABNORMALITIES

Growth. Small stature.

Skeletal. Cervicothoracic vertebral defects, especially from C5–T1 (80%), sometimes to the extent of being termed the Klippel-Feil malformation sequence.

Genitourinary. Absence of proximal two thirds of vagina and absence to hypoplasia of uterus (96%, but there is an ascertainment bias for this defect; sometimes referred to as the Rokitansky malformation sequence); renal agenesis or ectopy (88%).

OCCASIONAL ABNORMALITIES.

Moderate frequency of rib anomalies, upper limb anomalies, primarily reduction defects although duplicated thumb has occurred, and Sprengel scapular anomaly. Infrequent features include deafness, cerebellar cyst, external ear defects, facial asymmetry, cleft lip and palate, micrognathia, gastrointestinal defects, defects of laterality, abnormal lung lobation, and occipital encephalocele.

NATURAL HISTORY.

Most patients are ascertained because of primary amenorrhea or infertility associated with normal secondary sexual characteristics. Rarely, the MURCS association may be diagnosed in the course of an investigation for a renal malformation or because of multiple malformations. Small stature is frequent, with adult stature usually being less than 152 cm.

ETIOLOGY.

The etiology of this disorder is unknown; it is usually a sporadic disorder in an otherwise normal family.

COMMENT.

The Rokitansky malformation sequence, one of the defects that comprise the MURCS association, is characterized by an incomplete to atretic vagina and a rudimentary to bicornuate uterus. The fallopian tubes and ovaries are usually nearly normal with normal secondary sexual characteristics, except for a lack of menstruation. The lower vagina, which is derived from an outpouching from the urogenital sinus, is usually present as a blindly ending pouch. The cause is unknown. Although most cases are sporadic, approximately 4% of cases have been familial, with affected female siblings.

References

Rokitansky K: Über sog. Verdoppelung des Uterus. Med Jahrb des Osterreich Staates 26:39, 1838.

Byran AL et al: One hundred cases of congenital absence of the vagina. Surg Gynecol Obstet 88:79, 1949.

Duncan PA: Embryologic pathogenesis of renal agenesis associated with cervical vertebral anomalies (Klippel-Feil phenotype). Birth Defects 13(3D):91, 1977.

Duncan PA et al: The MURCS association: Müllerian duct aplasia, renal aplasia, and cervicothoracic somite dysplasia. J Pediatr 95:399, 1979.

Greene RA et al: MURCS association with additional congenital anomalies. Hum Pathol 17:88, 1986.

Mahajan P et al: MURCS association—a review of 7 cases. J Postgrad Med 38:109, 1992.

Suri M et al: MURCS association with encephalocele: Report of a second case. Clin Dysmorph 9:31, 2000.

Lopez AG-M et al: MURCS association with duplicated thumb. Clin Genet 61:308, 2002.

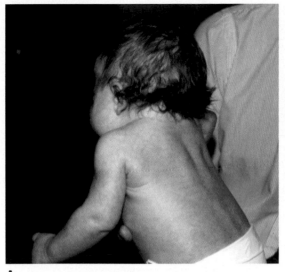

A

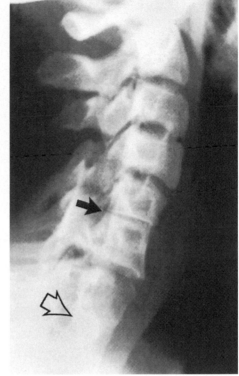

B

FIGURE 1. MURCS association. **A,** Child with short neck secondary to cervical vertebral defects. **B,** An example is depicted in the radiograph. Note the partial to complete cervical vertebral fusion (*arrows*).

ALPHABETICAL LISTING OF SYNDROMES

2 Approaches to Categorical Problems

Growth Deficiency, Mental Deficiency, Arthrogryposis, Ambiguous External Genitalia

Many patients with specific patterns of malformation may initially be evaluated by the clinician because of a categorical problem such as growth deficiency or mental deficiency. The physician is challenged to arrive at a specific overall diagnosis that will be of value in the management of and prognosis and counseling for that particular patient and family. This chapter sets forth approaches toward a specific diagnosis for several of the more common or more difficult categorical types of problems. It is designed to provide an overall diagnostic point of view, placing the patterns of malformation in relevant perspective to other types of disorders in which such a problem may occur.

Each categorical problem is considered from the standpoint of normal morphogenesis, mechanisms by which abnormal morphogenesis may occur, and the clinical manner of proceeding toward a specific overall diagnosis. These approaches are designed to be rational for the particular problem and germane for the specific patient.

APPROACH TO GROWTH DEFICIENCY

Normal Growth

Assuming proper skeletal organization and ossification, adult stature and the age at which it is achieved are the respective consequences of the following phenomena:

1. *Mitotic* rate and thereby rate of increasing cell number, especially in the epiphyses.
2. *Maturational* rate of the skeletal system toward final epiphyseal ossification, which can be assessed as "bone age."

Both of these processes are influenced by many genes (polygenic). Some of these genes are located on the sex chromosomes. For example, the XY male tends to be taller than the XX female, even in childhood, and the XYY individual is generally taller than the XY male. The XX female matures more rapidly and at a more consistent rate than the XY male and thus reaches the advent of adolescence and final height attainment at an earlier chronological age than the male. The genetically determined potential for stature and pace of maturation are dependent upon an adequate supply of certain nutrients, vitamins, hormones, and oxygen to the skeletal cells. The dramatic trend toward increasing size and pace of maturation during the past 100 years is most likely related to better nutrition and relatively less chronic disease during childhood.

Causes of Growth Deficiency

Growth deficiency, although a valuable clinical sign, is a highly nonspecific one. Five general categories of growth deficiency are presented subsequently, each having somewhat different overall characteristics in terms of growth pattern, mode of evaluation toward a specific diagnosis, prognosis for eventual stature, and management. The first two categories are variants of normal growth, and the other three represent abnormalities in the growth process. This classification, with the exception of prenatal growth deficiency, is summarized in Table 2-1.

Variants of Normal

Familial Short Stature

Familial short stature is characterized by an otherwise normal small child who is maturing at a normal rate, as indicated by "bone age," with a family history of small stature in otherwise normal close relatives. Such individuals are usually within normal limits for size at birth, have a consistently slow pace of linear growth during childhood, reach adolescence at a usual age, and are relatively short in final stature.

Familial Slow Maturation

Familial slow maturation is characterized by a slowly maturing child who is short for chronological age but not for maturational age (bone age), with a family history of slow maturation. The latter is indicated by late advent of adolescence and final height attainment in one or more close relatives. Such individuals are usually within normal limits for size at birth, with slowing in the pace of growth and maturation becoming evident during late infancy or early childhood. They have a late onset of normal adolescence and usually achieve a final height within the normal range, but at a late chronological age.

Abnormal Growth

Aside from the rare and rather obvious situation of sexual precocity leading to rapid growth and accelerated maturation with an early and relatively short final height attainment, the other growth deficiency disorders can be grouped into three general categories, which are presented subsequently.

Primary Skeletal Growth Deficiency

The implication for this category is that of a primary intracellular problem that affects the growth of the skeletal system. The growth deficiency is usually of prenatal onset and is often accompanied by malproportion or defects in skeletal molding. The same problem that affects cellular growth and morphogenesis in the skeleton may have affected other tissues as well. Thus the patient often presents with a *pattern* of multiple malformations, the recognition of which may allow for a concise overall diagnosis.

TABLE 2-1 CLASSIFICATION OF GROWTH DEFICIENCY

	NORMAL VARIANTS	
Features	**Familial Short Stature**	**Familial Slow Maturation**
Onset of growth deficiency	Postnatal	Postnatal (early childhood)
Rate of maturation	Normal	Slow
Family history	Short stature	Slow maturation
Final stature	Short	Normal limits
Therapy to increase eventual stature	None	None

	ABNORMALS*	
Features	**Primary Skeletal Growth Deficiency**	**Secondary Growth Deficiency**
Onset of growth deficiency	Usually prenatal	Usually postnatal
Rate of maturation	Variable, usually normal	Usually retarded
Associated anomalies	Frequent	Unusual, except when causative anomaly
Malproportionment	Frequent	Unusual, except for rickets
General modes of etiology	Chromosomal abnormalities	Environmental
	Mutant gene syndromes, including the osteochondrodysplasias	Defect in nonskeletal organ, including endocrine
	Syndromes of unknown etiology	Metabolic disorders
		Chronic infectious disease
Therapy to increase eventual stature	None usually[†,‡]	Specific treatment can result in "catch-up" growth

*Prenatal infectious disease, fetal alcohol syndrome, trisomy 18 syndrome, and other conditions resulting in early intrauterine growth restriction are not included.
[†]The Federal Drug Administration (FDA) has approved the use of recombinant human growth hormone (HGH) for children with Turner syndrome, Prader-Willi syndrome, idiopathic short stature, and intrauterine growth restriction whose height has not normalized by 2 years of age. HGH has also been used in treatment of achondroplasia and Noonan syndrome, among other conditions.
[‡]Limb lengthening procedures have been used to increase height in individuals with achondroplasia.

TABLE 2-2   SECONDARY GROWTH DEFICIENCY

PROBLEM	REASON FOR GROWTH DEFICIENCY	DIAGNOSTIC STUDIES

Nutritional
  a. Inadequate intake
  b. GI malformation
  c. Malabsorption
	Nutritional deficiency	Response to adequate intake
		Gastrointestinal imaging studies
		Measurements of absorption

Deprivation syndrome	Neglect, abuse, nutritional	Response to environmental change Home and family investigation
Mental deficiency, usually severe	Unknown	Exclude other causes of growth deficiency
Cardiac defect	Increased caloric requirement ?Hypoxia	Cardiac evaluation
Respiratory insufficiency	?Hypoxia Increased work of breathing	Pulmonary evaluation
Renal dysfunction	Acidosis	Renal imaging Renal function assessment
	Rickets	Calcium, phosphorus, alkaline phosphatase, radiographs

Pituitary growth hormone
  deficiency
	?Diminished lipolysis and amino
	  acid transport to cell
		Provocative testing

Hypothyroidism	Deficit in energy metabolism	Thyroid function testing, thyroid imaging

Chronic serious infectious
  disease (not upper-respiratory)
	Unknown, possible increased
	  caloric requirement	

Metabolic disorders such as hypercalcemia, hypophosphatemic rickets, hypokalemia, galactosemia, glycogen storage disease, salt-losing congenital adrenal hyperplasia. Workup specific to the presenting problem.

Postnatal growth generally proceeds at a consistently slow pace. Although the anomalous skeletal development may lead to difficulty in the interpretation of "bone age," maturation usually advances at a near-normal rate, and adolescence is achieved at a usual age. As yet, there is no known therapy for increasing the eventual stature of persons with most of the disorders within this category. Recombinant human growth hormone has been approved by the Food and Drug Administration for children with Turner syndrome and Prader-Willi syndrome. Human growth hormone has also been used to increase height in achondroplasia and Noonan syndrome among other conditions. Limb lengthening procedures have been used to increase height in individuals with achondroplasia.

The prognosis of stature can best be inferred with knowledge of the final height attainment of other patients with the same disorder. Many of the problems of malformation presented in this text have primary growth deficiency as one feature. These include chromosomal abnormality syndromes, osteochondrodysplasias and many other mutant gene syndromes, plus a number of syndromes of unknown etiology. For some of them, such as the Hurler syndrome and pseudoachondroplasia, the growth deficiency does not become manifest until months or years after birth.

Secondary Skeletal Growth Deficiency

The implication for this category is that the skeletal cells are normal. The growth deficiency is *secondary* to a problem outside the skeletal system that limits its capacity for growth. The problem may exist in the delivery of nutrients, hormones, or oxygen to the skeletal cells or in the maintenance of extracellular homeostasis. Specific types of secondary growth deficiency disorders are listed in Table 2-2. It is unusual for these types of problems to give rise to growth deficiency during fetal life,[*] and hence the onset of growth deficiency is usually *postnatal*. As illustrated in Figure 2-1, defects in the development and function of the brain, pituitary, thyroid, heart, lungs, liver, intestines, or kidneys seldom have a serious effect on prenatal growth but can cause postnatal growth deficiency. Because the growth problem is of postnatal onset, there usually are no associated malformations, except for an anomaly that may be responsible for the growth deficiency. Furthermore, the skeletal system is normally proportioned and modeled, except in the case of rickets.

---

[*]Mild degrees of prenatal secondary growth deficiency may occur with maternal toxemia, malnutrition, or heavy cigarette smoking.

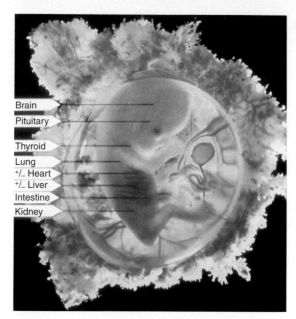

Brain
Pituitary
Thyroid
Lung
+/- Heart
+/- Liver
Intestine
Kidney

FIGURE 2-1. Serious problems in development and function of the listed tissues usually do not have an adverse effect on prenatal growth, whereas each problem can be the cause of serious postnatal secondary growth deficiency.

Skeletal maturation is usually retarded to about the same extent as linear growth, with the exception of primary hypothyroidism, in which case osseous maturation is usually relatively more retarded than is linear growth. Head circumference is usually spared.

When the cause of the secondary growth deficiency is recognized and rectified, one may witness the amazing phenomenon of catch-up growth, an acceleration of growth and maturation toward expectancy for chronologic age. This phenomenon dramatically emphasizes the fact that there is no primary growth problem within the skeletal system. The extent of catch-up growth varies in accordance with the age of onset, duration, and nature of the growth problem—plus the adequacy of therapy.

Prenatal Growth Deficiency

Certain disorders discussed in this text significantly impact prenatal growth through a variety of mechanisms including diminished cellular proliferation, decrease in the absolute number of cells, and interference with placental function. Among disorders to consider in a prenatally growth-retarded infant include chromosomal anomalies; exposure to a variety of human teratogens including alcohol, rubella, and cytomegalovirus; and recognized patterns of malformation with a major impact on growth. Typically such infants will have proportionate growth restriction (i.e., height, weight, and head circumference equally affected) or will demonstrate disproportionate impact on brain growth. Most children with these conditions remain small despite adequate caloric intake, remediation of associated medical condition, and surgical correction of associated malformations.

Clinical Approach to Growth Deficiency

Emphasis should be placed on the following:

1. Family history relative to stature and maturational rate.
2. History of patient's growth, plotted on normal grids. Of particular importance are the *age of onset* of growth deficiency and the *rate* of growth. Compare with normals for the mean parental stature when possible.
3. A complete physical evaluation should include height, weight, head circumference, and inspection for minor anomalies. Check closely for evidence of malproportion, including asymmetry. Measure span and upper-to-lower segment ratio when indicated.
4. Based on the findings, most patients can be separated into one of the following three categories:
   a. Normal for genetic background. No further studies indicated.
   b. Prenatal onset of growth deficiency. Strive to recognize a specific overall syndrome among the primary growth deficiency disorders presented in this text. Also consider prenatal infectious disease, the fetal alcohol syndrome, and other human teratogens.
   c. Postnatal onset of growth deficiency. Disproportionate growth (altered upper-lower segment ratio) is typically a consequence of an osteochondrodysplasia and should be evaluated with a dysmorphology bone survey. In normally proportioned children, obtain a bone age determination (hemiskeletal bone age before 2 years, usually just hand and wrist thereafter). Consider such secondary growth deficiency disorders as those set forth in Table 2-2.

APPROACH TO MENTAL DEFICIENCY

Much progress has been made since the 1960s regarding the causes of mental retardation. Table 2-3 summarizes categorical causes of mental retardation from various surveys in the literature. Advances in technology have dramatically improved the yield of diagnostic evaluation. However, there is to date no indication that a "shot-gun" approach to testing increases the diagnostic hit rate. The core evaluation of an individual with mental retardation continues to be a comprehensive history with specific focus on details of the pregnancy as well as developmental progress/regression, a three-generation pedigree, a detailed physical examination with attention to minor as well as major malformation, and longitudinal follow-up as the phenotype of many conditions evolves over time. The diagnostic rate is improved by a younger age at presentation (history is often lacking in adults), access to relatives for evaluation (helps distinguish familial variants of normal from features associated with hereditary syndromes), and the presence of structural abnormalities. A basic understanding of brain development is helpful in the approach to diagnosis.

TABLE 2-3   CAUSES OF MENTAL DEFICIENCY FROM LITERATURE SURVEYS

CAUSE	PERCENTAGE
Chromosomal anomalies	4–28
Recognizable patterns of malformation	3–7
Known single-gene disorders	3–9
Structural abnormalities of the brain	7–17
Complications of prematurity	2–10
Environmental/teratogenic causes	5–13
Culturo-familial mental retardation*	3–12
Provisionally unique syndromes	1–5
Metabolic/endocrine disorders	1–5
Unknown	30–50

*Defined by a family history of one or more relatives with mental retardation, no other identified cause, and no evidence for a single-gene disorder. Typically, economic disadvantage complicates the phenotype.

Anderson G, Schroer RJ, Stevenson RE: Mental retardation in South Carolina II: Causation. Proc Greenwood Genet Ctr 15:32, 1996.

Modified after Curry CJ, Stevenson RE, Aughton D, et al, of the American College of Medical Genetics: Evaluation of mental retardation: Recommendations of a consensus conference. Am J Med Genet 72:468, 1997.

Normal Development of Central Nervous System

At 18 days of fetal development, the thickened neural plate becomes a neural groove, the margins of which join to form the neural tube, which is completely closed by 28 days. Rapid growth takes place anteriorly with formation of the primitive brain vesicles: the prosencephalon (forebrain), mesencephalon (midbrain), and rhombencephalon (hindbrain). By 23 days, the optic outpouchings are occurring from the prosencephalon, and by 33 days, its lateral outpouchings (i.e., the early cerebral hemispheres) are evident. Major brain morphogenesis continues for many months; the cerebellum does not begin its major period of morphogenesis until 4 to 5 fetal months. Within the cerebral hemispheres, the inner layer of neuro-epithelial cells differentiates to become neuroblasts, which migrate outward in successive waves to form the cortical mantle layers. By 10 weeks, the cerebral cortex is quite thin, with only one outer cortical layer in contrast with the relatively large size of the lateral ventricles, as shown in Figure 2-2. Cell numbers are increasing rapidly, with a major addition of neurons at approximately 4 to 5 fetal months. New cells are being added well into postnatal life, as indicated in Figure 2-3. Although most of the neurons are present at birth, a major addition of glial cells occurs during the first 6 post-natal months. Most of the myelinization process, the responsibility of glial cells, occurs during the first year. The "wiring" of the axon networks, so integral to advancing and integrated function, is also occurring; however, less is known about critical periods for these interconnections between neurons. The functional consequences of this rapid brain growth and integration of neurons are reflected in the orderly progression of advancing performance during this time. Brain growth is almost complete by 2 years, with the organ reaching approximately 80% of its adult size by this age.

Approach to Problems in Which Mental Deficiency Is a Feature

Clinical Evaluation of Mental Deficiency Relative to Diagnostic Studies

Most population studies demonstrate that the likelihood of arriving at a diagnosis is greatest in the most severely delayed individuals although this notion has been recently challenged.[9] Many

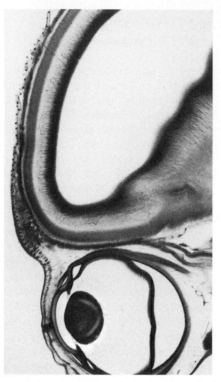

FIGURE 2-2. Sagittal section of a fetal brain at the level of the eye at 10 weeks of development. Note the single cortical zone of the cerebral cortex and the relatively large ventricular space. (From Smith DW, Gong BT: Teratology 9:17, 1974. Copyright © 1974. Reprinted with permission of Wiley-Liss, Inc., a subsidiary of John Wiley & Sons, Inc.)

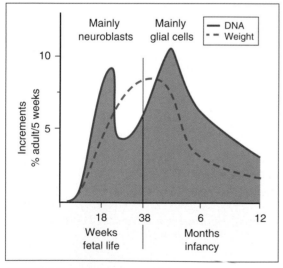

FIGURE 2-3. Rate of brain growth in terms of new cells (DNA) and weight during the most critical period of brain morphogenesis. (Adapted from Dobbin J: Am J Dis Child 120:411, 1970, with permission.)

children with milder degrees of mental deficiency, having intelligence quotients (IQs) in the range of 50 to 70, come from families impacted by poverty with delay in other relatives ("culturofamilial" mental retardation). Both genetic and environmental factors play a role. The mild mental retardation group also includes some XXY boys; an occasional XXX girl; some children with malformation syndromes; some children with the fragile X syndrome or the fetal alcohol syndrome; some patients with inborn errors of metabolism; and some children with milder defects of central nervous system (CNS) development or residual central nervous system insults. Among the more severely mentally deficient patients, with IQs less than 50, it is possible to arrive at a precise overall diagnosis in roughly two thirds of patients.

Diagnostic Studies in Patients with Mental Deficiency—Their Rational Usage

Studies That May Resolve the Diagnosis

CHROMOSOME STUDIES

In populations of patients in whom the cause of mental retardation remains unknown after history and physical examination, chromosome testing elucidates the diagnosis in 3% to 12%. The presence of minor malformations increases the yield in testing. The American College of Medical Genetics consensus conference recommended a minimum band level of 500 on a G-banded karyotype. Chromosome testing is recommended in most practice guidelines for children with otherwise unexplained mental retardation.

FRAGILE X STUDIES

Fragile X syndrome has been estimated to be the most common inherited cause of mental retardation. A prevalence of roughly 3% has been documented in populations with undiagnosed developmental delay. Autistic features may increase the diagnostic yield. Preselection using a seven-item screen including a positive family history of mental retardation, characteristic facies, large/protuberant ears, hyperextensible joints, soft/loose skin on the hands, enlarged testes, characteristic personality changes doubled the detection rate in males.[11] Because of the familial implications of this condition, testing should be considered in the absence of another obvious etiology for developmental delay.

FLUORESCENCE IN SITU HYBRIDIZATION STUDIES

Fluorescence in situ hybridization (FISH) testing is used in two contexts. The first involves the use of specific FISH probes to confirm the diagnosis of a recognized pattern of malformation for which molecular testing is available. A strong clinical suspicion of the condition is necessary to prompt request for the appropriate test. Specific probes are available for velocardiofacial/DiGeorge syndrome, Williams syndrome, deletion 4p syndrome, and others. More recently, molecular screening for sub-telomeric rearrangements using FISH has become clinically available. This testing is expensive and labor-intensive, yet studies have documented a roughly 7% detection rate among individuals with moderate-to-severe mental retardation. A five-item checklist has been suggested to increase the yield of testing.[12] This includes a positive family history of mental retardation, prenatal growth deficiency, postnatal growth deficiency or overgrowth, two or more dysmorphic facial features, and one or more nonfacial minor or major anomalies.

COMPARATIVE GENOMIC HYBRIDIZATION

Comparative genomic hybridization (CGH) is an emerging technology currently applied in cancer diagnosis that is rapidly moving into the arena of constitutional chromosomal abnormalities. Chromosomes from the individual to be tested are tagged with fluorochrome-labeled DNA probes that cover the genome and saturate areas of potential clinical interest. Chromosomes from a reference (normal) are spotted on an array labeled with identical probes tagged with a different colored fluorochrome. Gain or loss of information is detected through color change. The assay is automated. Probes can be designed to assess any area of potential interest. Currently available CGH assays cover all of the telomeres, all of the known clinical microdeletion areas (e.g., 22q11.2), and enough segments of each chromosome to detect monosomy and trisomy. Balanced chromosome rearrangements are not detected by this methodology. Whereas it is unlikely that CGH will completely replace routine cytogenetics in all of its applications, it may offer an excellent alternative to FISH-based testing.

TESTING FOR INBORN ERRORS OF METABOLISM

Patients with mental deficiency due to an inborn error of metabolic function often have one or more additional clues besides mental deficiency alone. Some of these are set forth in Table 2-4. Most appear normal at birth, and then diffuse non-lateralizing evidence of central nervous system

TABLE 2-4 EXAMPLES OF FEATURES IN ADDITION TO MENTAL DEFICIENCY THAT OFTEN OCCUR POSTNATALLY IN CERTAIN INBORN ERRORS OF METABOLISM

DISORDER	FEATURES
Phenylketonuria, classic; autosomal recessive	Light pigmentation, eczema (33%); poor coordination, seizures (25%), autistic behavior
Sanfilippo syndrome (MPS III); autosomal recessive	Developmental lag after 1 yr with deterioration toward restless behavior, clumsiness by age 6–7 yr, development of coarse facies and hair by 2–3 yr, gum hypertropy, mild limitation in finger extension
Hurler syndrome (MPS I); autosomal recessive	Developmental lag after 6–10 mo, with deterioration and growth deficiency, coarse facies, stiff joints, gibbus, hepatosplenomegaly, cloudy corneas, rhinitis
Hunter syndrome (MPS II), severe type; X-linked recessive	Developmental lag after 6–12 mo, with growth deficiency, coarse facies, stiff joints, hepatosplenomegaly; no gibbus or cloudy corneas
Galactosemia, severe type; autosomal recessive	Development in early infancy (on cow's milk feeding) of lethargy, hypotonia, heptomegaly, icterus, hypoglycemia, cataract, with failure to thrive
Lesch-Nyhan syndrome; X-linked recessive	Development after 6–8 mo of spasticity, choreoathetosis, self-mutilation, autistic behavior, growth deficiency; tophi in late childhood
Homocystinuria; autosomal recessive	Mild arachnodactyly, pectus, genu valgus, pes cavus, mild limitation of finger extension; downward lens dislocation, usually by age 10 yr; wide facial pores, malar flush; thrombotic phenomena, contributing to CNS problems
Argininosuccinicaciduria; autosomal recessive	Onset in first 1–2 yr of growth deficiency, mild hepatomegaly, skin lesions, dry brittle hair with trichorrhexis nodosa, seizures

deficit or deterioration of function develops at a variable postnatal age. Intermittent lapses of consciousness, inanition, unexplained hypoglycemia, or recurrent acidosis are potential clues to an inborn error of metabolism. Most reviews have documented an extremely low yield for nontargeted metabolic screening in the evaluation of mental retardation.

STUDIES FOR PRENATAL INFECTIOUS DISEASE

Patients with mental deficiency as the result of congenital rubella, cytomegalic inclusion disease, or toxoplasmosis usually also have one or more of the following features: microcephaly, chorioretinitis, prenatal onset growth deficiency, hepatosplenomegaly, neonatal petechiae, jaundice, and deafness. Patients with congenital rubella may also have cataract, cardiac defect, and other anomalies. The diagnosis of congenital infection is best pursued in the immediate newborn period through cultures for the offending agent, antibody titers, and placental evaluation.

THYROID STUDIES

Congenital hypothyroidism may account for 3% to 4% of mental retardation in areas without comprehensive newborn screening programs. Most affected individuals have obvious symptoms. Thyroid studies are not indicated in the patient with mental deficiency and short stature who does not show any other clinical indication of having hypothyroidism particularly if that patient has been screened as a neonate.

Ancillary Studies That May Assist in the Diagnosis

Neuroimaging has been recommended as part of the diagnostic evaluation of mental retardation.[16] Magnetic resonance imaging of the brain is generally preferable to computed tomography. In several recent studies, roughly half of affected individuals had abnormalities documented on neuroimaging. Improvements in imaging equipment will likely increase this number. In some instances, imaging is helpful with respect to etiologic diagnosis. In others, it merely documents another physical finding for the clinician. Microcephaly, macrocephaly, abnormalities of cranial contour, and focal neurologic findings increase the yield of this modality of testing.

Skeletal radiographs may be indicated by clinical findings such as disproportionate short stature or other malformation suggesting skeletal anomalites. Bone surveys are often diagnostic in skeletal dysplasias. In other instances, these radiographs identify bony features to assist in recognition of the pattern of malformation and in management. They are seldom diagnostic.

Electroencephalograms are rarely helpful with specific diagnoses but are useful in management if a seizure disorder is suspected.

APPROACH TO ARTHROGRYPOSIS (PRENATAL ONSET OF JOINT CONTRACTURES)

Normal Development of Joints

Joint development begins secondarily within the early mesenchymal condensations of the precartilaginous bone at approximately $5\frac{1}{2}$ weeks. By 7 weeks, many joint spaces exist, and by 8 weeks, there is movement of the limbs. Figure 2-4 shows the early development. Motion is essential for the normal development of the joints and their contiguous structures.

Problems That Can Cause Congenital Joint Contractures

Joint contractures can be secondary to factors that are intrinsic to the developing fetus, such as early onset of neurologic, muscle, and joint problems, or to factors that are extrinsic to the developing fetus, such as fetal crowding and constraint (Fig. 2-5).

1. *Neurologic abnormality* has been the most common cause of arthrogryposis in the experience of the author. The neurologic disorders that may be responsible for the secondary arthrogryposis include meningomyelocele; anterior motor horn cell deficiency; prenatal spasticity; and certain gross brain defects such as anencephaly, hydranencephaly, and holoprosencephaly.
2. *Muscle problems* such as muscle agenesis, rare fetal myopathies, and occasionally myotonic dystrophy.
3. *Joint and contiguous tissue problems* such as synostosis, lack of joint development, aberrant fixation of joints as in diastrophic dysplasia, aberrant laxity of joints with

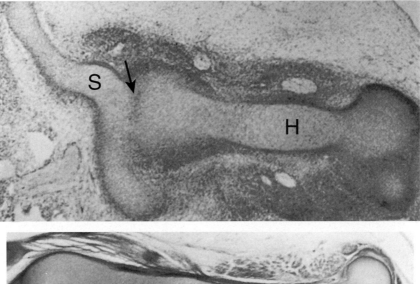

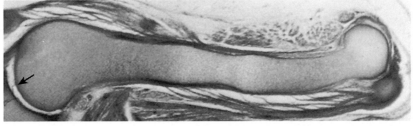

FIGURE 2-4. Development of scapulo (*S*) -humoral (*H*) shoulder joint (*arrow*) at 38 days of development (*top*) and at approximately 47 days (*bottom*). Note that joint morphogenesis occurs secondarily. By the time the joint is formed, functional muscle has differentiated.

dislocations as in the Larsen syndrome, and aberrant soft tissue fixations as in the popliteal pterygium syndrome.

4. *Fetal crowding and constraint* as with multiple births or with oligohydramnios in disorders such as renal agenesis or early persisting leakage of amniotic fluid.

Methods of Evaluation

1. *History*. The history relative to arthrogryposis should include information on the onset and character of fetal movements (often diminished), mode of delivery (often breech), and amniotic fluid (oligohydramnios) may give rise to fetal crowding while polyhydramnios secondary to decreased fetal swallowing is sometimes seen in situations associated with neurologic abnormalities).

2. *Total pattern of anomalies*. Non–joint-related anomalies may indicate that the arthrogryposis is part of a multiple defect syndrome such as the trisomy 18 syndrome.

3. *Joint and skeletal evaluation*. Physical and radiologic assessment of joints and skeletal system is indicated. Determine whether the joint fixation is a result of an anatomic anomaly, such as lack of development of a joint or synostosis, or a deficit in functional movement with no primary structural cause. Always check for scoliosis and for hip dislocation.

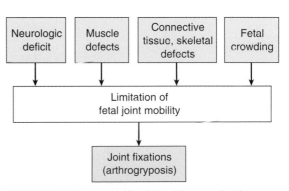

FIGURE 2-5. The types of problems that can lead to prenatal joint contractures.

4. *Evaluation of hand and foot creases.* The palmar and finger creases and the sole creases represent the planes of early flexional function and are evident by 11 to 12 weeks of fetal age. Absent or abnormal creases are secondary to aberrant form or function in the early hand or foot development. They also provide a historical

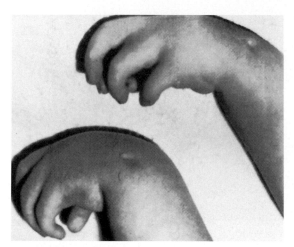

FIGURE 2-6. Dimples on the dorsum of the wrists, indicating that the aberrant positioning of the hands had been present from early in fetal life. The joint contractures in this infant were considered to be secondary to neurologic deficiency. (Courtesy of Dr. Michael Cohen, Dalhousie University, Halifax, Nova Scotia.)

record of the flexional planes of function that have existed and thus facilitate decisions relative to rehabilitation of existing function.

5. *Search for dimples.* When close fetal contact between bone and overlying skin has occurred, there may be failure in the development of subcutaneous and adipose tissue at that locale, thereby causing a dimple. The finding of aberrant dimples implies an early fetal onset of the problem, resulting in aberrant cutaneous-osseous approximation, as shown in Figure 2-6.

6. *Cautious neurologic and muscle assessment.* Attempts to determine whether there is a primary neurologic or muscle problem can be most difficult, since deficit in either one can lead to aberrant function of the other. Electromyographic studies occasionally may be of value. In the great majority of patients with arthrogryposis who have abnormal study results, the evidence points toward neuropathy and rarely to a myopathy. Muscle biopsy may only occasionally be of value, because it is difficult to determine whether muscle hypoplasia, fibrosis, or both are a primary or secondary phenomenon.

7. *Distinction between joint contractures caused by a problem intrinsic to the fetus versus those due to intrauterine constraint* (Fig. 2-7). Intrinsically derived contractures

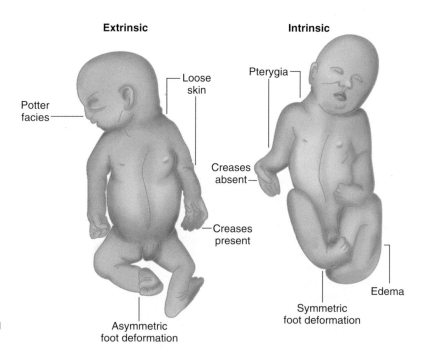

FIGURE 2-7. Differentiation between extrinsically and intrinsically derived deformational defects.

are symmetric and polyhydramnios is often present. The skin is taut and pterygia cross the joints. Flexion creases are lacking. By contrast, the infant with extrinsically derived contractures has positional limb anomalies, large ears, and loose skin. Flexion creases are normal or often exaggerated. Distinction between these two categories is important for the family, because children with extrinsically derived constraint-related arthrogryposis have an excellent prognosis and a low recurrence risk, while both recurrence risk and prognosis are dependent on the etiology of the joint contractures when they are intrinsically derived.

Comment and Management

When a particular diagnosis can be delineated, the management should be specific for that disorder. There remain a number of patients with multiple congenital joint contractures for whom no specific diagnosis can presently be clearly determined. Based on a study of over 350 patients with congenital contractures of joints, Judith Hall, University of British Columbia, Vancouver, has made the most significant contribution to our understanding of this problem as well as to an approach to its etiology.[21,22]

APPROACH TO AMBIGUOUS (PARTIALLY MASCULINIZED) EXTERNAL GENITALIA

Normal Development

Over the past several years, much has been learned about the genes that control male and female sexual differentiation. This information has come from the study of mouse models as well as detailed evaluation of human phenotypes. Primordial germ cells are activated in the epiblast by bone morphogenetic protein 4 (BMP4) secreted by the extraembyronic ectoderm. The germ cells migrate along the hindgut into the urogenital ridge from which the gonad eventually forms. Development of the urogenital ridge from intermediate mesoderm is influenced by a variety of genes including Emx2, GATA-4, Lim1, and Lhx9, mutations of which result in abnormal gonads in mice. No human counterparts have yet been identified. Also critical to ridge development are the genes WT1 (Wilms tumor suppressor gene), Sf-1 (steroidogenic factor 1), and DAX 1 (duplicated in adrenal hypoplasia congenita). WT1 is critical to both gonadal and renal development. Specific mutations in WT1 are associated with Fraser syndrome, a condition with nephrotic syndrome and gonadal dysgenesis. XY individuals have sex reversal because lack of WT1 affects downstream targets necessary for testicular development. Other mutations in WT1 produce Denys-Drash syndrome with glomerular and mesangial sclerosis and ambiguous genitalia in the XY individual with incomplete testicular differentiation and function. Sf-1 knockout mice die at birth with no adrenal glands and no gonads. DAX 1 is an X-linked gene that suppresses testicular differentiation. It is hypothesized to play some role in mixed gonadal dysgenesis. The gene SRY on the distal short arm of the Y chromosome is the major determinant of testicular differentiation. SRY interacts with SOX9 (SRY homeobox 9), activating the transcription of müllerian-inhibiting substance in the male. Mutations in SOX9 are responsible for campomelic dysplasia, a short limb dwarfing condition in which sex reversal occurs in the male. Both SRY and SOX9 are necessary for normal testicular development.

At approximately 8 weeks' gestation, the testis begins producing testosterone, actively causing masculinization of the external genitalia, with fusion of the labioscrotal folds to form a scrotum, enlargement of the phallus, and fusion of the labioscrotal folds into a penile urethra, as shown in Figure 2-8. The testes descend into the scrotum by 7 to 8 fetal months.

Early in development, both males and females have mesonephric (wolffian) ducts, which form the vas deferens, seminal vesicles, epididymides, and paramesonephric (müllerian) ducts, which give rise to the uterus, fallopian tubes, and upper third of the vagina. A number of genes are responsible for the development and maintenance of these structures including PAX2, Wnt-4, and homeobox transcription factors 9, 10, 11, and 13. Mutations in several of these genes have produced human phenotypes, most of which are not associated with ambiguous genitalia. The normally functioning testis produces two hormones that influence the duct system. Testosterone causes the wolffian ducts to develop while müllerian-inhibiting substance induces involution of müllerian structures. In the absence of these signals, duct development is reversed. Mutations in the gene coding for müllerian-inhibiting substance or its receptor when present in an XY individual result in males with persistence of müllerian duct structures, undescended testes, and crossed testicular ectopia.

Dihydrotestosterone is the most potent, locally active androgen. A number of errors in the choles-

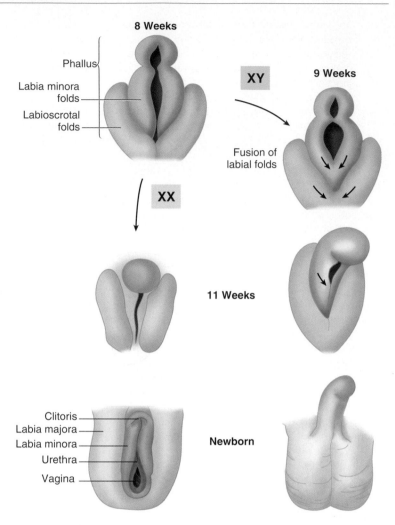

8 Weeks

Phallus

Labia minora folds

Labioscrotal folds

XY

9 Weeks

Fusion of labial folds

XX

11 Weeks

FIGURE 2-8. Normal morphogenesis of external genitalia. The normal male development is induced by testosterone derived from the fetal testicle. (Illustrations adapted from photographs supplied by Dr. Jan Jirásek, Prague, Czech Republic.)

Clitoris
Labia majora
Labia minora
Urethra
Vagina

Newborn

terol biosynthetic pathway may reduce the amount of dihydrotestosterone, resulting in incomplete masculinization of an XY individual. Conversely, inborn errors in steroid biosynthesis that result in diminished cortisol and aldosterone production induce overproduction of androgens, virilizing an XX individual.

Methods of Evaluation

In evaluation of the child with ambiguous genitalia, the focus should be to establish an etiologic diagnosis as rapidly as possible so that sex of rearing can be assigned confidently and metabolic complications of some of the potential diagnoses can be treated promptly.

With respect to sex of rearing, the vast majority of affected children can be raised in concordance with their genetic sex. An exception may be those

XY individuals who have inadequate masculinization on the basis of androgen insensitivity. Migeon and colleagues introduced the concept of the genitalia as a bioassay for androgen action, suggesting that the degree of undervirilization is proportionate to the degree of androgen deficiency regardless of the cause (underproduction versus failure to respond).[27] These authors suggested that the most undervirilized would best be raised as females, whereas the most virilized would optimally be raised as males. They, however, recognized the importance of an etiologic diagnosis in the assignment of gender. In the past, XY infants with severe perineal malformations who had insufficient tissue to allow reconstruction of a phallus (e.g., exstrophy of the cloaca) have been assigned female sex of rearing. These individuals make normal amounts of testosterone to which the brain is exposed prenatally. Long-term follow-up of individuals so managed suggests that many eventually identify themselves as male. Balancing what is surgically possible with the androgen imprint of the brain is clearly challenging.

The approach outlined in Figure 2-9 is predicated on determining if the infant is an XY individual who is incompletely masculinized or an XX individual who is virilized. Central to the diagnosis is determination of genetic sex usually by peripheral blood chromosomes. FISH or molecular analysis for SRY with polymerase chain reaction testing may be helpful adjuncts to diagnosis but are not usually part of the initial evaluation unless the turn-around time for cytogenetic testing is unduly long.

A complete physical examination is extremely helpful in determining genetic sex. The presence of associated nongenital anomalies rules out the various types of congenital adrenal hyperplasia and usually indicates that the affected child has either a defect in the mesodermal primordia that form the external genitalia or incomplete masculinization from inadequate follicle-stimulating hormone and/or luteinizing hormone production, inadequate production of cholesterol precursor for steroid hormone synthesis, or a genital malformation as part of an overall pattern of malformation, some of which are due to a chromosome abnormality. The majority of multiply malformed infants with

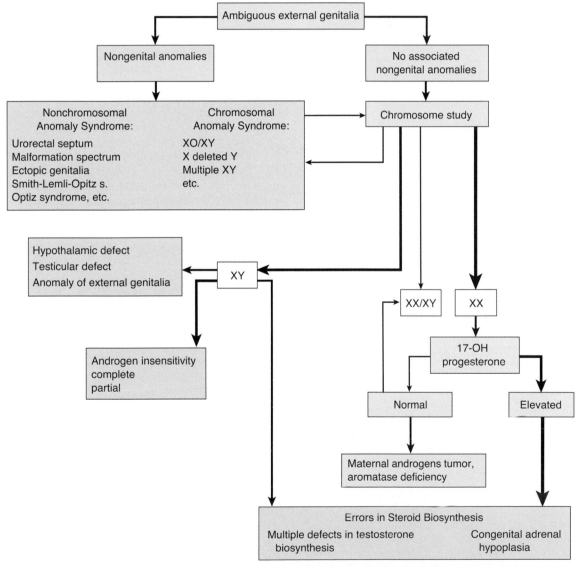

FIGURE 2-9. Approach toward arriving at a specific overall diagnosis in the patient who has ambiguous external genitalia.

ambiguous genitalia are XY. The only pattern of malformation that is likely to present confusion is the XX infant with the urorectal septum malformation sequence (see Chapter 1). These infants are readily identified by the lack of defined structures on the perineum (e.g., imperforate anus, no labioscrotal folds, an ill-defined phallus with or without a single perineal opening).

The algorithm in Figure 2-9 outlines the approach to the child with ambiguous external genitalia who has associated nongenital anomalies versus the child with ambiguous external genitalia who lacks associated nongenital anomalies.

Ambiguous External Genitalia with Associated Nongenital Anomalies

For infants with the urorectal septum malformation sequence or ectopically positioned genital parts, search should be made for defects in other mesodermally derived structures. For infants with incomplete masculinization manifest by perineal hypospadias and/or a shawl scrotum, evaluation of serum 7-dehydrocholesterol to rule out Smith-Lemli-Opitz syndrome should be performed and other multiple malformation syndromes associated with ambiguous external genitalia should be considered. For infants with ambiguity as manifest by micropenis and cryptorchidism, the hypothalamic axis and brain need to be evaluated. It is important to recognize, however, that most patients who present with an otherwise normally formed micropenis, cryptorchidism, or both lack associated nongenital anomalies. However small the phallus, a normal position of the male urethra indicates that testosterone secretion early in development was normal, an important factor in determining gender assignment.

Ambiguous External Genitalia without Associated Nongenital Anomalies

For this group of infants, determination of the following features of the genital anatomy can often provide strong evidence for genetic sex while chromosomes are pending.

Gonads

If no gonads are found in the scrotal area, place a finger over the inguinal canal to prevent the ascent of any inguinal gonad and palpate the inguinal areas carefully, ideally with three fingers. If one or more gonads are found, it is highly unlikely that the patient is a partially masculinized female, because

inguinal or lower gonads are usually testes. Only in the situation of inguinal hernia may one find an ovary in the inguinal area.

Phallus

If it is a relatively thin phallus, the patient is unlikely to be a female with congenital adrenal hyperplasia, because she would be under "active" androgen stimulation with increased caliber to the phallus. If there is a single opening at the base of the phallus and also a small "pit" on the glans, the former represents the urethral opening and the latter is of no significance.

Urogenital Sinus or Urethra; Vagina

When there is only a single opening at the base of the phallus, insert a relatively stiff catheter or sterile probe into it. Direct the catheter tip downward in the direction of the anal opening. If it goes in that direction easily and can be palpated beneath the perineal skin, there is probably a urogenital sinus with both urethral and vaginal orifices, as in the female with congenital adrenal hyperplasia. If it is "penile" urethra, the catheter will usually go cephalad and cannot be easily palpated in the perineal area. Inject radiopaque material into the single opening under pressure and obtain a lateral roentgenogram to demonstrate whether there is a vaginal pouch. If a vaginal opening is evident, insert a catheter into it and determine its depth.

Uterus

Do a cautious rectal examination with the little finger, feeling for a uterine body. When removing the finger in the neonate, stroke the anterior rectal area outward. If there is a vagina, this maneuver will often result in the extrusion of vagina mucus from the single urogenital opening. The majority of diagnoses that cause inadequate virilization of the external genitalia in an XY individual do not interfere with production of müllerian-inhibiting factor. Thus on rectal examination, no cervix or uterus should be palpable. In addition, pelvic ultrasound should not demonstrate müllerian derivatives.

XX Individuals Who Are Masculinized

These infants either have been exposed to exogenous androgen or have defects in adrenal steroid biosynthesis that cause them to produce endogenous androgen. The former may be identified on questioning the mother regarding medication intake and evaluating the mother for virilization (as should be seen with androgen-secreting tumors and placental aromatase deficiency). A 17-OH progesterone level is the most useful screen for the latter, because it will be elevated in the most common inborn error (21-hydroxylase deficiency). A more extensive panel including 17-OH pregnenolone and DHEA may be necessary to detect 3β-OH steroid dehydrogenase deficiency.

XY Individuals Who Are Inadequately Masculinized

These infants fall into one of three categories: (1) those with globally inadequate androgen production either on a central (hypothalamic) or peripheral (testis) basis; (2) those with inborn errors of testosterone biosynthesis; or (3) those with androgen resistance. Because testosterone levels in the first month of life in XY individuals are usually near adult levels, measurement of follicle-stimulating hormone, luteinizing hormone, testosterone, and its precursors can usually separate infants in category 1 (low testosterone and low precursors) from categories 2 (low testosterone and elevated precursors) and 3 (normal to high testosterone). Defining the etiology of inadequate androgen production frequently involves assessment of the gonad itself. Separating patients in categories 2 and 3 may require more specific assay of genital skin fibroblasts, although category 3 patients may have a history of maternal female relatives with infertility. Using this approach, it is usually possible to reach a diagnosis with a minimum of laboratory testing and a high degree of diagnostic certainty.

References
Growth Deficiency
1. Bryant J, Cave C, Mihaylova B, et al: Clinical effectiveness and cost-effectiveness of growth hormone in children: A systematic review and economic evaluation. Health Technol Assess 6:1, 2002.
2. Faulkner F (ed): Human Development. Philadelphia: WB Saunders, 1966.
3. Gardner LI (ed): Endocrine and Genetic Diseases of Childhood and Adolescence, 2nd ed. Philadelphia: WB Saunders, 1975.
4. Garn SM, Rohmann CG: Interaction of nutrition and genetics in the timing of growth and development. Pediatr Clin North Am 13:353, 1966.
5. Smith DW: Growth and Its Disorders: Basics and Standards, Approach and Classifications, Growth Deficiency Disorders, Growth Excess Disorders, Obesity. Philadelphia: WB Saunders, 1977.
6. Tanner JM, Goldstein H, Whitehouse RH: Standards for children's height at ages two to nine years allowing for height of parents. Arch Dis Child 45:755, 1970.
7. Wilson TA, Rose SR, Cohen P, et al, The Lawson Wilkins Pediatric Endocrinology Society Drug and Therapeutics Committee: Update of guidelines for the use of growth hormone in children: The Lawson Wilkins Pediatric Endocrinology Society Drug and Therapeutics Committee. J Pediatr 143:415, 2003.

Mental Deficiency
8. Anderson G, Schroer RJ, Stevenson RE: Mental retardation in South Carolina II: Causation. Proc Greenwood Genet Ctr 15:32, 1996.
9. Battaglia A, Carey JC: Diagnostic evaluation of developmental delay/mental retardation: An overview. Am J Med Genet 117C:3, 2003.
10. Curry CJ, Stevenson RE, Aughton D, et al, of the American College of Medical Genetics: Evaluation of mental retardation: Recommendations of a consensus conference. Am J Med Genet 72:468, 1997.
11. de Vries BBA, Mohkarnsing S, van den Ouweland AMW, et al: Screening for the Fragile X syndrome among the mentally retarded: A clinical study. J Med Genet 36:467–470, 1999.
12. de Vries BBA, White SM, Knight SJL, et al: Clinical studies on submicroscopic subtelomeric rearrangements: A checklist. J Med Genet 38:145, 2001.
13. Hunter AGW: Outcome of the routine assessment of patients with mental retardation in a genetics clinic. Am J Med Genet 90:60, 2000.
14. O'Rahilly R, Gardner E: The timing and sequence of events in the development of human nervous system during the embryonic period proper. Z Anat Entwicklungsgesch 34:1, 1971.
15. Park V et al: Policy Statement: American College of Medical Genetics. Fragile X syndrome: Diagnostic and carrier testing. Am J Med Genet 53:380, 1994.
16. Shevell M, Ashwal S, Donley D, et al: Practice parameter: Evaluation of the child with global developmental delay: Report of the quality standards subcommittee of the American Academy of Neurology and the Practice Committee of the Child Neurology Society. Neurology 60:367, 2003.
17. Smith DW, Bostian KD: Congenital anomalies associated with idiopathic mental retardation. J Pediatr 65:189, 1964.
18. Smith DW, Simons FER: Rational diagnostic evaluation of the child with mental deficiency. Am J Dis Child 129:1285, 1975.
19. Stevenson RE: Mental retardation: Overview and historical perspective. Proc Greenwood Genet Ctr 15:19, 1996.

Arthrogryposis
20. Fisher RL et al: Arthrogryposis multiplexed congenita: A clinical investigation. J Pediatr 76:255, 1970.
21. Hall JG, Reed SD, Driscoll EP: Part I. Amyoplasia: A common sporadic condition with congenital contractures. Am J Med Genet 15:571, 1983.
22. Hall JG, Reed SD, Greene D: The distal arthrogryposes: Delineation of new entities—review and nosologic discussion. Am J Med Genet 11:185, 1982.
23. Jones MC: Intrinsic versus extrinsically derived deformational defects: A clinical approach. Semin Perinatol 7:237, 1983.

Ambiguous External Genitalia
24. American Academy of Pediatrics, Committee on Genetics, Section on Endocrinology, Section on Urology: Evaluation

of the newborn with developmental anomalies of the external genitalia. Pediatrics 106:138, 2000.

25. Guthrie RD, Smith DW, Graham CB: Testosterone treatment for the micropenis during early childhood. J Pediatr 83:247, 1973.

26. MacLaughlin DT, Donahoe PK: Sex determination and differentiation. N Engl J Med 350:367, 2004.

27. Migeon CJ, Wisniewski AB, Brown TR, et al: 46,XY Intersex individuals: Phenotypic and etiologic classification, knowledge of condition, and satisfaction with knowledge in adulthood. Pediatrics 110(3): 2002. Available at: http://www.pediatrics.org/cgi/content/full/110/3/e32.

28. Migeon CJ, Wisniewski AB, Gearhart JP, et al: Ambiguous genitalia with perineoscrotal hypospadias in 46,XY individuals: Long-term medical, surgical, and psychosocial outcome. Pediatrics 110(3): 2002. Available at: http://www.pediatrics.org/cgi/content/full/110/3/e31.

29. Rangecroft, L, on behalf of the British Association of Paediatric Surgeons Working Party on the Surgical Management of Children Born with Ambiguous Genitalia: Surgical management of ambiguous genitalia. Arch Dis Child 88:799, 2003.

30. Sultan C, Paris F, Jeandel C, et al: Ambiguous genitalia in the newborn. Semin Reprod Med 20:181, 2002.

3 Morphogenesis and Dysmorphogenesis

Knowledge of normal morphogenesis may assist in the interpretation of structural defects, and the study of structural defects may assist in the understanding of normal morphogenesis. Each anomaly must have a logical mode of development and cause. When interpreting a structural defect, the clinician is looking back to an early stage in development with which he or she has often had little acquaintance. This chapter sets forth some of the phenomena of morphogenesis and the normal stages in early human development, followed by the types of abnormal morphogenesis and the relative timing of particular malformations.

NORMAL MORPHOGENESIS

Phenomena of Morphogenesis

The genetic information that guides the morphogenesis and function of an individual is all contained within the zygote. After the first few cell divisions, differentiation begins to take place, presumably through activation or inactivation of particular genes, allowing cells to assume diverse roles. The entire process is programmed in a timely and sequential order with little allowance for error, especially in early morphogenesis.

Although little is known about the fundamental processes that control morphogenesis, it is worthwhile to mention some of the normal phenomena that occur and to give examples of each.

Cell Migration

The proper migration of cells to a predestined location is critical in the development of many structures. For example, the germ cells move from the yolk sac endoderm to the urogenital ridge, where they interact with other cells to form the gonad.

Control over Mitotic Rate

The size of particular structures, as well as their form, is largely the consequence of control over the rates of cell division.

Interaction between Adjacent Tissues

The optic cup induces the morphogenesis of the lens from the overlying ectoderm, the ureteric bud gives rise to the development of the kidney from the adjacent metanephric tissue, the notochord is essential for normal development of the overlying neural tissue, and the prechordal mesoderm is important for the normal morphogenesis of the overlying forebrain. These are but a few examples of the many interactions that are essential features in morphogenesis.

Adhesive Association of Like Cells

In the development of a structure such as long bone, the early cells tend to aggregate closely in condensations, a membrane comes to surround them, and only later do they resemble cartilage cells. The association of like cells is dramatically demonstrated by admixing trypsinized liver and kidney cells in vitro and observing them reaggregate with their own kind.

Controlled Cell Death

Controlled cell death plays a role in normal morphogenesis. Examples include death of tissue between the digits resulting in separation of the fingers and recanalization of the duodenum. The dead cellular debris is engulfed by large macrophages, leaving no trace of the tissue.

Hormonal Influence over Morphogenesis

Androgen effect is one example of a hormonal influence over morphogenesis—in this case, that of the external genitalia. Normally, the individual with a Y chromosome has testosterone from the fetal testicle that induces enlargement of the phallus, closure of the labia minora folds to form a penile urethra, and fusion of the labioscrotal folds to form a scrotum. Before 8 weeks' gestation, the genitalia appear female in type and will remain so unless androgenic hormone is present.

Mechanical Forces

Mechanical forces play a major role in morphogenesis. The size, growth, and form of the brain and its early derivatives, for example, have a major function in the formation of the calvarium and upper face. The alignment of collagen fibrils and bone trabeculae relates directly to the direction of forces exerted on these tissues. The role of mechanical factors in development is covered in the text *Smith's Recognizable Patterns of Human Deformation.*

Normal Stages in Morphogenesis

The general steps in normal morphogenesis as set forth here are illustrated in Figures 3-1 to 3-16. The first week is a period of cell division without much enlargement, the conceptus being dependent on the cytoplasm of the ova for most of its metabolic needs. By 7 to 8 days, the zona pellucida is gone, and the outlying trophoblast cells invade the endometrium and form the early placenta that must function both to nourish the parasitic embryo and to maintain the pregnancy via its endocrine function. During this time, a relatively small inner cell mass has become a bilaminar disk of ectoderm and endoderm, each with its own fluid-filled cavity, the amniotic sac and yolk sac, respectively. By the end of the second week, a small mound, a primitive node, has developed in the ectoderm, and behind it a primitive streak forms. The embryo now has an axis to which further morphogenesis will relate. Cells migrate forward from the node between the ectoderm and endoderm to form an elastic cord, the notochord, which temporarily provides axial support for the embryo as well as influencing the adjacent morphogenesis. Ectodermal cells migrate through the node and the primitive streak to specific areas between the ectoderm and endoderm, becoming the mesoderm. One of the early mesodermal derivatives is a circulatory system; during the third week, the heart begins to develop, vascular channels form in situ, and blood cells are produced in the yolk sac. By the end of the third week, the heart is pumping, a neural groove has formed anterior to the node, the para-axial mesoderm has begun to be segmented into somites, the anterior and posterior regions of the embryo have begun to curl under, and the foregut and hindgut pouches become distinct. The stage is now set for the period of major organogenesis, which is best considered in relation to individual structures.

Early morphogenesis is set forth in the accompanying figures. As noted in the illustrations found on the inside front cover and inside back cover of this book, each stage of development represents a synchronous syndrome of characteristics.

Text continued on p. 793

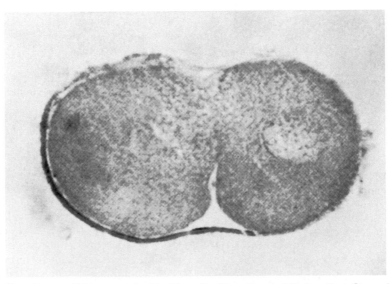

FIGURE 3-1. Two-cell specimen, within zona pellucida. (From the Department of Embryology, Carnegie Institution of Washington, DC, Baltimore.)

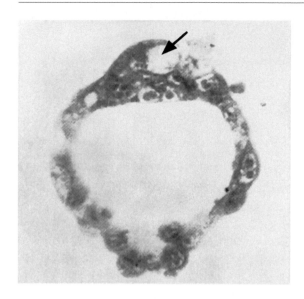

FIGURE 3-2. A 4- to 5-day-old blastocyst. The embryonic cell mass (*arrow*). (From the Department of Embryology, Carnegie Institution of Washington, DC, Baltimore.)

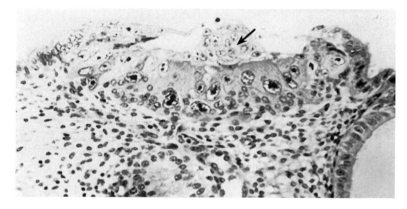

FIGURE 3-3. Seven days. The major part of the conceptus, the cytotrophoblast, has invaded the endometrium, and the embryo (*arrow*) is differentiating into two diverse cell layers, the ectoderm and endoderm. The amniotic cavity is beginning to form. (From the Department of Embryology, Carnegie Institution of Washington, DC, Baltimore.)

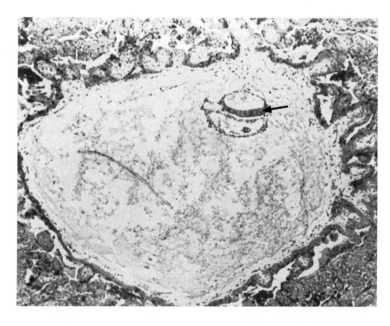

FIGURE 3-4. Fourteen to sixteen days. The thicker ectoderm (*arrow*) has its continuous amniotic sac, whereas the underlying endoderm has its yolk sac. Major changes will now begin to take place.

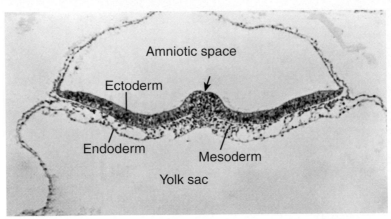

FIGURE 3-5. Seventeen to eighteen days. Mesoblast cells migrate from the ectoderm through the node (the hillock marked by the *arrow*) and the primitive streak to specific locations between the *ectoderm* and *endoderm*, constituting the highly versatile *mesoderm*. Anterior to the node the notochordal process develops, providing axial support and influencing subsequent development such as that of the overlying neural plate.

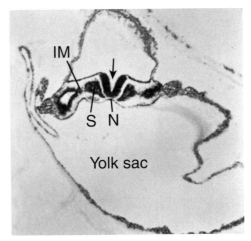

FIGURE 3-6. Twenty-one to twenty-three days. The midaxial ectoderm has thickened and formed the neural groove (*arrow*), partially influenced by the underlying notochordal plate (*N*). Lateral to it, the mesoblast has now segmented into somites (*S*), intermediate mesoderm (*IM*), and somatopleure and splanchnopleure as intervening steps toward further differentiation. Vascular channels are developing in situ from mesoderm, blood cells are being produced in the yolk sac wall, and the early heart is beating. Henceforth, development is extremely rapid, with major changes each day.

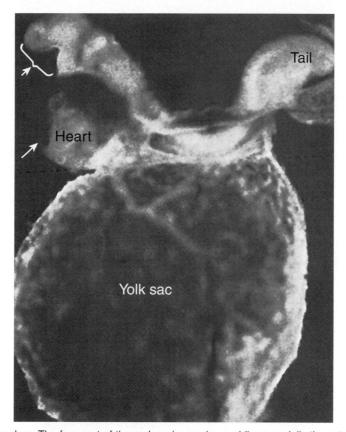

FIGURE 3-7. Twenty-four days. The fore part of the embryo is growing rapidly, especially the anterior neural plate. The cardiac tube (*long arrow*), under the developing face (*short arrow*), is functional. (From the Department of Embryology, Carnegie Institution of Washington, DC, Baltimore.)

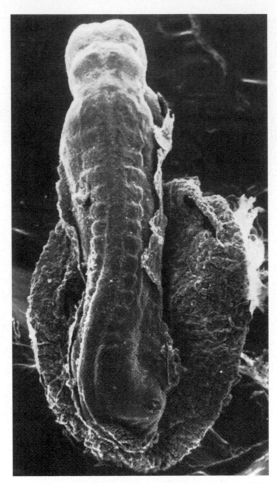

FIGURE 3-8. Scanning electron microscope photograph of human embryo of about 23 to 25 days' gestation, with the amnion largely stripped away. This dorsal view beautifully shows the developing brain (anterior) and spinal cord just after neural tube formation and the orderly bilateral segmentation of the somites. (Courtesy of Dr. Jan E. Jirásek, Prague, Czech Republic.)

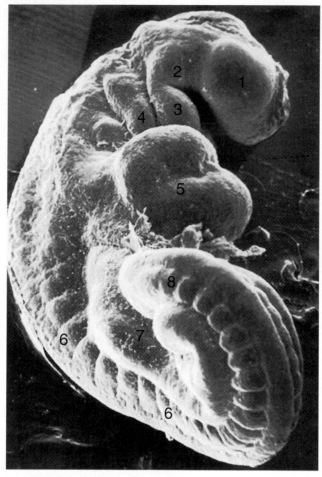

FIGURE 3-9. Scanning electron microscope photograph of a 28- to 30-day-old human embryo with the amnion removed, showing the following features: *1*, early optic vesicle outpouching; *2*, maxillary swelling; *3*, mandibular swelling; *4*, hyoid swelling; *5*, heart; *6*, somites, with adjacent spinal cord; *7*, early rudiments of upper limb bud; and *8*, tail. (Courtesy of Dr. Jan E. Jirásek, Prague, Czech Republic.)

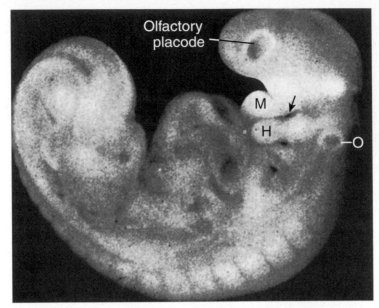

FIGURE 3-10. Twenty-eight to thirty days. The optic cup has begun to invaginate. Between it and the mandibular process is the area of the future mouth, where the buccopharyngeal membrane, with no intervening mesoderm, has broken down. Within the recess of the mandibular (*M*) and hyoid (*H*) processes, the future external auditory meatus will develop (*arrow*), and dorsal to it the otic vesicle (*O*) forms the inner ear. The relatively huge heart must pump blood in the yolk sac and developing placenta as well as to the embryo proper. Foregut outpouchings and evaginations will now begin to form various glands and the lung and liver primordia. Foregut and hindgut are now clearly delineated from the yolk sac. The somites, which will differentiate into myotomes (musculature), dermatomes (subcutaneous tissue), and sclerotomes (vertebrae), are evident on into the tail bud.

FIGURE 3-11. Approximately 30 to 31 days. The brain is rapidly growing, and its early cleavage into bilateral future cerebral hemispheres is evident in the telencephalic outpouching of the forebrain (*FB*). To the right of this is the developing eye with the optic cup (*arrow*) and the early invagination of the future lens from surface ectoderm. The limb swellings (*L*) have developed from the somatopleura. The loose mesenchyme of the limb bud, interacting with the thickened ectodermal cells at its tip, carries all the potential for the full development of the limb. The liver is now functional and will be a source of blood cells. The mesonephric ducts, formed in the mesonephric ridges, communicate to the cloaca, which is beginning to become septated, and the yolk sac is regressing.

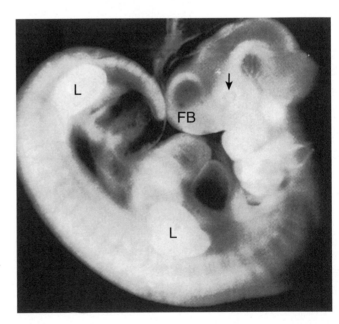

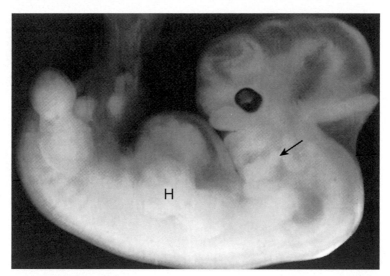

FIGURE 3-12. Thirty-six days. The retina is now pigmented, still incompletely closed at its inferomedial margin. Closure of the retinal fissure is nearly complete. The auricular hillocks are forming the early auricle (*arrow*) from the adjacent borders of the mandibular and hyoid swellings. The hand plate (*H*) has formed with condensation of mesenchyme into the five finger rays. The lower limb lags behind the upper limb in its development. The ventricular septum is partitioning the heart. The ureteral bud from the mesonephric duct has induced a kidney from the mesonephric ridge, which is also forming gonads and adrenal glands. Cloacal septation is nearly complete; the infraumbilical mesenchyme has filled in all the cloacal membrane except the urogenital area; and the genital tubercles are fused, whereas the labioscrotal swellings are unfused. The gut is elongating, and a loop of it may be seen projecting out into the body stalk.

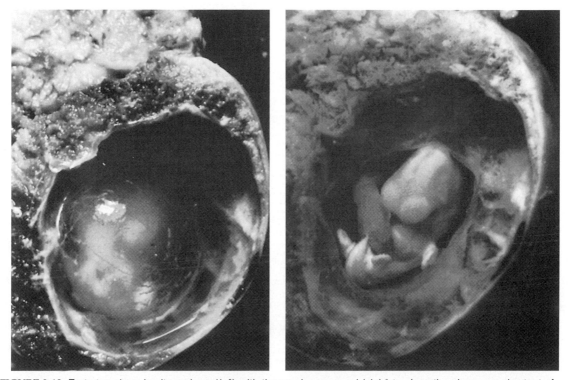

FIGURE 3-13. Forty-two days. In situ embryo (*left*) with the amnion removed (*right*) to show the phenomenal extent of early brain development with formation of the cerebral hemispheres, large heart, still "paddle-like" limbs, and the regressing tail. (Courtesy of Dr. Jan E. Jirásek, Prague, Czech Republic.)

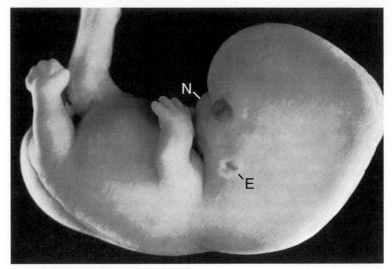

FIGURE 3-14. Forty-five days. The nose (*N*) is relatively flat, and the external ear (*E*) is gradually shifting in relative position as it continues to grow and develop. A neck area is now evident, the anterior body wall has formed, and the thorax and abdomen are separated by the septum transversum (diaphragm). The fingers are now partially separated, and the elbow is evident. The major period of cardiac morphogenesis and septation is complete. The urogenital membrane has now broken down, yielding a urethral opening. The phallus and lateral labioscrotal folds are the same for both sexes at this age.

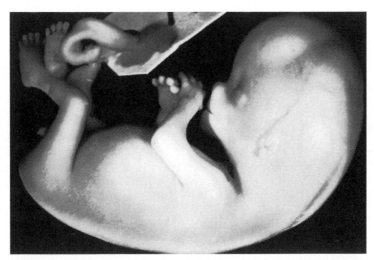

FIGURE 3-15. A 10-week-old boy. The eyelids have developed and fused, not to reopen until 4 to 5 months. Muscles are developed and functional, normal morphogenesis of joints is dependent on movement, and primary ossification is occurring in the centers of developing bones. In the male, the testicle has produced androgen and masculinized the external genitalia, with enlargement of the genital tubercle, fusion of the labioscrotal folds into a scrotum, and closure of the labia minora folds to form a penile urethra, these structures being unchanged in the female. The testicle does not descend into the scrotum until 8 or 9 months.

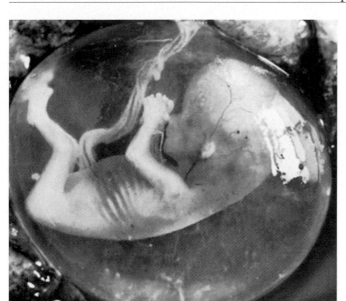

FIGURE 3-16. A 3½-month-old male fetus. The fetus is settling down for the last two thirds of prenatal life. The morphogenesis of the lung, largely solid at this point in development, will not have progressed to the capacity for aerobic exchange for another 3 to 4 months. The skin is increasing in thickness, and its accessory structures are differentiating. The form of the palmar surface of the hand and foot, especially the character of the prominent apical and other pads, will influence the patterning of parallel dermal ridges that form transversely to the relative lines of growth stress on the palms and soles between 16 and 19 weeks. Subcutaneous tissue is thin, and adipose tissue does not develop until 7 to 8 months.

ABNORMAL MORPHOGENESIS

As mentioned in the introduction, there are four general types of developmental pathology leading to structural defects. The first type is malformation, which is poor formation of the tissue. The second is deformation caused by altered mechanical forces on a normal tissue. Deformation may be secondary to extrinsic forces, such as uterine constraint on a normal fetus, or to intrinsic forces related to a more primary malformation. The third type of pathology is disruption, which is a result of the breakdown of a previously normal tissue. An example of this is porencephalic cyst of vascular causation. The fourth mechanism of abnormal morphogenesis is dysplasia, in which there is a lack of normal organization of cells into tissue. Hamartomas are examples of this mechanism. These anomalies represent an organizational defect leading to an abnormal admixture of tissues, often with a tumor-like excess of one or more tissues. Some have malignant potential. Examples of hamartomas are hemangiomas, melanomas, fibromas, lipomas, adenomas, and some strange admixtures that defy traditional classification.

Extrinsic deformation is set forth in a separate text, *Smith's Recognizable Patterns of Human Deformation*. A few disruption patterns of anomaly are considered in this book, as well as some dysplasias, with the major emphasis being on patterns of malformation, including malformation sequences. However, it is very important for the reader to appreciate that many of the anomalies in a given malformation sequence or syndrome are actually deformations that are engendered by the altered mechanical forces resulting from the more primary malformation. For example, most minor anomalies represent deformations, often secondary to a malformation.

Malformations may be broken down into a number of subcategories in terms of the nature of the poor formation.

Types of Malformation

Incomplete Morphogenesis

These are anomalies that represent incomplete stages in the development of a structure; they include the following subcategories, with one example listed for each:

Lack of development: renal agenesis secondary to failure of ureter formation.
Hypoplasia: micrognathia.
Incomplete separation: syndactyly (cutaneous).
Incomplete closure: cleft palate.
Incomplete septation: ventricular septal defect.
Incomplete migration of mesoderm: exstrophy of bladder.
Incomplete rotation: malrotation of the gut.
Incomplete resolution of early form: Meckel diverticulum.
Persistence of earlier location: cryptorchidism.

TABLE 3-1 RELATIVE TIMING AND DEVELOPMENTAL PATHOLOGY OF CERTAIN MALFORMATIONS

TISSUES	MALFORMATION	DEFECT IN	CAUSES PRIOR TO	COMMENT
Central nervous system	Anencephaly	Closure of anterior neural tube	26 days	Subsequent degeneration of forebrain
	Meningomyelocele	Closure in a portion of the posterior neural tube	28 days	80% lumbosacral
Face	Cleft lip	Closure of lip	36 days	42% associated with cleft palate
	Cleft maxillary palate	Fusion of maxillary palatal shelves	10 weeks	
	Branchial sinus or cyst	Resolution of branchial cleft	8 weeks	Preauricular and along the line anterior to sternocleidomastoid
Gut	Esophageal atresia plus tracheoesophageal fistula	Lateral septation of foregut into trachea and foregut	30 days	
	Rectal atresia with fistula	Lateral septation of cloaca into rectum and urogenital sinus	6 weeks	
	Duodenal atresia	Recanalization of duodenum	7–8 weeks	Associated incomplete or aberrant mesenteric attachments
	Malrotation of gut	Rotation of intestinal loop so that cecum lies to the right	10 weeks	
	Omphalocele	Return of midgut from yolk sac to abdomen	10 weeks	
	Meckel diverticulum	Obliteration of vitelline duct	10 weeks	May contain gastric or pancreatic tissue
	Diaphragmatic hernia	Closure of pleuroperitoneal canal	6 weeks	
Genitourinary system	Exstrophy of bladder	Migration of infraumbilical mesenchyme	30 days	Associated müllerian and wolffian duct defects
	Bicornuate uterus	Fusion of lower portion of müllerian ducts	10 weeks	
	Hypospadias	Fusion of urethral folds (labia minora)	12 weeks	
	Cryptorchidism	Descent of testicle into scrotum	7–9 months	
Heart	Transposition of great vessels	Directional development of bulbus cordis septum	34 days	
	Ventricular septal defect	Closure of ventricular septum	6 weeks	
	Patent ductus arteriosus	Closure of ductus arteriosus	9–10 months	
Limb	Aplasia of radius	Genesis of radial bone	38 days	Often accompanied by other defects of radial side of distal limb
	Syndactyly, severe	Separation of digital rays	6 weeks	
Complex	Cyclopia, holoprosencephaly	Prechordal mesoderm development	23 days	Secondary defects of midface and forebrain

Aberrant Form

An occasional anomaly may be interpreted as an aberrant form that never exists in any stage of normal morphogenesis. An example is the pelvic spur in the nail-patella syndrome. Such an anomaly may be more specific for a particular clinical syndrome entity than anomalies of incomplete morphogenesis.

Accessory Tissue

Accessory tissue such as polydactyly, preauricular skin tags, and accessory spleens may be presumed to have been initiated at approximately the same time as the normal tissue, developing into finger rays, auricular hillocks of His, and spleen, respectively.

Functional Defects

Function is a necessary feature in joint development; hence joint contractures, such as clubfoot, may be caused by a functional deficit in the use of the lower limb resulting from a more primary malformation.

RELATIVE TIMING OF MALFORMATIONS

Malformations resulting from incomplete morphogenesis usually have their origin *before* the time when normal development would have proceeded beyond the form represented by the malformation. This type of developmental timing should not be construed as indicating that something happened *at* a particular time; all one can say is that a problem existed *before* a particular time. Serious errors in early morphogenesis seldom allow for survival; hence, only a few malformation problems are seen that can be said to have occurred before 23 days. The cyclopia-cebocephaly type of defect appears to be the consequence of a defect in the prechordal mesoderm, and presumably developed before 23 days. Aside from this example, the vast majority of serious malformations represent errors that occur after 3 weeks of development.

Table 3-1 sets forth the relative timing as well as the presumed developmental error for some of the malformations that appear to represent incomplete stages in morphogenesis.

References

Ebert JD, Sussex I: Interacting Systems in Development. New York: Holt, Rinehart & Winston, 1970.

Gilbert SF: Developmental Biology, 7th ed. Sunderland, Mass: Sinauer Associates, 2003.

Graham JM: Smith's Recognizable Patterns of Human Deformation, 2nd ed. Philadelphia: WB Saunders, 1988.

Hamilton WJ, Boyd JD, Mossman HW: Human Embryology. Baltimore: Williams & Wilkins, 1962.

Millen JW: Timing of human congenital malformations. Dev Med Child Neurol 5:343, 1963.

Moore KL, Persaud TVN: The Developing Human: Clinically Oriented Embryology, 7th ed. Philadelphia: WB Saunders, 2004.

Moore KL, Persaud TVN, Shiota K: Color Atlas of Human Embryology. Philadelphia: WB Saunders, 1994.

Nilsson L, Ingelman-Sundberg A, Wirsen C: A Child Is Born. New York: Dell Books, 1986.

O'Rahilly R, Muller F: Human Embryology and Teratology. New York: Wiley-Liss, 1992.

Sadler TW: Langman's Medical Embryology, 9th ed. Baltimore: Williams & Wilkins, 2004.

Streeter GL: Developmental Horizons in Human Embryo: Age Groups XI to XXIII. Washington, DC: Carnegie Institute of Washington, 1951.

Willis RA: The Borderland of Embryology and Pathology. Washington, DC: Butterworth, 1962.

4 Genetics, Genetic Counseling, and Prevention

The basic process of morphogenesis is genetically controlled. However, the ability of an individual to reach his or her genetic potential with respect to structure, growth, or cognitive development is impacted by environmental factors in both prenatal and postnatal life. Review of the etiologies of those structural abnormalities and syndromes for which an etiology is known indicates that the majority of malformations and syndromes appear to be genetically determined. The purpose of this chapter is to outline the most prevalent mechanisms through which genetic abnormalities impact morphogenesis, to suggest genetic counseling strategies for each, and to discuss approaches to prevention.

The structure and function of a human being is determined by roughly 30,000 genes, which come in pairs. The great majority of these genes are distributed in the 46 chromosomes that are found in the nucleus of the cell. A few genes reside in the cytoplasm inside the mitochondria, the energy-producing apparatus of the cell. Genetic abnormalities may be grossly divided into those that affect gene dosage (chromosomal abnormalities), those that involve changes in the actual genes themselves (single-gene disorders), and those that create a susceptibility to developmental errors that is then modified by factors in the environment (multifactorial inheritance). The frequency with which each of these genetic mechanisms contributes to malformation and disease depends on the time in development at which inquiry is made. For example, roughly half of all first-trimester miscarriages are a consequence of chromosomal abnormalities, whereas only 6 of 1000 live-born infants are similarly affected. Figure 4-1 provides a perspective as to the frequency with which each mechanism contributes to birth defects or human disease over the lifetime of a population. Each of these problems is considered separately as it relates to malformation, especially multiple defect syndromes. Recommended genetic counseling is presented at the end of each section.

GENETIC IMBALANCE CAUSED BY GROSS CHROMOSOMAL ABNORMALITIES

The 46 normal chromosomes consist of 22 homologous pairs of autosomes plus an XX pair of sex chromosomes in the female or an XY pair in the male. Normal development is not only dependent on the gene content of these chromosomes but on the gene balance as well. An altered number of chromosomes most commonly arises because of fault in chromosome distribution at cell division. During the gametic meiotic reduction division (Fig. 4-2), one of each pair of autosomes and one of the sex chromosomes are distributed randomly to each daughter cell, whereas during mitosis (Fig. 4-3), each replicated chromosome is separated longitudinally at the centromere so that each daughter cell receives an identical complement of genetic material.

Figure 4-4 shows the natural appearance of the stained chromosomes at early, middle, and later stages of mitosis. It would obviously be difficult to count these chromosomes or to distinguish their individual structure from such preparations. To obtain adequate preparations for the study of chromosome number and morphology, the cultured cells are treated with an agent that blocks the spindle formation and thus leads to the accumulation of cells at the metaphase of mitosis. These cells are then exposed to a hypotonic solution that spreads the unattached chromosomes, allowing for preparations such as those shown in Figure 4-5. Various techniques, such as trypsin treatment and Giemsa staining, can be used to allow for the identification of individual chromosomes. The development of synchronized culture techniques that allow evaluation of chromosomes in prophase and prometaphase have greatly enhanced the ability to detect subtle abnormalities and have expanded our understanding of the impact of chromosomal rearrangement on morphogenesis. A chromosome

Gene dosage effects	Chromosomal maldistribution	Aneuploidy, Trisomies 21, 18, 13, 45, X XXX, XXY, XYY	
	Chromosomal rearrangments	Translocations, fragility, duplications, deletions, submicroscopic deletions	
Major mutant genes	Autosomal dominant	Over 6000 individually rare disorders	
	Autosomal recessive		
	X-linked		
	Mitochondrial		
Multifactoral inheritance	Major and minor genes determining susceptibility interacting with the environment	Common isolated malformations, schizophrenia, coronary artery disease, hypertension, diabetes mellitus, other common disorders	

0   1%   10%

FIGURE 4-1. The scale at the base represents the percentage of individuals born who have, or will have, a problem in life secondary to a genetic difference. The three categories of genetic aberration are depicted to the left. The *dots* within the chromosomes represent "normal" genes, the *bar* represents a dominant mutant gene, the *hash-bar* represents a recessive mutant gene, and the *triangles* denote major and minor genes that confer susceptibility to a given process.

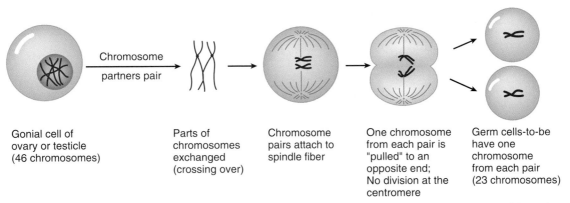

Gonial cell of ovary or testicle (46 chromosomes) → Chromosome partners pair → Parts of chromosomes exchanged (crossing over) → Chromosome pairs attach to spindle fiber → One chromosome from each pair is "pulled" to an opposite end; No division at the centromere → Germ cells-to-be have one chromosome from each pair (23 chromosomes)

FIGURE 4-2. Meiotic reduction division in development of gametes (sex cells). One pair of chromosomes is followed through the cycle.

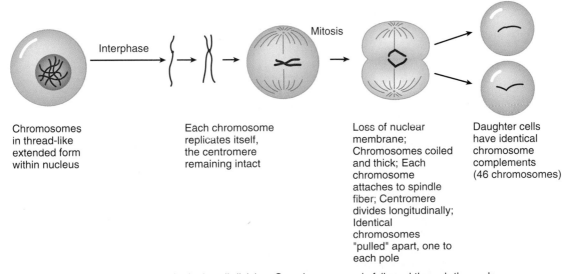

Chromosomes in thread-like extended form within nucleus → Interphase → Each chromosome replicates itself, the centromere remaining intact → Mitosis → Loss of nuclear membrane; Chromosomes coiled and thick; Each chromosome attaches to spindle fiber; Centromere divides longitudinally; Identical chromosomes "pulled" apart, one to each pole → Daughter cells have identical chromosome complements (46 chromosomes)

FIGURE 4-3. Normal mitotic cell division. One chromosome is followed through the cycle.

797

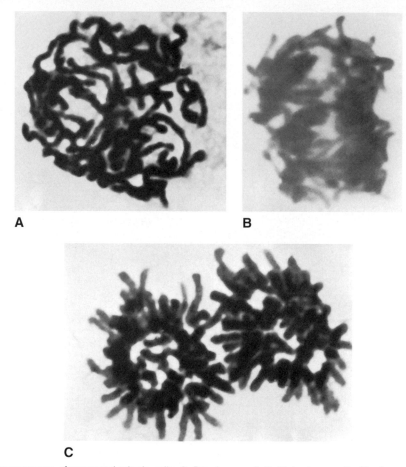

FIGURE 4-4. Chromosomes of untreated mitotic cells. **A,** Prophase cell. **B,** Metaphase cell with chromosomes attached to the spindle fibers and beginning to separate. **C,** Anaphase cell with identical chromosomal complements having been "pulled apart" toward the development of two daughter cells.

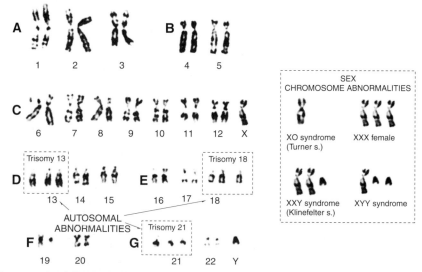

FIGURE 4-5. Giemsa-stained chromosomes arranged into a karyotype by letter grouping and number designation on the basis of length of the chromosome, position of the centromere, and banding patterns. The most common types of aneuploidy are shown within the boxes.

analysis using this technique is a high-resolution analysis (Fig. 4-6).

Two newer technologies that allow detection of more subtle changes in copy number in the genome are fluorescence in situ hybridization (FISH) and comparative genomic hybridization (CGH). In FISH, fluorescent-labeled probes of known DNA sequence are hybridized to chromosomes that are fixed on a slide and denatured in place (in situ), allowing the probe to attach to its complementary sequence. When viewed with a wavelength of light that excites the fluorescent dye, a colored signal is generated, allowing localization of the probe. FISH probes may consist of contiguous genomic sequences, parts of chromosomes, or whole chromosomes. Whole chromosome probes are known as "painting" probes. Depending on the probe and the clinical question, FISH may be performed on interphase instead of metaphase cells offering advantages in some clinical situations such as pre-natal diagnosis. Comparative genomic hybridization is based on FISH technology. DNA from one sample is labeled with a red fluorescent dye while DNA from a another is labeled in green. The two are mixed in equal amounts and used as a chromosome painting probe on normal human chromosomes. The ratio of red-to-green fluorescence along each chromosome is measured. Deviations from the expected 1:1 ratio of red to green will be detected as a change in the color signal in that region documenting gain or loss of copy number. CGH is often

done on whole human chromosomes; however, the technique can be modified (using known DNA sequences rather than whole chromosomes) to accommodate chip technology. This modification is called array CGH. Although CGH is currently primarily applied in cancer diagnosis, chips for constitutional abnormalities have recently become available.[45,56]

Figure 4-7 illustrates some of the mechanisms that can lead to genetic imbalance (too many or too few copies of normal genes) as a consequence of chromosomal rearrangement and maldistribution. Such abnormalities occur in at least 4% of recognized pregnancies. Most of these imbalances have such an adverse effect on morphogenesis that the conceptus does not survive. Figure 4-8 summarizes the frequency and types of chromosomal abnormalities found in newborns and spontaneous abortuses. Approximately 50% of these have a chromosome abnormality compared to 0.5% of liveborn babies. The nature of the abnormalities detected in live-born infants differs from those seen in abortuses, with sex chromosomal aneuploidy and trisomy 21 (Down syndrome) accounting for most of the anomalies observed in live-born infants because these are least likely to have an early lethal effect. It has been estimated that only approximately 1 in 500 45,X conceptuses survives to term compared to 4% of trisomies 18 and 13, and 20% of trisomy 21 conceptuses. There are some data to suggest that survival is impacted by the presence of a normal as well as an aneuploid cell line (mosaicism). The Human Genome Project has identified that the genome is in clumps with some chromosomes (such as 19 with 1621 known genes) being gene-rich and others (such as the Y with 251 genes) gene-poor. Interestingly, autosomes 21, 18, and 13 are relatively gene-poor, perhaps contributing to their in-utero survival.[22]

Although much is being learned about the etiology of faulty chromosomal distribution, one clear recognized factor is older maternal age.[25] This applies especially to the autosomal trisomy syndromes and to the sex chromosome aneuploidy, XXX and XXY. Figure 4-9 shows the progressive increase in the frequency of live-born infants with the Down syndrome during the later period of a woman's reproductive life. The frequency of aneuploidy detected by amniocentesis at 14 to 16 weeks' gestation is appreciably higher because some of the aneuploid conceptuses detected at this early stage in gestation would normally abort spontaneously or die in utero later in pregnancy.

The timing of the error in chromosome distribution can seldom be stated with assurance from a routine karyotype, although molecular techniques,

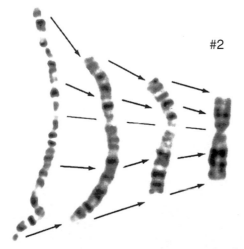

#2

FIGURE 4-6. Giemsa-stained chromosome number 2 harvested at different points in the cell cycle. The prometaphase appearance is on the left, while the metaphase is on the right. Note the dramatic increase in detail visible in the prometaphase chromosome. (Courtesy of Dr. James T. Mascarello, Children's Hospital, San Diego.)

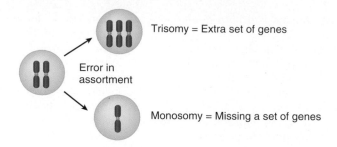

Chromosomal Maldistribution

Trisomy = Extra set of genes

Error in assortment

Monosomy = Missing a set of genes

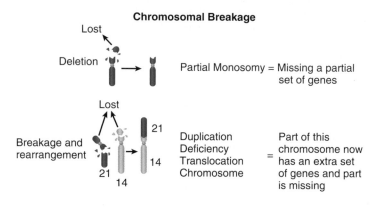

Chromosomal Breakage

Lost

Deletion → Partial Monosomy = Missing a partial set of genes

Lost

Breakage and rearrangement

21

14

21

14

Duplication
Deficiency
Translocation
Chromosome

= Part of this chromosome now has an extra set of genes and part is missing

Maldivision at Centromere

Lost

Abnormal plane of centromere division

Duplication
Deficiency
Isochromosome

= Extra long arm, missing short arm

Usual plane of centromere division at mitosis

FIGURE 4-7. Types of chromosomal abnormalities leading to genetic imbalance.

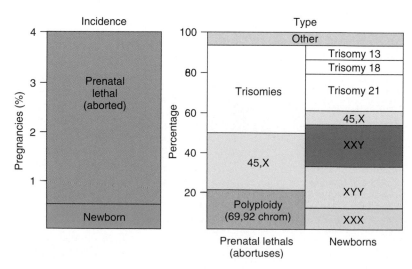

FIGURE 4-8. Incidence and types of chromosomal abnormalities.

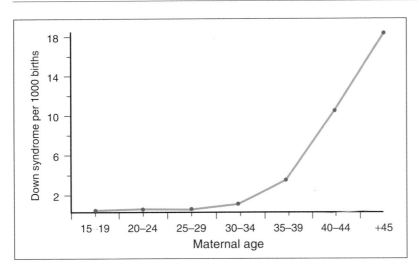

FIGURE 4-9. Increasing incidence of the Down syndrome during the later portion of a woman's reproductive period. (From Smith DW: Am J Obstet Gynecol 90:1055, 1964, with permission.)

as is discussed subsequently, have permitted detailed investigation of this issue in certain aneuploidy states. Numerical errors may result from altered chromosomal segregation in the cells that will give rise to the germ cells (gonadal mosaicism), or in either the first or second division of meiosis leading to an abnormal chromosome number in the egg or sperm (nondisjunction), or during the first divisions of the newly formed zygote. Errors in the assortment of chromosomes may also occur later in embryogenesis, giving rise to somatic mosaic individuals who have two populations of cells from the standpoint of chromosome number. Mosaicism also develops when a trisomic conceptus "self-corrects" and loses one copy of the trisomic chromosome in early cell division, thus establishing a normal along with the aneuploid cell line. This process has been termed trisomic rescue. Individuals who are mosaic for a condition show every gradation of the phenotype associated with that chromosomal abnormality, from a pattern indistinguishable from complete aneuploidy to near normal appearance and function. In general, the degree of mosaicism present in the peripheral blood is not, in and of itself, that helpful in predicting prognosis. Detection of mosaicism may require the sampling of more than one tissue such as assessment of cultured fibroblasts from a skin biopsy.

New molecular techniques that allow identification of the parent of origin of individual chromosomes have shed some light on the source of the extra or deleted chromosome and the stage of cell division during which accidents leading to aneuploidy occur. In conceptuses and live-born individuals with 45,X, the chromosome that is deleted is usually paternal in origin.[26] This is consistent with the observation that maternal age is not related to a 45,X karyotype in the fetus. By contrast, the extra chromosome in trisomy 21 is of maternal origin in 95% of cases.[1] Most of the maternal errors involve nondisjunction in meiosis I. Of the paternally derived chromosomes, most represent errors in meiosis II. Similarly, the extra X chromosome in 47,XXX females is usually maternally derived. In 47,XXY the source of the extra chromosome appears to be equally divided.[36] In those cases of 47,XXY and XXX with a maternally derived extra chromosome, increasing maternal age correlated with errors in the first meiotic cell division but not with errors in meiosis II or in postzygotic events. The precise etiology of nondisjunction is unknown; however, evidence is accumulating that mammalian trisomies may be a consequence of abnormal levels or positioning of meiotic cross-overs (recombination events).[28] Between 1% and 5% of sperm from chromosomally normal men are aneuploid. Indirect estimates from spontaneous abortions and studies of embryos from in-vitro fertilization clinics have suggested an aneuploidy rate of nearly 25% in oocytes.[25]

In addition to errors in chromosome number, genetic imbalance can result from chromosomal rearrangement (see Fig. 4-7). A break in one chromosome may result in loss or gain of information (deletion or duplication). If more than one chromosome breaks, rearrangement of the resulting pieces may take place, creating a translocation. An individual can have a translocation between chromosomes with no evident problem as long as he or she has a balanced set of genes. However, as illustrated in Figure 4-10, a balanced carrier of a translocation has a significant risk of producing unbalanced germ cells during the meiotic reduction division, meiosis I. Should a germ cell receive the translocation chromosome as well as the normal 21 chromosome from the same parent, the resulting zygote would be trisomic for most of chromosome 21. Such individuals generally have Down syndrome. About 4% of patients with Down syndrome have 46 chromosomes, with the extra set being attached to another chromosome. Similarly, a small proportion of patients with the trisomy 18 or trisomy 13 syndromes have the extra set of genes attached as part of a translocation chromosome.

Less commonly, a pattern of malformation will result from a deletion (or duplication) of chromosomal material in which the missing (or extra) piece is so small that routine chromosome analysis cannot detect the abnormality. Such conditions are referred to as microdeletion (microduplication) syndromes to denote the fact that the phenotype is a consequence of imbalance in dosage of several

genes that lie next to each other along a chromosome. FISH and array-CGH are techniques used to identify these rearrangements.

The major reason for doing chromosome studies on individuals with autosomal trisomy syndromes, beyond confirmation of the clinical diagnosis, is to determine whether the patient has an unbalanced translocation chromosome rather than the more usual complete trisomy. If a translocation is identified, then both parents should be studied to determine whether either of them is a balanced translocation carrier with a consequent increased risk of having affected offspring. Fortunately, many unbalanced translocations represent de novo events with a low risk for recurrence.

Surveys of the incidence of chromosomal abnormalities in newborns have documented that roughly 1 in 520 normal individuals has a balanced structural chromosomal rearrangement, whereas 1 in 1700 newborns has an unbalanced rearrangement. Systematic surveys of undiagnosed children with mental retardation and multiple structural defects

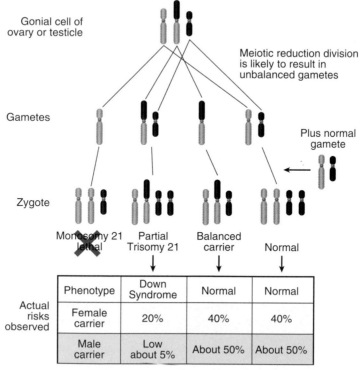

	Phenotype	Down Syndrome	Normal	Normal
Actual risks observed	Female carrier	20%	40%	40%
	Male carrier	Low about 5%	About 50%	About 50%

FIGURE 4-10. Potential inheritance from balanced translocation carrier using a 21/14 translocation as an example. Only chromosomes 21 and 14 are depicted. The translocation could be constitutional (in all the cells in the body) or a fresh occurrence in the gonial cell (gonadal mosaicism). The illustration shows the theoretical risk for balanced and unbalanced offspring. The table beneath lists the actual observed risks by sex of the carrier parent. For many rare translocations, this type of empiric information is not available. The example documents how difficult it is to predict the actual outcome in the offspring of translocation carriers.

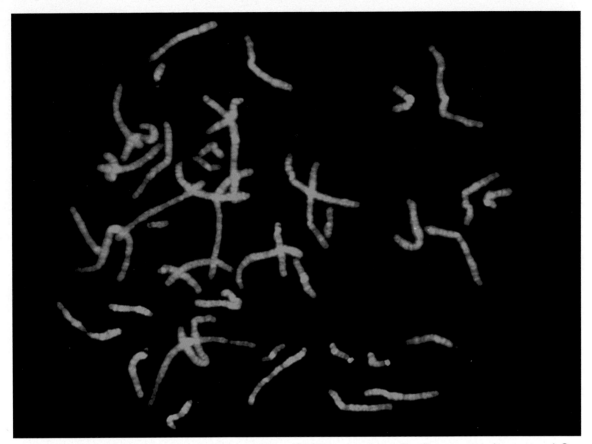

FIGURE 4-11. FISH analysis for elastin locus in a patient with Williams syndrome. Two fluorescent probes are used. One hybridizes with the telomere of chromosome 7, allowing ready identification of both chromosomes. The second probe identifies the elastin locus. In this patient only one signal is visible, consistent with a submicroscopic deletion in the other chromosome. (Courtesy of Dr. James T. Mascarello, Children's Hospital, San Diego.)

have documented an 8% incidence of chromosome abnormalities.[50] In a survey of mentally retarded individuals in South Carolina, chromosome abnormalities including Down syndrome occurred in 12% of the population.[44] With the use of high-resolution chromosome analysis, subtle abnormalities, which would have escaped detection on a routine study, will be identified in an additional 1.1% of patients evaluated for similar indications.[38] Several studies demonstrate an increased detection rate for submicroscopic chromosome rearrangements among individuals with mental retardation of unknown etiology using FISH probes that recognize the unique subtelomeric sequences of each chromosome (telomere FISH) and more recently array-CGH; however, most of the populations studied have been enriched by virtue of a suggestive family history or a complex pattern of malformation.[18,34] The utility of this technology as a "first round" test has yet to be established; however, with appropriate screening, detection rates of up to 20% have been suggested.[11,55]

In clinical situations in which a specific disorder is known to be associated with a characteristic but subtle cytogenetic abnormality (microdeletion syndrome), a focused chromosome analysis may be recommended to address the question. High-resolution methods are imperative for this type of evaluation. Increasingly high-resolution analysis is being replaced by FISH-based testing, which is clinically available for all of the microdeletion disorders discussed in Chapter 1 including deletion 22q11.2 syndrome, Prader-Willi syndrome, and Williams syndrome among others (Fig. 4-11). FISH is most useful when there is a high index of clinical suspicion. Chip-based array-CGH may soon offer a panel of microdeletion probes as well as subtelomeres on the same analysis.

Another type of chromosomal abnormality that can lead to genetic imbalance is maldivision or breakage at the centromere during mitosis, leading to the formation of an isochromosome (see Fig. 4-7). The cell receiving the isochromosome has an extra dose of the long arm of the parent chromosome and is missing the set of genes on the short arm. Occasionally, autosomal trisomy syndromes may be found to have an isochromosome of the long arm (21, 13, or 18) accounting for the imbalance. Also, isochromosome X accounts for roughly 10% of the cases of Turner syndrome in live-born female infants.

GENETIC COUNSELING FOR CHROMOSOMAL ABNORMALITIES

Autosomal Trisomy Syndromes

Chromosomal studies are warranted on all individuals suspected of having an autosomal trisomy syndrome to determine whether full trisomy (47 chromosomes) or an unbalanced translocation is involved. If a full trisomy is identified, the risk for recurrence is roughly 1%. For women 35 years of age and older, the risk is based upon the maternal age at delivery in the subsequent pregnancy. For trisomy 21, parental karyotypes are suggested *only* if a second child in the same sibship has an identical trisomy. In this rare circumstance, mosaicism in one of the parents may be detected in as many as 38% of families if a diligent search is made. The presence of a second- or third-degree relative with a similar trisomy can be accounted for by chance alone and does not appear to increase the risk for recurrence.[43]

Should an unbalanced translocation be identified, both parents must be evaluated to determine if either one is a balanced translocation carrier, a finding in approximately one third of cases. The recurrence risk for parents with normal chromosomes is very small (probably less than 1%) and reflects the unlikely possibility of gonadal mosaicism that cannot be identified by peripheral blood karyotype. The recurrence risk for a carrier parent is obviously greater, but is often less than the theoretical possibilities might indicate (see Fig. 4-10).

Informing parents that their child has an autosomal trisomy is best accomplished in as straightforward yet compassionate a manner as possible. Knowledge of the natural history of the specific trisomy should serve as a guideline for anticipatory guidance; however, it is best to approach the child as an individual with respect to such issues as survival (in trisomy 18 and 13) and intellectual

potential (in trisomy 21). The karyotype does not predict either of these issues with complete accuracy. There is no substitute for clinical correlation and longitudinal follow-up.

Other Chromosomal Disorders

45X Syndrome

Suspicion of Turner syndrome should lead to a chromosome study. Although a wide variety of chromosomal rearrangements are known to produce the phenotype (including X/XX and X/XY mosaicism, X, iso X, or X, deleted X), the recurrence risk for these arrangements is low to negligible.

Any Case with a Deletion, Duplication, or Unbalanced Translocation

In this situation, chromosome studies should be done on both parents to rule out a rearrangement such as a pericentric inversion or balanced translocation that could predispose to recurrence of the abnormality. If parental karyotypes are normal, as is the case in the majority of families, the recurrence risk is low. If a parental rearrangement is identified, the theoretical risk for recurrence is increased. For some of the more common rearrangements, empiric risk figures are available in the literature. The actual risks often do not coincide with the theoretical risk as has been previously reviewed (see Fig. 4-10).

Microdeletion Syndromes

Although microdeletion syndromes are chromosomal abnormalities because the problem that produces the phenotype is genetic imbalance rather than genetic mutation and because the abnormality is identified using cytogenetic methodology, from a counseling standpoint the conditions behave like dominantly inherited Mendelian disorders. The majority of cases represent de novo events that carry a negligible risk for recurrence for unaffected parents and a 50% risk for the affected individual's offspring. Evaluation of parents using FISH analysis or focused high-resolution cytogenetics is recommended, since vertical transmission of microdeletion syndromes is reported. However, the overwhelming majority of parents who are identified to have deletions also express the phenotype to some degree. Recurrence risk for these individuals is 50% for each subsequent pregnancy.

GENETIC IMBALANCE CAUSED BY SINGLE-GENE DISORDERS

Genes located on the X chromosome are referred to as X-linked genes and those on the autosomes as autosomal genes. Man is a diploid organism with two sets of chromosomes, one set being derived from each parent. Each pair of chromosomes will have comparable gene determinants located at the same position on each chromosome pair. The pair of genes may be referred to as *alleles*, or partners, which normally work together. Thus with the exception of the genes of the X and Y chromosomes in the male, each genetic determinant is present in two doses, one from each parent. A mutant gene indicates a changed gene. A major mutant gene is herein defined as a genetic determinant that has changed in such a way that it can give rise to an abnormal characteristic. If a mutant gene in single dose produces an abnormal characteristic despite the presence of a normal allele (partner), it is referred to as dominant because it causes abnormality even when counterbalanced by a normal gene partner. A mutant gene that causes an abnormal characteristic when present in double dosage (or single dosage without a normal partner, as for an X-linked mutant gene in the male) is referred to as recessive. These principles, set forth diagrammatically in Figure 4-12, reflect Mendelian laws of inheritance, which equate the presence of an altered gene or pair of genes with a phenotype or trait. As more is learned about the molecular biology of mutant genes, the distinction between dominant and recessive genes becomes blurred. In general, however, mutations in genes that code for structural proteins, in which an abnormal product is made, tend to function in a dominant fashion, since the abnormal product often has the capacity to

Normal
Except for the XY, there is a pair of genes for each function, located at the same loci on sister chromosomes. One pair of normal genes is represented as dots on a homologous pair of chromosomes.

Dominant
A single mutant (changed) gene is dominant if it causes an evident abnormality. The chance of inheritance of the mutant gene (▬▬) is the same as the chance of inheriting a particular chromosome of the pair: 50 per cent.

Heterozygous Recessive
A single mutant gene is recessive (◤) if it causes no evident abnormality, the function being well covered by the normal partner gene (allele). Such an individual may be referred to as a *heterozygous* carrier.

Homozygous Recessive
When both genes are recessive mutant (◤), the abnormal effect is expressed. The parents are generally carriers, and their risk of having another affected offspring is the chance of receiving the mutant from one parent (50 per cent) times the chance from the other parent (50 per cent), or 25 per cent for each offspring.

An X-linked recessive will be expressed in the male because he has no normal partner gene. His daughters, receiving the X, will all be carriers, and his sons, receiving the Y, will all be normal.

X-linked Recessive   X   Y

An X-linked recessive will not show overt expression in the female because at least part of her "active" X's will contain the normal gene. The risk for affected sons and carrier daughters will each be 50 per cent.

X   X

FIGURE 4-12. Normal and major mutant gene inheritance (Mendelian inheritance).

interfere with the function of the product of the normal partner. The various forms of osteogenesis imperfecta are good examples of dominant mutations. Because collagen is a triple helical molecule, mutations that give rise to one abnormal procollagen molecule will impact the final assembly process. Recessive mutations often serve to reduce the quantity of product made by half; however, many biologic systems are forgiving of quantitative decrease in enzyme function, hence the silence of recessive mutations when present in single copy. Hurler syndrome is an example. Half of the normal amount of activity of alpha-iduronidase has no effect on the individual with the altered gene; however, the enzyme deficiency resulting from a double dose of the altered gene produces a severe phenotype.

Expression is a term used to indicate the extent of abnormality that is due to a genetic aberration. The expression may be stated as severe, usual, mild, or no expression, the last being synonymous with lack of penetrance in an individual who has the genetic aberration. Individuals with the same genetic aberration frequently show variance in expression, especially with respect to structural defects.

Traditionally, the mutant gene disorders have been categorized into those caused by genes located on the autosomes (autosomal dominant and autosomal recessive) and those caused by genes on the X chromosome (X-linked dominant and X-linked recessive).

Autosomal Dominant Disorders

Autosomal dominant disorders show a wide variation in expression among affected individuals both between families and among affected family members, presumably because of differences in the normal allele (partner) of the mutant gene as well as other differences in the genetic and environmental background of the affected individual. Figure 4-13 demonstrates the variation in expression for an autosomal dominant disorder, ectrodactyly. The risk of the single mutant gene being passed to a given offspring is 50%, yet the risk of a severe defect of hand development is less than 50% because of variation in expression. To use the example of Waardenburg syndrome, the risk of inheritance of the mutant gene from an affected individual is 50%, yet only about 20% of affected individuals have deafness, the most disturbing expression of the mutant gene. Hence, the risk of deafness in offspring of a parent with the Waardenburg syndrome is the risk of receiving the mutant gene (50%) times the likelihood of expression for deafness in the disorder (20%), or 10%.

This dichotomy between the risk of receiving the gene and the risk of a particular expression of the disorder must be utilized in counseling, especially for autosomal dominant conditions. A significant proportion of autosomal dominant patterns of malformation appear to represent fresh gene mutations in the individuals who express the condition. In reproductive counseling for the family, it is impor-

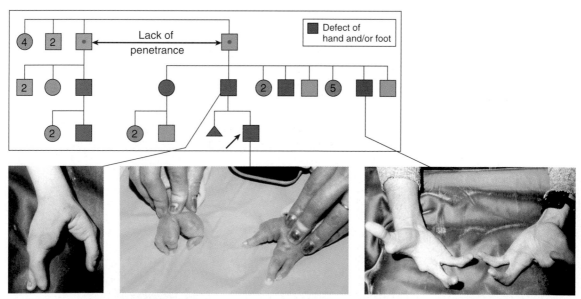

FIGURE 4-13. Variation in expression for autosomal dominant ectrodactyly among various related individuals. Note also the *intraindividual* asymmetry of expression in the propositus (*arrow*).

tant to try to distinguish between lack of expression in the parent caused by variability and fresh gene mutation in the child. Knowledge of both the natural history and the clinical variability of the disorder is extremely helpful in these determinations. Fresh gene mutation is more likely at older paternal age, as has been shown for at least 12 autosomal dominant multiple malformation syndromes.[30] Hence, paternal age should always be noted in the evaluation of disorders that may be the consequence of a single mutant gene.

Autosomal Recessive Disorders

Autosomal recessive disorders generally have less variation in expression among family members than do dominant syndromes. The inheritance is from clinically normal parents who both have the same, or an allelic, recessive mutant gene in single dose. The likelihood of this occurring is enhanced if the parents are related. Hence, the possibility of consanguinity should always be addressed in disorders known to be autosomal recessive as well as when evaluating patterns of malformation of unknown cause.

X-Linked Disorders

Mutations on the X chromosome may be dominant or recessive in nature. Dominant mutations produce obvious clinical effects in XX females and either severe or lethal effects in the XY male who has no normal gene to lessen the impact of the mutation. By contrast, X-linked recessive mutations usually have minimal to no impact on the XX (carrier) female, whereas XY males demonstrate a phenotype.

Parent-of-Origin Effects

Although it has been assumed that genes inherited from mother and father are equally weighted in terms of expression and effect, observations in a variety of clinical settings have led to the appreciation that this is not invariably the case. Triploid conceptuses, who have an entire extra complement of genes, provide graphic illustration of this point.[39] When triploidy is produced by one maternal and two paternal sets of chromosomes, the pregnancy consists of a large hydatidiform placenta with a small, malformed but proportionate fetus. If two maternal and one paternal set of chromosomes are responsible, the fetus is disproportion-

ately growth-retarded and the placenta is usually extremely small, confirming observations in mouse embryos that paternal genes contribute to placental development, whereas maternal genes tend to define the embryo.

Genomic *imprinting* is a phenomenon first described in mice whereby certain genes are marked differently during male versus female germ cell formation so that apparently identical genes possess dissimilar function depending upon whether they are passed from the mother or the father. Imprinting commonly serves to "turn off" a gene or reduce its expression. Imprinting has been shown to play a role in a number of human syndromes including Prader-Willi syndrome, Angelman syndrome, and Beckwith syndrome. For example, Prader-Willi syndrome occurs if the paternal copy of genes in the q11 region of chromosome 15 are missing through deletion of that region or disomy as discussed subsequently. The inference from this observation is that the maternally inherited genes at this locus are normally imprinted or turned off. Absence for whatever reason of the paternally derived copies produces the phenotype. Current understanding suggests that imprinting involves allele-specific epigenetic modification through a variety of mechanisms including cytosine methylation and histone acetylation. These modifications are erased in the germ cells and re-established in early embryogenesis.[54] A redundant series of five elements acting in *cis* (along the same chromosome) has recently been shown to control imprinting at the Prader-Willi-Angelman syndrome locus in mice, which shows a high degree of homology to humans at this locus.[33]

Uniparental *disomy* is a term that indicates that both members of a chromosome pair or both alleles of a gene pair come from the same parent. This situation usually occurs when an embryo, initially trisomic for a certain chromosome, "self-corrects" by eliminating one of the extra chromosomes. In one third of such cases, the remaining two chromosomes will have the same parent of origin, resulting in uniparental disomy for the genes on that chromosome. The impact of uniparental disomy on morphogenesis is just beginning to be understood. Uniparental disomy for chromosome 16 has been documented in several growth-retarded fetuses in whom mosaicism for trisomy 16 was confined to the placenta.[32] Moreover, uniparental disomy may account for some of the phenotypic effects observed in individuals with apparently balanced Robertsonian translocations involving chromosome 14.[13] The implication is that certain chromosomes contain genes that are either paternally or maternally imprinted. Two copies from one parent would disturb the gene balance required for normal development. Uniparental disomy from correction of a trisomic conceptus is one mechanism that is known to produce Prader-Willi syndrome.

Unstable DNA Mutations

Throughout the human genome there are a number of sites in which short triplet repeated sequences of nucleotides normally occur. Although the purpose of these triplet repeats is not always known, the number of repeats at a given site is usually transmitted in a stable fashion from one generation to the next. An unstable DNA mutation occurs when the number of copies of a repeated sequence becomes increased. Expansion in the number of repeats at a locus may produce disease directly or it may create what has been termed a premutation. The latter indicates that the expanded sequence has no clinical effects on the individual; however, the sequence is likely to be unstable during meiosis (germ cell formation), resulting in offspring with clinical abnormalities. Although unstable DNA mutations usually expand further during meiosis, contraction of unstable sequences is documented. Unstable DNA mutations account for some observations that seem to defy the laws of single-gene inheritance such as anticipation (a condition getting worse in successive generations) and unaffected transmitting males in X-linked recessive disorders.[9] Parent-of-origin effects are common in unstable mutations, with some expanding only when transmitted through the mother and others showing paternal effects. Several classes of trinucleotide repeat disorders are recognized.[10] Fragile X syndrome is the prototype for conditions caused by expansion of trinucleotide repeats in the noncoding region of the responsible gene. Such expansions typically cause loss of function of the involved gene. Myotonic dystrophy has a similar pathogenesis. A second class of conditions, typically with midlife onset neurodegeneration, is caused by much smaller expansions of a polyglutamine $(CAG)_n$ track within the exon of a gene. The altered protein resulting from these mutations disrupts protein turnover within the cell, an effect that worsens over time. Strand slippage during DNA replication is thought to be the likely mechanism of formation for these classes of repeats.[46] More recently, expansion within a polyalanine tract has been shown to account for a variety of disorders including synpolydactyly type II, cleidocranial dysplasia (one family), and holoprosencephaly 5.[5] These expansions typically occur in genes that code for transcription factors. Mutations produce defects by altering the function of downstream target genes.

Mitochondrial Mutations

The DNA of the normal mitochondrion is a circular molecule that contains 37 genes encoding 22 types of transfer RNA, two types of ribosomal RNA, and 13 structural proteins, which are all subunits of the respiratory chain complexes involved in oxidative phosphorylation. Any given cell may contain from a hundred to several thousand mitochondria. Because the mitochondria are the energy-producing apparatus of the cell, most mitochondrial disorders described present postnatally with visual loss, progressive myopathy, seizures, encephalopathy, or diabetes presumably as a consequence of insufficient energy production in a critical tissue. The effects of mitochondrial mutation appear to worsen over time.[53] The impact of these abnormalities on morphogenesis is unknown.

GENETIC COUNSELING FOR SINGLE-GENE DISORDERS

For single-gene disorders, it is a good general rule to consult the literature directly before counseling families or affected individuals regarding the availability of testing as it pertains to carrier detection, presymptomatic diagnosis, and prenatal diagnosis, because the nature of the workup that is required to address many of these questions changes dramatically as the level of the understanding of the genetic abnormality becomes more refined. Increasingly, molecular diagnosis is available for single-gene disorders. The GeneTests web site (http://www.genetests.org/) is an excellent source of information regarding laboratories offering testing on both a clinical and research basis.

Autosomal Dominant Disorders

The parents and siblings of the affected individual should be examined to determine whether any of them show any features of the disorder in question. The nature of the "examination" to exclude the effects of an altered gene varies by disorder from simple assessment of parental stature in achondroplasia to cutaneous examination plus eye evaluation plus cranial and renal imaging in tuberous sclerosis. If neither parent shows any features of the condition, it is appropriate to counsel the family that the condition in the child likely represents a fresh gene mutation (gene change in one of the germ cells that went to make the baby) for which the risk for recurrence is negligible. More distant relatives need have no concern of having affected children. As molecular testing becomes more readily available and progressively less costly, direct DNA testing for the pathogenic mutation in single-gene disorders may be more commonly performed to allow molecular testing of relatives regarding their carrier status.

The risk for an *affected* individual having an affected child is 50% for each offspring. This number represents the risk for vertical transmission of the altered gene; however, it does not predict the severity of the effect in offspring who inherit the mutation. Knowledge of the frequency of various features in affected individuals is helpful in outlining not only the risk for transmission but also the likelihood of particular complications.

In the uncommon circumstance in which a dominant condition is the result of an unstable mutation in DNA, the likelihood of anticipation (increasing severity in subsequent generations) should be addressed if the affected parent is of the gender in which expansion of the unstable sequence is known to occur. For example, congenital myotonic dystrophy occurs only when the altered gene is transmitted through the mother.

Explanation of how the phenotype relates to the effects of the single altered gene is often helpful in outlining the natural history of the condition and need for follow-up of certain specific issues.

Autosomal Recessive Disorders

Inheritance is from clinically normal parents who both have the same, or an allelic, recessive mutant gene in single dose. The risk is obviously enhanced if the parents are related. The possibility of consanguinity should always be addressed in disorders known to be autosomal recessive and when evaluating patterns of malformation of unknown cause. Autosomal recessive disorders generally have less variation in expression among members of the same family than autosomal dominant conditions.

Recurrence risk from the same parentage is 25% for each subsequent pregnancy. The risk of any relative having an affected child may be calculated by multiplying their risk of being a heterozygote (carrier) times the risk of marrying a heterozygote (the general carrier frequency for that gene in the population) times one fourth (the chance of two heterozygotes having an affected offspring).

In counseling parents of individuals with recessive disorders, it is helpful to emphasize that most people have several altered genes that cause no problem because each is balanced by a normal partner. They happen to have one altered gene in common. The normal children of carrier parents have a two of three chance of being carriers as well. However, their risk of randomly marrying another carrier is low, thus their risk for affected offspring is low.

X-Linked Recessive Disorders

The X-linked genes in the XY male are present in a single dose with no partner gene. Hence, a single copy of a mutant gene on the X chromosome will express a full recessive disorder. The chance of an XX female having a pair of such X-linked recessive genes and expressing the same disorder as the XY male is very small. The following generalizations apply to this pattern of inheritance: with rare exception, only males are affected; transmission is through unaffected or mildly affected (carrier) females; male-to-male transmission does not occur.

X-linked disorders in the male often represent fresh gene mutation. These disorders present a problem in determining the generation in which the gene mutation arose, for it could be in the patient alone or in the mother or even further back in the family, having been silently passed through carrier females. For some X-linked disorders, such as hypohidrotic ectodermal dysplasia, this dilemma can be resolved by demonstrating the presence or absence of mild (carrier) expression in the females in question. Older paternal age has been noted to be a factor in fresh X-linked mutation; however, the older age effect is seen in the father of the mother (maternal grandfather) of the first affected XY male rather than the boy's father from whom he does not receive his X.[27]

For unstable X-linked mutations, such as those that account for the fragile X syndrome, counseling needs to incorporate knowledge of parent-of-origin effects. Unstable X-linked mutations tend to expand when passed through the mother, accounting for a more severe phenotype in offspring of carrier women who inherit the altered gene.

If the mother is not a carrier, the risk for recurrence is low. If the mother is a carrier, she has a 50% risk that any future male will be affected. Normal sons cannot transmit the disorder. All sons of affected males are normal. All daughters of affected males are usually clinically normal carriers.

In general, all daughters of carrier mothers will be clinically normal, although 50% will carry the altered gene and have themselves a risk for vertical transmission. The major exception is the case of unstable DNA mutation in which daughters of carrier mothers who inherit an expanded mutation often show clinical effects.

X-Linked Dominant Inheritance

X-linked dominant disorders show expression in the XX female, usually with more severe, often lethal, effects in the XY male. This type of inheritance is most commonly confused with autosomal dominant inheritance from which it may be discriminated in the following ways: males are more severely affected than females, although affected males are underrepresented in large kindreds, reflecting the male lethality of X-linked dominant conditions; male-to-male transmission is not observed; instead, affected males have normal sons and all of their daughters are affected.

Affected females have a 50% risk for affected daughters. Although the risk that an XY fetus will inherit the gene is also 50%, the probability of a live-born affected male is usually significantly less because of the selection pressure against affected XY conceptuses. Males born to affected women are usually normal. The affected males represent early miscarriages.

Mothers of daughters with X-linked dominant conditions should be examined closely for evidence of clinical effect. If the mother is normal, fresh gene mutation in the offspring is likely and the risk for recurrence is negligible. If not, counseling is the same as that for affected females mentioned previously.

Mitochondrial Inheritance

Because mitochondria are exclusively maternally inherited, males with disorders caused by mitochondrial mutations have no risk for affected offspring. Females, on the other hand, have a risk that approaches 100%, because the human egg is the source of all of the mitochondria for the offspring. Most affected women have both normal and abnormal mitochondria; thus, any given egg will have both types in different proportions. Random distribution of mitochondria in dividing cells in the early embryo creates different proportions of abnormal to normal mitochondria in different tissues. A clinical phenotype occurs only when a threshold of abnormal to normal mitochondria is exceeded in a critical tissue. Thus, all offspring of affected women may be assumed to have inherited some abnormal mitochondria; however, not all will manifest disease. Clinically unaffected daughters

of affected women also have a risk for vertical transmission, because lack of clinical disease does not preclude the possibility that some of the daughter's mitochondria might harbor the mutation.

MULTIFACTORIAL INHERITANCE

In the mid-1960s, a model was advanced to explain the findings emerging from a variety of epidemiologic studies, which suggested that a broad number of common malformations including cleft lip and palate, isolated cleft palate, neural tube defects, clubfoot, and pyloric stenosis among others tended to cluster in families, although the pattern of inheritance did not conform to the laws of gene transmission as set forth by Mendel.[7] The model involved the concept of genetic liability or susceptibility to a given characteristic, governed by many different genes, and a threshold, determined by both genetic and environmental factors. Individuals lying beyond the threshold exhibited the phenotype, whereas those who did not were phenotypically normal. The model converted the normal distribution of a morphogenetic process within a population into an "all-or-none" expression of a structural defect. As initially proposed, the many genes contributing to susceptibility were given equal weight. The multifactorial/threshold model makes several predictions that in large measure are in accord with the clinical and epidemiologic observations regarding given malformations:

1. *Familial clustering is observed.* As stated previously, clustering is observed among family groups. In addition, many common malformations have different birth frequencies in different populations. Because numerous subtle genetic differences are presumed to account for some of the normal variation observed among ethnic groups, it is hypothesized that some of these differences may confer susceptibility for certain developmental problems. Thus, the model would predict variation in the prevalence of certain malformations by ethnic groups, a finding that is well documented in population surveys.

2. *The risk for first-degree relatives (parents, siblings, and offspring) approximates the square root of the population risk.* Table 4-1 lists the frequency of recurrence of the same defect in offspring of normal parents who have had one affected child. For the majority of defects, the risk is 2% to 5%, which is 20 to 40 times the frequency of the problem in the general population. The

TABLE 4-1 RECURRENCE RISKS FOR SOME DEFECTS[30,31]

Defect	Normal Parents of One Affected Child	RECURRENCE RISK FOR Future Males	Future Females
Cleft lip with or without cleft palate	4–5%*		
Cleft palate alone	2–6%		
Cardiac defect (common type)	3–4%		
Pyloric stenosis	3%	4%	2.4%
Hirschsprung anomaly	3–5%		
Clubfoot	2–8%		
Dislocation of hip	3–4%	0.5%	6.3%
Neural tube defects—anencephaly, meningomyelocele	3–5%		
Scoliosis	10–15%		

*Range of recurrence risks observed.

figures in Table 4-1 are derived from direct observations in clinical populations and correlate well with the numbers predicted by the model.

3. *Second-degree relatives (uncles, aunts, half-siblings) have a sharply lower risk than first-degree relatives.* This characteristic differentiates multifactorial inheritance from autosomal dominant inheritance in which the risk drops only by half with each degree of relational distance from the affected individual and from autosomal recessive inheritance in which the major risk is for full siblings.

4. *The greater the number of affected family members, the greater the risk for recurrence.* This pattern of recurrence of multifactorial traits is in contrast to both dominant and recessive inheritance in which the risk for future offspring remains unchanged despite recurrences.

5. *Consanguinity increases the risk.* This concept relates to the fact that inbreeding increases the number of "susceptibility genes," thus making a developmental problem more likely.

6. *The more severe the malformation, the greater the risk for recurrence.* This presumes that the severity of the malformation reflects a greater adverse genetic influence, thereby increasing the risk from the same parentage. Certainly with cleft lip and palate, data support the hypothesis, because the risk for recurrence in subsequent children when an offspring has a severe bilateral cleft lip and palate is 5.7% as contrasted with a 2.5% recurrence risk when the offspring has a less severe degree of defect.[4,8,47]

7. *The risk for recurrence will be increased for relatives of the least affected gender, if gender differences are noted.* The gender difference between the XX and XY genetic background has an appreciable effect on the occurrence of many malformations (Fig. 4-14). Some of the gender differences in malformation occurrence may be explained as the direct effects of structural genital differences, such as hypospadias in the

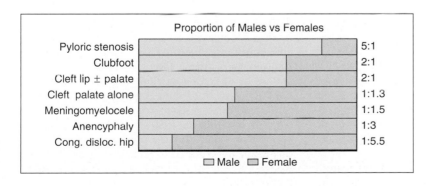

FIGURE 4-14. Relative gender incidence of single common malformations.

male. Similarly, the marked male predominance of the urethral obstruction sequence may be explained by the fact that the most common site of urethral obstruction is the prostatic urethra.[3] The humoral impact of testosterone, which makes connective tissue tougher in the male, may explain the preponderance of dislocation of the hip, related to connective tissue laxity, in the female. Also, testosterone, which is produced by the male during the first few postnatal months, may enhance the likelihood of muscle hypertrophy and thereby increase the tendency to develop hypertrophic pyloric stenosis.[3] The gender differences related to the incidence of other structural defects would appear to imply that genes on the X or Y chromosome may increase the likelihood of particular anomalies developing during morphogenesis.

One indirect manner in which the genetic background of XX versus XY may influence the frequency of structural defects at birth is simply the growth rate in utero. Thus, with the exception of anomalies related to joint laxity, most late uterine constraint-induced deformations are more common in the male, who is normally growing faster in the last trimester of gestation than the female.[20]

The hypothesis reasons that if it takes more genetic factors to give rise to an anomaly in the female, then the affected female should pass on more of these genetic factors to her offspring, who would have a higher frequency of the anomaly than would offspring of affected males. Observational studies in pyloric stenosis documenting a 24% risk of transmission from affected mothers compared to 6% from affected fathers bear this out.

8. *Concordance in twins.* If both twins have a defect, they are concordant for the anomaly. If one twin has the defect and the other does not, they are discordant. The frequency of concordance and discordance in monozygotic and dizygotic twins has been used to argue both for environmental and for single-gene causation of common malformations. For most of these defects, the incidence of concordance in dizygotic twins is similar to that of siblings born of separate pregnancies, arguing against both a single-gene etiology and a major environmental influence.

Over the past 15 years, numerous investigators have reanalyzed previously published data sets for specific "multifactorial" malformations with respect to a variety of alternative hypotheses. For cleft lip with or without cleft palate, it now seems likely that susceptibility is determined by a small number (two to eight genes) acting in a multiplicative fashion and interacting with environmental factors.[16,40,41] Genes conferring susceptibility for clefting have been identified through a variety of strategies including linkage or association studies, cloning of chromosomal break points, Mendelian models, animal models, and human and mouse expression studies.[49] Among these genes are the following:

PVRL1 (homozygous mutations cause Margarita Island ectodermal dysplasia[51]; whereas heterozygous mutations appear to increase the risk for nonsyndromic clefting)[48]

MSX1 (mutations in this gene cause Witkop syndrome[31] as well as increased susceptibility to clefting)[29]

FGFR1 (inactivating mutations in this gene cause autosomal dominant Kallman syndrome associated with cleft lip, cleft palate and hypodontia)[12]

TBX22 (responsible for X-linked cleft palate with ankyloglossia[42] as well as susceptibility to nonsyndromic cleft palate)[37]

IRF6 (mutations in this gene account for Van der Woude syndrome,[35] but also confer susceptibility for nonsyndromic clefting)[57]

Similar strategies are being used to identify genes that define susceptibility to other common "multifactorial" malformations.

Despite the accumulating evidence that suggests that the multifactorial model is probably not biologically true, the empiric data obtained from the observational studies used to construct the model remain the basis for genetic counseling of families. Molecular testing for susceptibility genes is not yet available.

That environmental influences play a role in the determination of common malformations is born out by many studies such as those of anencephaly and meningomyelocele that document that social class is a variable that impacts birth frequency.[14] Birth order influences have also been noted, with congenital dislocation of the hip and pyloric stenosis being more likely to occur in firstborn children.[7] One obvious environmental factor is fetal in utero constraint leading to deformation. Such constraint is more common in the firstborn who is the first to distend the uterus and the abdominal wall.[20] Environmental factors such as this probably explain the greater frequency of dislocation of the hip as well as most other deformations in the firstborn.

Studies in experimental animals have dramatically illustrated the profound influence that genetic background may have on the likelihood of a given environmental teratogen causing malformation. For example, Fraser[17] could regularly produce cleft palate in mouse embryos of the A/Jax strain by giving the mothers a high dose of cortisone during early gestation, whereas the same treatment in a different strain led to only 17% affected offspring. In humans, genetic susceptibility to hydantoin-induced teratogenesis appears to correlate with the genetically determined activity levels of epoxide hydrolase, one of the enzymes necessary for the metabolism of hydantoin.[6] Expression of the phenotype requires both genetic susceptibility and drug exposure.

The search for environmental factors that allow for expression of a single malformation is ongoing. However, just as the genetic differences that contribute to susceptibility are multiple and difficult to characterize, so environmental factors are likely to be multiple and incremental in effect. The total factors combine to approach the threshold for a particular error in morphogenesis, a threshold predominantly set by the genetic makeup of the individual.

GENETIC COUNSELING FOR DEFECTS THAT ARE A RESULT OF MULTIFACTORIAL INHERITANCE

For many common single defects, empiric risk figures relative to recurrence of the problem in a subsequent pregnancy are available.[24] The risk is 3% to 5% or less for most of the common single defects, with the exception of scoliosis (see Table 4-1). The risk figures may be slightly increased when the defect in the affected individual is severe in degree, and decreased when the anomaly is mild in degree. If the gender of the child impacts the condition (such as in pyloric stenosis and hip dislocation), gender-specific risks for recurrence may be appropriate. If two offspring are affected, the risk for the next child is two to three times greater, or approximately 10% to 15%. Because recurrence risk figures address the risk for first-degree relatives, the risk that an affected individual will have affected offspring is similar in magnitude to that of the sibling risk (or 3% to 5%). As the factors that influence both genetic and environmental susceptibility to multifactorial traits become elucidated, it is expected that more precise counseling will be possible.

The multifactorial model is useful in explaining common malformations to parents, as it dictates that the genetic factors that contribute come from both sides of the family. It is helpful to explain the developmental pathology of the defects so that parents can appreciate that there was only a single localized problem in the early development of their child. A discussion that the localized problem in development must have occurred before a particular time in gestation may be helpful in dispelling any concerns over later gestational events that are likely to have had no impact on the occurrence on the particular malformation. The prognosis of multifactorial traits depends on the amenability of the specific malformation to surgical intervention or, in the case of constraint-related problems, to postural intervention. The prognosis is poor for certain neural tube defects, but may be quite good for cardiac malformations and other defects in which advances in therapy have improved both morbidity and mortality.

PRENATAL DIAGNOSIS

Technologic advancement as well as progress in the understanding of the etiology and pathogenesis of many disorders have made the possibility for prenatal diagnosis an increasing reality for many families. For a very few conditions, fetal therapy may be available; however, most prenatal diagnosis is offered to allow parents options for managing their reproductive risk. The subsequent sections present some of the techniques for early fetal evaluation along with indications for their application.

Screening Approaches for the General Pregnant Population

Chromosomal Abnormalities

Because the risk for many chromosomal aneuploidy states increases with advancing maternal age, a variety of approaches have been developed to assess fetal karyotypes in older mothers. The most accurate way to address this issue is with direct assessment of the fetal chromosomes, which requires a sample of fetal cells. The traditional method by which this is done is *amniocentesis* at 15 to 18 weeks of pregnancy. Although highly accurate,[19] the procedure carries a roughly 1 in 200 risk for miscarriage, which is a deterrent to some couples. *Chorionic villus sampling* (CVS) affords the advantage of earlier diagnosis, as the procedure is done at 11 to 12 weeks of pregnancy. The test carries a slightly increased risk for miscarriage even correcting for the earlier gestational age at which testing is done. In addition, mosaicism in the sampled placental cells is documented in approximately 1% of cases, causing counseling dilemmas. Noninvasive serum screening using a triple marker screen (maternal age, alpha fetoprotein, human chorionic gonadotropin, and unconjugated estriol) or quad screening (triple markers plus dimeric inhibin A) is a useful way to modify the age-related risk for Down syndrome to determine which women in the general population are at high enough risk that more invasive testing should be offered.[23] Noninvasive first-trimester screening using ultrasound measurement of nuchal translucency with serum marker analysis (pregnancy-associated plasma protein A) is gaining popularity. With combined first- and second-trimester screening results (integrated testing), an 85% Down syndrome detection rate is possible with a less than 1% false-positive rate.[52]

Single-Gene Disorders

Carrier screening is available for a number of single-gene disorders that are inherited in an autosomal recessive fashion and that have a high prevalence in certain populations. Examples include Tay-Sachs disease, sickle cell anemia, and cystic fibrosis. For most of the conditions in this book, approaches for carrier screening in the general population have not been developed.

Multifactorial Conditions

The only multifactorial conditions for which population screening is specifically available are the neural tube closure defects. Elevation of alpha-fetoprotein both in the amniotic fluid and in maternal serum has been associated with the presence of an open defect in the fetus. Serum screening in conjunction with thorough ultrasound evaluation should detect over 90% of affected pregnancies.

Ultrasonography is also an increasingly useful screening tool for a number of other malformations. However, variations in equipment and operator experience make this an imperfect technique as it is currently practiced.[15]

Prenatal Diagnostic Approaches for Specific Disorders

Chromosomal Abnormalities

Amniocentesis or chorionic villus sampling should be offered in the following situations:

1. Previous child with trisomy 21.
2. Parental balanced translocation.
3. Affected parent with a microdeletion syndrome.
4. Any de novo abnormality in which the parents, although chromosomally normal, are interested, because this is the only way to exclude recurrence from gonadal mosaicism.

Single-Gene Disorders

Prenatal testing for single-gene disorders is more difficult because the approach that is used for any given condition depends upon, among other things, the level of understanding of the molecular basis of the disorder in question. Testing can be done at the level of the gene (DNA), the message (RNA), the product (biochemical analysis), or the phenotype produced (gross morphology). Even in situations in which the gene that causes a specific condition is known, direct analysis of the gene is not always the easiest, least costly, and most reliable approach to prenatal testing. The rapidity with which changes occur in this arena dictates that the literature be reviewed at the time prenatal diagnosis is requested. Information available in textbooks will be out of date for some conditions at the time of publication.

1. For conditions in which the specific gene mutation is known, prenatal diagnosis is often possible using amniocentesis or chorionic villus sampling to collect fetal cells for direct mutation analysis. If a common mutation accounts for the majority of the cases (such as achondroplasia) the approach can be relatively straightforward. By contrast, in conditions such as Marfan syndrome in which multiple different mutations within the same gene produce the same phenotype, prenatal diagnosis using direct DNA analysis is possible only if the family's specific mutation is known.
2. For disorders in which the location of the gene is known, linkage analysis may be useful. This technique dictates that DNA samples be obtained on multiple family members and often requires a confirmed diagnosis in more than one family member. Nonpaternity is occasionally discovered in the course of this type of investigation.
3. Biochemical studies may be diagnostic in conditions in which the approach is based on analysis of gene product. Some tests are performed on amniotic fluid directly. Other

studies demand cultured fetal cells for enzyme analysis requiring amniocentesis or chorionic villus sampling.

4. For X-linked conditions in which neither direct DNA analysis nor linkage are available, prenatal gender determination may be an option. However, 50% of the male offspring of carrier women would be expected to be normal.

5. For conditions in which the diagnosis is made on the clinical phenotype, prenatal diagnosis is dependent upon the ability of ultrasound to visualize specific features of the condition such as severe limb shortening in some of the skeletal dysplasias.

Multifactorial Conditions

For conditions that have neither a chromosomal or genetic marker, prenatal diagnosis is entirely dependent on the amenability of the specific structural defects to ultrasound imaging. For example, holoprosencephaly is readily visualized with prenatal imaging, whereas isolated cleft palate is not at this time. It is important that clinicians be aware of the limitations of ultrasound. The Eurofetus Study regarding the accuracy of ultrasound detection of fetal malformations in an unselected population documented a roughly 60% overall detection rate, which is also to say that 40% of defects were missed.[21] This is not to downplay the usefulness of ultrasound imaging, but rather to foster realistic expectations among families and physicians when this method is used.

References

1. Antonarakis SE, and the Down Syndrome Collaborative Group: Parental origin of the extra chromosome in trisomy 21 using DNA polymorphism analysis. N Engl J Med 324:872, 1991.
2. Antonarakis SE et al: The meiotic stage of non-disjunction in trisomy 21: Determination by using DNA polymorphisms. Am J Hum Genet 50:544, 1992.
3. Arenas F, Smith DW: Sex liability to single structural defects. Am J Dis Child 132:970, 1978.
4. Bixler D: Genetics and clefting. Cleft Palate J 18:10–18, 1981.
5. Brown LY, Brown SA: Alanine tracts: The expanding story of human illness and trinucleotide repeats. Trends Genet 20:51–58, 2004.
6. Buehler BA, Delimont D, van Waes M, et al: Prenatal prediction of risk of the fetal hydantoin syndrome. N Engl J Med 322:1567, 1990.
7. Carter CO: The inheritance of common congenital malformations. Progr Med Genet 4:59, 1965.
8. Carter CO, Evans K, Coffey R, et al: A three generation family study of cleft lip with or without cleft palate. J Med Genet 19:246–261, 1982.
9. Caskey CT, Pizzuti A, et al: Triplet repeat mutations in human disease. Science 256:784, 1991.
10. Cummings CJ, Zoghbi HY: Fourteen and counting: Unraveling trinucleotide repeat diseases. Hum Mol Genet 9:909–916, 2000.
11. Dawson AJ, Putnam S, Schultz J, et al: Cryptic chromosome rearrangements detected by subtelomere assay in patients with mental retardation and dysmorphic features. Clin Genet 62:488–494, 2002.
12. Dodé C, Levilliers J, Dupont J-M, et al: Loss-of-function mutations in FGFR1 cause autosomal dominant Kallmann syndrome. Nat Genet 33:463–465, 2003.
13. Donnai D: Robertsonian translocations: Clues to imprinting. Am J Med Genet 46:681, 1993.
14. Edwards JH: Congenital malformations of the central nervous system in Scotland. Br J Prev Soc Med 12:115, 1958.
15. Ewigman BG, Crane JP, Frigoletto FE, et al: Effect of prenatal ultrasound screening on perinatal outcome. N Engl J Med 329:821, 1993.
16. Farrall M, Holder SE: Familial recurrence pattern analysis of cleft lip with or without cleft palate. Am J Hum Genet 50:270, 1992.
17. Fraser FC: The use of teratogens in the analysis of abnormal developmental mechanisms. First International Conference on Congenital Malformations. Philadelphia: JB Lippincott, 1961.
18. Ghaffari SR, Boyd E, Tolmie JL, et al: A new strategy for cryptic telomeric translocation screening in patients with idiopathic mental retardation. J Med Genet 35:225–233, 1998.
19. Golbus MS, Loughman WD, Epstein CJ, et al: Prenatal genetic diagnosis in 3000 amniocenteses. N Engl J Med 300:157, 1979.
20. Graham JM: Smith's Recognizable Patterns of Human Deformation, 2nd ed. Philadelphia: WB Saunders, 1988.
21. Grandjean H, Larroque D, Levi S: The performance of routine ultrasonographic screening of pregnancies in the Eurofetus Study. Am J Obstet Gynecol 181:446–454, 1999.
22. Guttmacher AE, Collins FS: Genomic medicine: A primer. N Engl J Med 347:1512–1520, 2002.
23. Haddow JE, Palomake GE, Knight GJ, et al: Reducing the need for amniocentesis in women 35 years of age or older with serum markers for screening. N Engl J Med 330:1114, 1994.
24. Harper P: Practical Genetic Counseling, 5th ed. Oxford: Butterworth-Heinemann, 1998.
25. Hassold T, Hunt P: To err (meiotically) is human: The genesis of human aneuploidy. Nat Rev Genet 2:280–291, 2001.
26. Hassold T, Pettay D, Robinson A, Uchida I: Molecular studies of parental origin and mosaicism in 45,X conceptuses. Hum Genet 89:647, 1992.
27. Herrmann J: Ein Einfluss des zeugungsalters auf die Mutationen zu Hamophilie A. Humangenetik 3:1, 1966.
28. Hunt PA, Hassold TJ: Sex matters in meiosis. Science 296:2181–2183, 2002.
29. Jezewski PA, Vieira AR, Nishimura C, et al: Complete sequencing shows a role for MSX1 in nonsyndromic cleft lip and palate. J Med Genet 40:399–407, 2003.
30. Jones KL et al: Older paternal age and fresh gene mutation. J Pediatr 86:84, 1975.
31. Jumlongras D, Bei M, Stimson JM, et al: A nonsense mutation in MSX1 causes Witkop syndrome. Am J Hum Genet 69:67–74, 2001.
32. Kalousek DK, Langlois S, Barrett I, et al: Uniparental disomy for chromosome 16 in humans. Am J Hum Genet 52:8, 1993.
33. Kantor B, Makedonski K, Green-Finberg Y, et al: Control

elements within the PWS/AS imprinting box and their function in the imprinting process. Hum Mol Genet 13:751–762, 2004.

34. Knight SJ, Regan R, Nicod A, et al: Subtle chromosomal rearrangements in children with unexplained mental retardation. Lancet 354:1676–1681, 1999.

35. Kondo S, Schutte BC, Richardson RJ, et al: Mutations in IRF6 cause Van der Woude and popliteal pterygium syndromes. Nat Genet 32:285–289, 2002.

36. MacDonald M, Hassold T, Harvey J, et al: The origin of 47,XXY and 47,XXX aneuploidy: Heterogeneous mechanisms and role of aberrant recombination. Hum Mol Genet 3:1365, 1994.

37. Marçano ACB, Doudney K, Braybrook C, et al: TBX22 mutations are a frequent cause of cleft palate. J Med Genet 41:68–74, 2004.

38. Mascarello JT, Hubbard V: Routine use of methods for improved G-band resolution in a population of patients with malformations and developmental delay. Am J Med Genet 38:37, 1991.

39. McFadden DE, Kalousek DK: Two different phenotypes of fetuses with chromosomal triploidy: Correlation with parental origin of the extra haploid set. Am J Med Genet 38:535, 1991.

40. Mitchell LE, Christensen K: Analysis of the recurrence patterns for nonsyndromic cleft lip with or without cleft palate in the families of 3,073 Danish probands. Am J Med Genet 61:371, 1996.

41. Mitchell LE, Risch N: Mode of inheritance of nonsyndromic cleft lip with or without cleft palate: A reanalysis. Am J Hum Genet 51:323, 1992.

42. Moore GE, Ivens A, Chambers J, et al: Linkage of an X-chromosome cleft palate gene. Nature 326:91–92, 1987.

43. Pangalos CG et al: DNA polymorphism analysis in families with recurrence of free trisomy 21. Am J Hum Genet 51:1015, 1992.

44. Phelan MC, Crawford EC, Bealer DM: Mental retardation in South Carolina. III. Chromosome aberrations. Proc Greenwood Genet Center 15:45–60, 1996.

45. Shaw CJ, Shaw CA, Yu W, et al: Comparative genomic hybridisation using a proximal 17p BAC/PAC array detects rearrangements responsible for four genomic disorders. J Med Genet 4:113–119, 2004.

46. Sinden RR, Potaman VN, Oussatcheva EA, et al: Triplet repeat DNA structures and human genetic disease: Dynamic mutations from dynamic DNA. J Biosci 27:53–65, 2002.

47. Smith DW, Aase JM: Polygenic inheritance of certain common malformations. J Pediatr 76:653, 1970.

48. Sözen MA, Suzuki K, Tolarova MM, et al: Mutation of PVRL1 is associated with sporadic, nonsyndromic cleft lip/palate in northern Venezuela. Nat Genet 29:141–142, 2001.

49. Spritz RA: The genetics and epigenetics of orofacial clefts. Curr Opin Pediatr 13:556–560, 2001.

50. Summitt R: Cytogenetics in mentally retarded children with anomalies: A controlled study. J Pediatr 74:58, 1969.

51. Suzuki K, Hu D, Buston T, et al: Mutations of PVRL1, encoding a cell-cell adhesion molecule/herpes receptor, in cleft lip/palate-ectodermal dysplasia. Nat Genet 25:427–429, 2000.

52. Wald NJ, Rodeck C, Hackshaw AK, Rudnicka A: SURUSS in perspective. Br J Obstet Gynecol 111:521–531, 2004.

53. Wallace DC: Mitochondrial defects in neurodegenerative disease. Ment Retard Dev Disabil Res Rev 7:158–166, 2001.

54. Walter J, Paulsen M: Imprinting and disease. Sem Cell Dev Biol 14:101–110, 2003.

55. Walter S, Sandig K, Hinkel GK, et al: Subtelomeric FISH in 50 children with mental retardation and minor anomalies, identified by a checklist, detects 10 rearrangements including a de novo balanced translocation of chromosomes 17p13.3 and 20q13.33. Am J Med Genet 128A:364–373, 2004.

56. Yu W, Ballif BC, Kashork CD, et al: Development of a comparative genomic hybridization microarray and demonstration of its utility with 25 well-characterized 1p36 deletions. Hum Mol Genet 12:2145–2150, 2003.

57. Zuccero TM, Cooper ME, Maher BS, et al: Interferon regulatory factor 6 (IRF6) gene variants and the risk of isolated cleft lip or palate. N Engl J Med 351:769–779, 2004.

5 Minor Anomalies

Clues to More Serious Problems and to the Recognition of Malformation Syndromes

Minor anomalies are herein defined as unusual morphologic features that are of no serious medical or cosmetic consequence to the patient. The value of their recognition is that they may serve as indicators of altered morphogenesis in a general sense or may constitute valuable clues in the diagnosis of a specific pattern of malformation. Those who want a more detailed discussion of this subject or those who desire information on a minor malformation not addressed in this chapter are referred to the elegant text by Jon M. Aase, *Diagnostic Dysmorphology*.[2]

Regarding the general occurrence of minor anomalies detectable by surface examination (except for dermatoglyphics), Marden and colleagues[9] found that 14% of newborn babies had a single minor anomaly. This was of little concern because the frequency of major defects in this group was not appreciably increased. However, only 0.8% of the babies had two minor defects, and in this subgroup, the frequency of a major defect was five times that of the general group. Of special importance were the findings in babies with three or more minor anomalies. This was found in only 0.5% of babies,[10] and 90% of them had one or more major defects as well, as depicted in Figure 5-1.

In two additional studies, Mehes and colleagues[10] and Leppig and colleagues[8] demonstrated that 26% and 19.6% of newborn infants with three or more minor anomalies, respectively, had a major malformation, a much lower incidence than that documented in the study by Marden and colleagues and most likely related to differences in study design. Based on these studies, it is concluded that any infant with three or more minor anomalies should be evaluated for a major malformation, many of which are occult.

These minor external anomalies are most common in areas of complex and variable features, such as the face, auricles, hands, and feet. Before ascribing significance to a given minor anomaly in a patient, it is important to note whether it is found

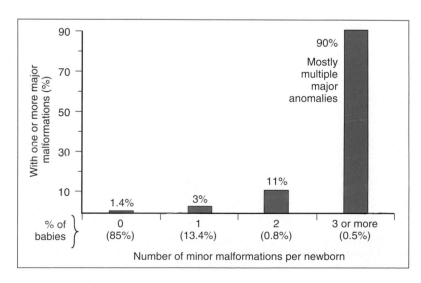

FIGURE 5-1. Frequency of major malformations in relation to the number of minor anomalies detected in a given newborn baby. (From Marden PM, Smith DW, McDonald MJ: J Pediatr 64:357, 1964, with permission.)

817

in other family members. Almost any minor defect may occasionally be found as a usual feature in a particular family, as noted in Figure 5-2.

The following figures illustrate certain minor anomalies and allude to their developmental origin and relevance (Figs. 5-3 to 5-8). Many, if not most, minor anomalies represent deformations caused by altered mechanical forces affecting the develop-ment of otherwise normal tissue. The reason for the deformation may be purely external uterine con-straint. Thus, most minor anomalies of external ear formation at birth are constraint-induced. However, the minor deformational anomaly may be the result of a more primary malformation, and this is the presumed reason for the association between minor anomalies and major malformations.

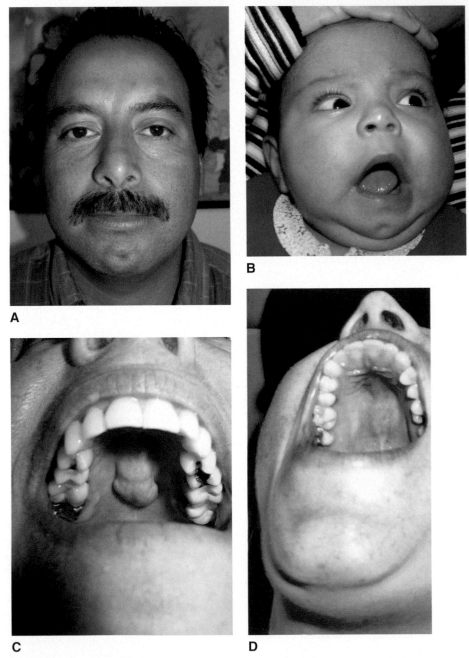

FIGURE 5-2. An otherwise normal father (**A**) and daughter (**B**) with a pit on the chin. An otherwise normal mother (**C**) and daughter (**D**) with a torus deformity of the palate. A family history should be obtained before ascribing significance to a given minor anomaly.

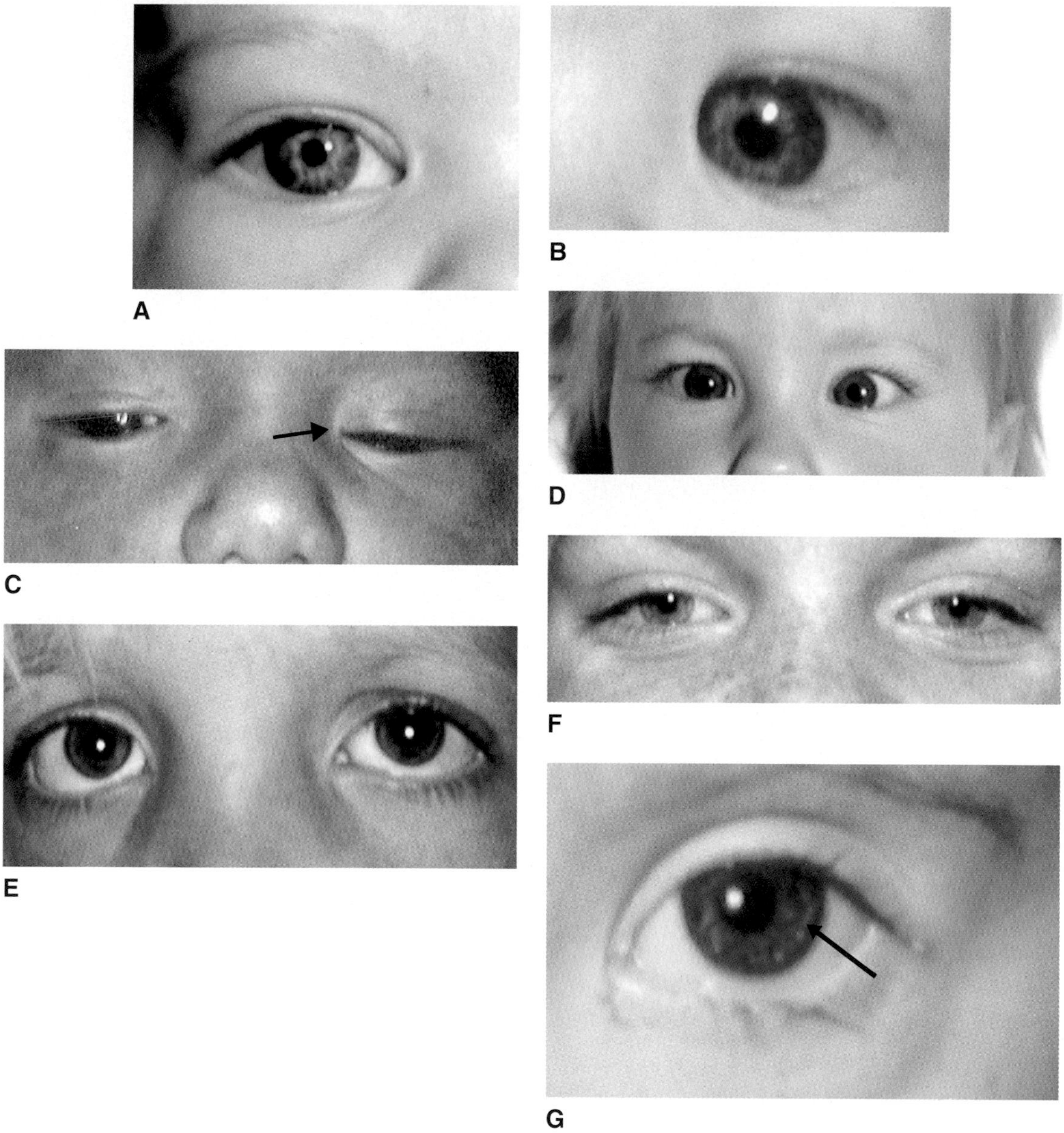

FIGURE 5-3. Minor anomalies of the ocular region. **A** and **B,** Inner epicanthal folds appear to represent redundant folds of skin, secondary to either low nasal bridge (most common) or excess skin, as in cutis laxa. Minor folds are frequent in early infancy, and as the nasal bridge becomes more prominent, they are obliterated. **C,** A unilateral epicanthal fold (*arrow*) is indicative of torticollis. (**C,** From Jones MC: J Pediatr 108:707, 1986, with permission.) Slanting of the palpebral fissures seems to be secondary to the early growth rate of the brain above the eye versus that of the facial area below the eye. For example, the patient with upslanting (**D**) had mild microcephaly with a narrow frontal area, resulting in the upslant; the patient with downslanting (**E**) had maxillary hypoplasia, resulting in the downslant. Mild degrees of upslant were noted in 4% of 500 normal children. **F,** Ocular hypertelorism refers to widely spaced eyes. A low nasal bridge will often give rise to a visual impression of ocular hypertelorism. This should always be determined by measurement. Measurement of inner canthal distance, coupled with the visual distinction of whether telecanthus is present, is usually sufficient. **G,** Brushfield spots are speckled rings about two thirds of the distance to the periphery of the iris. There is relative lack of patterning beyond the ring. These spots are found in 20% of normal newborn babies, but they are found in 80% of babies with Down syndrome.

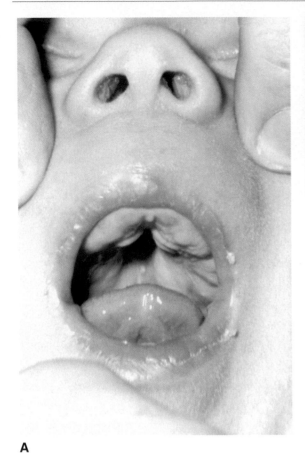

A

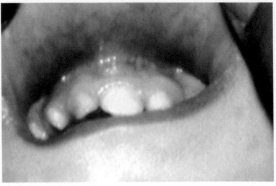

B

FIGURE 5-4. Minor anomalies of the oral region. **A,** Prominent lateral palatal ridges may be secondary to a deficit of tongue thrust into the hard palate, allowing for relative overgrowth of the lateral palatal ridges. This ridge may be a feature in a variety of disorders, especially those with hypotonia and with serious neurologic deficits related to sucking. As such, it can be a useful sign of a long-term deficit in function. **B,** Lack of lingular frenulum and single central incisor. Indicative of holoprosencephaly.

CALVARIUM

The presence of unusually *large fontanels* (see standards in Chapter 6) may be a nonspecific indicator of a general lag in osseous maturation.[13] It may, for example, lead to the detection of congenital hypothyroidism in the newborn or young infant, as shown in Figure 5-9.[16] The finding of a large posterior fontanel is especially helpful in this regard, because the posterior fontanel is normally fingertip size or smaller in 97% of full-term neonates. Large fontanels may also be a feature in certain skeletal dysplasias and can, of course, be a sign of increased intracranial pressure.

DERMAL RIDGE PATTERNS (DERMATOGLYPHICS)

The parallel dermal ridges on the palms and soles form between the 13th and 19th fetal weeks. Their patterning appears to be dependent on the surface contours at the time, and the parallel dermal ridges tend to develop transversely to the planes of growth stress.[11] Curvilinear arrangements occur when there was a surface mound, for example, over the fetal pads that are prominently present during early fetal life on the fingertips, on the palm between each pair of fingers, and occasionally in the hypothenar area. Indirect evidence suggests that a high fetal fingertip pad tends to give rise to a whorl pattern, a low pad yields an arch pattern, and an intermediate pad produces a loop, as illustrated in Figure 5-10*B*. The dermal ridge patterning thereby provides an indelible historical record that indicates the form of the early fetal hand (or foot). Mild to severe alterations in hand morphology occur in a variety of syndromes, and hence it is not surprising that dermatoglyphic alterations have been noted in numerous dysmorphic syndromes. These alterations have seldom been pathognomonic for a particular condition. Rather, they simply provide additional data that, viewed in relation to the total pattern of malformation, may enhance the clinician's capac-

Text continued on page 826

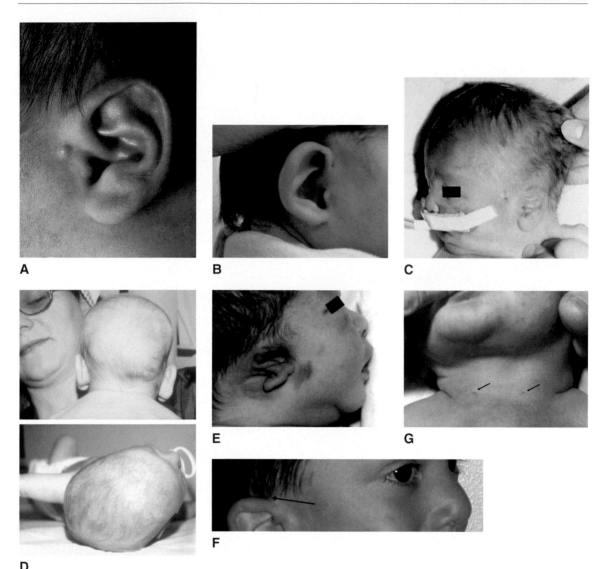

FIGURE 5-5. Minor anomalies of the auricular region. **A,** Preauricular tags, which often contain a core cartilage, appear to represent accessory hillock of His, the hillocks that normally develop in the recess of the mandibular and hyoid arches and coalesce to form the auricle. **B,** Preauricular pits may be familial, are twice as common in females than in males, and are more common in blacks than in whites. Both pits and tags should initiate evaluation of hearing. **C,** Large ears are often due to intrauterine constraint as in this child with oligohydramnios. Asymmetric ear size can be secondary to torticollis as in **D**. The child's head was positioned constantly on his right side, leading to plagiocephaly and enlargement of the right ear. **E,** Microtia. This defect should always initiate evaluation for hearing loss. Eighty-five percent of children with unilateral microtia have an ipsilateral hearing loss and 15% have a contralateral hearing loss as well. **F,** Low-set ears: This designation is made when the helix meets the cranium at a level below that of a horizontal plane that may be an extension of a line through both inner canthi. This plane may relate to the lateral vertical axis of the head. Ears slanted: This designation is made when the angle of the slope of the auricle exceeds 15 degrees from the perpendicular. Note that the findings of low placement and slanted auricle often go together and usually represent a lag in morphogenesis, since the auricle is normally in that position in early fetal life. It is important to appreciate that deformation of the head secondary to in utero constraint may temporarily distort the usual landmarks.[15] **G,** Branchial cleft sinuses.

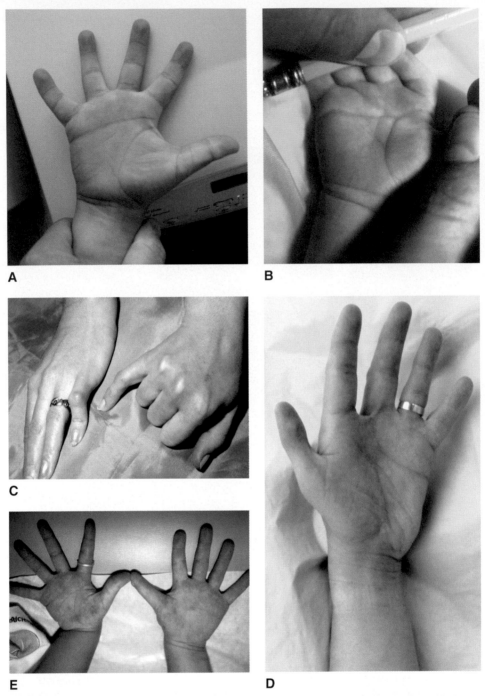

FIGURE 5-6. Minor anomalies of the hands. A and **B,** Creases represent the planes of folding (flexion) of the thickened volar skin of the hand. As such, they are simply deep wrinkles. The finger creases relate to flexion at the phalangeal joints, and if there has been no flexion, as in **B**, there is no crease.[7] Camptodactyly (contracted fingers), depicted in **B** and **C**, most commonly affects the fifth, fourth, and third digits in decreasing order of frequency. It is presumably the consequence of relative shortness in the length of the flexor tendons with respect to the growth of the hand. The thenar crease is the consequence of oppositional flexion of the thumb; hence, if there is no oppositional flexion, there will be no crease, as in **D** and **E**. The slanting upper palmar crease reflects the palmar plane of folding related to the slope of the third, fourth, and fifth metacarpophalangeal joints. The midpalmar crease is the plane of skin folding between the upper palmar crease and the thenar crease. Any alteration in the slope of the third, fourth, and fifth metacarpophalangeal planes of flexion, or relative shortness of the palm, may give rise to but a single midpalmar plane of flexion and thereby the *simian crease,* as in **A**. This is found unilaterally in approximately 4% of normal infants and bilaterally in 1%. Davies[6] found the incidence to be 3.7% in newborn babies and noted that the simian crease is twice as common in males as in females. All degrees are found between the normal and the simian crease, including the bridged palmar crease. The creases are evident by 11 to 12 weeks of fetal life; hence, any gross alteration in crease patterning is usually indicative of an abnormality in form or function of the hand prior to 11 fetal weeks.[7]   *Continued*

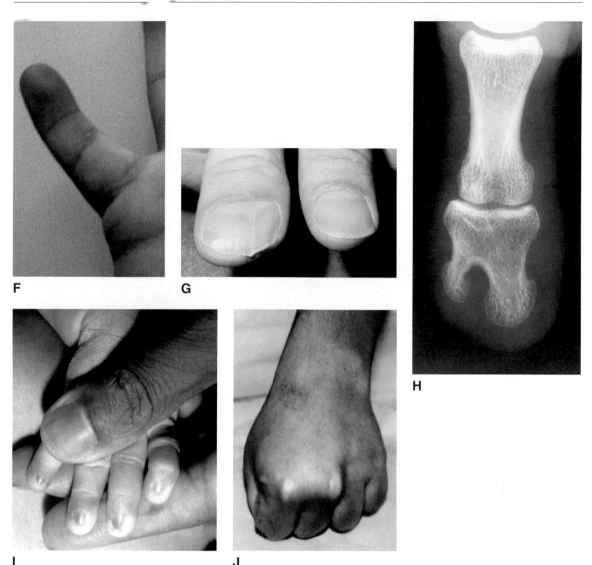

Fig. 5-6, cont'd. Clinodactyly (curved finger) (**F**) is most common in the fifth finger and is the consequence of hypoplasia of the middle phalanx, normally the last digital bone to develop. Up to 8 degrees of inturning of the fifth finger is within normal limits. Regardless of which digits are affected (fingers or toes), there is usually incurvature toward the area between the second and third digits. Partial cutaneous syndactyly represents an incomplete separation of the fingers and most commonly occurs between the third and fourth fingers and between the second and third toes. The *nails* generally reflect the size and shape of the underlying distal phalanx; hence, a bifid nail (**G**) reflects dimensions of the underlying respective phalanges (**H**), as does a hypoplastic nail seen in **I**. Malproportionment or disharmony in the length of particular segments of the hand is not uncommon. The most common is a short middle phalanx of the fifth finger with clinodactyly. **F,** Another is relative shortness of the fourth or fifth metacarpal or metatarsal bone. This is best appreciated in the hand by having the patient make a fist and observing the position of the knuckles, as shown in **J**. The altered alignment of these metacarpophalangeal joints may result in an altered palmar crease, especially the simian crease. It may also yield the impression of partial syndactyly between the third, fourth, and fifth fingers. Such relative shortness of the fourth and fifth metacarpals *may develop* postnatally by earlier than usual fusion of the respective metacarpoepiphyseal plates. When this occurs, it tends to do so in the center of the epiphyseal plate first, yielding the radiographic appearance of a cone-shaped epiphysis. This is a nonspecific anomaly that may occur by itself or as one feature of a number of syndromes.

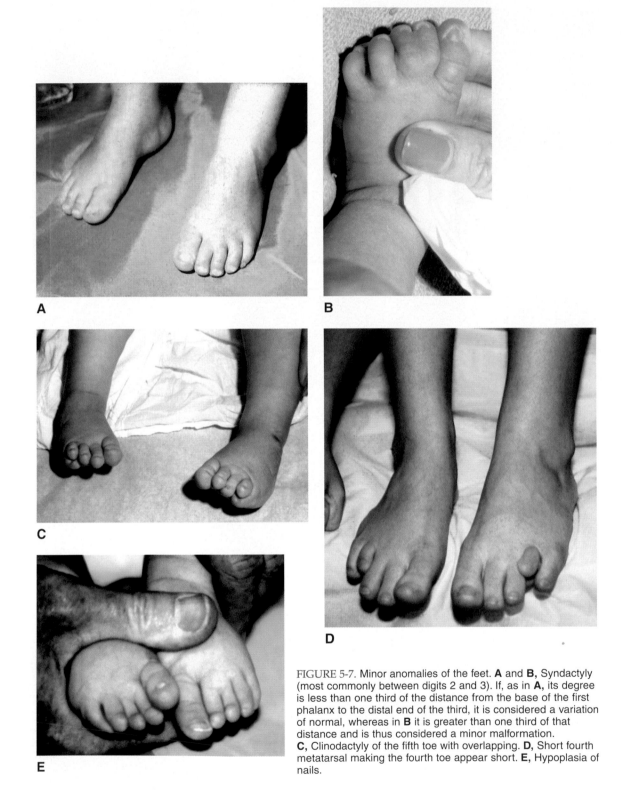

FIGURE 5-7. Minor anomalies of the feet. **A** and **B,** Syndactyly (most commonly between digits 2 and 3). If, as in **A,** its degree is less than one third of the distance from the base of the first phalanx to the distal end of the third, it is considered a variation of normal, whereas in **B** it is greater than one third of that distance and is thus considered a minor malformation. **C,** Clinodactyly of the fifth toe with overlapping. **D,** Short fourth metatarsal making the fourth toe appear short. **E,** Hypoplasia of nails.

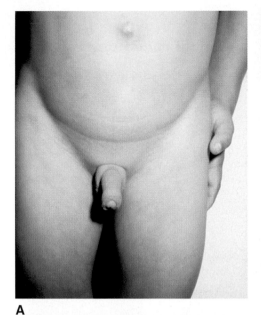

A

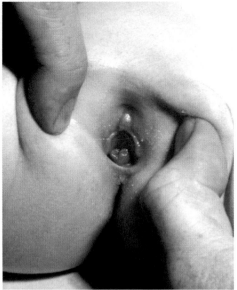

B

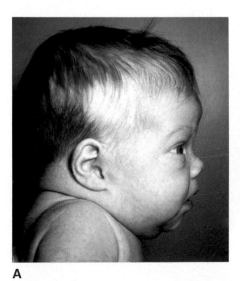

C

FIGURE 5-8. Minor anomalies of genitalia. **A,** Shawl scrotum appears to represent a mild deficit in the full migration of the labial-scrotal folds and as such may be accompanied by other signs of incomplete masculinization of the external genitalia. This photo shows a patient with the Aarskog syndrome. **B,** Hypoplasia of the labia, which may in some cases give rise to the false visual impression of a large clitoris. **C,** Median raphe is due to testosterone-induced fusion of the labioscrotal folds in a normal male. It is never seen in a 46,XX individual unless there has been abnormal secretion of androgen.

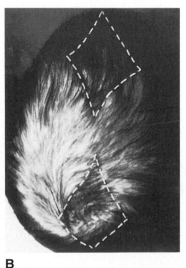

A

B

FIGURE 5-9. **A** and **B,** Unusually large fontanels, especially the posterior fontanel, in a 6-week-old baby with athyrotic hypothyroidism. The fetal onset of retarded osseous maturation is also evident in the immature facial bone development. (From Smith DW, Popich G: J Pediatr 80:753, 1972, with permission.)

ity to arrive at a specific overall diagnosis. Dermal ridge patterning may be evaluated with a seven-power illuminated magnifying device such as an otoscope or a stamp collector's flashlight, which has a wider field of vision. Permanent records may be obtained by a variety of techniques.[3,5,17] There are two general categories of dermatoglyphic alterations: an *aberrant pattern* and *unusual frequency* or *distribution of a particular pattern on the fingertips*.

Aberrant Patterning

Distal Axial Palmar Triradius

Triradii occur at the junction of three sets of converging ridges (Fig. 5-10*A*). There are usually no triradii between the base of the palm and the interdigital areas of the upper palm. However, patterning in the hypothenar area often gives rise to a distal axial triradius located, by definition, greater

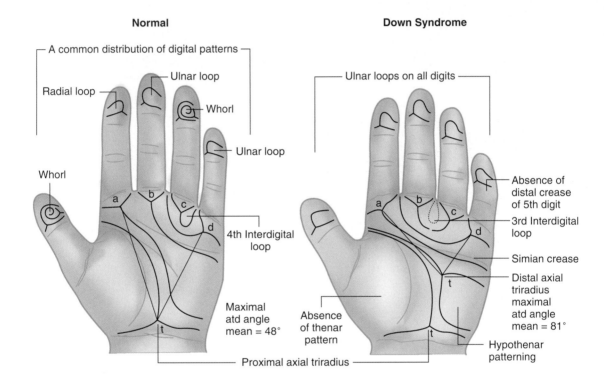

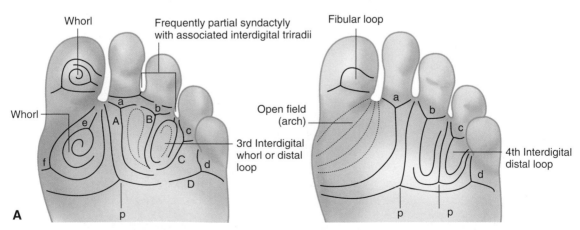

FIGURE 5-10. **A,** The *solid lines* and *dotted lines* denote the dermal ridge configurations. (**A,** Courtesy of Dr. M. Bat-Miriam; prepared by Mr. R. Lee of the Kennedy-Galton Center near St. Albans, England.) *Continued*

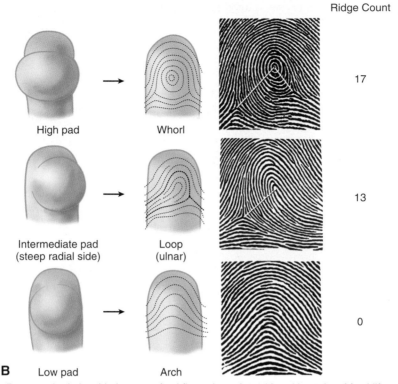

Ridge Count

High pad → Whorl   17

Intermediate pad → Loop   13
(steep radial side)   (ulnar)

B Low pad → Arch   0

Fig. 5-10, cont'd. B, Presumed relationship between fetal fingertip pads at 16 to 19 weeks of fetal life and the fingertip dermal ridge pattern, which develops at that time. Technique for dermal ridge counting: A line is drawn between the center of the pattern and the more distal triradius, and the number of ridges that touch this line is the fingertip ridge count. The sum of the ten fingertip ridge counts is the total ridge count; this average is 144 in the male and 127 in the female. (**B,** From Holt S: Br Med Bull 17:247, 1961, with permission.)

than 35% of the distance from the wrist crease to the crease at the base of the third finger. This alteration, found in approximately 4% of whites, is a frequent feature in a number of patterns of malformation.

Open Field in Hallucal Area (Arch Tibial)

Open field simply means that there is a relative lack of complexity in patterning, and it thereby implies a low surface contour in that area at the time that ridges developed (see Fig. 5-10*A*). The hallucal area of the sole usually has a loop or whorl pattern, and a lack of such a pattern is unusual in the normal individual; however, it is found in approximately 50% of patients with the Down syndrome and as an occasional feature in other syndromes.

Lack of Ridges

The failure of development of ridges in an area, most commonly the hypothenar region of the palm,

is an occasional but nonspecific feature in the deLange syndrome.

Other Patterns

There are a number of other unusual patterns, especially in the upper palmar, hypothenar, and thenar areas, which may be of clinical significance, but these are so rarely of value in an individual case that they will not be discussed.

Unusual Frequency or Distribution of Patterns on the Fingertips

High Frequency of Low-Arch Configurations

It is unusual to find a normal person with more than six of ten fingertips having a low-arch configuration; however, this is a frequent feature in the trisomy 18 syndrome and the XXXXY syndrome, presumably reflecting hypoplasia of the fetal fingertip pads in these disorders. High frequency of low arches is nonspecific, being an occasional finding in certain other syndromes and in approximately 0.9% of normal individuals.

High Frequency of Whorl Patterning

It is unusual to find nine or more fingertip whorls in an individual (3% in normal persons). Excessive patterning, presumably reflecting prominent fetal pads, is more likely to be found in the 45X syndrome, the Smith-Lemli-Opitz syndrome, occasionally in other patterns of malformation, and in some normal individuals.

Unusual Distribution, Especially of Radial Loop Patterns

Loops opening to the radial side of the hand are unusual on the fourth and fifth fingers. Radial loop patterns on these fingers are more common in people with Down syndrome (12.4%) than in individuals who are normal (1.5%).

HAIR: ORIGIN AND RELEVANCE OF ABERRANT SCALP AND UPPER FACIAL HAIR PATTERNING AND GROWTH

The origin and relevance of hair directional patterning and aberrant hair growth[15] will be considered individually.

Hair Directional Patterning

Normal Development and Relevance

The origin of the sloping angulation of each hair follicle, which determines the surface hair directional patterning, is derived from the direction of stretch on the surface skin during the time the hair follicle is growing down from it into the loose underlying mesenchyme, as shown in Figure 5-11. Over the scalp and upper face, this directional patterning reflects the plane of growth stretch on the surface skin that was exerted by the growth of underlying structures during the period of hair follicle downgrowth, which takes place from 10 to 16 weeks of fetal life. Thus the parietal hair whorl, or crown, is interpreted as representing the focal point from which the posterior scalp skin was under growth tension exerted by the dome-like outgrowth of the early brain during this fetal period (Fig. 5-12). Its location is normally several cen-

timeters anterior to the position of the posterior fontanel. Fifty-six percent of single parietal hair whorls are located to the right of the midline; 30% are left-sided, and 14% are midline in location. Five percent of normal individuals have bilateral parietal hair whorls. From the posterior whorl, the parietal hair stream flares out progressively, sweeping anteriorly to the forehead. Over the frontal region, the growth of the forebrain and the upper face results in bilateral frontal hair streams that emanate from the fixed points of the ocular puncta and tend to arc outward in a lateral direction, thereby affecting eyebrow hair directional patterning (Fig. 5-13). The anterior parietal hair stream normally converges with the upsweeping frontal hair stream on the forehead, resulting in a variety of forehead hair patterning, such as converging whorls and quadriradial patterns. If the frontal hair stream meets the parietal hair stream above the forehead, there may be an anterior upsweep of the scalp hair, known as a "cowlick." Mild-to-moderate lateral upsweep or central upsweep of the scalp hair occurs in 5% of normal individuals.

Defects of the calvarium, such as primary craniosynostosis, have not been noted to affect hair patterning, because the calvarium is not yet developed at the time of hair follicle downgrowth.

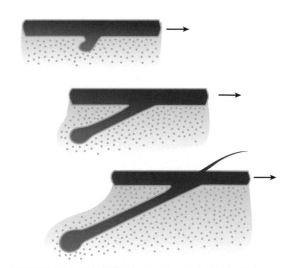

FIGURE 5-11. Hair follicles over the scalp begin their downgrowth into the loose underlying mesenchyme at 10 fetal weeks. The slope of each hair follicle and thereby the hair directional patterning is determined by the direction of growth stretch (*arrows*) exerted on the surface skin by the development of underlying tissues. For the scalp hair, the patterning relates to the growth in size and form of the underlying brain during the period of 10 to 16 weeks. By 18 weeks, when hairs are extruded onto the surface, their patterning is set. (From Smith DW, Gong BT: Teratology 9:17, 1974. Copyright © 1974. Reprinted with permission of Wiley-Liss, Inc., a subsidiary of John Wiley & Sons, Inc.)

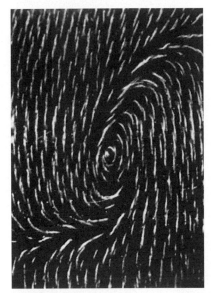

FIGURE 5-12. Parietal hair whorl at 18 weeks. This appears to be the fixed focal point from which the skin is being stretched by the dome-like outgrowth of the brain between 10 and 16 weeks. (From Smith DW, Gong BT: Teratology 9:17, 1974. Copyright © 1974. Reprinted with permission of Wiley-Liss, Inc., a subsidiary of John Wiley & Sons, Inc.)

which occurs from 10 to 16 weeks of fetal development.

Hair Growth Patterns

Normal Development and Relevance

At 18 fetal weeks, when hair first emerges, it grows on the entire face and scalp. Later, the eyebrows and scalp hair predominate, and the growth of hair over the remainder of the face is apparently suppressed. Studies imply that there is a periocular zone of hair growth suppression.

Nature and Relevance of Aberrant Facial Hair Growth Patterns

The V-shaped midline, downward projection of the scalp hair, known as the "widow's peak," is considered to represent an upper forehead intersection of the bilateral fields of periocular hair growth suppression.[14] This may occur because the fields are widely spaced, as in ocular hypertelorism, or

Relevance and Nature of Aberrant Scalp and Upper Facial Hair Directional Patterning

Abnormal size or shape of the brain and upper facial area during the 10- to 16-week fetal period can apparently result in aberrant hair patterning. Severe microcephaly may lead to a lack of a parietal hair whorl (25%) or a frontal upsweep of the scalp hair (70%), as shown in Figure 5-14. This feature appears to relate to the individual who has a narrow and smaller frontal area of the brain.

The parietal whorl is more likely to be midline and posteriorly located in patients with microcephaly, as shown in Figure 5-15. In a variety of other gross defects of early brain development, the hair directional patterning may be secondarily altered. In each case, the aberrant scalp hair patterning reflects the altered shape or growth of the early fetal brain. Gross aberrations of hair patterning often imply a serious degree of mental deficiency, because the brain is at such an early stage of development at 10 to 16 weeks (Fig. 5-16). Abnormal eyebrow patterning, such as the unusual outflaring of the medial eyebrows of the patient shown in Figure 5-17, implies that there was abnormal shape or growth in the upper midface before or during the period of hair follicle downgrowth,

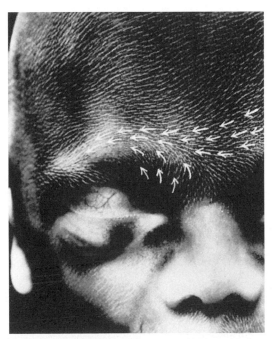

FIGURE 5-13. Frontal hair stream at 18 weeks, arcing laterally from the ocular punctum to meet with the downsweeping parietal hair stream. The frontal hair stream has been influenced by the growth of the underlying upper facial structures and the forebrain. (From Smith DW, Gong BT: Teratology 9:17, 1974. Copyright © 1974. Reprinted with permission of Wiley-Liss, Inc., a subsidiary of John Wiley & Sons, Inc.)

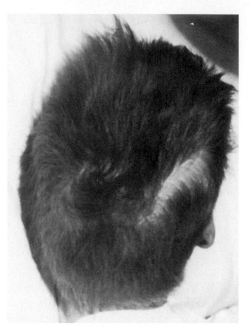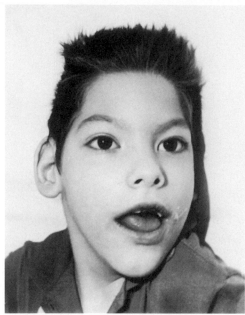

FIGURE 5-14. Hair patterning in a patient with primary microcephaly. The posterior scalp shows a lack of concise whorl, and the anterior scalp shows a marked frontal upsweep. These findings are interpreted as being the consequence of a deficit in growth of the brain before and during the period of hair follicle development and thus imply an early defect in morphogenesis of the brain before 10 to 16 weeks. (From Smith DW, Gong BT: Teratology 9:17, 1974. Copyright © 1974. Reprinted with permission of Wiley-Liss, Inc., a subsidiary of John Wiley & Sons, Inc.)

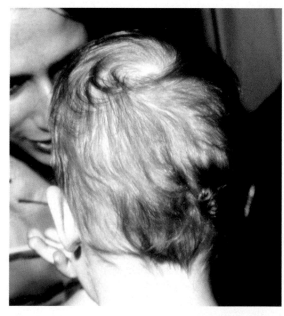

FIGURE 5-15. Posterior scalp hair of the type more commonly found in mild microcephaly, in this instance, the Down syndrome. The parietal whorl tends to be more central and posterior than usual, being over the former position of the posterior fontanel. This is considered secondary to the brain having been smaller and more symmetric than usual at 10 to 16 weeks, the time when the hair follicles develop. (From Smith DW, Gong BT: Teratology 9:17, 1974. Copyright © 1974. Reprinted with permission of Wiley-Liss, Inc., a subsidiary of John Wiley & Sons, Inc.)

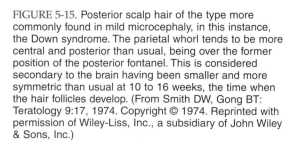

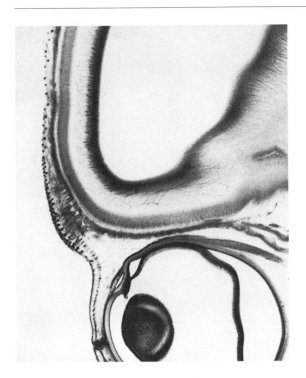

FIGURE 5-16. Sagittal section of forebrain area of a 10-week-old fetus, showing the early stage of cerebral cortical development and the lack of any organized calvarium at the time the hair follicles are beginning their downgrowth. (From Smith DW, Gong BT: Teratology 9:17, 1974. Copyright © 1974. Reprinted with permission of Wiley-Liss, Inc., a subsidiary of John Wiley & Sons, Inc.)

because the ocular fields of hair growth suppression are smaller with a low-scalp hairline and low position of intersection, as illustrated in Figure 5-18. In the presence of cryptophthalmos, there may be an abnormal projection of scalp-like hair growth toward the ocular area (Fig. 5-19). The auricle appears to influence hair growth in the region anterior to the ear. With absence of the auricle, there is usually absence of hair growth in the sideburn area (Fig. 5-20) anterior to the ear. When there is a rudimentary ear, such as is often found in Treacher Collins syndrome, there may be an aber-

rant tongue of hair growth projecting onto the cheek area.

Usually, a short neck or webbed neck may be associated with the secondary feature of a low posterior hairline, especially at the lateral borders, as shown in Figure 5-21.

Whether the facial body hirsutism found in patients with the de Lange syndrome and in a variety of failure to thrive growth deficiency disorders represents a more generalized failure of normal growth suppression in these conditions remains to be determined.

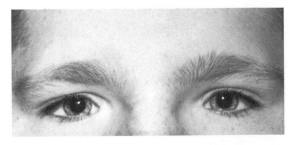

FIGURE 5-17. Aberrant mid-eyebrow patterning, which implies an aberration in growth or form of underlying facial structures by 10 to 16 fetal weeks. This patient has the Waardenburg syndrome, in which aberrant mid-upper facial development is a usual feature.

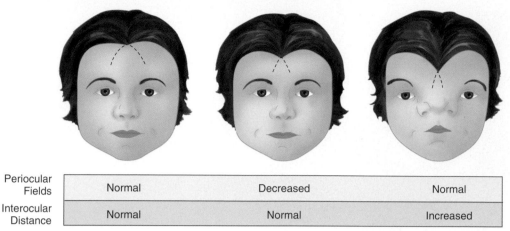

Periocular Fields	Normal	Decreased	Normal
Interocular Distance	Normal	Normal	Increased

FIGURE 5-18. If the eyes are widely spaced, or the area of periocular hair growth suppression is smaller than usual, the bilateral zones of periocular hair growth suppression may overlap at a lower point than usual, allowing for the presence of a widow's peak. The drawing on the right is of a patient with the frontonasal dysplasia anomaly. (From Smith DW, Cohen MM Jr: Lancet 2:1127, 1973, with permission.)

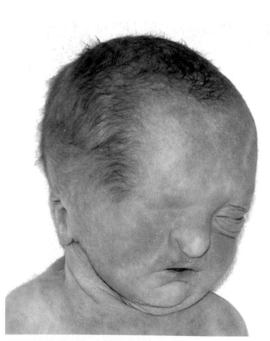

FIGURE 5-19. Aberrant growth of hair in lateral forehead area, related to the cryptophthalmos anomaly. (From Bergsma D, McKusick VA [eds]: National Foundation—Birth Defects. Baltimore: Williams & Wilkins, 1973, p 27, with permission.)

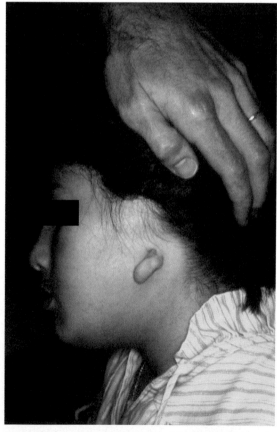

FIGURE 5-20. Lack of preauricular (sideburn) hair growth in relation to a deficit of auricular development.

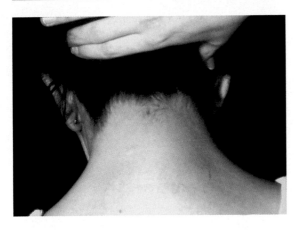

FIGURE 5-21. Low posterior hairline, usually related to either a short or webbed neck.

OTHER CUTANEOUS ANOMALIES

Cutaneous features such as unusual dimples and punched-out scalp lesions are shown in Figure 5-22. The skin normally grows in response to the growth of the structure that it invests. Tangential traction on the skin produced by external constraint can lead to redundant skin (Fig. 5-23).[1] Differentiation between talipes equinovarus caused by intrauterine constraint and talipes equinovarus caused by a neurologic problem that limits joint mobility can sometimes be made by observing the skin, which in the latter situation is taut and thin secondary to early onset of lack of movement in a fetus that has had ample space to move.

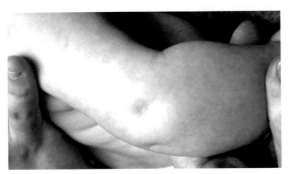

A

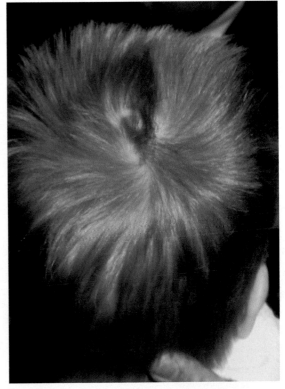

B

FIGURE 5-22. **A,** Unusual dimples may occur at a location where there has been a closer than usual proximity between the skin and underlying bony structures during fetal life, resulting in deficient development of subcutaneous tissue at that locus. Such dimples may be secondary either to a deficit in early subcutaneous tissue or to an aberrant bony promontory. They tend to occur at the elbows, at the knees, over the acromion promontories, and over the lower sacrum.
B, Punched-out scalp lesions are most commonly found toward the midline in the posterior parietal scalp area. The skin is usually totally lacking, but the crater becomes covered with scar tissue postnatally. The developmental pathology for these lesions is unknown.

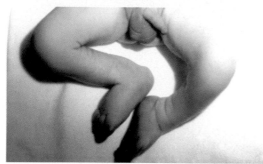

A

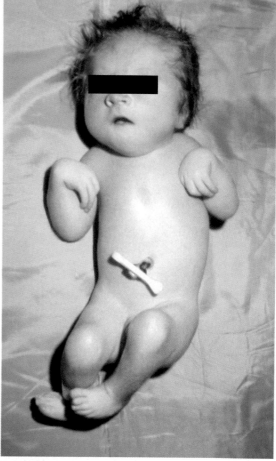

B

FIGURE 5-23. Redundant skin (**A**) is indicative of tangential traction produced by external constraint. Compare the redundant skin in **A** to the tight, thin skin over the joints in **B**, which is indicative of early onset lack of mobility secondary to neurologic impairment.

References

1. Aase JM: Structural defects as a consequence of late intrauterine constraint: Craniotabes, loose skin and asymmetric ear size. Semin Perinatol 7:237, 1983.
2. Aase JM: Diagnostic Dysmorphology. New York: Plenum Medical, 1990.
3. Aase JM, Lyons RB: Technique for recording dermatoglyphics. Lancet 1:32, 1971.
4. Davies P: Sex and the single transverse crease in newborn singletons. Dev Med Child Neurol 8:729, 1966.
5. Ford-Walker N: Inkless methods of finger, palm and sole printing. J Pediatr 50:27, 1957.
6. Graham JM: Recognizable Patterns of Human Deformation, 2nd ed. Philadelphia: WB Saunders, 1988.
7. Jones MC: Unilateral epicanthal folds: Diagnostic significance. J Pediatr 108:702, 1986.
8. Leppig KA et al: Predictive value of minor anomalies: Association with major malformations. J Pediatr 110:530, 1987.
9. Marden PM, Smith DW, McDonald MJ: Congenital anomalies in the newborn infant, including minor variations. J Pediatr 64:357, 1964.
10. Mehes K et al: Minor malformation in the neonate. Helv Pediatr Acta 28:477, 1973.
11. Mulvihill J, Smith DW: Genesis of dermal ridge patterning. J Pediatr 75:1969.
12. Popich GA, Smith DW: The genesis and significance of digital and palmar hand creases: Preliminary report. J Pediatr 77:1917, 1970.
13. Popich GA, Smith DW: Fontanels: Range of normal size. J Pediatr 80:479, 1972.
14. Smith DW, Cohen MM Jr: Widow's peak scalp anomaly, origin and relevance to ocular hypertelorism. Lancet 2:1127, 1973.
15. Smith DW, Gong BT: Scalp hair patterning as a clue to early fetal brain development. J Pediatr 83:374, 1973, and Teratology 9:17, 1974.
16. Smith DW, Popich GA: Large fontanels in congenital hypothyroidism: A potential clue toward earlier recognition. J Pediatr 80:753, 1972.
17. Uchida IA, Soltan HC: Evaluation of dermatoglyphics in medical genetics. Pediatr Clin North Am 10:409, 1963.

6 Normal Standards

The following compilation of normal measurements is set forth as an aid in determining whether or not a given feature is abnormal. Such data may be especially useful when the visual impression is potentially misleading. For example, when the nasal bridge is low, the visual impression may falsely suggest ocular hypertelorism, and when the patient is obese, the hands may *appear* to be small. Besides comparing patient measurements with these normal cross-sectional population standards, it may be important to contrast the findings of the patient with those of his parents or siblings in an attempt to determine whether or not a given feature is unusual for that particular family.

These measurements have been predominantly obtained from whites; hence they may not be accurate for other racial groups. Separate data are presented for males and females, except for features that do not show significant differences between the sexes. For paired structures, the measurements are given for the right side. Many of the charts were kindly supplied by Dr. Murray Feingold from his Boston study of normal measurements. For normal measurements of structures not included in this chapter, the reader is referred to the excellent reference by Hall and colleagues, *Handbook of Normal Physical Measurements.*[1]

STANDARDS FOR HEIGHT AND WEIGHT

The growth charts for children (Figs. 6-1 to 6-12) were developed by the National Center for Health Statistics in collaboration with the National Center for Chronic Disease Prevention and Health Promotion.

Notes on Use

1. *Weight* is preferably taken in the nude; otherwise, the estimated weight of clothing is subtracted before plotting.
2. When a child is born earlier than 37 weeks' gestation preterm, the birth weight is plotted at the appropriate number of weeks on the preterm growth chart. Subsequent weights are plotted in relation to this "conception age"; thus, for a child born at 32 weeks, the 8-weeks-after-birth weight is plotted at B (birth) on the scale, the 12-week weight at 4 weeks after B, and so on. Length is plotted in the same manner.
3. *Supine length* (up to age 2.0 years) should be taken with the infant lying on a measuring table constructed for this purpose. One person holds the infant's head so that he looks straight upward (the lower borders of the eye sockets and the external auditory meati should be in the same vertical plane) and pulls very gently to bring the top of the head into contact with the fixed measuring board. A second person, the measurer, presses the infant's knees down into contact with the board, and, also pulling gently to stretch the infant out, holds the infant's feet, with the toes pointing directly upward. He brings the movable footboard to rest firmly against the infant's heels and reads the measurement to the last completed 0.1 cm.
4. *Standing height* should be taken without shoes, the child standing with heels and back in contact with an upright wall or preferably a statometer made for this purpose. [†]His head is held so that he looks straight forward, with the lower borders of the eye sockets on the same horizontal plane as the external auditory meati (i.e., head not with nose tipped upward). A right-angled block (preferably counterweighted) is slid down the wall until its bottom surface touches the child's head, and a scale fixed to the wall is read. During this measurement, the child should be told to stretch his neck to be as tall as possible, although care must be taken to prevent his heels from coming off the ground. The measurer should apply gentle but firm upward pressure under the mastoid processes to help the child stretch. In this way, the variation in height from morning to evening is minimized. Standing

height should be recorded to the last completed 0.1 cm.

OTHER STANDARDS

The reader will find charts showing normal measurements for head circumference, chest, hand, foot, inner and outer canthal distances, palpebral fissure length, fontanel, ear, penis, and testis (Figs. 6-13 to 6-25) after the growth charts.

Reference
1. Hall JG et al: Handbook of Normal Physical Measurements. New York: Oxford University Press, 1989.

CDC Growth Charts: United States

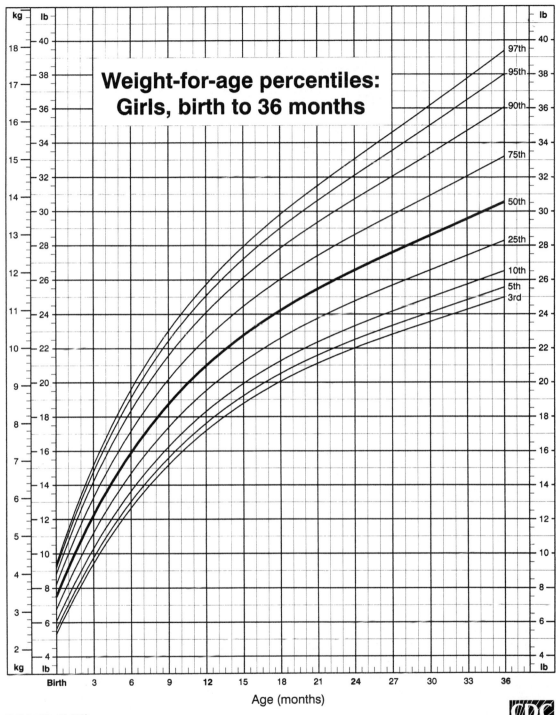

Weight-for-age percentiles: Girls, birth to 36 months

Age (months)

Published May 30, 2000.
SOURCE: Developed by the National Center for Health Statistics in collaboration with
the National Center for Chronic Disease Prevention and Health Promotion (2000).

SAFER·HEALTHIER·PEOPLE™

FIGURE 6-1. Weight-for-age percentiles: girls, birth to 36 months. (Developed by the National Center for Health Statistics in collaboration with the National Center for Chronic Disease Prevention and Health Promotion [2000].)

CDC Growth Charts: United States

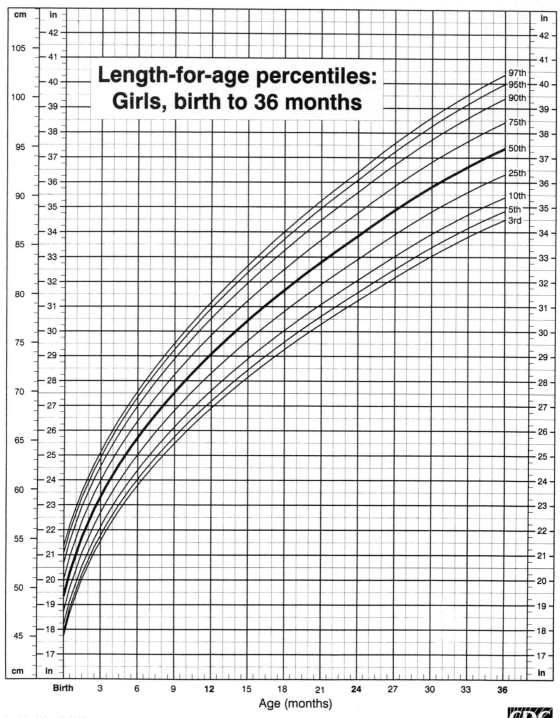

Length-for-age percentiles: Girls, birth to 36 months

Published May 30, 2000.
SOURCE: Developed by the National Center for Health Statistics in collaboration with
the National Center for Chronic Disease Prevention and Health Promotion (2000).

FIGURE 6-2. Length-for-age percentiles: girls, birth to 36 months. (Developed by the National Center for Health Statistics in collaboration with the National Center for Chronic Disease Prevention and Health Promotion [2000].)

CDC Growth Charts: United States

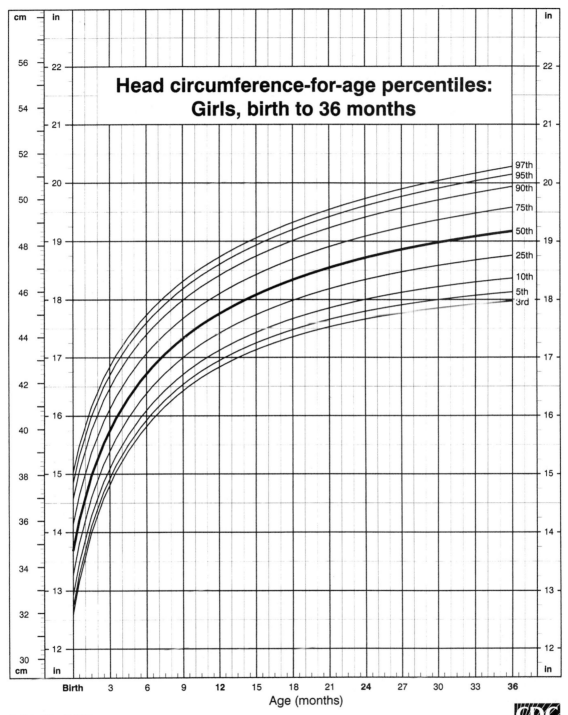

FIGURE 6-3. Head circumference-for-age percentiles: girls, birth to 36 months. (Developed by the National Center for Health Statistics in collaboration with the National Center for Chronic Disease Prevention and Health Promotion [2000].)

CDC Growth Charts: United States

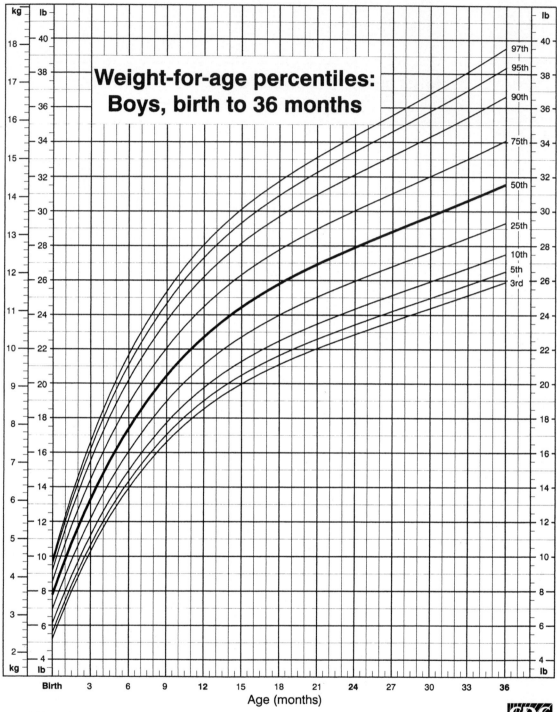

Weight-for-age percentiles: Boys, birth to 36 months

Published May 30, 2000.
SOURCE: Developed by the National Center for Health Statistics in collaboration with
the National Center for Chronic Disease Prevention and Health Promotion (2000).

SAFER・HEALTHIER・PEOPLE™

FIGURE 6-4. Weight-for-age percentiles: boys, birth to 36 months. (Developed by the National Center for Health Statistics in collaboration with the National Center for Chronic Disease Prevention and Health Promotion [2000].)

CDC Growth Charts: United States

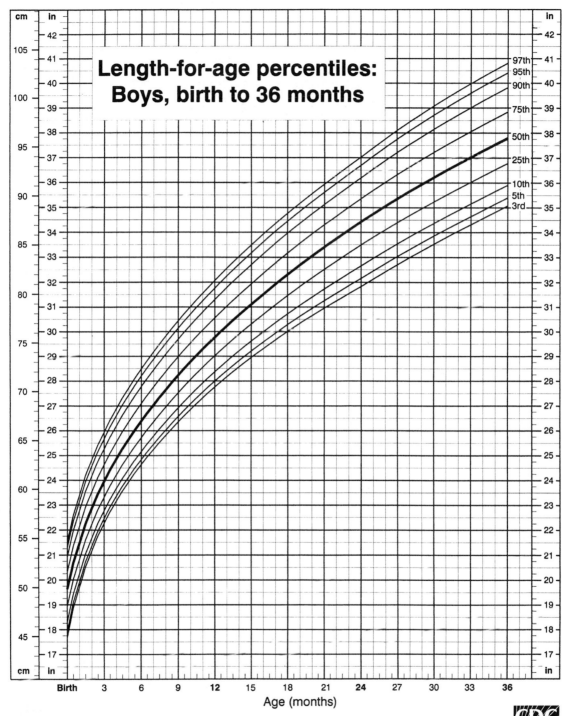

FIGURE 6-5. Length-for-age percentiles: boys, birth to 36 months. (Developed by the National Center for Health Statistics in collaboration with the National Center for Chronic Disease Prevention and Health Promotion [2000].)

CDC Growth Charts: United States

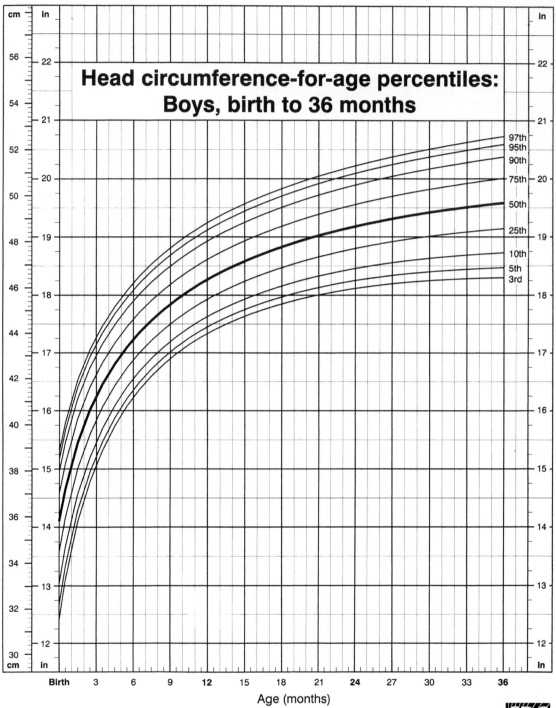

FIGURE 6-6. Head circumference-for-age percentiles: boys, birth to 36 months. (Developed by the National Center for Health Statistics in collaboration with the National Center for Chronic Disease Prevention and Health Promotion [2000].)

CDC Growth Charts: United States

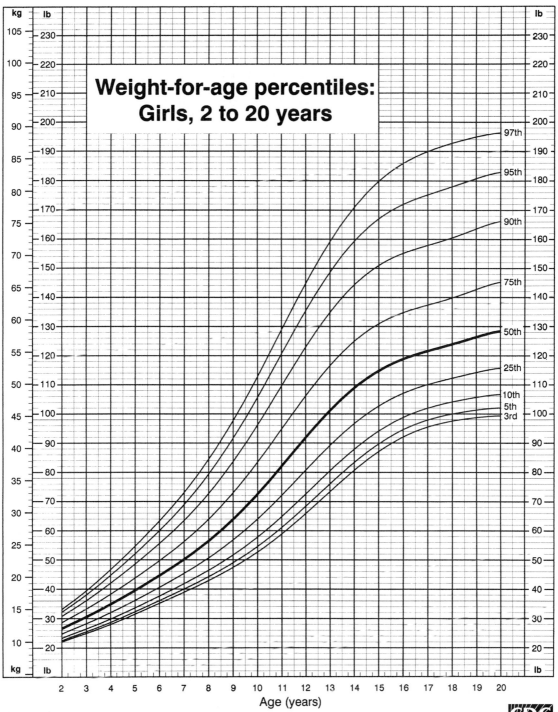

Weight-for-age percentiles: Girls, 2 to 20 years

Published May 30, 2000.
SOURCE: Developed by the National Center for Health Statistics in collaboration with the National Center for Chronic Disease Prevention and Health Promotion (2000).

FIGURE 6-7. Weight-for-age percentiles: girls, 2 to 20 years. (Developed by the National Center for Health Statistics in collaboration with the National Center for Chronic Disease Prevention and Health Promotion [2000].)

CDC Growth Charts: United States

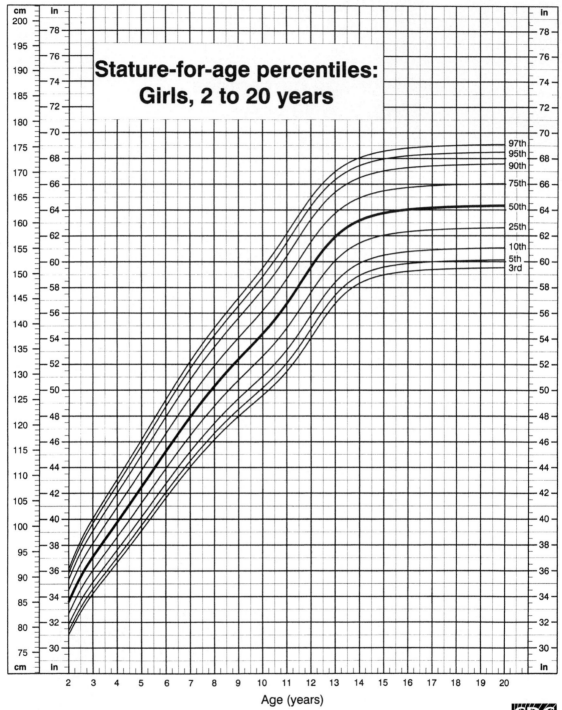

**Stature-for-age percentiles:
Girls, 2 to 20 years**

Age (years)

Published May 30, 2000.
SOURCE: Developed by the National Center for Health Statistics in collaboration with
the National Center for Chronic Disease Prevention and Health Promotion (2000).

SAFER·HEALTHIER·PEOPLE™

FIGURE 6-8. Stature-for-age percentiles: girls, 2 to 20 years. (Developed by the National Center for Health Statistics in collaboration with the National Center for Chronic Disease Prevention and Health Promotion [2000].)

CDC Growth Charts: United States

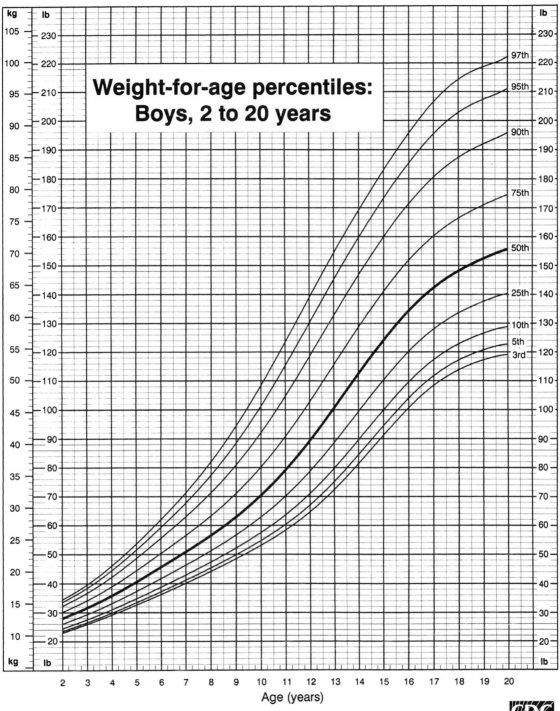

FIGURE 6-9. Weight-for-age percentiles: boys, 2 to 20 years. (Developed by the National Center for Health Statistics in collaboration with the National Center for Chronic Disease Prevention and Health Promotion [2000].)

CDC Growth Charts: United States

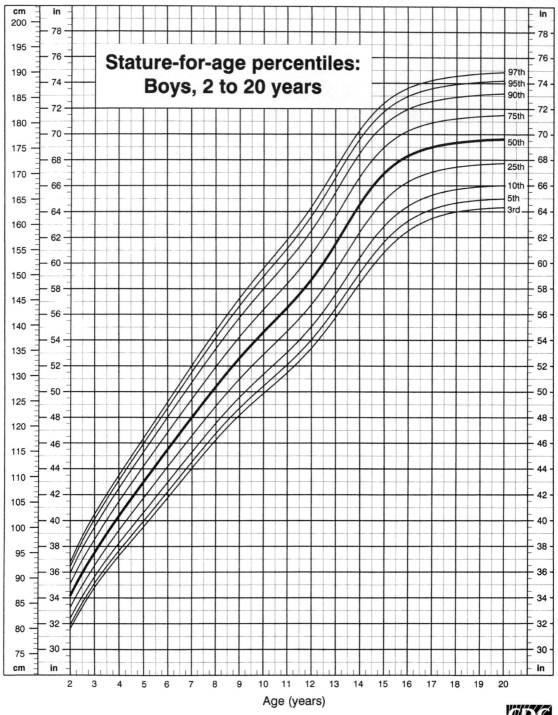

Published May 30, 2000.
SOURCE: Developed by the National Center for Health Statistics in collaboration with the National Center for Chronic Disease Prevention and Health Promotion (2000).

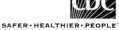

SAFER·HEALTHIER·PEOPLE™

FIGURE 6-10. Stature-for-age percentiles: boys, 2 to 20 years. (Developed by the National Center for Health Statistics in collaboration with the National Center for Chronic Disease Prevention and Health Promotion [2000].)

CDC Growth Charts: United States

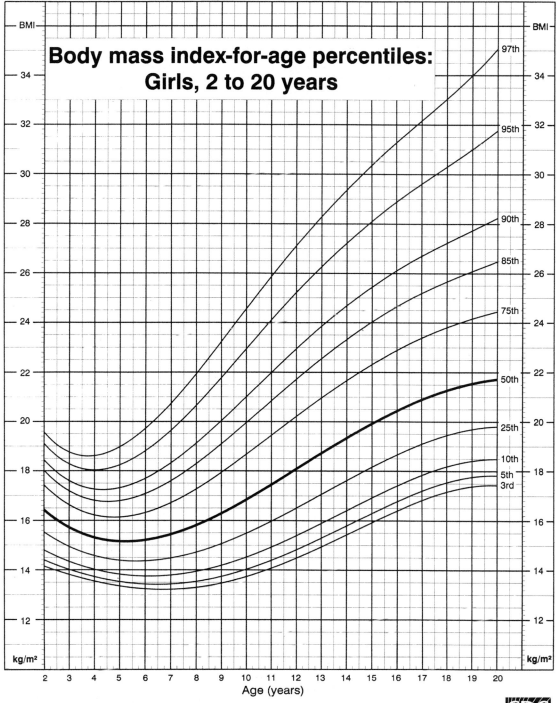

FIGURE 6-11. Body mass index-for-age percentiles: girls, 2 to 20 years. (Developed by the National Center for Health Statistics in collaboration with the National Center for Chronic Disease Prevention and Health Promotion [2000].)

CDC Growth Charts: United States

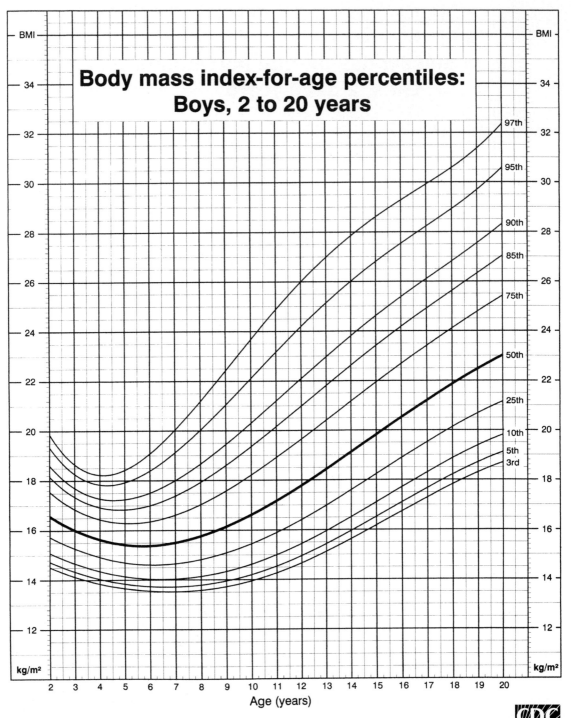

FIGURE 6-12. Body mass index-for-age percentiles: boys, 2 to 20 years. (Developed by the National Center for Health Statistics in collaboration with the National Center for Chronic Disease Prevention and Health Promotion [2000].)

HEAD CIRCUMFERENCES

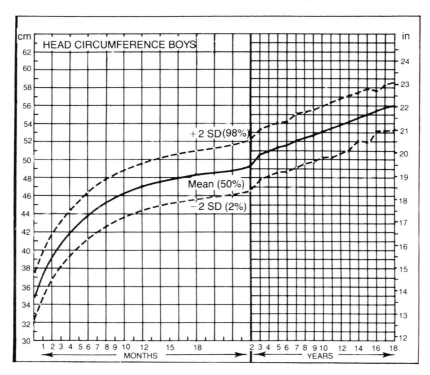

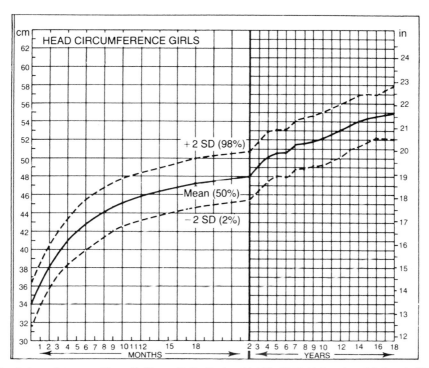

FIGURE 6-13. Head circumferences. (From Nellhaus G: Pediatrics 41:106, 1968. University of Colorado Medical Center Printing Services.)

CHEST MEASUREMENTS

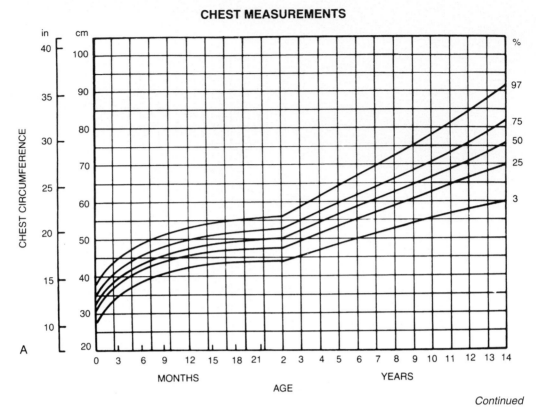

Continued

FIGURE 6-14. Chest circumference (**A**) and internipple distance (**B**). (From Feingold M, Bossert WH: Birth Defects 10[Suppl 13], 1974. With permission of the copyright holder, March of Dimes Birth Defects Foundation.)

CHEST MEASUREMENTS

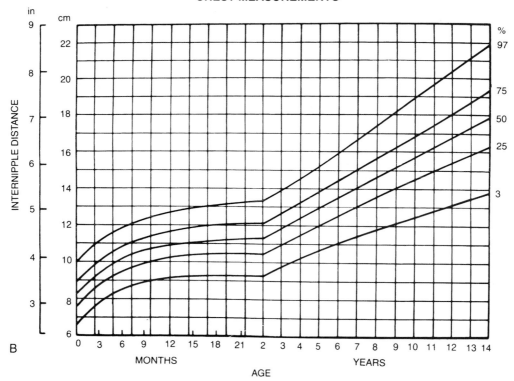

B

Fig. 6-14, cont'd.

HAND MEASUREMENTS

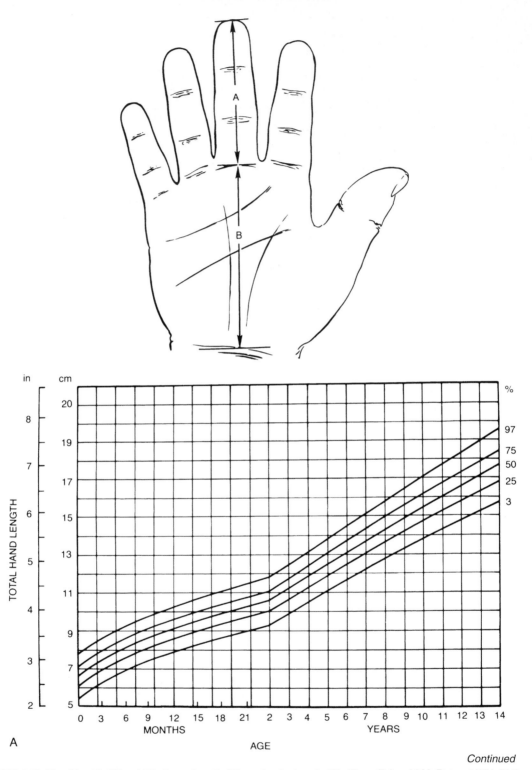

FIGURE 6-15. Hand length (**A**), middle finger length (**B**), and palm length (**C**). (From Feingold M, Bossert WH: Birth Defects 10[Suppl 13], 1974. With permission of the copyright holder, March of Dimes Birth Defects Foundation.)

Continued

HAND MEASUREMENTS

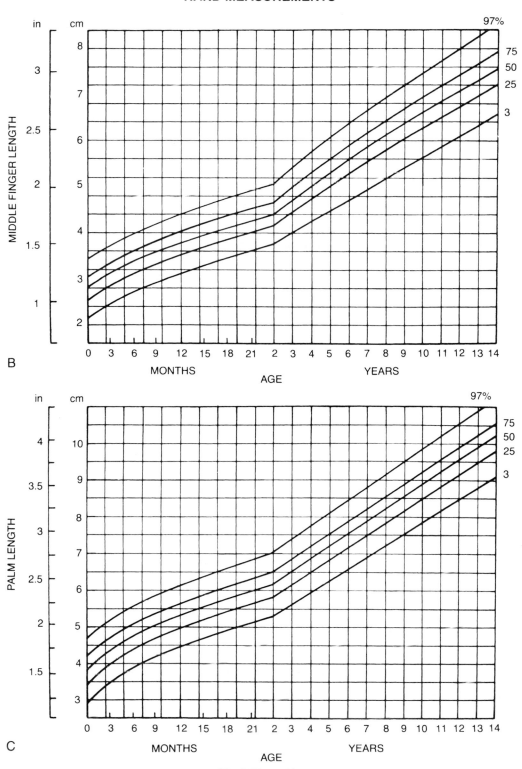

Fig. 6-15, cont'd.

HAND MEASUREMENTS

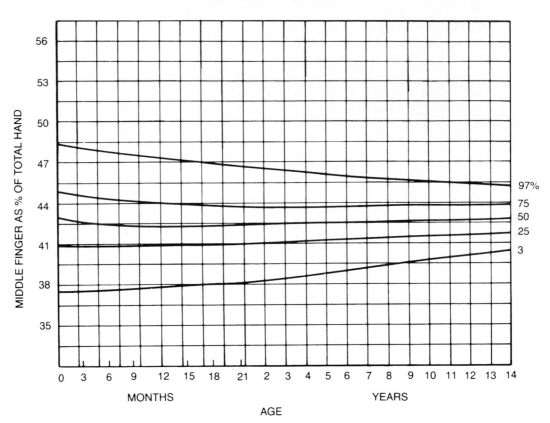

FIGURE 6-16. Proportion (percent) of middle finger to hand length. (From Feingold M, Bossert WH: Birth Defects 10[Suppl 13], 1974. With permission of the copyright holder, March of Dimes Birth Defects Foundation.)

FOOT LENGTH

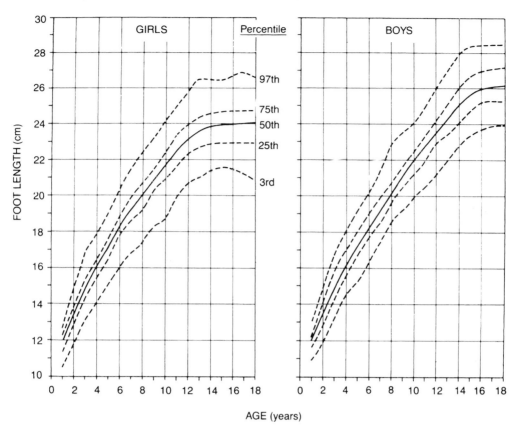

AGE (years)

FIGURE 6-17. Mean and percentile values for foot length. Note that because the adolescent growth spurt of the foot usually begins prior to the general linear growth spurt and ends before final height attainment, the foot growth spurt is a good early indicator of adolescence. (Adapted from Blais MM, Green WT, Anderson M: J Bone Joint Surg 38-A:998, 1956, with permission.)

FACIAL MEASUREMENTS

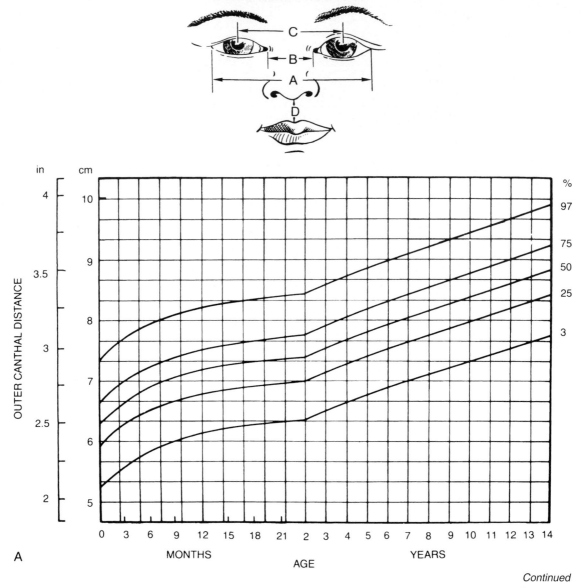

A

Continued

FIGURE 6-18. Outer canthal (**A**), inner canthal (**B**), and interpupillary (**C**) measurements. (From Feingold M, Bossert WH: Birth Defects 10[Suppl 13], 1974. With permission of the copyright holder, March of Dimes Birth Defects Foundation.)

FACIAL MEASUREMENTS

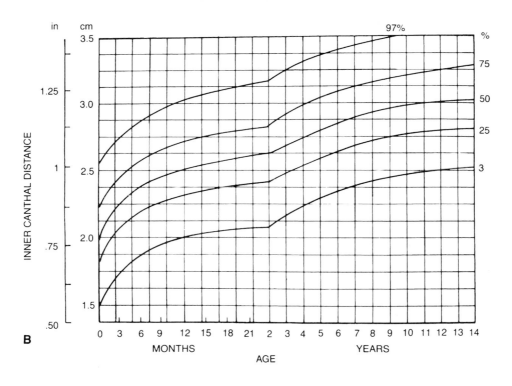

B

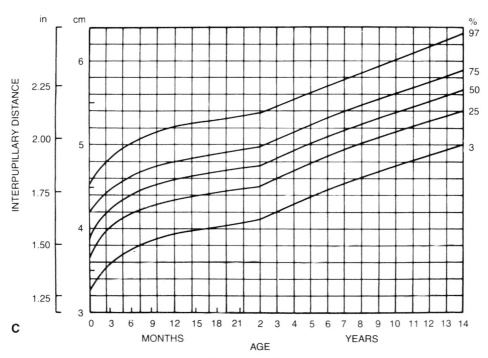

C

Fig. 6-18, cont'd.

EYE MEASUREMENTS

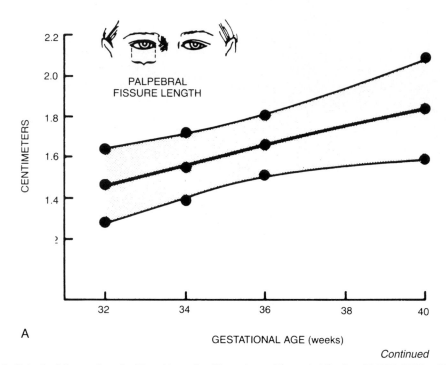

A

Continued

FIGURE 6-19. **A,** Palpebral fissure length, 32 to 40 weeks. (From Jones KL et al: J Pediatr 92:787, 1978, with permission.) **B,** Relationship of palpebral fissure length to age in white American children. (From Thomas IT, Gaitantzis YA, Frias JL: J Pediatr 111:267–268, 1987, with permission.)

PALPEBRAL FISSURE LENGTH

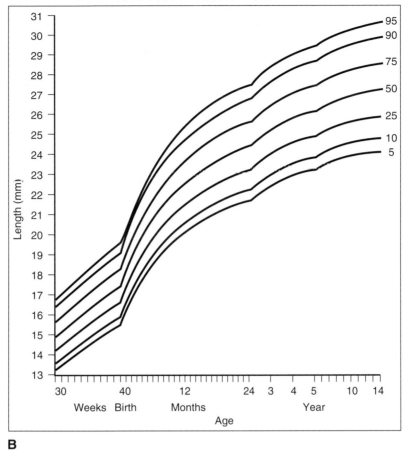

B

Fig. 6-19, cont'd.

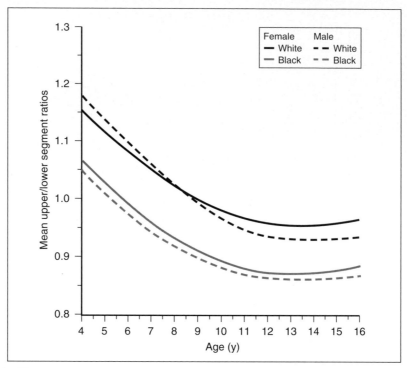

FIGURE 6-20. Ethnic differences in mean upper-to-lower segment ratios. (Data from McKusick VA: Heritable Disorders of Connective Tissue, 4th ed. St. Louis: Mosby, 1971.)

EAR LENGTH

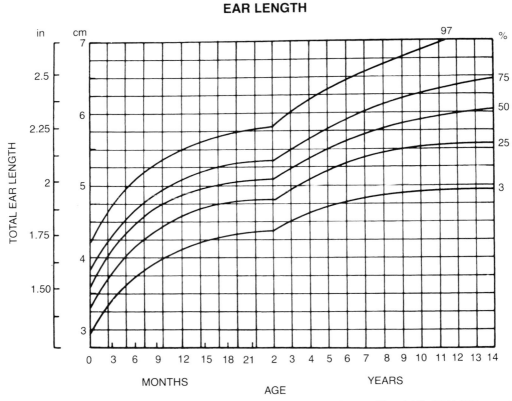

FIGURE 6-21. Maximum ear length. (From Feingold M, Bossert WH: Birth Defects 10[Suppl 13], 1974. With permission of the copyright holder, March of Dimes Birth Defects Foundation.)

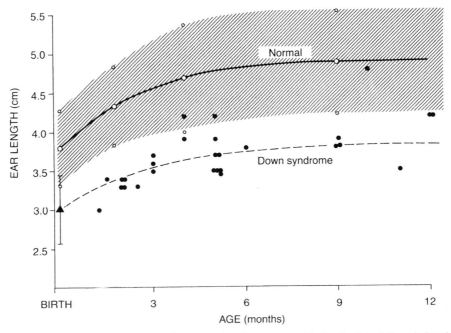

FIGURE 6-22. Ear length in normals during the first year, showing mean and 2 standard deviations in hatched area, as contrasted with ear length in Down syndrome, showing mean and 2 standard deviations for 26 affected newborns and individual values (*black dots*) during the first year. (From Aase JM et al: J Pediatr 82:845, 1973, with permission.)

PENILE LENGTH

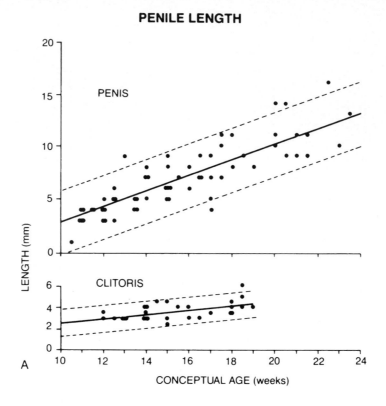

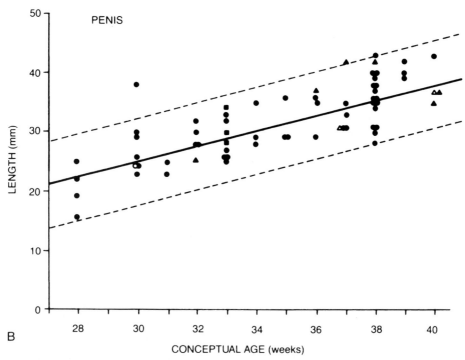

FIGURE 6-23. **A,** Growth of the penis contrasted with growth of the clitoris from formalin-fixed fetuses. **B,** Penile stretched length (from pubic bone to tip of glans) in the newborn. The mean full-term length is 3.5 cm with a 2 standard deviation range, from 2.8 to 4.2 cm. The *solid line* approximates the mean values, and the *broken lines* the 2 standard deviation values. (From Feldman KW, Smith DW: J Pediatr 86:395, 1975, with permission.)

PENILE AND TESTICULAR GROWTH

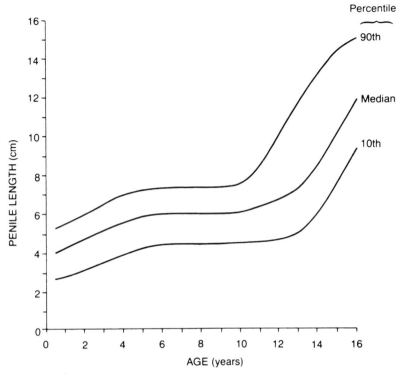

FIGURE 6-24. Penile growth in stretched length (from the pubic ramus to the tip of the glans) from infancy into adolescence. (From Schonfeld WA: Am J Dis Child 65:535, 1943, with permission.)

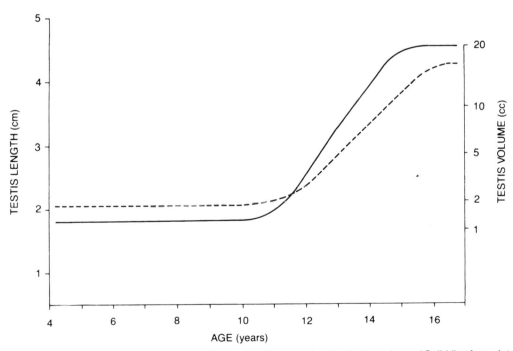

FIGURE 6-25. Testicular growth in length, adapted from normal standards of testicular volume. (*Solid line* from data of A. Prader, Zurich; *broken line* from data of Laron A, Zilka E: J Clin Endocrinol Metab 29:1409, 1969.)

APPENDIX I:

Pattern of Malformation Differential Diagnosis by Anomalies

The following lists were developed from the syndromes delineated in Chapter 1. Listed for each anomaly are the syndromes in which this defect is a frequent feature, as well as those syndromes in which it is an occasional feature. Characteristics such as mental or growth deficiency are not considered because they are frequent features in a large number of disorders.

The anomalies are set forth under the following headings:

1. Central Nervous System Dysfunction Other Than Mental Deficiency
2. Deafness
3. Brain: Major Anomalies
4. Cranium
5. Scalp and Facial Hair Patterning
6. Facies
7. Ocular Region
8. Eye
9. Nose
10. Maxilla and Mandible
11. Oral Region and Mouth
12. Teeth
13. External Ears
14. Neck, Thorax, and Vertebrae
15. Limbs
16. Limbs: Nails, Creases, Dermatoglyphics
17. Limbs: Joints
18. Skin and Hair
19. Cardiac
20. Abdominal
21. Renal
22. Genital
23. Endocrine and Metabolism
24. Immune Deficiency
25. Hematology-Oncology
26. Unusual Growth Patterns

1. CENTRAL NERVOUS SYSTEM DYSFUNCTION OTHER THAN MENTAL DEFICIENCY

Hypotonicity

Frequent in

Achondroplasia	390
Acrocallosal S.	252
Angelman S.	220

Bannayan-Riley-Ruvalcaba S.	610
Blepharophimosis S. (variable)	260
Börjeson-Forssman-Lehmann S.	668
Cardio-Facio-Cutaneous (CFC) S.	131
Cerebro-Oculo-Facio-Skeletal (COFS) S.	190
Coffin-Lowry S.	312
Coffin-Siris S.	666
Cohen S.	228
Deletion 3p S.	32
Deletion 4p S.	36
Deletion 9p S.	44
Deletion 18p S.	60
Deletion 4q S.	38
Deletion 11q S.	54
Deletion 18q S.	62
Deletion 22q11.2 S.	298
Down S.	7
Ehlers-Danlos S.	558
FG S.	316
Generalized Gangliosidosis S., Type I (Severe Infantile Type)	518
Hypophosphatasia	442
Johanson-Blizzard S.	106
Kabuki S.	118
Killian/Teschler-Nicola S. (infancy)	230
Lenz Microphthalmia S.	306
Langer-Giedion S.	324
Marden-Walker S.	248
Marfan S.	546
Marshall-Smith S.	172
Miller-Dieker S.	208
Mowat-Wilson S.	686
Mulibrey Nanism S.	98
1p36 Deletion S.	234
Opitz G/BBB S.	140
Osteogenesis Imperfecta S., Type II	565
Prader-Willi S. (infancy)	223
Rieger S.	680
Shprintzen-Goldberg S.	554
Simpson-Golabi-Behmel S.	178
Sotos S.	163
Spondyloepiphyseal Dysplasia Congenita	407
Stickler S.	318
Thanatophoric Dysplasia	382
Toriello-Carey S.	684
3C S.	254
22q13 Deletion S.	218

X-Linked α-Thalassemia/Mental
  Retardation (ATR-X) S. (infancy)   314
XXXXY S.   70
Zellweger S.   238

Occasional in

Atelosteogenesis, Type III   374
Blepharophimosis S.   260
Deletion 5p S.   40
Fetal Aminopterin/Methotrexate S.   658
Fragile X S.   160
Hyperthermia-Induced Spectrum of
  Defects   664
Multiple Endocrine Neoplasia,
  Type 2b   614
Myotonic Dystrophy S.   244
Tricho-Rhino-Phalangeal S.   328
Trisomy 13 S.   18
Weaver S.   168
Williams S.   120

Hypertonicity

Frequent in

Brachmann–de Lange S.   82
Deletion 18p S.   60
Hunter S.   532
Menkes S.   216
Schinzel-Giedion S.   250
Smith-Lemli-Opitz S.   114
Trisomy 18 S.   13
Weaver S.   168
X-Linked α-Thalassemia/Mental
  Retardation (ATR-X) S.   314

Occasional in

Cardio-Facio-Cutaneous (CFC) S.   131
Fragile X S.   160
Incontinentia Pigmenti S.   580
Oculodentodigital S.   302
Sturge-Weber Sequence   572
Trisomy 13 S.   18
Wiedemann-Rautenstrauch S.   150
Xeroderma Pigmentosa S.   642
X-Linked Hydrocephalus Spectrum   202

Ataxia

Frequent in

Angelman S.   220
Ataxia-Telangiectasia S. (onset 1 to 5 years)   213
Cockayne S.   154

Occasional in

Oculodentodigital S.   302
Xeroderma Pigmentosa S.   642
XXY S.   68

Seizures

Frequent in

Acrocallosal S.   252
Angelman S.   220
Autosomal Recessive Chondrodysplasia
  Punctata   440
Coffin-Siris S.   666
Deletion 4p S.   36
Deletion 9p S.   44
Deletion 11q S.   54
DiGeorge Sequence   714
Duplication 3q S.   34
Encephalocraniocutaneous Lipomatosis   604
Fetal Varicella S.   662
FG S.   316
Generalized Gangliosidosis S., Type I
  (Severe Infantile Type)   518
Hypomelanosis of Ito   584
Killian/Teschler-Nicola S.   230
Linear Sebaceous Nevus Sequence   576
Menkes S.   216
Miller-Dieker S.   208
Neurocutaneous Melanosis Sequence   574
1p36 Deletion S.   234
Schinzel-Giedion S.   250
Sturge-Weber Sequence   572
Trisomy 13 S.   18
Tuberous Sclerosis S.   586
X-Linked α-Thalassemia/Mental
  Retardation (ATR-X) S.   314
Zellweger S.   238

Occasional in

Adams-Oliver S.   356
Ataxia-Telangiectasia S.   213
Atelosteogenesis, Type III   374
Baller-Gerold S.   492
Bannayan-Riley-Ruvalcaba S.   610
Börjeson-Forssman-Lehmann S.   668
Cardio-Facio-Cutaneous (CFC) S.   131
Cat-Eye S.   64
Catel-Manzke S.   322
Cerebro-Oculo-Facio-Skeletal
  (COFS) S.   190
Cockayne S.   154
Cohen S.   228
Crouzon S.   478
de Lange S.   82

Occasional in

2. DEAFNESS

Frequent in

3. BRAIN: MAJOR ANOMALIES

Anencephaly/Meningomyelocele

Occasional in

Encephalocele

Frequent in

Occasional in

Holoprosencephaly

Frequent in

Occasional in

Monozygotic (MZ) Twinning and Structural
    Defects—General   748
Pallister-Hall S.   200
Smith-Lemli-Opitz S.   114
Triploidy S.   28

Lissencephaly

Frequent in

Acrocallosal S. (polymicrogyria)   252
Adams-Oliver S.   356
Kabuki S. (polymicrogyria)   118
Killian/Teschler-Nicola S. (polymicrogyria)   230
Miller-Diekcr S.   208
Neu-Laxova S.   194
Seckel S. (polymicrogryia)   108
Sturge-Weber Sequence   572
Walker-Warburg S.   260

Dandy-Walker Malformation

Frequent in

3C S.   254
Walker-Warburg S.   206

Occasional in

Branchio-Oculo-Facial S. (agenesis of vermis)   274
Chondroectodermal Dysplasia   422
Coffin-Siris S.   666
Fetal Warfarin S.   656
Fryns S.   236
Jeune Thoracic Dystrophy   386
Laterality Sequences   698
Marden-Walker S.   248
Meckel-Gruber S.   198
Neurocutaneous Melanosis Sequence   574
Neu-Laxova S.   194
Opitz G/BBB S. (hypoplastic vermis)   140
Oral-Facial-Digital S., Type VI   292
Oto-Palato-Digital S., Type II   310
Pallister-Hall S.   200
Radial Aplasia–Thrombocytopenia S.
    (hypoplastic vermis)   364
Retinoic Acid Embryopathy   660
Short Rib–Polydactyly S., Type II
    (Majewski Type) (small vermis)   380
Simpson-Golabi-Behmel S. (hypoplastic
    vermis)   178
Sotos S. (hypoplastic vermis)   163
Toriello-Carey S.   684
Trisomy 9 Mosaic S.   26
XXXXX S.   74

XYY S.   66
Yunis-Varon S. (hypoplastic vermis)   466

Agenesis of Corpus Callosum

Frequent in

Acrocallosal S.   252
Cerebro-Oculo-Facio-Skeletal (COFS) S.   190
FG S.   316
Fryns S.   236
Marden-Walker S.   248
Meckel-Gruber S.   198
Microphthalmia–Linear Skin Defects S.   626
Miller-Dieker S.   208
Neu-Laxova S.   194
Septo-Optic Dysplasia Sequence   708
Toriello-Carey S.   684
Walker-Warburg S.   206
Zellweger S.   238

Occasional in

Apert S.   474
Baller-Gerold S.   492
Carpenter S.   484
Cerebro-Costo-Mandibular S.   688
Coffin-Siris S.   666
Congenital Microgastria–Limb Reduction
    Complex   744
Crouzon S.   478
Deletion 11q S.   54
Deletion 22q11.2 S.   298
Fanconi Pancytopenia S.   362
Fetal Alcohol S.   646
Fetal Warfarin S.   656
FG S.   316
45X S.   76
Frontonasal Dysplasia Sequence   268
Gorlin S.   616
Greig Cephalopolysyndactyly S.   486
Hydrolethalus S.   204
Lenz-Majewski Hyperostosis S.   458
Lenz Microphthalmia S.   306
Marshall-Smith S.   172
Mowat-Wilson S.   686
Oculo-Auriculo-Vertebral Spectrum   738
Opitz G/BBB S.   140
Oral-Facial-Digital S.   292
Peters'-Plus S.   682
Radial Aplasia–Thrombocytopenia S.   364
Rubinstein-Taybi S.   88
Seckel S.   108
Simpson-Golabi-Behmel S.   178
Smith-Lemli-Opitz S.   114
Trisomy 8 S.   22

Hydrocephalus

Frequent in

Occasional in

Microcephaly

Frequent in

Macrocephaly

Frequent in

Occasional in

Occasional in

Frontal Bossing or Prominent Central Forehead

Frequent in

Occasional in

5. SCALP AND FACIAL HAIR PATTERNING

Anterior Upsweep, Scalp

Frequent in

Occasional in

Posterior Midline Scalp Defects

Frequent in

"Coarse" Facies

Frequent in

Occasional in

7. OCULAR REGION

Hypotelorism

Frequent in

Occasional in

Hypertelorism

Frequent in

Short Palpebral Fissure

Frequent in

Occasional in

Lateral Displacement of Inner Canthi (Giving Rise to Short Palpebral Fissures)

Frequent in

Occasional in

Inner Epicanthal Folds

Frequent in

Frontometaphyseal Dysplasia (down) 450
Greig Cephalopolysyndactyly S. (down) 486
Hallermann-Streiff S. (down) 110
Levy-Hollister S. (down) 360
Peters'-Plus S. (up) 682
Prader-Willi S. (up) 223
Smith-Magenis S. (up) 210
Toriello-Carey S. (down) 684
Trisomy 13 S. (up) 18
Trisomy 18 S. (up) 13

Shallow Orbital Ridges

Frequent in

Apert S. 474
Cardio-Facio-Cutaneous (CFC) S. 131
Carpenter S. 484
Crouzon S. 478
Deletion 9p S. 44
Dubowitz S. 100
Fetal Aminopterin/Methotrexate S. 658
Marshall-Smith S. 172
Osteogenesis Imperfecta S., Type II 565
Roberts-SC Phocomelia 334
Saethre-Chotzen S. 468
Schinzel-Giedion S. 250
Trisomy 18 S. 13
Zellweger S. 238

Occasional in

Trisomy 13 S. 18

Prominent Supraorbital Ridges

Frequent in

Alagille S. 670
Börjeson-Forssman-Lehmann S. 668
Coffin-Lowry S. 312
Craniometaphyseal Dysplasia 448
Frontometaphyseal Dysplasia 450
Gorlin S. 616
Hypohidrotic Ectodermal Dysplasia 628
Langer-Giedion S. 324
Metaphyseal Dysplasia, Jansen Type 434
Oto-Palato-Digital S., Type I 308

Prominent Eyes

Frequent in

Anencephaly Sequence 704
Antley-Bixler S. 488
Apert S. 474

Beckwith-Wiedemann S. 174
Cardio-Facio-Cutaneous (CFC) S. 131
Craniometaphyseal Dysplasia 448
Crouzon S. 478
Fetal Aminopterin/Methotrexate S. 658
Fibrochondrogenesis 372
Floating-Harbor S. 144
GAPO S. 638
Kniest Dysplasia 410
Lenz-Majewski Hyperostosis S. 458
Mandibuloacral Dysplasia 692
Marshall S. 282
Marshall-Smith S. 172
Melnick-Needles S. 674
Metaphyseal Dysplasia, Jansen Type 434
Neu-Laxova S. 194
Pena-Shokeir Phenotype 188
Roberts-SC Phocomelia 334
Robinow S. 136
Schinzel-Giedion S. 250
Sclerosteosis 456
Seckel S. 108
Shprintzen-Goldberg S. 554
Stickler S. 318

Occasional in

de Lange S. 82
Langer-Giedion S. 324
Pfeiffer S. 472

Periorbital Fullness of Subcutaneous Tissue

Frequent in

Athyrotic Hypothyroidism Sequence 710
GAPO S. 638
Leroy I-Cell S. 520
Williams S. 120

Eyebrows Extending to Midline (Synophrys)

Frequent in

de Lange S. 82
Deletion 3p S. 32
Deletion 9p S. 44
Duplication 3q S. 34
Hajdu-Cheney S. 444
Sanfilippo S. 536
Smith-Magenis S. 210
Waardenburg S. 278

Occasional in

Unusual Flare of Medial Eyebrow

Frequent in

Ptosis of Eyelid or Blepharophimosis

Frequent in

Occasional in

Lacrimal Defects

Frequent in

Occasional in

Strabismus

Frequent in

Nystagmus

Frequent in

Occasional in

Occasional in

8. EYE

Myopia

Frequent in

Bardet-Biedl S.	676
Branchio-Oculo-Facial S.	274
Coffin-Siris S.	666
Cohen S.	228
Down S.	7
Kniest Dysplasia	410
Marfan S.	546
Marshall S.	282
Menkes S.	216
Noonan S.	124
Rubinstein-Taybi S.	88
Schwartz-Jampel S.	246
Shprintzen-Goldberg S.	554
Smith-Magenis S.	210
Spondyloepiphyseal Dysplasia Congenita	407
Stickler S.	318

Occasional in

Angelman S.	220
Beals S.	552
de Lange S.	82
Deletion 5p S.	40
Deletion 18q S.	62
Ehlers-Danlos S.	558
Fetal Alcohol S.	646
Frontometaphyseal Dysplasia S.	450
Fragile X S.	160
Geleophysic Dysplasia	420
Noonan S.	124
1p36 Deletion S.	234
Proteus S.	600
Scheie S.	528
XXXXY S.	70

Blue Sclerae

Frequent in

Marshall-Smith S.	172
Osteogenesis Imperfecta S., Type I	562
Osteogenesis Imperfecta S., Type II	565
Roberts-SC Phocomelia	334
Russell-Silver S.	92

Occasional in

Aarskog S.	134
Ehlers-Danlos S.	558
45X S.	76

Hallermann-Streiff S.	110
Hypophosphatasia	442
Incontinentia Pigmenti S.	580
Kabuki S.	118
Marfan S.	546
Trisomy 18 S.	13

Microphthalmos

Frequent in

Branchio-Oculo-Facial S.	274
Cerebro-Oculo-Facio-Skeletal (COFS) S.	190
CHARGE S.	276
Deletion 4p S.	36
Deletion 13q S.	56
Duplication 10q S.	49
Frontonasal Dysplasia Sequence	268
Goltz S.	622
Hallermann-Streiff S.	110
Hydrolethalus S.	204
Lenz Microphthalmia S.	306
Meckel-Gruber S.	198
Microphthalmia–Linear Skin Defects S.	626
Oculodentodigital S.	302
Triploidy S.	28
Trisomy 13 S.	18
Walker-Warburg S.	206

Occasional in

Adams-Oliver S.	356
Albright Hereditary Osteodystrophy	516
Aniridia–Wilms Tumor Association	52
Blepharophimosis S.	260
Cat-Eye S.	64
Chondrodysplasia Punctata, X-Linked Dominant Type	437
Cohen S.	228
Congenital Microgastria–Limb Reduction Complex	744
Deletion 18q S.	62
Distichiasis-Lymphedema S.	696
Dubowitz S.	100
Duplication 3q S.	34
Encephalocraniocutaneous Lipomatosis	604
Fanconi Pancytopenia S.	362
Fetal Alcohol S.	646
Fetal Valproate S.	654
Fetal Varicella S.	662
Fetal Warfarin S.	656
Fraser S.	270
Fryns S.	236
Hyperthermia-Induced Spectrum of Defects	664
Incontinentia Pigmenti S.	580
Linear-Sebaceous Nevus Sequence	576

Marden-Walker S.	248
Neu-Laxova S.	194
Oculo-Auriculo-Vertebral Spectrum	738
Pallister-Hall S.	200
Proteus S.	600
Roberts-SC Phocomelia	334
Smith-Lemli-Opitz S.	114
Treacher Collins S.	280
Trisomy 9 Mosaic S.	26
Trisomy 18 S.	13

Colobomata of Iris

Frequent in

Aniridia–Wilms Tumor Association (aniridia)	52
Branchio-Oculo-Facial S.	274
Cat-Eye S.	64
CHARGE S.	276
Deletion 4p S.	36
Deletion 13q S.	56
Goltz S.	622
Rieger S.	680
Triploidy S.	28
Trisomy 13 S.	18
Walker-Warburg S.	206

Occasional in

Beals S.	552
Cohen S.	228
Crouzon S.	478
Deletion 4p S.	36
Deletion 11q S.	54
Deletion 18q S.	62
Dubowitz S.	100
Duplication 3q S.	34
Duplication 10q S.	49
Fetal Hydantoin S.	652
Frontonasal Dysplasia Sequence	268
Gorlin S.	616
Langer-Giedion S.	324
Linear Sebaceous Nevus Sequence	576
Marfan S.	546
Microphthalmia–Linear Skin Defects S.	626
Meckel-Gruber S.	198
Mulibrey Nanism S.	98
Noonan S.	124
Oculo-Auriculo-Vertebral Spectrum	738
1p36 Deletion S.	234
Pallister-Hall S.	200
Rubinstein-Taybi S.	88
Smith-Lemli-Opitz S.	114
Smith-Magenis S.	210
Sturge-Weber Sequence	572
3C S.	254

Trisomy 18 S.	13
XXXXX S.	74

Iris, Unusual Patterning or Coloration

Frequent in

Angelman S. (pale blue)	220
Down S. (Brushfield spots)	7
Ectrodactyly–Ectodermal Dysplasia–Clefting S. (blue)	330
Fragile X S. (pale blue)	160
Nail-Patella S. ("cloverleaf")	504
Marfan S. (hypoplastic)	546
Neurofibromatosis S. (Lisch nodules)	590
Oculodentodigital S. (fine, porous)	302
Smith-Magenis S. (brushfield spots)	210
Sotos S. (hypoplastic)	163
Waardenburg S. (heterochromia)	278
Williams S. (stellate)	120

Occasional in

Hypomelanosis of Ito	584
Klippel-Trenaunay S. (heterochromia)	598
Mowat-Wilson S.	686
Prader-Willi S. (blue)	223
Smith-Lemli-Opitz S.	114
Smith-Magenis S. (Brushfield spots)	210
Sturge-Weber Sequence (heterochromia)	572
Triploidy S. (heterochromia)	28
XXXY S. (Brushfield spots)	70
Zellweger S. (Brushfield spots)	238

Glaucoma

Frequent in

GAPO S.	638
Kniest S.	410
Marshall S.	282
Peters'-Plus S.	682
Rieger S.	680
Stickler S.	318

Occasional in

Aase S.	366
Aniridia–Wilms Tumor Association	52
Bardet-Biedl S.	676
Chondrodysplasia Punctata, X-Linked Dominant Type	437
Duplication 3q S.	34
Ehlers-Danlos S.	558
Gorlin S.	616
Hallermann-Streiff S.	110

Large Cornea

Frequent in

Occasional in

Keratoconus, Microcornea

Frequent in

Occasional in

Corneal Opacity

Frequent in

Occasional in

Cataract, Lenticular Opacities

Frequent in

Lens Dislocation

Frequent in

Occasional in

Retinal Pigmentation

Frequent in

Occasional in

9. NOSE

Low Nasal Bridge

Prominent Nasal Bridge

Broad Nasal Bridge

Broad Nasal Root

Frequent in

Small or Short Nose, with or without Anteverted Nostrils

Frequent in

Occasional in

Hypoplasia of Nares and/or Alae Nasi

Frequent in

Prominent Nose (Relative)

Choanal Atresia

10. MAXILLA AND MANDIBLE

Malar Hypoplasia

Maxillary Hypoplasia, Often with Narrow or High-Arched Palate

Micrognathia

Prognathism

Frequent in

Occasional in

11. ORAL REGION AND MOUTH

Cleft Lip with or without Cleft Palate

Frequent in

Occasional in

Abnormal Philtrum

Frequent in

Prominent Full Lips

Frequent in

Occasional in

Lower Lip Pits

Frequent in

Occasional in

Downturned Corners of Mouth

Frequent in

Microstomia

Frequent in

Occasional in

Macrostomia

Frequent in

Cleft Palate or Bifid Uvula without Cleft in Lip

Frequent in

Oral Frenula (Webs)

Frequent in

Occasional in

Cleft or Irregular Tongue

Frequent in

Occasional in

Macroglossia

Frequent in

Occasional in

Microglossia

Frequent in

Oromandibular-Limb Hypogenesis Spectrum	742

Occasional in

Distal Arthrogryposis S., Type II	184
Freeman-Sheldon S.	242
Hydrolethalus S.	204
Lenz-Majewski Hyperostosis S.	458
Moebius Sequence	258
Mulibrey Nanism S.	98
Pallister-Hall S.	200
Short Rib–Polydactyly, Type II (Majewski Type)	380
Smith-Lemli-Opitz S.	114

Hypertrophied Alveolar Ridges

Frequent in

Costello S.	128
Generalized Gangliosidosis S., Type I (Severe Infantile Type)	518
Hunter S.	532
Hurler S.	524
Leroy I-Cell S.	520
Menkes S.	216
Robinow S.	136
Shprintzen-Goldberg S.	554

Occasional in

Killian/Teschler-Nicola S.	230

Broad Secondary Alveolar Ridges

Frequent in

Fetal Hydantoin S.	652
Miller-Dieker S.	208
Oculodentodigital S.	302
Simpson-Golabi-Behmel S.	178
Smith-Lemli-Opitz S.	114
Sotos S.	163
Yunis-Varon S.	466

Abnormalities of Larynx

Frequent in

Fraser S. (atresia)	270
Hydrolethalus S. (hypoplasia)	204
Multiple Endocrine Neoplasia, Type 2b (neuromata)	614

Opitz G/BBB S. (cleft)	140
Pallister-Hall S. (cleft)	200
Pfeiffer S.	472
Robin Sequence (glossoptosis)	262
Short Rib–Polydactyly S., Type II (Majewski Type) (hypoplasia)	380
Toriello-Carey S.	684

Occasional in

Apert S. (tracheal)	474
Atelosteogenesis, Type I	374
Campomelic Dysplasia	388
Cerebro-Costo-Mandibular S. (trachea)	688
Chondrodysplasia Punctata, X-Linked Dominant Type (tracheal stenosis)	437
Deletion 22q11.2 S. (web)	298
Diastrophic Dysplasia (stenosis)	424
Fetal Valproate S.	654
Fraser S. (subglottic stenosis)	270
Frontometaphyseal Dysplasia (subglottic narrowing)	450
Geleophysic Dysplasia (tracheal stenosis)	420
Larsen S. (mobile arytenoid cartilage)	498
Levy-Hollister S. (hypoplastic epiglottis)	360
Marshall-Smith S.	172
Meckel-Gruber S. (cleft epiglottis)	198
Nager S. (hypoplasia)	288
Oculo-Auriculo-Vertebral Spectrum	738
Pachyonychia Congenita S. (obstructed)	640
Smith-Lemli-Opitz S.	114
Smith-Magenis S.	210
Sternal Malformation–Vascular Dysplasia Spectrum	746
Treacher Collins S. (hypoplasia)	280
Ulnar-Mammary S.	342
VATERR Association (stenosis)	756
Wiedemann-Rautenstrauch S. (laryngomalacia)	150
Yunis-Varon S. (glossoptosis)	466

12. TEETH

Anodontia (Aplasia)

Frequent in

Albright Hereditary Osteodystrophy	516
Chondroectodermal Dysplasia	422
Cleidocranial Dysostosis	462
Ectrodactyly–Ectodermal Dysplasia–Clefting S.	330
Frontometaphyseal Dysplasia	450
GAPO S. (pseudo-anodontia)	638
Hallermann-Streiff S.	110
Hay-Wells S. of Ectodermal Dysplasia	332

Occasional in

Hypodontia (including Conical Teeth)

Frequent in

Occasional in

Enamel Hypoplasia

Frequent in

Occasional in

Carious

Frequent in

Early Loss of Teeth

Frequent in

Occasional in

Irregular Placement of Teeth

Frequent in

Occasional in

Late Eruption of Teeth

Frequent in

Occasional in

Neonatal Teeth

Frequent in

Occasional in

Dental Cysts

Frequent in

Other Teeth Anomalies

Frequent in

Occasional in

13. EXTERNAL EARS

Low-Set Ears

Frequent in

Occasional in

Malformed Auricles

Frequent in

Occasional in

Preauricular Tags or Pits

Frequent in

Occasional in

14. NECK, THORAX, AND VERTEBRAE

Web Neck or Redundant Skin

Frequent in

Occasional in

Short Neck

Frequent in

Nipple Anomaly

Frequent in

Hypoplasia of Clavicles

Frequent in

Other Clavicular Anomalies

Frequent in

Acromesomelic Dysplasia (high, curved)	404
Ehlers-Danlos S., Type IX (short, broad)	558
Escobar S. (long, hooked)	346
Fibrochondrogenesis (thin)	372
Fryns S. (broad medial)	236
Hurler S. (wide-medial end)	524
Lenz-Majewski Hyperostosis S. (thick)	458
Lenz Microphthalmia S.	306
Oto-Palato-Digital S., Type II (thin, wavy)	310
Pyknodysostosis (dysplasia of acromion)	460
Restrictive Dermopathy (dysplastic)	196
Saethre-Chotzen S. (short)	468
Schinzel-Giedion S. (long)	250
Sclerosteosis	456
Short Rib–Polydactyly S., Type II (Majewski Type) (high)	380
Shprintzen-Goldberg S.	554
3-M S. (horizontal)	96

Occasional in

Aase S. (agenesis)	366
Albright Hereditary Osteodystrophy	516
Craniofrontonasal Dysplasia	482
Deletion 4p S.	36
Deletion 9p S.	44
Floating-Harbor S. (pseudarthrosis)	144
Holt-Oram S.	358
Nail-Patella S. (prominent)	504
Progeria S.	146
Radial Aplasia–Thrombocytopenia S.	364
Toriello-Carey S.	684
Trisomy 18 S. (incomplete ossification)	13

Pectus Excavatum or Carinatum

Frequent in

Aarskog S.	134
Beals S.	552
Bannayan-Riley-Ruvalcaba S.	610
Coffin-Lowry S.	312
Deletion 18p S.	60
Duplication 10q S.	49
Duplication 15q S.	58
Dyggve-Melchior-Clausen S.	412
45X S.	76
Marden-Walker S.	248
Marfan S.	546
Meier-Gorlin S.	508
Melnick-Needles S.	674
Morquio S.	538
Mucopolysaccharidosis VII	544

Multiple Endocrine Neoplasia, Type 2b	614
Multiple Lentigines S.	620
Noonan S.	124
Osteogenesis Imperfecta S., Type I	562
Oto-Palato-Digital S., Type I	308
Oto-Palato-Digital S., Type II	310
Schwartz-Jampel S.	246
Simpson-Golabi-Behmel S.	178
Shprintzen-Goldberg S.	554
Spondyloepiphyseal Dysplasia Congenita	407
Spondylometaphyseal Dysplasia, Kozlowski Type	414
3-M S.	96
XYY S.	66

Occasional in

Cardio-Facio-Cutaneous (CFC) S.	131
Catel-Manzke S.	322
Down S.	7
Fragile X S.	160
Geleophysic Dysplasia	420
Gorlin S.	616
Hallermann-Streiff S.	110
Holt-Oram S.	358
Kabuki S.	118
Miller S.	286
Mohr S.	296
Multiple Synostosis S.	494
Peters'-Plus S.	682
Proteus S.	600
Rieger S.	680
Robinow S.	136
Simpson-Golabi-Behmel S.	178
Stickler S.	318
Toriello-Carey S.	684
Tricho-Rhino-Phalangeal S.	328
Williams S.	120
XXXXY S.	70

Short Sternum

Frequent in

Sternal Malformation–Vascular Dysplasia Spectrum	746
Trisomy 18 S.	13

Occasional in

Coffin-Lowry S.	312
Coffin-Siris S.	666
de Lange S.	82
Marshall-Smith S.	172
Multiple Synostosis S.	494
Popliteal Pterygium S.	344
Schinzel-Giedion S.	250

Small Thoracic Cage

Frequent in

Occasional in

Rib Defects Other Than Small Thorax

Frequent in

Occasional in

Scoliosis

Frequent in

Occasional in

Other Vertebral Defects (Usually as Part of Generalized Bone Disorder)

Frequent in

Other Vertebral Defects (Primarily Segmentation Defects)

Frequent in

Occasional in

Odontoid Hypoplasia/Cervical Spine Instability

Frequent in

Occasional in

15. LIMBS

Arachnodactyly

Frequent in

Occasional in

Fractures

Frequent in

Occasional in

Short Limbs

Frequent in

Occasional in

Limb Reduction, Moderate to Gross

Frequent in

Occasional in

Small Hands and Feet, including Brachydactyly

Frequent in

Occasional in

Clinodactyly of Fifth Fingers

Frequent in

Occasional in

Thumb Hypoplasia to Aplasia, Triphalangeal Thumb

Frequent in

Occasional in

Radius Hypoplasia to Aplasia

Frequent in

Occasional in

Metacarpal Hypoplasia—All Metacarpals

Frequent in

Metacarpal Hypoplasia—Third, Fourth, and/or Fifth

Metacarpal Hypoplasia—First Metacarpal with Proximal Placement of Thumb

Metatarsal Hypoplasia

Polydactyly

Broad Thumb and/or Toe

Frequent in

Occasional in

Syndactyly, Cutaneous or Osseous

Frequent in

Occasional in

Fetal Aminopterin/Methotrexate S.
(synostosis) 658
Fetal Hydantoin S. 652
Fibrodysplasia Ossificans Progressiva S.
(short hallux with synostosis) 568
Hallermann-Streiff S. 110
Hay-Wells S. of Ectodermal Dysplasia 332
Hydrolethalus S. 204
Hyperthermia-Induced Spectrum of Defects 664
Hypomelanosis of Ito 584
Incontinentia Pigmenti S. 580
Klippel-Trenaunay S. 598
Langer-Giedion S. 324
Levy-Hollister S. 360
Limb–Body Wall Complex 736
McKusick-Kaufman S. 678
Meckel-Gruber S. 198
Moebius Sequence 258
Multiple Synostosis S. 494
Nager S. (toes) 288
Neurofibromatosis S. 590
Oromandibular-Limb Hypogenesis Spectrum 742
Osteogenesis Imperfecta S., Type I 562
Oto-Palato-Digital S., Type I 308
Peters'-Plus S. 682
Popliteal Pterygium S. 344
Prader-Willi S. 223
Radial Aplasia–Thrombocytopenia S. 364
Rapp-Hodgkin Ectodermal Dysplasia 632
Rubinstein-Taybi S. 88
Russell-Silver S. 92
Schinzel-Giedion S. 250
Thanatophoric Dysplasia 382
3C S. 254
Townes-Brocks S. 290
Tricho-Rhino-Phalangeal S. 328
Trisomy 13 S. 18
Trisomy 18 S. 13
22q13 Deletion S. (second and third toes) 218
Yunis-Varon S. 466

Elbow Dysplasia and Cubitus Valgus

Frequent in

Antley-Bixler S. (fused) 488
Apert S. (synostosis) 474
Cerebro-Costo-Mandibular S. 688
Cohen S. 228
Costello S. 128
de Lange S. 82
45X S. 76
Larsen S. 498
Multiple Synostosis S. 494
Nail-Patella S. 504
Noonan S. 124

Oto-Palato-Digital S., Type I 308
Trisomy 8 S. 22
Weaver S. 168
XXXX S. 72
XXXXY S. 70
XXY S. (mild) 68

Occasional in

Aarskog S. 134
Acrodysostosis 514
Albright Hereditary Osteodystrophy 516
Crouzon S. (subluxed) 478
Deletion 18p S. 60
Marden-Walker S. (synostosis) 248
Melnick-Needles S. 674
Miller S. (synostosis) 286
Nager S. (synostosis) 288
Oculodentodigital S. 302
Peters'-Plus S. 682
Pfeiffer S. (synostosis) 472
Proteus S. 600
Saethre-Chotzen S. (synostosis) 468
Spondylocarpotarsal Synostosis S. 496
XYY S. 66
Zellweger S. 238

Patella Dysplasia

Frequent in

Coffin-Siris S. 666
Escobar S. 346
Meier-Gorlin S. 508
Multiple Epiphyseal Dysplasia 428
Nail-Patella S. 504

Occasional in

Baller-Gerold S. 492
Beals S. 552
Carpenter S. 484
Diastrophic Dysplasia 424
Rothmund-Thomson S. 157
Tibial Aplasia–Ectrodactyly S. 354
Trisomy 8 S. 22

16. LIMBS: NAILS, CREASES, DERMATOGLYPHICS

Nail Hypoplasia or Dysplasia

Frequent in

Acromesomelic Dysplasia (short) 404
Adams-Oliver S. (small) 356
Antley-Bixler S. (narrow) 488

Occasional in

Single Crease (Simian), Upper Palm

Frequent in

Occasional in

Distal Palmar Axial Triradius

Frequent in

Low-Arch Dermal Ridge Pattern on Majority of Fingertips

Whorl Dermal Ridge Pattern on Majority of Fingertips

Prominent Fingertip Pads

17. LIMBS: JOINTS

Joint Limitation and/or Contractures; Inability to Fully Extend (Other Than Foot)

Clubfoot—Especially Equinovarus Deformity, including Metatarsus Adductus

Frequent in

Occasional in

Clenched Hand: Index Finger Tending to Overlie the Third and the Fifth Finger Tending to Overlie the Fourth

Frequent in

Occasional in

Joint Hypermobility and/or Lax Ligaments

Frequent in

3-M S.	96
XXXXY S.	70

Occasional in

Bannayan-Riley-Ruvalcaba S.	610
Cardio-Facio-Cutaneous (CFC) S.	131
Dubowitz S.	100
Fragile X S. (hands)	160
Goltz S.	622
Killian/Teschler-Nicola S.	230
Langer-Giedion S.	324
Multiple Lentigines S.	620
Robinow S. (hands)	136
Toriello-Carey S.	684

Joint Dislocation

Frequent in

Atelosteogenesis, Type I	374
Campomelic Dysplasia	388
Coffin-Siris S. (elbow)	666
Distal Arthrogryposis S. (hip)	184
Dyggve-Melchior-Clausen S. (hip)	412
Ehlers-Danlos S.	558
Fetal Hydantoin S. (hip)	652
45X S. (hip)	76
Hajdu-Cheney S.	444
Langer-Giedion S.	324
Larsen S. (elbow, knee, hip)	498
Leri-Weill Dyschondrosteosis (wrist, elbow)	510
Oto-Palato-Digital S., Type I (elbow, hip)	308
Oto-Palato-Digital S., Type II (elbow, knee)	310
Trisomy 9 Mosaic S. (hip, knee, elbow)	26
XXXY and XXXXY S. (hip)	70
Yunis-Varon S. (hip)	466

Occasional in

Amyoplasia Congenital Disruptive Sequence (hip)	180
Autosomal Recessive Chondrodysplasia Punctata	440
Carpenter S. (fingers)	484
Catel-Manzke S.	322
Cat-Eye S. (hip)	64
Cerebro-Costo-Mandibular S. (hip)	688
Chondrodysplasia Punctata, X-Linked Dominant Type (patella)	437
Deletion 18p S. (hip)	60
Diastrophic Dysplasia (elbow, hip, knee)	424
Duplication 9p S. (hip, knee, elbow)	46
Escobar S. (hip)	346
Fanconi Pancytopenia S. (hip)	362

Fetal Aminopterin/Methotrexate S. (hip)	658
Freeman-Sheldon S. (hip)	242
Hurler S. (hip)	524
Kabuki S. (hip)	118
Killian/Teschler-Nicola S. (hip)	230
Lenz-Majewski Hyperostosis S. (hip)	458
Melnick-Needles S. (hip)	674
Miller S. (hip)	286
Nager S. (hip)	288
Nail-Patella S.	504
Neurofibromatosis S. (elbow)	590
Oculodentodigital S.	302
Oligohydramnios Sequence (hip)	726
1p36 Deletion S. (hip)	234
Osteogenesis Imperfecta S., Type I	562
Pallister-Hall S.	200
Popliteal Pterygium S.	344
Proteus S. (hip)	600
Radial Aplasia–Thrombocytopenia S. (hip, knee)	364
Robinow S. (hip, fingers)	136
Rubinstein-Taybi S. (radial head)	88
Russell-Silver S.	92
Schwartz-Jampel S. (hip)	246
Seckel S. (hip)	108
Shprintzen-Goldberg S.	554
Simpson-Golabi-Behmel S. (hip)	178
Smith-Lemli-Opitz S. (hip)	114
Spondyloepiphyseal Dysplasia Congenita (hip)	407
Stickler S. (hip)	318
3-M S.	96
XXXXX S.	74

18. SKIN AND HAIR

Loose Redundant Skin

Frequent in

Acrodysostosis (hands)	514
Acromesomelic Dysplasia (hands)	404
Cerebro-Costo-Mandibular S.	688
CHILD S.	348
Costello S.	128
Diastrophic Dysplasia	424
Early Urethral Obstruction Sequence	718
Ehlers-Danlos S. (hyperelastic)	558
45X S.	76
GAPO S. (drooping forehead)	638
Langer-Giedion S.	324
Lenz-Majewski Hyperostosis S.	458
Oligohydramnios Sequence	726
Pyknodysostosis (hands)	460
Weaver S.	168

Edema of Hands and Feet

Altered Skin Pigmentation, Melanomata

Thin Skin, Skin Defects

Thick or Ichthyotic

Frequent in

Cardio-Facio-Cutaneous (CFC) S.	131
CHILD S.	348
Chondrodysplasia Punctata, X-Linked Dominant Type	437
Clouston S.	636
Geleophysic Dysplasia	420
Hunter S. (nodular lesions)	532
Hurler S.	524
Hurler-Scheie S.	530
Leroy I-Cell S.	520
Neu-Laxova S.	194
Pachyonychia Congenita S.	640
Restrictive Dermopathy	196
Senter-KID S.	644
Wiedemann-Rautenstrauch S.	150

Occasional in

Autosomal Recessive Chondrodysplasia Punctata	440
Bloom S.	102
Deletion 11q S.	54
Deletion 18q S.	62
Maroteaux-Lamy Mucopolysaccharidosis S.	542
Menkes S.	216
Oral-Facial-Digital S.	292
Simpson-Golabi-Behmel S.	178
Werner S. (stiff)	152

Cutis Marmorata, Unusual

Frequent in

Adams-Oliver S.	356
Athyrotic Hypothyroidism Sequence	710
de Lange S.	82
Trisomy 18 S.	13

Occasional in

Cardio-Facio-Cutaneous S.	131
Down S.	7
Klippel-Trenaunay S.	598

Eczema

Frequent in

Cardio-Facio-Cutaneous (CFC) S.	131
Dubowitz S.	100

Occasional in

Deletion 18q S.	62
Hypohidrotic Ectodermal Dysplasia	628
Incontinentia Pigmenti S.	580
Shwachman S.	436

Hemangiomata and Vascular Malformations

Frequent in

Amyoplasia Congenita Disruptive Sequence (glabellar hemangioma)	180
Ataxia-Telangiectasia S. (telangiectases)	213
Beckwith-Wiedemann S. (glabellar hemangioma)	174
Bloom S. (telangiectases)	102
Branchio-Oculo-Facial S.	274
Goltz S.	622
Hereditary Hemorrhagic Telangiectasia (telangiectases)	612
Klippel-Trenaunay S.	598
Lethal Multiple Pterygium S. (glabellar hemangioma)	192
Maffucci S. (hemangiomata)	606
Occult Spinal Dysraphism Sequence	706
Pallister-Hall S. (glabellar hemangioma)	200
Proteus S.	600
Roberts-SC Phocomelia	334
Robinow S. (glabellar hemangioma)	136
Rothmund-Thomson S. (telangiectases)	157
Sternal Malformation–Vascular Dysplasia Spectrum	746
Sturge-Weber Sequence	572
Tuberous Sclerosis S.	586
Xeroderma Pigmentosa S.	642

Occasional in

Antley-Bixler S.	488
Baller-Gerold S. (facial hemangioma)	492
Bannayan-Riley-Ruvalcaba S.	610
Cardio-Facio-Cutaneous (CFC) S.	131
Coffin-Siris S.	666
Diastrophic Dysplasia (midface)	424
Fetal Alcohol S. (hemangiomata)	646
45X S.	76
Generalized Gangliosidosis S., Type I (Severe Infantile Type) (angiokeratomas)	518
Leroy I-Cell S. (hemangiomata)	520
Radial Aplasia–Thrombocytopenia S. (glabellar hemangioma)	364
Rubinstein-Taybi S.	88

Schinzel-Giedion S. (facial hemangioma)   250
Simpson-Golabi-Behmel S.
   (hemangiomatosis)   178
Trisomy 13 S. (hemangiomata)   18
Trisomy 18 S.   13

Photosensitive Dermatitis

Frequent in

Bloom S.   102
Cockayne S.   154
Rothmund-Thomson S.   157
Xeroderma Pigmentosa S.   642

Occasional in

Prader-Willi S.   223

Deep Sacral Dimple, Pilonidal Cyst

Frequent in

Bloom S.   102
Carpenter S.   484
Chondrodysplasia Punctata, X-Linked
   Dominant Type   437
Deletion 4p S.   36
Fetal Hydantoin S.   652
FG S.   316
Robinow S.   136
Smith-Lemli-Opitz S.   114

Occasional in

Dubowitz S.   100
Miller-Dieker S.   208
Zellweger S.   238

Other Dimples

Frequent in

Amyoplasia Congenita Disruptive Sequence   180
Campomelic Dysplasia   388
Caudal Dysplasia Sequence (buttock)   730
Deletion 18q S.   62
Distal Arthrogryposis S.   184
Duplication 9p S.   46
Freeman-Sheldon S. (chin)   242
Hypophosphatasia   442
Pena-Shokeir Phenotype   188

Unusual Acne

Frequent in

Apert S.   474
Pseudo-Hurler Polydystrophy S.   522
XYY S.   66

Occasional in

Gorlin S. (milia)   616
Oral-Facial-Digital S. (milia)   292

Hirsutism

Frequent in

Berardinelli Lipodystrophy S.   694
Cerebro-Oculo-Facio-Skeletal S.   190
Coffin-Siris S.   666
de Lange S.   82
Duplication 3q S.   34
Fetal Hydantoin S.   652
Frontometaphyseal Dysplasia   450
Generalized Gangliosidosis S., Type I
   (Severe Infantile Type)   518
Hajdu-Cheney S.   444
Hunter S.   532
Hurler S.   524
Hurler-Scheie S.   530
Marshall-Smith S.   172
Scheie S.   528
Schinzel-Giedion S.   250
Trisomy 18 S.   13

Occasional in

Bardet-Biedl S.   676
Bloom S.   102
Costello S.   128
Fetal Alcohol S.   646
Floating-Harbor S.   144
45X S.   76
Greig Cephalopolysyndactyly S.   486
Hypomelanosis of Ito   584
Rubinstein-Taybi S.   88

Alopecia (Sparse to Absent Hair)

Frequent in

CHILD S.   348
Clouston S.   636
Cockayne S.   154
Coffin-Siris S. (sparse scalp hair)   666

Costello S. 128
Dubowitz S. 100
Encephalocraniocutaneous Lipomatosis (focal) 604
GAPO S. 638
Hallermann-Streiff S. 110
Hay-Wells S. of Ectodermal Dysplasia 332
Hypohidrotic Ectodermal Dysplasia 628
Incontinentia Pigmenti S. 580
Johanson-Blizzard S. 106
Killian/Teschler-Nicola S. 230
Langer-Giedion S. 324
Lenz-Majewski Hyperostosis S. (infancy) 458
Linear Sebaceous Nevus Sequence (spotty alopecia) 576
Menkes S. 216
Metaphyseal Dysplasia, McKusick Type 432
Mowat-Wilson S. 686
Oculodentodigital S. 302
Progeria S. 146
Rapp-Hodgkin Ectodermal Dysplasia 632
Tricho-Rhino-Phalangeal S. 328
Wiedemann-Rautenstrauch S. 150
Werner S. 152
Yunis-Varon S. 466

Occasional in

Cardio-Facio-Cutaneous (CFC) S. 131
Chondrodysplasia Punctata, X-Linked Dominant Type 437
Chondroectodermal Dysplasia 422
Deletion 18p S. 60
Down S. 7
FG S. 316
Goltz S. 622
Hypomelanosis of Ito 584
Linear Sebaceous Nevus Sequence 576
Neu-Laxova S. 194
Oral-Facial-Digital S. 292
Pachyonychia Congenita S. 640
Popliteal Pterygium S. 344
Rapp-Hodgkin Ectodermal Dysplasia 632
Roberts-SC Phocomelia 334
Rothmund-Thomson S. 157
Seckel S. 108
Senter-KID S. 644
Toriello-Carey S. 684

Assorted Abnormalities of Hair

Frequent in

Aarskog S. (widow's peak) 134
Angelman S. (blonde) 220
Branchio-Oculo-Facial S. (prematurely gray) 274
Cardio-Facio-Cutaneous (CFC) S. (curly) 131
Cervico-Oculo-Acoustic S. (low hairline) 284
Chondrodysplasia Punctata, X-Linked Dominant Type 437
Costello S. (curly) 128
de Lange S. (long lashes) 82
Deletion 22q11.2 S. (abundant on scalp) 298
Down S. (straight) 7
Ectrodactyly–Ectodermal Dysplasia–Clefting S. (light, sparse, thin, wiry) 330
Fetal Hydantoin S. (coarse, profuse, low hairline) 652
FG S. (fine) 316
Floating-Harbor S. (low hairline) 144
45X S. (low hairline) 76
Fraser S. (growth on lateral forehead) 270
Frontonasal Dysplasia Sequence (widow's peak) 268
Hajdu-Cheney S. (thick, straight) 444
Hallermann-Streiff S. (thin, light) 110
Hay-Wells S. of Ectodermal Dysplasia (wiry) 332
Klippel-Feil Sequence (low posterior hairline) 716
Menkes S. (twisted, fractured, light in color) 216
Metaphyseal Dysplasia, McKusick Type (fragile) 432
Myotonic Dystrophy S. (recession of scalp hair) 244
Oculo-Auriculo-Verterbal Spectrum (low posterior hairline) 738
Oculodentodigital S. (fine, slow growing) 302
Opitz G/BBB S. (widow's peak) 140
Oral-Facial-Digital S. (dry) 292
Prader-Willi S. (blonde) 223
Rapp-Hodgkin Ectodermal Dysplasia (fine) 632
Restrictive Dermopathy (absent eyebrows and lashes) 196
Retinoic Acid Embryopathy (abnormal hair pattern) 660
Rothmund-Thomson S. (thin, prematurely gray) 157
Rubinstein-Taybi S. (long lashes) 88
Treacher Collins S. (projection of scalp hair onto lateral cheek) 280
Tricho-Dento-Osseous S. (kinky) 634
Tricho-Rhino-Phalangeal S. (thin, hypopigmented) 328
Ulnar-Mammary S. 342
Waardenburg S. (white forelock) 278
Weaver S. (thin) 168
Werner S. (gray) 152
XXXXX S. (low hairline) 74

Altered Sweating

19. CARDIAC

Cardiac Malformation

Cardiomyopathy

Occasional in

Abnormal Connective Tissue/Storage

Frequent in

Occasional in

Arrhythmia/Abnormal EKG

Frequent in

Occasional in

20. ABDOMINAL

Inguinal or Umbilical Hernia

Frequent in

Occasional in

Incomplete Rotation of Colon (Malrotation)

Frequent in

Occasional in

Duodenal Atresia

Occasional in

Hirschsprung Aganglionosis

Frequent in

Occasional in

Tracheoesophageal-Fistula/ Esophageal Atresia

Frequent in

Occasional in

Diaphragmatic Hernia

Frequent in

Occasional in

Single Umbilical Artery

Frequent in

Occasional in

Short Umbilical Cord

Frequent in

Occasional in

21. RENAL

Kidney Malformation

Frequent in

Renal Insufficiency

Hypertension

22. GENITAL

Ambiguous Genitalia/ Hypospadias/Bifid Scrotum

Frequent in

Occasional in

Micropenis, Hypogenitalism, Other Than Conditions Previously Cited

Frequent in

Cryptorchidism

Hypoplasia of Labia Majora

Frequent in

Occasional in

Bicornuate Uterus and/or Double Vagina

Frequent in

Occasional in

Vaginal Atresia

Frequent in

Anal Defects or Anorectal Malformations

23. ENDOCRINE AND METABOLISM

Hypogonadism

Triploidy S. (adrenal hypoplasia)	28
Tuberous Sclerosis S. (sexual precocity)	586
Werner S. (hyperthyroidism, adrenal atrophy)	152
Wiedemann-Rautenstrauch S. (hyperprolactinemia, insulin resistance)	150
Williams S. (precocious puberty)	120
XXXXY S. (growth hormone deficiency)	70

Diabetes Mellitus

Frequent in

Berardinelli Lipodystrophy S. (insulin resistance)	694
Werner S.	152

Occasional in

Achondroplasia (abnormal glucose tolerance test)	390
Ataxia-Telangiectasia S. (insulin resistance)	213
Bannayan-Riley-Ruvalcaba S.	610
Bardet-Biedl S.	676
Bloom S.	102
45X S.	76
Johanson-Blizzard S.	106
Mandibuloacral Dysplasia (insulin resistance)	692
McCune-Albright S.	594
Myotonic Dystrophy S.	244
Prader-Willi S.	223
Sotos S. (abnormal glucose tolerance test)	163
XXY S.	68

Hypocalcemia

Occasional in

Albright Hereditary Osteodystrophy	516
Deletion 22q11.2 S.	298
DiGeorge Sequence	714
Linear Sebaceous Nevus Sequence	576
Osteopetrosis: Autosomal Recessive— Lethal	453
Retinoic Acid Embryopathy	660

Hypercalcemia

Occasional in

Athyrotic Hypothyroidism Sequence	710
Hypophosphatasia	442
Metaphyseal Dysplasia, Jansen Type	434
Williams S.	120

Various Calcifications

Frequent in

Albright Hereditary Osteodystrophy (subcutaneous, basal ganglia)	516
Autosomal Recessive Chondrodysplasia Punctata	440
Cerebro-Oculo-Facio-Skeletal S.	190
Chondrodysplasia Punctata, X-Linked Dominant Type	437
Encephalocraniocutaneous Lipomatosis (cranial)	604
Fetal Warfarin S. (epiphyses)	656
Fibrodysplasia Ossificans Progressiva S.	568
Gorlin S. (falx cerebri, cerebellum)	616
Linear Sebaceous Nevus Sequence (cerebral)	576
Sturge-Weber Sequence (cerebral)	572
Tuberous Sclerosis S. (subependymal)	586
Werner S.	152
Zellweger S.	238

Occasional in

Acrodysostosis (epiphyseal)	514
Cerebro-Costo-Mandibular S. (epiphyseal)	688
CHILD S. (epiphyseal)	348
Cockayne S. (cranial)	154
Klippel-Trenaunay S. (cranial)	598
Oculo-Auriculo-Vertebral Spectrum (falx cerebri)	738
Oculodentodigital S. (basal ganglia)	302
Smith-Lemli-Opitz S. (epiphyseal)	114
Trisomy 9 Mosaic S. (developing cartilage)	26

Lipoatrophy (Loss or Lack of Subcutaneous Fat)

Frequent in

Berardinelli Lipodystrophy S.	694
Cockayne S.	154
Fetal Alcohol S.	646
Lenz-Majewski Hyperostosis S.	458
Progeria S.	146
Werner S.	152

Occasional in

Klippel-Trenaunay S.	598
Mandibuloacral Dysplasia	692
Marfan S.	546

Hyperlipidemia

Frequent in

Alagille S. (cholesterol)	670
Berardinelli Lipodystrophy S.	694

Hyperthermia

Frequent in

Occasional in

24. IMMUNE DEFICIENCY

Immunoglobulin Deficiency

Frequent in

Occasional in

Cell-Mediated Immune Deficiency

Frequent in

Occasional in

25. HEMATOLOGY-ONCOLOGY

Anemia

Frequent in

Occasional in

Thrombocytopenia

Frequent in

Occasional in

Other Bleeding Tendency

Occasional in

Leukocytosis

Occasional in

Lymphoreticular Malignancy

Occasional in

Other Malignancies

Frequent in

Occasional in

26. UNUSUAL GROWTH PATTERNS

Obesity

Frequent in

Occasional in

Hydrops Fetalis

Frequent in

Achondrogenesis, Type I	368
Fibrochondrogenesis	372
45X S.	76
Monozygotic (MZ) Twinning and Structural Defects—General	748
Osteogenesis Imperfecta S., Type II	565

Occasional in

Achondrogenesis-Hypochondrogenesis, Type II	370
Chondrodysplasia Punctata, X-Linked Dominant Type	437
Down S.	7
Generalized Gangliosidosis S., Type I (Severe Infantile Type)	518
Lethal Multiple Pterygium S.	192
Morquio S.	538
Mucopolysaccharidosis VII	544
Noonan S.	124
Short Rib–Polydactyly S., Type II (Majewski Type)	380

Early Macrosomia, Overgrowth

Frequent in

Beckwith-Wiedemann S.	174
Berardinelli Lipodystrophy S.	694
Marshall-Smith S.	172
Simpson-Golabi-Behmel S.	178
Sotos S.	163
Weaver S.	168

Occasional in

Acrocallosal S.	252
Bannayan-Riley-Ruvalcaba S.	610
Fragile X S.	160
Fryns S.	236
Killian/Teschler-Nicola S.	230
Proteus S.	600
Sclerosteosis	456

Asymmetry

Frequent in

Cervico-Oculo-Acoustic S. (facial)	284
CHILD S. (limbs)	348
Chondrodysplasia Punctata, X-Linked Dominant Type (limbs)	437
Craniofrontonasal Dysplasia (craniofacial)	482
Diploid/Triploid Mixoploidy S. (limbs)	28
Encephalocraniocutaneous Lipomatosis (cranial)	604
Klippel-Feil Sequence (facial)	716
Klippel-Trenaunay S. (hemihypertrophy)	598
Linear Sebaceous Nevus Sequence	576
Oculo-Auriculo-Vertebral Spectrum (craniofacial)	738
Proteus S.	600
Russell-Silver S.	92
Saethre-Chotzen S. (facial)	468
Sclerosteosis (mandible)	456

Occasional in

Beckwith-Wiedemann S. (hemihypertrophy)	174
Deletion 4p S. (cranial)	36
Deletion 4q S. (facial)	38
Deletion 13q S. (facial)	56
Fanconi Pancytopenia S. (limbs)	362
Goltz S.	622
Incontinentia Pigmenti S. (hemiatrophy)	580
Maffucci S. (limbs)	606
McCune-Albright S. (facial)	594
Miller S. (facial)	286
MURCS Association (facial)	760
Neurofibromatosis S. (segmental hypertrophy)	590
Noonan S. (cranial)	124
Opitz G/BBB S. (cranial)	140
Oromandibular-Limb Hypogenesis Spectrum (facial)	742
Rothmund-Thomson S.	157
Seckel S. (facial)	108
X-Linked Hydrocephalus Spectrum (facial)	202
XYY S. (facial)	66

APPENDIX II:

Nomenclature for Chromosomal Syndromes

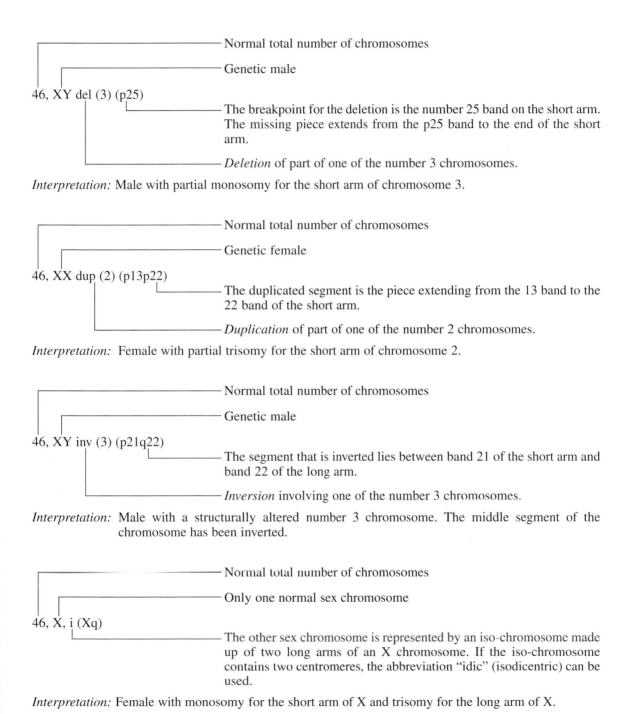

46, XY del (3) (p25)

- Normal total number of chromosomes
- Genetic male
- The breakpoint for the deletion is the number 25 band on the short arm. The missing piece extends from the p25 band to the end of the short arm.
- *Deletion* of part of one of the number 3 chromosomes.

Interpretation: Male with partial monosomy for the short arm of chromosome 3.

46, XX dup (2) (p13p22)

- Normal total number of chromosomes
- Genetic female
- The duplicated segment is the piece extending from the 13 band to the 22 band of the short arm.
- *Duplication* of part of one of the number 2 chromosomes.

Interpretation: Female with partial trisomy for the short arm of chromosome 2.

46, XY inv (3) (p21q22)

- Normal total number of chromosomes
- Genetic male
- The segment that is inverted lies between band 21 of the short arm and band 22 of the long arm.
- *Inversion* involving one of the number 3 chromosomes.

Interpretation: Male with a structurally altered number 3 chromosome. The middle segment of the chromosome has been inverted.

46, X, i (Xq)

- Normal total number of chromosomes
- Only one normal sex chromosome
- The other sex chromosome is represented by an iso-chromosome made up of two long arms of an X chromosome. If the iso-chromosome contains two centromeres, the abbreviation "idic" (isodicentric) can be used.

Interpretation: Female with monosomy for the short arm of X and trisomy for the long arm of X.

937

46, XY, r (6) (p24q26)

Normal total number of chromosomes

Genetic male

The breakpoints that have allowed formation of the ring are the 24 band on the short arm and the 26 band on the long arm. Genetic material distal to these breakpoints has been lost.

One of the number 6 chromosomes is represented by a ring chromosome.

Interpretation: Male with partial monosomy for both the distal long and distal short arms of chromosome 6.

46, XY/47, XY, + 21

One population of cells with a normal male karyotype

One population of cells with an extra chromosome 21

Interpretation: Male with mosaic trisomy 21.

45, XY, t (13;14) (p11;q11)

Reduced total number of chromosomes

Genetic male

The breakpoints that have allowed the translocation are the 11 band of the short arm of chromosome 13 and the 11 band of the long arm of chromosome 14. Both are adjacent to the centromeres.

Translocation between chromosomes 13 and 14. Because chromosomes 13 and 14 are composed almost exclusively of long arm material, breaks that occur adjacent to the centromere (see previous) with deletion of both short arms result in an insignificant loss of genetic information. The rearrangement creates a large fused chromosome and reduces the total number of chromosomes. This particular type of translocation is called Robertsonian. The triplet "rob" may be used in place of "t" to indicate this.

Interpretation: Male with a normal amount of genetic material but reduced number of chromosomes. One of the number 13 and one of the number 14 chromosomes are represented by a large chromosome that is the fusion product of 13 and 14.

46, XX, t (2;5) (p21;q31)

Normal total number of chromosomes

Genetic female

The breakpoints at which the trading of material has occurred are the 21 band on the short arm of chromosome 2 and the 31 band on the long arm of 5. The material distal to the breakpoints has been involved in a 1:1 trade.

Reciprocal translocation between chromosomes 2 and 5.

Interpretation: Female with balanced translocation in which the distal piece of the short arm of 2 is attached to the long arm of 5 and the distal piece of the long arm of 5 is attached to the short arm of 2. No genetic material has been lost or added.

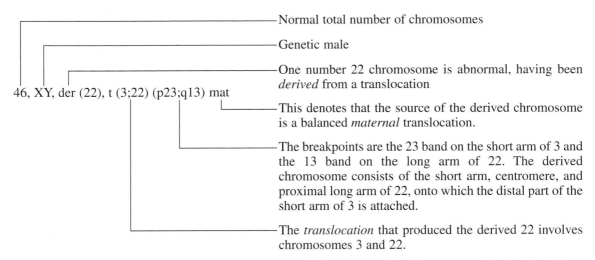

46, XY, der (22), t (3;22) (p23;q13) mat

Normal total number of chromosomes

Genetic male

One number 22 chromosome is abnormal, having been *derived* from a translocation

This denotes that the source of the derived chromosome is a balanced *maternal* translocation.

The breakpoints are the 23 band on the short arm of 3 and the 13 band on the long arm of 22. The derived chromosome consists of the short arm, centromere, and proximal long arm of 22, onto which the distal part of the short arm of 3 is attached.

The *translocation* that produced the derived 22 involves chromosomes 3 and 22.

Interpretation: Male with trisomy for the short arm of chromosome 3 and monosomy for the distal long arm of chromosome 22.

Index

Note: Page numbers followed by f indicate figures; those followed by t indicate tables.

FETAL DEVELOPMENT

AGE weeks	LENGTH cm		WT gm	GROSS APPEARANCE	CNS	EYE, EAR	FACE, MOUTH	CARDIO-VASCULAR	LUNG
	C-R	Tot.							
7½	2.8				Cerebral hemisphere ... Infundibulum, Rathke's	Lens nearing final shape	Palatal swellings ... Dental lamina, Epithel	Pulmonary vein into left atrium	
8	3.7				Primitive cereb. cortex ... Olfactory lobes Dura and pia mater	Eyelid Ear canals	Nares plugged Rathke's pouch detach. ... Sublingual gland	A-V bundle Sinus venosus absorbed into right auricle	Pleuroperitoneal canals close ... Bronchioles
10	6.0				Spinal cord histology ... Cerebellum	Iris Ciliary body Eyelids fuse Lacrimal glands Spiral gland different	Lips, Nasal cartilage Palate		Laryngeal cavity reopened
12	8.8				Cord—cervical & lumbar enlarged, Cauda equina	Retina layered Eye axis forward Scala tympani	Tonsillar crypts Cheeks ... Dental papilla	Accessory coats, blood vessels	Elastic fibers
16	14				Corpora quadrigemina Cerebellum prominent Myelination begins	Scala vestibuli ... Cochlear duct	Palate complete Enamel and dentine	Cardiac muscle condensed	Segmentation of bronchi complete
20						Inner ear ossified	Ossification of nose		Decrease in mesenchyme Capillaries penetrate linings of tubules
24	32	800			Typical layers in cerebral cortex Cauda equina at first sacral level		Nares reopen Calcification of tooth primordia		Change from cuboidal to flattened epithelium Alveoli
28	38.5	1100			Cerebral fissures and convolutions	Eyelids reopen Retinal layers complete Perceive light			Vascular components adequate for respiration
32	43.5	1600		Accumulation of fat		Auricular cartilage	Taste sense		Number of alveoli still incomplete
36	47.5	2600							
38	50	3200			Cauda equina, at L-3 Myelination within brain	Lacrimal duct canalized	Rudimentary frontal maxillary sinuses	Closure of foramen ovale, ductus arteriosus, umbilical vessels, ductus venosus	
First postnatal year +					Continuing organization of axonal networks Cerebrocortical function, motor coordination Myelination continues until 2-3 years	Iris pigmented, 5 months Mastoid air cells Coordinate vision, 3-5 months Maximal vision by 5 years	Salivary gland ducts become canalized Teeth begin to erupt 5-7 months Relatively rapid growth of mandible and nose	Relative hypertrophy left ventricle	Continue adding new alveoli